The Case Manager's Handbook

Fourth Edition

Catherine M. Mullahy, RN, BS, CRRN, CCM

Mullahy & Associates, LLC
Huntington, New York

JONES AND BARTLETT PUBLISHERS

Sudbury, Massachusetts

BOSTON   TORONTO   LONDON   SINGAPORE

World Headquarters

Jones and Bartlett Publishers
40 Tall Pine Drive
Sudbury, MA 01776
978-443-5000
info@jbpub.com
www.jbpub.com

Jones and Bartlett Publishers
Canada
6339 Ormindale Way
Mississauga, Ontario L5V 1J2
Canada

Jones and Bartlett Publishers
International
Barb House, Barb Mews
London W6 7PA
United Kingdom

Jones and Bartlett's books and products are available through most bookstores and online booksellers. To contact Jones and Bartlett Publishers directly, call 800-832-0034, fax 978-443-8000, or visit our website at www.jbpub.com.

Substantial discounts on bulk quantities of Jones and Bartlett's publications are available to corporations, professional associations, and other qualified organizations. For details and specific discount information, contact the special sales department at Jones and Bartlett via the above contact information or send an email to specialsales@jbpub.com.

The authors, editor, and publisher have made every effort to provide accurate information. However, they are not responsible for errors, omissions, or for any outcomes related to the use of the contents of this book and take no responsibility for the use of the products and procedures described. Treatments and side effects described in this book may not be applicable to all people; likewise, some people may require a dose or experience a side effect that is not described herein. Drugs and medical devices are discussed that may have limited availability controlled by the Food and Drug Administration (FDA) for use only in a research study or clinical trial. Research, clinical practice, and government regulations often change the accepted standard in this field. When consideration is being given to use of any drug in the clinical setting, the healthcare provider or reader is responsible for determining FDA status of the drug, reading the package insert, and reviewing prescribing information for the most up-to-date recommendations on dose, precautions, and contraindications, and determining the appropriate usage for the product. This is especially important in the case of drugs that are new or seldom used.

Production Credits
Publisher: Kevin Sullivan
Acquisitions Editor: Emily Ekle
Acquisitions Editor: Amy Sibley
Associate Editor: Patricia Donnelly
Editorial Assistant: Rachel Shuster
Associate Production Editor: Amanda Clerkin
Marketing Manager: Rebecca Wasley
V.P., Manufacturing and Inventory Control: Therese Connell
Composition: diacriTech, Chennai, India
Cover Design: Scott Moden
Cover Image Credit: © sprinter81/ShutterStock, Inc., © János Gehring/ShutterStock, Inc., © Dmitry Naumov/ShutterStock, Inc., © Andresr/ShutterStock, Inc., © Alexander Raths/ShutterStock, Inc., © Dmitriy Shironosov/ShutterStock, Inc.
Printing and Binding: Malloy, Inc.
Cover Printing: Malloy, Inc.

Library of Congress Cataloging-in-Publication Data

Mullahy, Catherine M.
    The case manager's handbook / Catherine M. Mullahy.–4th ed.
        p. ; cm.
Includes bibliographical references and index.
    ISBN 978-0-7637-7724-1 (alk. paper)
    1. Hospitals–Case management services–Handbooks, manuals, etc. I. Title.
    [DNLM: 1. Case Management. W 84.7 M958c 2010]
    RA975.5.C36M85 2010
    362.11–dc23
                        2009012326
6048

Printed in the United States of America
13 12 11 10 09   10 9 8 7 6 5 4 3 2 1

Table of Contents

Foreword . . . .   **xiii**

Preface . . . .   **xv**

Acknowledgments . . . .   **xviii**

PART I   PROFILE OF A CASE MANAGER **1**

Chapter 1   The Case Manager as Catalyst, Problem Solver,
                Educator **3**
                The Case Manager's Role   5
                Case Management Is Not Equivalent to Managed Care   6
                Medical Credentials and Expertise   9
                A Definition of Case Management   12
                Case Management Role and Functions   13
                Certification, Accreditation, and Standards of Practice   16

Chapter 2   The Case Manager's Universe **19**
                Important Contacts Among Healthcare Providers   19
                HMOs, PPOs, MCOs, IPAs, PHOs, IDSs, HCOs,
                  and EPOs   21
                Managed Care   23
                Managed Competition   26
                Complementary and Alternative Care   28
                Standards of Care   31

Chapter 3   Insurance Providers and Administrators **35**
                Basic Insurance and Administrative Company Players   36
                Administrative and Customized Services   39
                The Case Management Delivery System and Report Cards   40

Chapter 4   Insurance Lines and Health Benefit Plans **45**
Workers' Compensation   46
Auto Insurance   59
Indemnity Plans   59
Group Medical Plans   60
Disability Plans   61
Point-of-Service Plans   64
Consumer-Driven Healthcare Plans   65
Diagnosis-Specific Benefits   67
Traditional Insurance Versus Self-Funded Plans   68
Stop-Loss Insurance Plans   71
Multiple-Employer Benefit Plans and Trusts   72
Viatical Settlements   73
Nontraditional Policies   75
Riders to Life Insurance Policies   77
Coordination of Benefits   78

Chapter 5   Legal Responsibilities of the Case Management Profession **81**
Licensure and Liability   81
Patient Bill of Rights and Patient Confidentiality   85
Consent/Disclosure and Consent Authorization Forms   93
Medical Records   96
The Right to Know Versus the Need to Know   96
Disclosure Issues   97
Adequate Information   98
Contracts and Letters of Agreement   98
Legal Issues in Case Management   99
Legislation   108
Day-to-Day Practices   114
Getting Legal Information   115
Appendix 5–A: Written Agreement: Some Typical Provisions   118
Appendix 5–B: Legal Issues in Case Management Checklist   122
Appendix 5–C: AMA Evidence-Based Principles of Discharge
    and Discharge Criteria   126

**Chapter 6   Ethical Responsibilities of the Case Management
        Profession** **129**
Patient Rights and Case Manager Responsibilities   130
Codes of Ethical Conduct   143
Look to Your Resources   149
Appendix 6–A: CCMC Rules of Conduct   152
Appendix 6–B: Excerpts from the CCMC Code of Professional
    Conduct for Case Managers   161
Appendix 6–C: CMSA Ethics Survey   170

Chapter 7   **Case Manager Credentialing** **173**
     Certified Case Manager (CCM) 173
     The CCM Exam 174
     Before CCM, to the Wide Array of Credentials 175
     Certified Disability Management Specialist (CDMS) 176
     Certified Occupational Health Nurse (COHN) 177
     Certified Occupational Health Nurse–Specialist (COHN-S) 177
     Certified Occupational Health Nurse/Case Manager—COHN/
       CM and Certified Occupational Health Nurse–Specialist/
       Case Manager (COHN-S/CM) 177
     Certified Rehabilitation Counselor (CRC) 178
     Continuity of Care Certification, Advanced (A-CCC) 178
     Case Manager, Certified (CMC) 178
     Care Manager, Certified (CMC) 179
     Registered Nurse–Nurse Case Manager (RN-NCM) 180
     Certified Professional in Healthcare Quality (CPHQ) 180
     Case Management Administrator, Certified (CMAC) 180
     Certified Rehabilitation Registered Nurse (CRRN) 180
     Certified Social Work Case Manager (C-SWCM) 181
     Certified Managed Care Nurse (CMCN) 181
     Case Manager Associate (CMC-A) 182
     Other Credentials and Credentialing Groups 182

PART II   **CASE MANAGEMENT PROCESS** **185**

Chapter 8   **Communications** **187**
     Communicating with Physicians 187
     Stereotypes Become Reality 190
     Creative Collaboration 191
     Communications with Patients and Families 197
     Communications with Payer Sources 206
     Communications with Legal Professionals 210
     Communication Subtleties 212
     The Right Mind-Set 213
     Communications and Caring Overload: Burnout 213

Chapter 9   **The Case Management Work Format and Process** **217**
     Gathering and Assessing Information 220
     The R.I.P. Method of Conducting Interviews 220
     Talking with the Referral Source 221
     Case Finding and Targeting 233
     Talking with the Patient 236
     Talking with the Family 250
     Talking with the Treating Physician 258

Telephonic Case Management 264
Independent Medical and Second Opinion Exams 273
Talking with Other Professionals 278
Planning 287
Reporting 291
Obtaining Approval 300
Coordination: Putting the Plan into Action 308
Follow-Up 311
Evaluating the Plan 312
Repeating the Process 313
Specific Case Management Activities 314
Stay on Point 316
Case Management Scenarios 317
Appendix 9–A: CMSA Standards of Practice for
    Case Management 325

Chapter 10   Integrated Case Management: Preadmission, Concurrent
              Review, Utilization Review, Disease Management,
              and Case Management 329
              Introducing Utilization Review to Client Groups and
                  Plan Participants 332
              The Preadmission and Concurrent Review Process 340
              Timing Disease Management and Case Management
                  Intervention 345
              Preadmission and Concurrent Review Reports 347
              Establishing an Effective Preadmission Review,
                  Concurrent Review, Case Management,
                  and Disease Management System 349
              Preadmission Review, Concurrent Review, Disease
                  Management, and Case Management Checklist 368
              Fees: Capitated, Hourly, or per Case 370

Chapter 11   Working Effectively with Claims Departments:
              Case Managers in Consulting Roles 379
              Claims Department Structure and Operations 381
              Computerization 385
              Claims Issues 387
              Indicators for Case Management 387
              The Case Manager as Consultant 394
              Tracking Claims by Group 397
              Tracking Claims by Individual Claims Histories 402
              Moving into the Consultant Role 405

**PART III CASE MANAGEMENT ADMINISTRATION AND
OUTCOMES MANAGEMENT** **411**

Chapter 12 Financial and Quality Assurance Reporting **413**
Dollars and Health Care 414
Negotiating Skills 418
Nuances Between Negotiating with Providers and Payers 424
Negotiating in a Managed Care Environment 426
Documenting Negotiated Arrangements 428
Cost-Benefit Analysis Reports 434
The Cost-Benefit Analysis Summaries 441
Quality Assurance Programs 443
Explaining Difficult Situations 443
Feedback from Patients 447
Sharing Questionnaire Results 454
Communicating Success 456
Appendix 12–A: Program Questionnaire and Facility Review
for Case Managers 459
Appendix 12–B: Provider Service Agreements 465
Appendix 12–C: Expanded Cost-Benefit Analysis Summary 471
Appendix 12–D: Expanded Cost-Benefit Analysis Summary
for Self-Funded Plan 491

**Chapter 13 Managing a Case Management Department: Your Role as
Department Head or Independent Case Manager** **505**
Redefining Case Management 505
Becoming an Independent Case Manager 508
For Your Business or Department 510
Developing a Business Plan 510
Pricing the Market 513
Looking at the Competition 514
Networking and the Professional Community 517
The Business Community 520
Generating New Business 524
Hiring Additional Staff 532
The Search for Case Managers 539
Appendix 13–A: Sample Nurse Reviewer for Prenotification
Department Position Description 544
Appendix 13–B: Sample Medical Case Manager Position
Description 550
Appendix 13–C: Sample Director of Case Management
Services Position Description 556

Appendix 13–D: Interview Evaluation Form 562
Appendix 13–E: Summary Evaluation Scale 563
Appendix 13–F: Competencies for Unit-Based
    Nurse Case Manager 564

PART IV   EMERGING TRENDS AND OPPORTUNITIES **567**

Chapter 14   Obesity: The New Epidemic **569**
Obesity: A Simple Definition, a Complex Problem 570
Metrics to Determine Obesity 573
BMI 574
Etiology 575
Treatment Overview 576
Going Forward 588

Chapter 15   Our Nation's Multiculturalism and
    Challenges to Case Managers **591**
Changing Demographics 591
Cultural Competency 609
Case Managers Make a Difference 610
Developing Cultural Competency 611
Conclusion 615
Appendix 15–A: Communicating with Your
    Chinese Patient 617
Appendix 15–B: Communicating with Your American
    Indian/Alaska Native Patient 619
Appendix 15–C: Communicating with Your Latino Patient 621
Appendix 15–D: Communicating with Your Russian Patient 623

Chapter 16   Health Literacy and Adherence Issues **625**
Increased Need for Health Literacy 625
Economic Impact of Health Literacy 626
Literacy and Health Literacy 626
Day-to-Day Considerations 628
Health Literacy Manifestations 631
The Case Manager's Vital Role 634
Conclusion 637
Resources 637

Chapter 17   Pharmaceuticals: The Ever-Evolving World **641**
When Drugs Become Deadly 642
Marketing Drugs Direct to Consumers 645
Staying Abreast of Pharmaceuticals 646
Conclusion 649

Chapter 18   The Aging Population, Medical Advancements, and
New Case Management Considerations **651**
Our Graying Population 651
New Challenges 652
New Opportunities 654

Chapter 19   Dying in America **657**
A Personal Story 657
Death Is Not an Option 662
Examining Your Own Feelings 663
Addressing the Issue of Death 664
DNR Orders 668
Pain Management 670
Hospice Care 671
Palliative Care 671
CMSA's 2002 "Dying in America" Survey 672
Cultural Diversity and End-of-Life Issues 674
Conclusion 675
Endnote 675
Resources 678
Appendix 19–A: Deciding about CPR: Do-Not-Resuscitate
Orders (DNR): A Guide for Patients and Families 680
Appendix 19–B: End-of-Life Care: The Latino Culture 684
Appendix 19–C: End-of-Life Care: The Russian Culture 686
Appendix 19–D: End-of-Life Care: The Vietnamese Culture 688

Chapter 20   The Growing Need for Direct-to-Consumer, Community-Based
Case Managers: Our Changing Times **691**
Independent, Disciplined, Proactive 691
The Case Manager as Change Agent 692

Chapter 21   Behavioral Health **697**
Chronic Disease and Depression 698
Partnering Successfully with Behavioral Health Professionals 699
Behavioral Health Disease Management Programs 701
Resources 701

PART V   CASES IN PROFILE **703**

Chapter 22   Care at Home **705**
Consumer Demand—and Ambivalence 707
The Case Manager as a Pivotal Link 708
Cases in Profile 710
Ongoing Support at Home 715

Importance of Feedback and Communication 716
Payment Concerns 718

Chapter 23   Managing a Long-Term Case 723
Informing the Client 724
Level of Involvement 725
Importance of Ongoing Involvement 726
Changes in Long-Term Cases 728
Negotiating for Long-Term Care 729
Employing All Possible Resources 730
Long-Term Care of the Elderly 731
Implications of Long-Term Care for the Family 732
Implications of a Long-Term Case for the Case Manager 734
From Acute Care to Home Care: A Case History 736

Chapter 24   Public Sector Case Management 741
New Directions in Public Sector Case Management 741
Funding Sources for Public Sector Health Benefits 741
Economic Impact and Government Response 743
A Case Manager in the Public Sector 746
CMS Population Groups Challenge Managed
    Care Industry and Providers 748
Challenges for Case Managers 748
Complications That Remain 748
Nonmedical Challenges Influence Outcomes 751
Military Case Management 752
Conclusion 753

Chapter 25   Cases in Profile 755
High-Risk Pregnancy 755
Long-Term Case Management for Chronic
    Disease Management 757
Pediatric Asthma 760
AIDS Management 763
Diabetes 766
Oncology Management 769
Morbid Obesity/Gastric Bypass 772
Pediatric: Long-Term Feeding Disorder 777
Pediatric: Long-Term Rare Respiratory Disorder 782
Transplant Rejection of Small Bowel with
    Psychological Component 785

PART VI CONTINUUM CONCEPTS **789**

Chapter 26 **Continuum of Care Initiatives** **791**
Medical Home Model 791
Chronic Care Model 794
The Guided Care Model 795
The National Transitions of Care Coalition 797
Conclusion 798

Appendix A **Additional Resources** **799**

Appendix B **Glossary** **819**

Appendix C **Case Management and Healthcare Web Sites** **845**

Index **849**

Foreword

Unless someone like you cares a whole awful lot, nothing is going
to get better. It's not.
–Dr. Seuss
It's easy to make a buck. It's a lot tougher to make a difference.
–Tom Brokaw

Whether as expressed by Dr. Seuss or Tom Brokaw, if there is one single unifying factor for all of case management, it is to truly make a positive difference in the clients and families we serve through a professional caring relationship. As Tom Brokaw says, it is a lot tougher to make a difference. Those health professionals who take on that challenge are a very special and gifted group. Inspirational and best practice communication with case managers has been a hallmark of this author's career and is uniquely captured within these pages.

A dramatic shift in health care is placing increasing responsibility for health and financial management directly on the consumer. This fact alone opens opportunities for case managers and healthcare managers regardless of our practice settings. While technology has supported strides in data availability, efficiency and reporting, the professional interface between case manager and client has become exponentially more important. High tech demands high touch.

It is within the client–case manager relationship that the critical difference is made, that clients are heard, encouraged, educated, and supported in progress toward health and financial wellbeing. And it is that professional relationship that is the focus of this book.

The story of case management is told here with the passion that only an extraordinary service to the most medically vulnerable of our population can elicit. With clarity and sensitivity, Catherine describes the professional role that case managers engage when at their very best. In this way she becomes a mentor to each reader. Those who have heard her speak can almost "hear her words" as they read. She describes the best of technical performance and the heart of the caring professional in the various roles and specialties case managers face today.

Always the visionary, Catherine sees currently emerging opportunities as the most exciting yet for the practice of pure case management. The cultural diversity of our nation, the aging population, the increasing medical complexity, the challenges of transitions of care, the focus of our political leaders on changing healthcare delivery . . . all offer significant opportunities for case management professionals to provide the next generation of case management and healthcare management to an increasingly aware public.

The fourth edition of *The Case Manager's Handbook* goes far beyond previous editions. Some chapter titles remain the same but each chapter contains current and, in most cases, additional significant and critical new information. There are a number of new chapters in the book that mirror the transitions in our society. . . . Cultural Diversity, Obesity, Pharmaceuticals, Aging, Health Literacy and Direct to Consumer Case Management. Updated with emerging issues vital to today's case manager, *The Case Manager's Handbook* is a "cannot-live-without-book." In fact, with this fourth edition, *The Case Manager's Handbook* has become an encyclopedia of healthcare management and will be of great value to those crafting health care of the future.

This book stands on its own as the powerful premier industry reference and text while championing both the art of the caring heart and practice of the scientifically most advanced case management practice and healthcare management in the midst of changing healthcare practice.

Jeanne Boling, MSN, CCM
Executive Director, CMSA 1994–2006

Preface

Just as this fourth edition of *The Case Manager's Handbook* went to press, our nation ushered in its first African-American president whose platform and voice call for change. Within the case management field, voices of leadership and concern for our nation's failing healthcare system are also calling for change. What will be especially critical in this movement to reshape our healthcare system will be the voice of case managers. Just as their role has evolved over the past decades, so too must their commitment to be a greater voice and advocate for the patients they serve. Our troubled healthcare system requires it and our patients—now assuming more of the decision-making in their treatment plans—deserve it. But equally important, case managers have earned this heightened role and now need to start owning it.

This latest edition of *The Case Manager's Handbook* has as its central mission empowerment for case managers. It is a mission which—by providing the latest information on "Best in Class" practices, emerging trends, challenges and opportunities, the state-of-health care in America and a new domain for case managers—strives to engage more case managers, the rookies and veterans alike—to step up to the plate and take a swing at making a real difference for our patients specifically, and for our healthcare system in general.

While the "nuts and bolts" of the case manager's role and responsibilities within the context of insurance, the law, ethics and various settings remain the major contents of this edition, this information has been enhanced with current research, data and new real life experiences which will give case managers both the knowledge and insights they need to be true instruments of change in the delivery of better health care.

Among the new areas being covered in this fourth edition of *The Case Manager's Handbook* are the expanding obesity epidemic, the nation's increasing multiculturalism, health literacy, the graying of America, and the influx of new pharmaceuticals; all of which pose new challenges for case managers.

There's something else new to *The Case Manager's Handbook.* It is a discussion of an exciting new career path for case managers—that of the direct-to-consumer, community-based case manager. As the nation adopts a new consumer-driven healthcare model wherein consumers now are making their own choices in health insurance and are more involved in determining their prescription medicines and treatment options, case managers are needed to guide them in these decisions. By establishing a presence right in the community and being available and account-able directly to patients and their families, direct-to-consumer case managers can realize their full potential as true patient advocates *and* catalysts for change.

The fact is, to quote Bob Dylan, "For the times they are a-changin." With or without us, health care is evolving. It can evolve painfully slow or we can help it achieve a more speedy recovery. Education, ethics, credentials, adherence to high standards, and "Best in Class" practices are essential for case managers. But equally important will be their rising to the challenge of change—being willing to assume new responsibilities in our changing world and for our changing health-care system. The last section of this book speaks to one of the major challenges facing patients today, as well as case managers and other healthcare professionals who try to assist them. As our patients transition from one healthcare setting to another and receive care and services from countless providers, we know now that we have reason to be concerned about their safety. A direct response to this has been the development of several initiatives . . . all of which extend an open "invitation" to case managers. The Guided Care Model, the National Transitions of Care Coalition, and Medical Home Models need to have the voices, creativity, and commitment from case managers. Our patients need to feel safe; they need to trust that their care-providers are actually communicating with others about them . . . case managers are the essential components within these new care con-tinuum concepts to insure that this occurs.

Through *The Case Manager's Handbook,* case managers and others who aspire to better understand this critical field will gain access to time honored professional principles, leading-edge data, and practical "how to" advice on effective case management work formats, processes and communications with patients, physicians, providers, etc. It is the quintessential textbook and training manual for case managers in all phases of their careers. From those individuals curious to see if case management is a good career path, through the more experienced professional who wants to insure the maintenance of a cutting edge best-in-class practice, and on to those seeking to explore other practice settings, this book will provide the necessary information and insight.

The Case Manager's Handbook is also a motivational and inspirational writing which taps into the psyche of the caring heart of the case manager. It recognizes that most individuals who enter this one-of-a-kind field of case management are dedicated to helping patients and their families through one of life's most challenging episodes—that of a serious illness or chronic medical condition. To be the best beacon of hope and help to those patients and their families, it is critical that today's case managers recognize the intricacies of integrated case management and the skill set they need to be the consummate case manager. It means understanding the nuances of different cultures and how they influence a patient's healthcare decision. It means recognizing how the aging patient more often than not has multiple medical conditions that must be addressed through interface with multiple physicians and providers. It means understanding that physicians today are also grappling with the changing healthcare system and rather than be viewed as adversaries or "Gods of Medicine," they must be regarded as comrades in a mutual quest to help patients. It means that health literacy and patient safety are directly intertwined and that our roles as patient educators and advocates are more essential than ever before.

What does it mean to be a case manager in America today? *The Case Manager's Handbook* provides the answers through my own personal lens as a veteran healthcare professional; a nurse with diverse and extensive clinical experience; a case manager and entrepreneur who was founder, president, and CEO of a successful case management firm; and a case management industry leader having held top positions in the preeminent professional case management associations and standards boards. I share my experience with you in hopes that some of you who read this book will be inspired to follow a path that has fulfilled me and continues to inspire me.

So, "Come gather 'round people, wherever you roam. . . . For the times they are a-changin.'"

Author's Note: Because the majority of case managers are women, I have used the feminine pronoun throughout this book. No offense to our male colleagues is implied or intended. For your reference, terms of widely used healthcare field concepts that are abbreviated in the text are spelled out in the Acronyms and Abbreviations section of the book.

Acknowledgments

This edition of *The Case Manager's Handbook,* similar to the three that preceded it, was not created in a vacuum. There have been so many individuals in my life and along this special journey in case management who have allowed me the opportunity to share this experience with others. To everyone at Jones and Bartlett Publishers, especially Kevin Sullivan, who had confidence in this newest edition; Tricia Donnelly, for her patience, encouragement, and understanding—especially during my technologically challenged times; Linda McGarvey; Amanda Clerkin; and Rebecca Wasley.

Almost 5 years have passed since the last edition of this book, and once again the circle of life continues to influence me and remind me of the love and support that I have been blessed to receive. My mom passed away 3 years ago, and readers will hopefully appreciate how she contributed to my understanding of what's really important in life and, in her final days, how important our role, as case managers, can be. Although there was indeed some sadness in my life, there was joy as well with the addition of three more grandsons (totaling five!) to our family. Life continues to teach us lessons, some which are inevitable, some for which we are never quite prepared. My husband, John, had a few encounters with the excellence, anxiety, and confusion that are all part of today's healthcare delivery system. Fortunately, all is well; however, these experiences only served to further reinforce my vision for the direct-to-consumer community-based case manager role. In the years that I had owned my company Options Unlimited (1983–2003), it became my "laboratory." Our staff, client companies, patients, and their families provided the opportunities to create the kind of case management process that became the foundation for our other programs and for the many editions of this book. I am forever grateful for and miss that ongoing experience. Since the acquisition of my company by Matria Healthcare (which, along with Paradigm, is now part of Alere), Mullahy and Associates has been involved in the provision and, yes, the creation of other opportunities to enhance the role and contributions of case management. Jeannie Boling, past executive director of Case Management Society of America (CMSA), colleague, friend, and consummate professional, has joined with me for this next chapter of our professional careers. Her ongoing support and shared vision for the future of case management have been invaluable. As a reviewer for this edition of the book, and as partner in our consulting and educational endeavors, her perspective, insight, and, when needed, constructive input have been and continue to be deeply appreciated.

I also wish to thank Donna Autuori, who provided another voice as I continued my quest to expand the visibility of case management to consumers and to empower case managers with a real sense of their potential. As collaborative writing partner during these last few years, Donna has provided me with the enthusiastic energy, expertise, and assistance that I so needed, especially during the research and execution of this edition. Her ability to bring a sense of organization into chaos is much appreciated.

Colleagues in case management continue to be generous with their expertise and kind in contributing once again to this edition: Linda Chalmers, RN, BSN, CCM, WCLA, who shared her perspective and knowledge of workers' compensation case management from the corporate perspective and additionally provided a historical overview of the practice and the importance of communication; Tom Strickland, MA, CRC, who continues in his position as president and CEO of his regional company Systemedic Corporation and provided some important updates involving workers' compensation challenges encountered by his Arkansas-based staff and shared by case managers in other states as well; Christopher Wood, PhD, who sold his company and is now senior vice president of MCMC and who reviewed some of the trends he sees in workers' compensation and disability case management; and Dave Hubbard, RN, who is a disability case manager with Ft. Dearborn Life Insurance, and who provided valuable insights about challenges faced by those who provide disability management services.

The future of case management is certainly stronger today because of the many contributions of two of its early leaders who sadly departed this earth within months of each other in 2007. Mary Gambosh, RN, CDMS, CCM and Patricia McCollum, RN, MS, CRRN, CCM were gifted colleagues and dear friends who left their footprints so others could follow. Their stars shine brightly, as do their memories . . . rest in peace, job well done!

Other colleagues, although not direct contributors to this book, have been generous with their time, insight, and enthusiasm as the seeds of direct-to-consumer case management were gently scattered to take root across our nation. Thanks go to Anne Llwellyn, editor-in-chief of *Case in Point*, for her enthusiastic recognition and support through her interview of me in the "Meet the Leaders" special edition; another audio interview on the Web site and the publishing of an article provided me with a forum to share my vision for the future. To Suzanne Powell, editor of *Professional Case Management*, who also accepted one of my articles; to Dorothy Angelini, director of continuing education, and others with the Gannett Health Care Group, for sponsoring me at career fairs as well as at seminars—all of these have provided opportunities to grow the practice of case management and generate additional interest, especially in the direct-to-consumer model. Each of these individuals has my deep appreciation.

Another very special individual, Deborah Jensen, has been involved in all of the editions of *The Case Manager's Handbook*. She has been an incredibly valuable writer, communicator, and editor, and was so instrumental in helping me to communicate the essence and heart of case management for more than 15 years. Our paths have taken us in different directions, and although Deborah was not actively involved as an additional author for this edition, to be sure, her previous efforts made this one possible.

I would like to acknowledge some other very special individuals: my husband, John, for his love, good humor, and unending support and encouragement for the work that I do; our children, Michael and Aileen, and their spouses, Pam and Neal, and our five grandsons; and family and friends for their understanding of the time spent away from them as I continue this journey. And finally, my parents and first teachers, Mary and Tommy Lyons, who gave me so much over their lifetime, and in whose memory this book is dedicated.

Part I

Profile of a Case Manager

Chapter 1

The Case Manager as Catalyst, Problem Solver, Educator

Case management is not for the faint at heart. It is not for those seeking to avoid the stress of a hospital setting or the stretch of working with patients and families in distress. Providing intervention on behalf of the patient, medical provider, and payer (insurer), a case manager must place herself at the center of the confusion in today's healthcare delivery system and be willing and able to ask the tough questions. Is that surgical procedure appropriate and necessary? Can we do better on the pricing for the TPN (total parenteral nutrition) infusion or the out-of-network rehabilitation program? Can we honor this patient's wishes and enable him to live his last days at home? And because case management is a process, a case manager must have commitment to go the distance, offering ongoing, on-site, individualized services and becoming involved in finding medical treatment alternatives, monitoring results, solving problems, and revising the treatment plan as needed. A case manager is the catalyst who sifts through the array of possible paths, selects the most appropriate plan, and then coordinates the expertise and support of other professionals, family members, agencies, and suppliers. Case managers are concerned with every detail, from the minute—is the noise from the oxygen concentrator disruptive, preventing the patient from utilizing it?—to the major—can the family member, home health aide, or registered nurse in attendance handle a patient emergency? Is the family rejecting the needed hospital bed because they don't want their den to have a "sick look"?

It is not an easy professional specialty, but it is a tremendously rewarding one. As a discipline, case management requires an understanding of how various medical, insurance, government, and corporate mechanisms affect the healthcare delivery system. Each of these areas influences the type of care available and how it will be administered.

It is the case manager's responsibility to know the distinctions between acute hospitalization, subacute care, and specialized chronic care; the results and impact of federal legislation; and the coverage offered by different lines of insurance.

It is also the case manager's responsibility to make assessments and recommendations on an objective basis, having no vested interest in which rehabilitation facility or infusion service is selected. If it seems that case managers are held accountable not only for their academic credentials and work history, but also for their personal ethics, it is because they are. Often functioning without peer support or direction from an immediate supervisor, case managers must bring their own motivation, moral strength, independence, and confidence to each case. This is the personal profile needed to oversee a wide spectrum of activities with the sole focus of ensuring the best possible outcome for a patient in the most cost-effective manner.

The current nursing shortage has been widely reported and could reach as high as 500,000 by 2025.[1] Nurses are working more overtime or double shifts, and are responsible for a greater number of patients than before, meaning they have less time to spend with each patient and to complete all their tasks to the standards they feel are important to maintain. Turnover is increasing, especially among the more experienced nurses. Many hospital nurses are concerned that these conditions have the potential to affect their early detection of patient complications and their ability to maintain patient safety.

In this environment, the case manager's role becomes increasingly significant toward ensuring appropriate, quality care. Case management intervention addresses the needs that arise as hospital staff, for example, is stretched to its capacity. Conversations between case managers and acute care nurses were never relaxed coffee klatches, but now have become even quicker exchanges of information. To obtain background that might not have been communicated verbally, our staff has begun looking more closely at nurses' notes, especially when the things we're hearing don't match up; the patient is saying he's fine, but he's experiencing complications. The insights gained from these notes, where treatment changes and patient reaction are recorded, enhance our ability to spot potential problems or a lack of progress, so we can intervene and redirect, as considered necessary.

Aware of the higher possibility of infections due to understaffing, a case manager will be more proactive, and assess skin integrity, on-site or through conversation, to avoid the development of decubitus ulcers. On behalf of a stroke patient, she might ask if hand splints are in place to prevent contracture, which would decrease hand mobility and a return to strength.

Exacerbating the shortage, hospital-based RNs have also become more involved in and accountable for activities not associated with patient care, such as budgets, coding meetings, staffing issues, and usage of quality improvement tools. Each of these is of value to hospital administration, but does not contribute directly to patient care.

Similarly, case managers are vulnerable to revisions of their job descriptions and responsibilities as hospitals and healthcare organizations face both economic stresses and this shortage of qualified nurses. In an article in *The Case Manager*, trends noticed by CMSA (Case Management Society of America) members included: the delegation of clerical responsibilities to case managers, delegation of patient interactions to non-case managers, an increase in the clinical condition responsibilities now falling to case managers, and a rise in caseloads.[2] (A closer look at changes in caseloads is documented in the "Case in Point" (official magazine of CMSA) 2008 Salary and Trends Survey.) Each of these undermines the case manager's role by drawing her away from patient advocacy and coordinating care across the continuum, and siphoning off her time with secretarial duties, or loading up on her work responsibilities so that rushing through each task would be the only way to complete them all. This lessens the value and effectiveness of her contributions, and opens the door for complications. Would anyone knowingly hurry an analyst through reading a sonogram or a breast x-ray?

THE CASE MANAGER'S ROLE

Case managers are not the claims police. Ensuring cost-effective treatment does not mean that case managers are overrated number crunchers who review treatment alternatives simply to find the cheapest scenario. Case managers are coordinators, facilitators, impartial advocates, and educators. Their roles are as varied as the sites where they are employed and the job titles that designated their position in the past.

The case manager in an acute care facility may have been called a discharge planner a few years ago. In behavioral health facilities, the "Program Coordinator" or "Coordinator of Patient Services" may now carry the title "Case Manager."

Case managers in hospitals, rehabilitation facilities, home health agencies, and infusion care companies are in the provider sector of health services and may include nurses and social workers. They may oversee treatment while a patient is in a particular facility or receiving a certain type of service, such as infusion therapy, but not be involved with that same patient's care once the patient moves on to a different center or care program. Depending on the employer, a case manager may never make a home visit or manage care outside of a particular facility.

In the payer sector, both public and private, case managers may work through Third Party Administrators (TPAs), self-administered programs, health maintenance organizations (HMOs), preferred provider organizations (PPOs), point-of-service plans (POSs), military programs, or major insurance carriers. In these settings, case managers identify and track all hospital admissions and other events in which there is a likelihood of costly or high-exposure conditions. Although employer emphasis may seem to be on reducing overall costs, these case managers are also dedicated to assisting employees and their dependents in the utilization of services.

Because of financial organizational structure and administrative overhead, many organizations do not elect to maintain an in-house case management department or staff. This, coupled with the direct-to-consumer trend, is behind the growing and diverse opportunities for independent case managers. Those with strong expertise in neonatal, oncology, elder care, or organ transplants may find heightened demand for their services. One such source is stress-ridden baby boomers who call on independent case managers on behalf of their aging parents.

Independent case managers are outside both the medical care provider and the claims payer systems. All case managers are charged with the responsibility to make totally objective assessments and to coordinate a program of care. With no vested interest in the companies selected to provide this care or services, independent case managers can remain more impartial advocates for their clients and may have an advantage in exercising out-of-the-box thinking and solutions.

The focal point of case management in all of its roles is to empower patients, giving them and their families access to a greater understanding of their disability or disease, a larger voice in the delivery of their care, and more personalized attention to their particular needs. Obtaining data on the particulars of each patient's case, case managers enable patients and their families to make informed decisions. Through their role as advocates, they help patients deal with the complexities of the healthcare system.

CASE MANAGEMENT IS NOT EQUIVALENT TO MANAGED CARE

Managed care and *case management* are not interchangeable concepts. Managed care is a system of cost-containment programs; case management is a process. A global term, managed care consists of the systems and mechanisms utilized to control, direct, and approve access to the wide range of services and costs within the healthcare delivery system. Case management can be one of those mechanisms, one component in the managed care strategy.

Based on the use of cost-containment programs that include guidelines and criteria for healthcare delivery, managed care organizations (MCOs) incorporate a wide variety of options. These may include Pharmacy Benefits Management (PBM), POS plans, consumer-driven plans, HMOs, PPOs, direct contracting (in which an employer contracts directly with a hospital or other healthcare facility), bill audits, utilization review, preadmission authorization, concurrent review, retrospective review, second surgical opinions (SSOs), independent medical exams (IMEs), disease management, and case management. Whereas managed care programs strive to involve all potential users of healthcare services, case management focuses on certain individuals—the 3 to 5% of the patient population responsible for 60 to 70% of the expenditures in any health plan.[3]

Case management is a highly individualized process that aims to identify those most at-risk, vulnerable, or care- and cost-intensive patients; assess treatment options and opportunities to coordinate care; design treatment programs to improve quality and efficacy of care; control costs; and manage patient care to ensure the optimum outcome. Concentrating for the most part on catastrophic or chronic cases, case managers are called in to consult for diagnoses such as head injury, multiple trauma, cancer, AIDS, organ transplants, cardiovascular and respiratory disease, stroke, burns, spinal cord injury, premature infants, diabetes, and high-risk pregnancy.

In the Towers Perrin 2008 Health Care Cost Survey Report of Key Findings, employers are paying 39% more than they spent five years ago. ($5100 in 2003 versus $7,080 in 2008) and employees are spending 61% more ($1,284 in 2003 versus $2,064 in 2008).[4]

In a 2006 survey of 3,000 employer sponsored health plans, Mercer Health & Benefits found that about two-thirds of employers with 500 or more employees rated care management services as important or very important cost management strategy over the next five years. Only 37 percent believe that shifting costs to employees or scaling back benefits. The most prominent strategy in recent years . . . would be an important consideration.[5]

The trend toward greater use of case management is not new. In its 1996 Executive Opinion Poll (which introduced a new survey design and methodology), *Business & Health* asked respondents to name the management techniques applied by their healthcare plans, from a list including case management, utilization review, disease management, demand management, pharmacoeconomics, and outcomes research. Outcomes published in *"Business & Health* Executive Opinion Poll—1996" showed case management leading the other categories as the management technique most used by the healthcare plans of large and small companies combined (with 43% applying it) and by companies with 20 to 499 employees (with 42% applying it). Among larger companies employing more than 500 individuals, 73% of healthcare plans used case management techniques and 75% applied utilization review. In a note that should have been a wake-up call to chief executive officers (CEOs), even as it warmed the hearts of Third Party Administrators and insurers nationwide, the report mentioned that a substantial portion of respondents didn't know whether a particular technique was utilized by their healthcare plan(s). Nearly half of the respondents in many cases, and 60% of those asked about demand management, weren't certain whether that technique was being applied by their healthcare plan. This reinforced my concern (and continued amazement) that the majority of employers (those who ultimately pay for employees' healthcare coverage) do not know how that money, that resource, is being managed.

In 2005 URAC (originally incorporated under the name "Utilization Review Accreditation Commission," shortened to URAC, and now also known as the American Accreditation HealthCare Commission) conducted a national survey of more than 282 companies regarding trends and issues in medical management. Participants included HMOs, PPOs, stand-alone medical management companies, insurance carriers, and others. The study researched national trends and issues in medical management, and the white paper "Trends and Practices in Medical Management: 2005 Industry Profile" reported that more and more companies were utilizing a combination of utilization management (UM), disease management (DM), and case management (CM).[6]

Case managers have long expressed the benefits of combining CM, utilization review (UR)/UM, PreCert, and—as new concepts in healthcare came on the scene—disease management, in a coordinated system to best provide for the patient and limit employer and payer risks. Now it seems that this type of system is becoming a reality.

The positive piece that all case managers can embrace is that, within this comprehensive study, case management is perceived as a distinct role and function that is best applied in a coordinated program with UM, DM, discharge planning, and social work. Still, this collaborative model can be improved upon, and more information about case management needs to be communicated.

MEDICAL CREDENTIALS AND EXPERTISE

Agreed-upon credentials and criteria for what makes a good case manager and the level of preparation required to handle the usual responsibilities have long been established as part of the development of the Certified Case Manager (CCM) and other case management credentials. Predictably, the criteria caused an outcry from some individuals who claim to offer case management but discovered they are worlds apart from those case management practitioners who are eligible for certification. For example, there are individuals currently working as case managers who have no more experience than one year in a hospital and a weekend-obtained certificate in case management. Case management as a profession demands critical thinking skills, in-depth clinical knowledge, and extensive, diversified experience within the healthcare delivery system. It is an advanced practice, and as such, requires a high level of knowledge and competency.

Today's case managers come from diverse educational and clinical settings, many with broader backgrounds than a strict hospital environment. Generally, they are nurses, social workers, or rehabilitation counselors, and a number of them have had experience administering workers' compensation and disability cases involving catastrophic injury. Far beyond helping an individual recuperate and return to work, case managers address health and wellness within disease management and wellness programs, as well as the needs of those already experiencing costly medical conditions and their complications. They assist in everything from tertiary neonatal cases, premature babies, and healthy baby programs to geriatric cases, stroke victims, and living with diabetes. There is a need for broad clinical knowledge and standards of care for the less complicated conditions, and on to kidney failure and amputations, which is causing subtle shifts among case management practitioners.

Social welfare caseworkers, involved with programs like Medicare, originated some elements of case management procedures. They developed and perfected the skills involved in connecting people to their community resources and obtaining financial aid from federal and state agencies. Social workers will undoubtedly continue to make up a substantial portion of case managers. Although considerable supplementary training and experience might be required before they could manage complex medical cases, such as ventilator-dependent babies or an individual requiring infusion services, social workers with medical backgrounds can handle stable cases and provide assistance to our fast-growing "gray" population. They also take a significant role in behavioral health programs. And combining social workers and RNs in medical case management teams has already proven very effective, enabling speedier identification of solutions to patient problems. As professionals with a different focus, rehabilitation counselors have also become valuable members of such teams, with their emphasis on recuperation and the return to work.

Because of the medical problem solving and coordination responsibilities inherent in the case management role, the kind of experience and education that nurses possess becomes important. In addition to basic educational preparation—associate degree, diploma-school, or baccalaureate-level college—life experience counts for a great deal. But case management demands a greater depth and intensity of involvement than traditional nursing, as well as more advanced medical, psychological, and sociological training. Therefore, a case manager's educational process should be ongoing and, through continuing education studies or postgraduate work, should be directed toward achieving a master's degree in a clinical specialty, for example. Because continuing education is not mandated for updated RN certification in many states, a number of practicing case managers neglect their obligation to remain current in their field. Those selecting case management as a career owe it to their patients, their profession, and themselves to read, attend conferences, and sit in on seminars and lectures so as to broaden their knowledge base. The CCM designation requires case managers to take advantage of continuing education to maintain their credential status, as does the Care Manager Certified certification (CMC) and the Case Manager Associate (CMC-A) from the American Institute of Outcomes Case Management (AIOCM), the Certified Social Work Case Manager (C-SWCM) designation from the National Association of Social Workers, the RN-BC from American Nurses Credentialing Center and many others.

Due to the tendency of multiple conditions, sometimes comorbid, in the case management patient population, the kind of clinical experience of greatest value is that of a generalist. Although there are case managers with a single practice area, such as those who specialize in high-risk neonates, head trauma, organ transplants, oncology, or hematology, most case managers should have experience with a variety of age groups, treatment facilities, and medical conditions. The majority of case managers will receive referrals requiring knowledge of a wide spectrum of medical practice specialties, and they will need to acquire a diversified clinical background to meet the challenges. Ideal clinical preparation includes in-depth exposure to medical-surgical treatments, intensive care, critical care, home care, psychology, obstetrics, pediatrics, and neurological care. Case managers must be able to distinguish good care from bad care, understand potential complications, and evaluate alternate treatment options. Working in one hospital unit for one year does not provide the range of cases and insight required of a good case manager. Even comprehensive hospital experience alone is insufficient preparation. In most hospitals, equipment and supplies are readily available. Leaving the safety and support systems of the hospital environment, we can appreciate how vulnerable our patients can become when necessary services are fragmented. Further, case management requires self-direction, critical thinking, and independent functioning and judgment, skills honed more readily in nontraditional healthcare settings. Experience in home healthcare, walk-in clinics, and occupational health nursing can provide a beneficial view of community healthcare options.

Because the work requires financial savvy, a business background is also helpful. Hospital nurses do not have to cost out the care they are administering, but case managers must be financially accountable. If they cannot demonstrate the positive impact of case management to its stakeholders (payers, providers, patients), they undermine the value of their industry and, therefore, their future. They need to know, for example, the cost of infusion care treatment so they can question payment on a creatively submitted invoice. Forget that they can help improve employee morale, can help a disabled person get back to work faster to continue a rewarding career, can locate an appropriate facility 10 miles from home rather than 550 miles away for a child with a head injury; if they cannot combine their healing skills with practical business skills, they will lose the opportunity to practice.

Case management work often places individuals in situations in which patients and their families are devastated by health-related problems. Beyond facilitating healthcare decisions on behalf of other human beings, case managers also face the type of intense social/dynamic family issues that never become "easy" to handle but can be approached with more empathy and grace by practitioners who have become acquainted with the emotions encountered in marriage, divorce, illness, and death. Less experienced practitioners are likely to have difficulty appreciating the significance of such issues. Five or more years of clinical experience helps develop a maturity and depth that makes it easier to relate to patients and understand their emotional state.

Case managers need personal stamina and strength. Most caseloads include tragic cases. Case managers cannot make a terminal illness fade away. They cannot fully empower a patient if the family is too broken to accept the necessary responsibility. Case managers, therefore, need personal resources and support from friends and family to meet the challenges each day will present. A can-do mentality, a ready sense of humor, and the gift of levelheaded self-affirmation to take personal note of the small successes every day are among the traits that boost a case manager's effectiveness.

A DEFINITION OF CASE MANAGEMENT

The Commission for Case Manager Certification (CCMC) (www .ccmcertification.org) defines case management as follows: Case management is a collaborative process that assesses, plans, implements, coordinates, monitors, and evaluates the options and services required to meet the client's health and human service needs. It is characterized by advocacy, communication & resource management and promotes quality & cost-effective interventions & outcomes.[7]

The Case Management Society of America (www.cmsa.org) (CMSA) defines case management as "a collaborative process of assessment, planning, facilitation, and advocacy for options and services to meet an individual's health needs through communication and available resources to promote quality cost-effective outcomes."[8]

Although it is not in all the language referring to the role and function of case managers, and is not possible in all settings, for all case managers I would add that case management is most effective when provided across the continuum of care. When a case is opened and then worked as the patient moves from acute care hospital to a skilled nursing facility or rehabilitation center, and then home, case management can offer its greatest contributions to quality healthcare and the best use of healthcare dollars.

In the broadest sense, a case manager is the person who can make the healthcare system work, influencing both the quality of the outcome and the cost. In our country, healthcare delivery is fragmented and complex. Providers range from the walk-in clinics to exclusive provider organizations and centers of excellence, and care settings run the gamut from a patient's own bedroom, up through rehabilitation facilities, outpatient facilities, specialized long-term care sites, and nursing homes, to hospices, sub acute care facilities, and hospitals. It is no surprise patients are confused.

Working as an advocate for the patient (always searching for and moving toward the most medically appropriate solution), an empowering agent for the family, and a facilitator of communication among the patient, family, care providers, and payers, the case manager is a sentinel for quality assurance and cost-effectiveness. Perhaps the case manager can affect an earlier discharge, negotiate a better fee from a medical equipment supplier, or encourage the family to assume responsibility for a portion of the day-to-day care the patient needs. She can be a catalyst for change by seeking solutions that promote improvement or stabilization rather than simply monitoring patient status. If the case manager performs all these functions well, quality assurance and cost savings fall into place as a matter of course, prolonging the life of benefit dollars for individuals and helping to free up healthcare monies for the 47 million uninsured in the United States today.

CASE MANAGEMENT ROLE AND FUNCTIONS

To be effective, case managers require broad-based knowledge. They need to be part general practitioner, part social worker, part psychologist, and part minister or rabbi. Even if the case management role never requires going beyond the boundaries of this specialty, a case manager needs to be aware of the psychosocial, environmental, family, economic, and religious dynamics that can impact patients. She also must have a diverse medical background; being a clinician is not enough.

Areas of general knowledge and the understanding of healthcare treatments and systems required by case management practitioners were encompassed in the preliminary 1992 CCM credentialing report. Suggested general knowledge included theories of family functioning; the characteristics of various stages of physical and psychosocial development; the traits of functional and dysfunctional coping and their implications for health; and resources, eligibility for services, and referral procedures. In the area of healthcare, first-draft credentialing criteria called for comprehension of "home health resources; strategies to access medical records; medical terminology; pharmaceuticals and pharmacological management; levels of care in acute and rehabilitative treatment; adaptive equipment and assistive devices for various disabilities and illnesses; issues involving experimental treatments and protocols; and competitive cost for medical and healthcare services, aftercare and independent living resources,"[9] in addition to other healthcare factors. Because of the case manager's role as a communicator and liaison, she must also be familiar with certain elements within the insurance, legal, and vocational disciplines. For example, to interact successfully with insurance and funding sources, a case manager must be facile with insurance terminology, the preparation of cost-benefit analyses for payers, the reporting requirements of various healthcare reimbursement and government agencies, disability compensation systems, extended medical or indemnity payments, and the coordination of benefits. To practice ethically and safely, a case manager should also be familiar with legal terminology, liability issues, use of depositions, confidentiality laws, and the accepted procedures and requirements for releasing or sharing information. To best meet patient needs, one must be familiar with cultural issues, complementary and alternative care, herbal medications, end-of-life concerns such as pain management, and specialty areas of case management. And finally, vocational and legislative protocols will govern care options and benefit plan dollar availability for some individuals. These areas of knowledge will encompass resources for reentry into the labor force, work evaluation processes, job accommodation principles, affirmative action, the philosophy of workers' compensation, the Americans with Disabilities Act of 1990 (ADA), Medicaid and Medicare provisions, and the rights of individuals under federal and state law (both the state in which a case manager practices and the state in which a patient is undergoing treatment).

All this said, it must also be noted that case management usually is not a hands-on role. Case managers, while continuing to be actively practicing nurses, clinicians, or caregivers, do not diagnose an ailment, prescribe a medication, or set the course of treatment. They do offer their observations on a patient's status and use their expertise to plan and suggest alternative care options. Using on-site visits as fact-gathering missions, a case manager can make sure a noncompliant patient is following the treatment plan outlined by the physician or note the possible complications from the medication recommended by the patient's ear-nose-and-throat specialist but never mentioned to his or her cardiologist. Case managers are consultants, advisors, and facilitators.

Although the majority of case managers do not offer hands-on care, neither can they be truly effective if they act in a totally hands-off manner. Telephone work, which is a part of case management, is necessary for keeping open the lines of communication without driving up costs. It is particularly effective for preventive and case-screening measures as well as for tracking low-intensity patients or patients whose conditions have improved to the point where in-person case management is no longer needed. However, strict telephonic case management, in which all the communication between the case manager, patient, family, physician, and payer occurs over the phone, can lead to major oversights in care unless skillfully conducted, especially in cases in which the patient is noncompliant, undereducated, or poor. The vulnerability of the patient, combined with the legal and monetary exposure of the case manager, provider, and payer, often necessitates on-site interaction.

Case managers fulfill a role not provided for elsewhere in the healthcare system. They become the eyes and ears for others, a resource for physicians and other members of the healthcare team, insurance groups, employers, and particularly families. Because people tend to picture described situations in terms of their own experience, they tend to make incorrect assumptions. A telephonic case manager might envision a patient's "home" as complete with a stocked refrigerator, adequate room for the ventilator or the motorized wheelchair modified with respiratory equipment, and clean sheets on the bed. During an on-site home visit, a case manager will be able to note the empty refrigerator, the two toddlers careening around the couch and bumping into the infant's oxygen-supply tubing, the unopened medication bottles, and the family in need of respite. Let's review a real case in which a gentleman suffered a left-sided stroke leaving him with right-sided weakness. The physician assured the case manager that the patient was fine upon discharge and didn't require any equipment or support services. The case manager never asked the patient: Can you walk comfortably? Will you need a cane for support? Will you be able to walk around inside your home? In the weeks following discharge, the man experienced complications and difficulty maneuvering around his house. His wife was upset with the case manager and the physician for their lack of support. A more complete telephone conversation and the appropriate follow-up calls would have solved these problems. (For more information on telephonic case management, please see Chapter 9.)

Beyond the medical aspects lies another whole dynamic of an illness, the logistics of coping, which might require putting a caretaker's job on hold or a home up for sale. Here is where a case manager can help fill a void in the system by assisting the well persons in the family to deal with practical matters. The comatose patient does not need hand-holding, but the caretaker in the family might—or might need guidance from a person who can fully explain treatment options, a safe person to share emotions with, or someone to fill out the forms and help file the claims. When the claims department returns a form marked "incomplete," there is no note describing what information was omitted. Unfiled claims cannot be reimbursed, and the case manager can be the person to help pull the details together, to get the burned-out caretaker some part-time assistance, or to call the bank and request a payment plan for the home mortgage.

Again, once a basic assessment of the patient's condition and family and home setting has been completed, the case manager has established her role with the patient, treating physician, and nurses, and has set up the services to match the resources and needs of the patient and family, then the telephone can become a tremendous resource. The moment a case manager hears something during a telephone conversation that sets off an internal "red alert," an on-site visit ideally should be made. If the assigned case manager cannot accomplish this due to geographic or other restriction, and especially if patient safety and/or liability is an issue, then a home care nurse can serve as valuable eyes and ears.

CERTIFICATION, ACCREDITATION AND STANDARDS OF PRACTICE

CCMC publishes the *CCM Certification Guide*, revised periodically to meet the changing roles of case managers in numerous practice settings within the evolving managed care industry. Every five years, representatives from the entire field of case management practitioners across the continuum of care are canvassed, and their conclusions are incorporated into the CCM exam content and credentialing criteria, leading to appropriate updates in the CCM role and function information. In this way, the CCM exam remains an accurate reflection of the field. The results also indicate areas in which case managers might require additional educational support and reference materials.

The Case Management Society of America developed the first set of Standards of Practice for Case Management in 1995. In 2001, it became apparent that an update was needed to bring the standards in line with the evolution of the case manager's role, the process of case management, and practice settings as the healthcare delivery system changes to meet our times. Following a rigorous peer review of the standards, public comment, and research, drafts and final versions were developed. Published in 2002 by the CMSA, the revised Standards of Practice for Case Management lists the primary case manager role functions as assessment, planning, facilitation, and advocacy.

URAC, a leader in the accreditation of health and managed care organizations, has created the URAC Case Management Core Standards, which also speaks to case management staff development, organization ethics, processes, and other issues that are involved in the provision of case management services. Taken together, these three new documents offer a comprehensive, detailed description of the case manager's purpose, goals, role, function, experience, performance indicators, and more. (The most recent versions of each can be obtained by calling or e-mailing CMSA, CCMC, and URAC at the numbers/addresses listed in Appendix A at the back of this book and at their specific organizational websites.) The CCMC certification guide provides insight into the kind of education, clinical preparation, and life experience that will most benefit a case manager.

The guide's "Licensure/Certification Requirements" section includes the eligibility standards, education, licensure, and certification criteria that applicants for the CCM credential must satisfy prior to sitting for the CCM examination.

In addition to CCMC's education, licensure, and certification criteria, applicants must meet the qualification of one of three employment experience categories. Category 1 calls for "12 months of acceptable full-time case management employment experience supervised by a Certified Case Manager (CCM). Supervision is defined as the systematic and periodic evaluation of the quality of the delivery of the applicant's case management services." Under Category 2, "24 months of acceptable full-time case management employment experience" is required. Supervision by a CCM is not requisite in this category. Category 3 lists employment experience of "12 months of acceptable full-time case management employment experience as a supervisor of individuals who provide DIRECT case management services." Verification of this status varies.

According to the *CCM Certification Guide*, applicants must perform services which encompass the essential activities of case management including: assessment, planning, implementation, coordination, monitoring, evaluation and outcomes, and be able to demonstrate that they apply these essential activities within at least five of the six core components of case management (case management concepts, case management principles and strategies, psychosocial and support systems, healthcare management and delivery, healthcare reimbursement, vocational concepts and strategies) across the continuum of care that matches ongoing needs of the individuals being served, with the appropriate level and type of health, medical, financial, legal, and psychosocial care. The employment experience regarding core components must also "involve interactions with relevant components of the individual's healthcare system such as physicians, family members, third-party payers, and other healthcare providers," and deal with the individual's broad spectrum of needs. To clarify those health-related services that fit the description of acceptable case management employment as described in the guide, a flowchart is included. It delineates processes and services that clearly demonstrate the provision of case management activities applying the essential functions across five of the six core areas beyond a single episode of care.

In order to enhance the accountability, recognition & professionalism of case managers, certain initiatives were developed over time by individuals as well as organizations. Standards of Practice, a Code of Professional Conduct, Accreditation of organizations and certification of professionals are just a few. Alongside the CCM credential, there are several other popular case management credentials.

NOTES

1. Buerhaus PE, "The Future of the Nursing Workforce in the United States."
2. Boling J and Hoffmann L, "The Nursing Shortage and its Implications for Case Management," *The Case Manager* 12, no. 6 (2001):53.
3. Mullahy M and Jensen DK, "Case Management: The Cost-Containment, Quality and Employee Satisfaction Link for Self-Funded Employers," *The Self-Insurer* 19 (2002): 7.
4. Towers Perrin, *Towers Perrin 2002 Health Care Cost Survey Report of Key Findings* (New York, NY: 2003).
5. Mercer 2006:1—Survey.
6. Greenburg L with Carneal G, Hattwick M, "Trends and Practices in Medical Management: 2005 Industry Profile," URAC (2005).
7. Commission for Case Manager Certification, *CCM Certification Guide* (Rolling Meadows, IL: 2003).
8. Moreo K and Lamb G, "CMSA Updates Standards of Practice for Case Management," *The Case Manager* 14, no. 3 (2003): 54.
9. Certification of Insurance Rehabilitation Specialists Commission, *Case Management Role and Function: Knowledge of Health Care* (Rolling Meadows, IL: 1992).

Chapter 2

The Case Manager's Universe

IMPORTANT CONTACTS AMONG HEALTHCARE PROVIDERS

The list of healthcare providers a case manager needs to know is as varied as the places these individuals work. Among a case manager's major contacts are physicians, surgeons, medical specialists, physical therapists, psychiatrists, pharmacists, behavioral health specialists, practitioners of alternative and Eastern medicine, discharge planners, rehabilitation nurses, rehabilitation and job counselors, nurse case managers, social workers, home health aides, family counselors, and medical equipment and service providers.

An addition to the provider group is hospitalists, general internists who practice only in the hospital. The concept was to improve care for hospitalized patients by having one physician on-site full-time at the hospital, responsible for most of their care, allowing office-based physicians to focus on their outpatients. Critics decry the further fragmentation of the healthcare delivery system. Concerned patients worry that they will not be able to see their own physicians, who are more familiar with their needs and medical history. Advocates point to the benefits of being tended by a specialist in hospital care and to the realities of today's healthcare system, in which internists no longer follow a patient through hospital care and discharge but refer to critical care specialists. Both sides are waiting to see how the use of hospitalists evolves. While we wait, case managers need to include these specialists in the care and communications loop. The range of facility resources includes hospitals, hospices, subacute care facilities, skilled nursing facilities, outpatient rehabilitation centers, nursing homes, and facilities offering illness-specific, chronic, or catastrophic care.

Case managers must be conversant with providers of specialized care, including, for example, neonatal teams that treat high-risk newborns at hospitals offering tertiary-level care. Centers of Excellence, which are designated areas within major university centers or other facilities that insurers have approved as providers of treatment, also offer specialized care. Also among a case manager's vital resources are specialized hospitals. There are, for example, fully accredited pediatric care facilities such as Stanford Children's Hospital in California, Children's Memorial Hospital in Chicago, and Schneider Children's Hospital in New York. Cumberland Hospital for Children and Adolescents has an Eating Disorders Program for patients ages 2–22 who not only have medical conditions but also are experiencing emotional and behavioral problems. The Mayo Clinic is noted for its team approach to diagnostic work ups, while Memorial Sloan-Kettering Cancer Center in New York City is renowned for its cancer research and treatment. Located in Denver, National Jewish Hospital/National Asthma Center is a diagnostic, research, and education facility that specializes in the treatment of asthma and pulmonary conditions, offering both adult and pediatric pro-grams. Shriners Hospitals in Boston, Cincinnati, Galveston, and Sacra-mento have a threefold mission: treating severely burned children, conducting research and improving methods of burn treatment, and training and educating medical personnel in the care and treatment of burn injuries. Other specialized centers include Joslin Diabetes Clinic in Boston, Patricia Neal Stroke Center in Knoxville, Rusk Institute for Reha-bilitation Medicine (New York University Medical Center), Bascom Palmer Eye Institute in Miami, and the M.D. Anderson Hospital and Tumor Institute in Houston.

Beyond acute care centers, case managers need to maintain an updated database listing facilities with accredited expertise and specialized programs for organ transplants; rehabilitation following head or spinal cord injury, burns, amputation, loss of sight or hearing; and other disabilities and diseases. In recent years, postacute or subacute care facilities have gained recognition as lower-cost alternatives for those medically complex cases that do not require the depth of service offered by a hospital or specialized care center but demand more than home-based recuperation. Individuals who might benefit from treatment at a subacute facility include patients needing short-term care following surgery, patients with a chronic illness who require intravenous pain control and/or nutrition, patients needing extended or respite care due to permanent debilitating injuries, and patients in a transitional stage of rehabilitation therapy after a fracture, stroke, or amputation. Subacute care centers are designed for medically stable patients and generally offer services such as wound management, infusion therapies, respiratory care, nutritional management, dialysis, TPN, and physical, occupational, and speech therapy.

HMOS, PPOS, MCOS, IPAS, PHOS, IDSS, HCOS, AND EPOS

The growth of managed care in the U.S. was spurred by the enactment of the Health Maintenance Organization Act of 1973. HMOs and PPOs were originally developed as alternative healthcare delivery systems, cost management strategies in which services are packaged for a group of insureds. The hope was that by shifting from a fee-for-service system to the use of payment schedules for packaged services, providers would have greater incentive to consider the appropriateness and costs of care when suggesting treatment. Today, PPOs are more prevalent, whereas the traditional HMO model is less common.

In the HMO arrangement, the physicians or practitioners within the HMO group agree to provide set benefits as needed by voluntarily enrolled members for a fixed dollar amount per member. Generally taking one of a few forms—staff model, group model, network model, or independent practice arrangement (IPA) model—an HMO usually offers members the choice of a primary care physician or other specialist from among those participating in the HMO. This primary physician then coordinates all the individual's medical care as well as any needed referrals to specialists and hospitals. Because they were losing patients, HMOs also created a service version allowing participants greater flexibility in choosing specialists and scheduling office visits without a referral, for an extra fee. The group HMO physician is usually employed by the HMO or receives most of his or her patients from the HMO. Staff-model HMO physicians limit their practice to the HMO and are salaried employees. In the IPA model, the HMO arranges contracts with physicians who also maintain their fee-for-service practice and who are paid a blend of fee for service and fixed fee. In a network model, two or more independent physician groups contract with an HMO to supply medical services. The HMO pays an established fee per employee per month, and the physicians or physician groups determine how those fees are split.

Most HMO services are generally covered in full or subject to co-payment. Limitations, restrictions, or nonreimbursement provisions come into play when services are sought outside of the HMO's geographical region of coverage or when medical treatment is obtained from nonparticipating providers. Waivers are usually granted if care given by a nonparticipant was received following an accident or the sudden acute onset of a life-threatening disease. The HMO will then retrospectively review the nonparticipant services and may provide coverage if the appropriateness of the care can be verified.

In the past fifteen years managed care became the predominant form of healthcare in the United States. More than 70 million Americans have been in HMO's and almost 90 million are enrolled in the more popular PPO's. In 2007, 21% of employees with healthcare coverage were in HMO's; 57% are in PPO's. Conventional indemnity plans continue to decline at 3% and Consumer-Directed Health Plans are experiencing an increase in enrollments with 12.5 million in 2007—up 25% from the 10 million in 2006.[1]

A PPO basically consists of a "limited provider panel," healthcare providers selected for their cost-effective style of practice. These providers also agree to lower their fees for services provided to PPO members. PPOs can be sponsored by medical providers, investors, or insurers. Some large national employers have created PPOs (and HMOs and HMO-PPO mixes) as nationwide networks of healthcare providers for their employees. In a PPO, members can choose to receive care from a provider outside of the PPO network, accepting reimbursement at levels similar to those received from traditional insurance coverage. (Network services may be provided with no deductible or for a lower co-payment than traditional insurance-covered services. Nonnetwork services may be subject to a deductible and higher coinsurance.) Nonnetwork emergency needs may be reimbursed at rates comparable to those for network services.

MCO (managed care organization) is a generic term that encompasses a variety of managed care plan types, such as an HMO, PPO, IPA, integrated delivery system (IDS), or an exclusive provider organization (EPO).

An IPA is a group holding a contract with a managed care plan to provide services in return for a single capitation rate. The IPA then arranges with individual providers to deliver the services on a capitation or a fee-for-service basis. Typically, an IPA encompasses all specialties, but one can be organized for primary care alone or another such specialty. An IPA may also exist as the "PO" element of a physician-hospital organization (PHO).

Often created to contract with managed care plans, PHOs are legal or informal arrangements that link hospitals with their attending staff as business entities. In some cases, any staff member may apply for inclusion in the PHO, or the organization may be closed to staff members who do not qualify or who are part of an overrepresented specialty.

The IDS is loosely defined as a system of healthcare providers organized to span a broad range of healthcare services. It is also referred to as an integrated healthcare delivery system, an integrated delivery network (IDN), an integrated delivery and financing system (IDFS), or an integrated delivery and financing network (IDFN). Anyone else have a headache now? This IDS is established to select from the broad healthcare provider market to "optimize cost and clinical outcomes, accept and manage a full range of financial arrangements to provide a set of defined benefits to a defined population, align financial incentives of the participants (including physicians), and operate under a cohesive management structure."[2]

Healthcare organizations (HCOs) are an outgrowth of California's 1993 workers' compensation reforms, which created a certification process for managed care companies, and seek to concentrate on applying the benefits of managed care strategies to work-related injuries. Disability insurers, HMOs, and other medical groups and providers may apply to become certified HCOs; the certification is not required to treat work-related injuries. HCOs are required to provide case management and return-to-work services.

An exclusive provider organization or EPO resembles an HMO; primary physicians are often gatekeepers, providers are often capitated, its provider group is often limited, and an authorization system is applied to care. The word "exclusive" is used to denote that members must remain within the network to receive benefits. Unlike HMOs, EPOs are usually regulated by insurance statutes.

MANAGED CARE

While HMO's continue to decline, and PPO's now enrolling more than 165 million Americans, there are an estimated 247 million enrolled in managed care plans. With the increasing popularity of CDHP (Consumer Director Health Plans), managed care continues to evolve, as a health-care service and as a business.[3] Many new provider organizations have developed (dental care providers are among those moving into managed care networks), and case managers have significantly more entities to sort out and address, as players and "rules" change and the system becomes more convoluted.

Numerous and significant mergers and acquisitions among providers have blurred previous distinctions. In the past, hospitals were entities unto themselves and physicians maintained private practices. Doctors would hang out their shingles and determine the type of practice they would build and how they would treat patients. Today, to capture larger markets and to position themselves as one-stop providers offering a broad range of services, hospitals and physician groups have merged or formed partnerships, just as healthcare companies and durable medical equipment companies have joined. As hospitals scoop up physician practices, combining them into larger organizations that span communities, we move away from a traditional arrangement in which the physician had greater control over his or her business and often maintained close ties to a local hospital. The balance of power in medicine has shifted from the insurance companies to the large providers.

From the case manager's perspective, such mergers raise quality-of-care and negotiation issues. Case managers are aware of the strengths and weaknesses of the hospitals in their communities. A signed contract establishing a hospital network does not automatically upgrade the technical capabilities or medical expertise of the weaker hospitals. Although advertising slogans assure patients that they will receive the same quality care, in some cases prestigious, university, or teaching hospitals are carrying smaller, less accomplished hospitals.

Decreased competition also affects quality of care. Instead of a variety of providers, we have two or three major players, or less. In our area, for example, smaller religious hospitals are considering a merger with a nonsectarian group to combat a rival medical "dynasty." As providers seek advantageous alignments, care can be inadvertently leveraged out. We once had hospitals and their respective boards of directors responding to the particular medical, social, welfare, economic, or language problems of the community and developing the structure to serve those needs. Now, we have healthcare monoliths attempting to run "lean and mean." What chance does the smaller hospital's wonderful high-risk pregnancy management program have of being sustained if management perceives it as a duplication of services?

I've also found that case managers have lost some of the opportunity we had to negotiate certain services, and our ability to work with local hospitals is somewhat curtailed. We hear that as part of ABC Healthcare Corporation, the hospital doesn't negotiate with anybody. Visiting a hospital where we had enjoyed a good rapport and friendly relationship with the administration becomes a confusion of red tape. We call a discharge planner and are told that we have to go through ABC corporate, or there is a completely new system in place to navigate. It's very difficult for case managers (as well as physicians and others), and I question whether patients are really being as well-served as some facilities would have us believe.

The burgeoning PPOs and networks are another challenge for case managers. What guarantees that the PPO group in New York maintains the same criteria and credentialing standards as the network in Massachusetts? Case managers need to be aware that while working with one network may seem easier than dealing with numerous providers, we still have a responsibility to know the people we're dealing with, from the physicians to the hospitals to the home care companies. We have a responsibility to look beyond the recognized logo and ads for quality of service. The more complicated the system is, the more on notice we have to be.

Working state to state, case managers may be involved with in-network providers, out-of-network providers, and out-of-state providers. A company may employ many individuals across a state where there are no network providers, or it may use one network in three states, a second network in another five states, plus out-of-network services in all states. A case manager working in a centralized location would find it extremely difficult to sort out and coordinate among these plans. Adding to the challenge are the physicians, home care providers, physical therapists, etc., who may have been accepted to the network or switched to another network within the past months. The networks cheerfully suggest that case managers call them to check on the status of network members, not realizing that the request is an overwhelming administrative task.

For example, an employer group we have worked with for four years uses a network, and we work with its doctors, physical therapists, and others. In one region of a northeast state, the network mandated that all precertification (precert) calls and case management services go through the network staff, rather than the Third Party Administrator (TPA) staff as is customary for employee precert calls in every other region of every other state. We were working a case only to find that it was to have been a network case; we shouldn't have gotten that case. A case manager who is part of a large company that offers its employees many plan options, or a case manager working with 30 different employer groups, each with its own arrangements, faces a huge managerial problem. She must track the employer group, plan, or network, as well as the division of labor within the network.

One major telecommunications group offers its employees a choice among eight different healthcare plans. Within each plan are options for indemnity coverage, an HMO, a PPO with point-of-service arrangements, and more. Each plan's overall benefits are the same, but the several providers have individual claims processing formats, and they pay claims separately. How can the telecommunications company, concerned with quality-of-care issues and wise allotment of monies, possibly know what is going on when so many different players are spending its dollars? It's an administrative nightmare and extremely difficult for the case managers providing outcomes tracking and cost-benefit analysis reports.

I see the evolution of managed care and the trend of narrowing down providers creating more problems. Patients have less to select from, and already there seems to be less response to certain population groups. The one-size-fits-all concept doesn't work with healthcare.

As an absolute acknowledgment of the increasing convictions within the healthcare delivery and payer systems, and the growing frustrations of employers and their employees another player is in our midst! Health advocates, integrators or navigators as they are also termed. We have responded and grown to address concerns and resolve problems. Through these services, employees have access to independent medical and insurance experts. Often former healthcare administrators, counselors and nurses who assist them with health plan and medical issues.[4]

MANAGED COMPETITION

Managed competition refers to the very real competition that HMOs, PPOs, and other managed care entities face in getting and maintaining business. Managed competition introduces new criteria for healthcare decision making and price evaluation, and puts control back in the hands of the purchaser. Within the last few years, the availability of outcomes data has made it possible to review and select a health provider facility based on quality of service and patient outcomes as well as pricing. It is no longer good enough to be price competitive; service providers have to demonstrate effective pricing and good outcomes without sacrificing the satisfaction of patients and their families.

When the term *managed* competition was first coined in the late 1970s by Alain Enthoven, he mentioned "sponsors," agencies that acted as brokers by examining all the health plan possibilities in the field and negotiating with those plans to help a client get the best mix of care and price based on the client's needs. More recently, the term *health insurance purchasing cooperative* (HIPC) has gained acceptance as a way of referring to brokering organizations that serve small employers and individuals. (In some managed care models, there is only one HIPC per geographical region, and all individuals purchase health insurance through that HIPC.) HIPCs and sponsors relate to that version of managed competition that is still in the theory stage. Yet, managed competition is already here, as is evident from the description of the managed competition model that follows.

It is generally agreed that there are four stages of managed competition. In the first, independent hospitals and physicians maintain profitable businesses without any organized purchasing payers. Provider networks begin to form in the second stage, called loose framework. Payments are structured in the form of discounts and per diems. The next stage, called consolidation, signals the emergence of a few large sophisticated purchasers and systems, and fewer private practices. In the fourth and last stage—managed competition—hospitals, physicians, and insurance companies form integrated networks to manage patient populations. Several large providers generally dominate markets. The rest of the providers have either sold their practices, merged with larger groups, or closed up shop.

Managed competition is here today in the form of managed care organizations. The PPOs that are successful are the ones that are able to deliver quality and good outcomes while holding down costs. At their origin, some argued that HMOs benefited from adverse risk selection, that healthier people usually opt for HMOs based on a belief they will not need catastrophic coverage. They are attracted by the lower premiums or have young children whom they can take to the doctor for a small fee per visit— a prime concern during the winter chickenpox-sniffles-and-strep school season. It was thought that the sicker people would tend to stay in the more flexible plans, PPOs, POS (point-of-service), and indemnity plans, which offer the most freedom of choice regarding physician selection, varying sites for care, different levels of co-payment, and reimbursement of customary fees. The challenge for HMOs became clear when the government, one of the nation's largest payer/providers through its Medicare and Medicaid programs, moved its sick and elderly into managed care plans. One can argue that a disproportionate share of high-cost patients was enrolled in HMOs, which reacted by restricting access. The biggest HMOs are the ones that are able to penetrate the market, and those that were and are well-managed are the ones that have survived.

Employer coalitions and business alliances are buying services and getting discounting arrangements from providers of prescriptions and durable medical equipment or from local rehab facilities. They say, "We'll send all of our people to you. What can you do for us?" Employers, insurance carriers, brokers, and TPAs are managing care and cost; they are being aggressive negotiators because of the law of supply and demand.

These changes signal the total management of the health delivery system, with employers sponsoring different levels of plans and consumers and providers sharing responsibilities for risk and choice, specifically in consumer-driven healthcare (CDH) plans, discussed in Chapter 4. Even when risk, which influences the payments an employer group makes, is a consideration, the employer group still has an edge. For instance, if a company has a high incidence of a particular disease, that is factored in to how the company is rated and the premiums it has to pay. But the company now has an ability to choose from a variety of health insurance programs and health providers and facilities, whether its health insurance network includes an HMO, a PPO, or whatever.

COMPLEMENTARY AND ALTERNATIVE CARE

The use of complementary and alternative care treatments is still considered controversial or "unorthodox" in some quarters; however, especially given the increased cultural diversity of our patient populations, they are among the most appropriate healing techniques for certain patients. Classified as mind/body/spirit treatment, holistic medicine, and Eastern medicine, these alternative approaches can refer to acupuncture, guided imagery, dietary therapy, Chinese medicine, spiritual healing, herbal remedies, homeopathy, meditation, craniosacral therapy, chiropractic care, massage including Reiki, fertility treatments, paranormal healing, Tai Chi, and Yoga, among others.

Premature infants are being aided by "kangaroo care" or skin-to-skin care. Mothers and fathers hold their baby, wearing a diaper, against their bare chests. These babies gain weight and thrive, and are also able to go home sooner in many cases.

The National Center for Complementary and Alternative Medicine (http://nccam.nih.gov/) offers insight into treatments, resources for additional information, studies in progress and completed, and fraud issues. Included in the resources the site suggests are CAMline, the Complementary Medical Association, the Alternative Medicine Foundation, and Alternative Health News Online. (I especially like its note on the last references as one that helps us to separate the hogwash from the promising therapies in alternative medicine.)

Case managers also need to know about alternative treatment facilities and programs, such as residential and experiential programs for teenagers. Aspen Achievement Academy in southern Utah combines an outdoor therapy program with traditional mental health therapeutic interventions for 13- to 18-year-olds who suffer from psychiatric, emotional, and substance abuse disorders. Working with emotionally disturbed youths aged 10 to 17, the Eckerd Alternative Treatment Program blends reality therapy, behavior modification, individualized mental health services, group therapy, and problem-solving sessions in a wilderness camp setting. In addition, there are camps designed to meet the needs of patient populations, such as Western Pennsylvania Hospital's Summer Camp for Burned Children, held at the Emma Kaufmann Camp in the Blue Ridge Mountains; Camp Barnabas, near Monett, Missouri, for children 7 years old or older with terminal or serious, chronic diseases; and facilities like Gilda's Club in New York City, for men, women, and families coping with cancer. In the San Bernardino Mountains of southern California is the World's Greatest Camp, created for the families of children with cancer. The Adaptive Sports Center at Crested Butte, Colorado, offers outdoor recreation to people with developmental and physical difficulties. Instruction and equipment includes skiing, snowboarding, snowshoeing, ice dancing, dogsledding, snowmobiling, downhill mountain biking, hand cycling, canoeing, multiday river trips, white-water rafting, hiking, camping, and fishing. Designed for children between 5 and 21 who have mild to moderate neurological and developmental impairments, Camp Le Mar is an accredited coed facility in Pennsylvania. Teaching youths with diabetes to maintain good habits for a healthier lifestyle while having a great time is Camp Sweeney in Gainesville, Texas. The Double 'H' Hole in the Woods Ranch in the Adirondacks was founded for children with cancer, hemophilia, sickle-cell anemia, spina bifida, and AIDS. The Imus Ranch in New Mexico is a 4,000-acre working cattle ranch where children suffering from cancer or serious blood disorders, and children who've lost brothers and sisters to Sudden Infant Death Syndrome (SIDS) complete daily chores, are responsible for a horse, and are required to pitch in caring for the other animals.

Located near Malibu, Camp Bloomfield was created for visually impaired and multidisabled blind children ages 5 to 18. Dating from 1868, Vacation Camp for the Blind in Spring Valley, New York, is a year-round facility providing a rich array of sports, cultural, rehabilitation, and educational programs for blind and visually impaired adults and children with disabilities.

KidSource online (www.kidsource.com) lists resources and guides from associations and private organizations, such as Easter Seals and the Hemophilia Association. *Summer Fun: The Parents' Complete Guide to Day Camps, Overnight Camps, Specialty Camps, and Teen Tours* by Marian Edelman Borden is recommended by *Library Journal*.

Other resources case managers need to be aware of include nursing services, home health agencies, infusion and respiratory care companies, counseling centers, surgical supply firms, and a host of local, state, and federal agencies and associations targeting problems such as aging, learning disabilities, and physical disabilities. There are national organizations for most major diseases, and it is the case manager's responsibility to know about them. As an example, the National Head Injury Foundation will send on request a state-by-state listing of facilities treating head injuries at various levels, from the catastrophic stage through transitional stage to rehabilitative care. National organizations are invaluable for assistance in another area: education. The American Lung Association and the American Heart Association are two prime providers of free educational materials. The Alzheimer's Foundation offers articles on estate planning, Medicaid law, long-term care insurance, and other topics written by the foundation's legal advisory board. The YMCA runs a healthy back program and is willing and able to provide informational pamphlets.

Where can a case manager begin to locate these legions of specialists, services, and support personnel? *The Case Management Resource Guide*, updated annually, includes information on mail-order pharmaceutical companies, pediatric home care, hand rehabilitation centers, hotlines for physical and mental disorder, and auto remodelers that can fit a car for a wheelchair ramp. A national guide, it is divided into four regional volumes and is published by Dorland Healthcare Information (A Contexo Media Company) and available from Amazon.

Other resource volumes include *How to Find the Best Doctors*, which includes hospitals, medical centers, specialties, specialists, and physician rating references. This series by John J. Connolly, Sandra Gainer, and others, offers editions for various parts of the country, updated on a rotating basis and published by Castle Connolly Medical Ltd. In addition, look for *America's Top Doctors: The Best in American Medicine*, second edition (by Castle Connolly Staff, Compiler, *et al.*, Castle Connolly Medical Ltd.), *Consumer's Guide to Top Doctors* (by Center for the Study of Services Consumer's Checkbook Magazine Staff), *America's Best Hospitals* (by editors of *U.S. News & World Report* with the National Opinion Research Center at the University of Chicago, J. Wiley & Sons), and *The Best Hospitals in America*, second edition (by John W. Wright, Linda Sunshine, Gale Group), and *Voluntary Health Organizations: A Guide to Patient Services* (Labe Scheinberg, Demos Medical Publishing; out of print but available). Also check for regional volumes that cover the array of facilities and services in your area.

As a case manager weighs the best solution for an individual, she must remember to examine all alternatives the patient is entitled to as well as possible overlapping resources. For example, if the case manager can refer a patient to one of the Lighthouse sites supervised by the Association for the Blind in the state, dollars may be conserved for insurer-provided care. For additional information on medical facility and service directories, please refer to Appendix A at the end of the book.

STANDARDS OF CARE

How does one distinguish the professionals from the we-do-that-toos? One method of evaluating an organization is to check whether there is a governing body or written standards of care. Today, there is a much greater emphasis on standards of care, facility accreditation, and the good standing of medical practitioners than existed a decade ago. For instance, rehabilitation facilities are accredited by the Commission on Accreditation of Rehabilitation Facilities (CARF). The National Committee for Quality Assurance (NCQA) provides accreditation for healthcare organizations, and for managed care organizations in particular. The Health Plan Employer Data and Information Set (HEDIS) is sponsored, supported, and maintained by the NCQA. It is a set of standardized, quality performance measures to help employers and other purchasers evaluate health plan operations.

We now have evidence-based medicine, and guidelines for care, and it is the case manager's responsibility to bring each patient as close as possible to these standards. It is our role to ensure that patients have access to information and can choose a physician, facility, and health plan, and evaluate them in light of others of the same class, to judge the methods and measures that have proven most effective. We want to move our patients into systems in which standards of care are utilized effectively.

When there are no recognized standards of care or when an individual is being evaluated, the best strategy is to combine available performance criteria information with a personal critique. Some case managers create their own facility or individual review form to separate core quality from showcase dressing. Questions might include these: How does the specialist or medical facility director answer questions—directly or by responding with his or her own questions? Is the facility truly open to sharing information on its programs or is it reciting the five-minute marketing speech? Is a request to attend a team conference met by resistance or a welcome? An individual or a group trying to control access to or hide background information should set off an alarm. The case manager should begin to suspect that getting complete reports on a patient's progress will be an onerous task.

Individual specialists should be board-certified in their field, have teaching experience, an active license, and a strong hospital or facility affiliation. Because there are subpar credentials, check the certifying agency. For example, in New York, the Medical Society of the State of New York has published a medical directory that lists credentialed practitioners in a number of specialties. The State Education Department can provide information on whether the physician is currently licensed and registered in New York State.

National medical societies can offer guidance on how to verify credentials. One can compare and research physicians at www .healthgrades.com, or contact the Board of Medical Specialties to confirm whether a physician is board-certified and to get the number of individual specialty boards. The Board can be reached at 1-800-275-2267 or www.abms.org. Found in the reference sections of most libraries, *The Directory of Physicians in the United States 40th Edition* (by the American Medical Association, 2008) and *The Official Abms Directory of Board-Certified Medical Specialists,* hardcover and CD ROM (by American Board of Medical Specialties, W. B. Saunders, & Elsevier, 2008) list qualifications of individual physicians, including where the physician attended medical school and received residency training, board certification, hospital affiliations, type of practice, and other information. At HealthGrades, located at www.healthgrades.com, one can find a physician, physician in a specialty, and information on hospital outcomes, nursing homes, home health agencies, hospice, and other services.

Whether reviewing a person or an agency, ask for names and phone numbers of references. If a home health agency provides dated information—case managers it last worked with when an actor was in the White House—question its capabilities. If a physician is unwilling to give references, question his or her reliability (the same goes for an agency). Medical "report cards" for physicians and facilities exist for each state.

Another way case managers can educate themselves on the appropriate levels of expertise and service to expect from providers and suppliers is to become members of local and national associations. Meetings planned by professionals working within separate disciplines and condition- or illness-specific conferences are excellent sources of information and resources. At conferences with exhibitors, case managers should talk with adaptive equipment vendors, marketers of oxygen-supply devices, prosthetics designers—and ask every question that comes to mind, including costs of equipment and services. Then, when reviewing bids from suppliers, they will have enough background to spot the inclusion of unnecessary equipment or overzealous billing. They will be more savvy and capable of providing improved advocacy for patients and more effective use of resources.

NOTES

1. "Employer Health Benefits, 2007," Section 5, Kaiser Family Foundation.
2. Kongstvedt PR, *Managed Care: What It Is and How It Works*, 2nd ed. Sudbury, MA: Jones and Bartlett Publishers, Inc., 2002.
3. "Consumer-Directed Health Plans Continue to Grow as Popular Vehicles to Bring Choice, Flexibility & Access to Consumers," Press Release from American AASN of Preferred Provider Organizations 3.24.08.
4. Wells SJ, "Health Advocates" H.R. Magazine – August 2006, Vol. 51, No 8.

3

Insurance Providers and Administrators

When considering the world of insurance, including insurance companies, reinsurance companies, indemnity providers, self-insured firms, and self-insured/self-administered corporations, case managers are tempted to ask, "Who are those guys? What are the differences in their services and why is it important for me to distinguish between them?" Good questions.

The role of the case manager becomes more complex the larger the company that is insuring and the larger the group that is being insured. Size and type of both the insurer and the insurance administrative arm will impact the autonomy of the case management role, influence (if not dictate) the format and frequency of communications, and affect the case manager's ability to obtain approval for allowances or exceptions in coverage should the need arise. In a CIGNA or Aetna fully insured plan, a company customarily pays premiums based on expected case incidences and outcomes. Conversely, case managers often work with patients whose needs are not considered in the typical premium structure. Further, when employer groups are blended into larger groups (PPOs, multiple employer trusts, or business alliances, for example) to increase their purchasing power, case managers find themselves layers away from the decision makers—the chief executive officers (CEOs) and employers—who sometimes can help speed the approval process when plan dollars need to be utilized in a nontraditional fashion. A case manager might have more flexibility and success working with local or regional insurers and employers because of the closer contact with those capable and willing to make decisions regarding reimbursement.

Insurance companies vary in how they work with case managers. Some firms have in-house or affiliated case management capabilities (e.g., CIGNA has Intracorp and UnumProvident Corp. has GENEX

Services, Inc.). Other insurers contract with several case management entities across the country by region, using one for all cases in the Northeast, for example, and another for cases on the West Coast. Another insurer might contract by specialty, clinical expertise, or by market niche. The larger the insurer, the less likely it will employ an independent case management provider, unless the insurer is sophisticated and already has an in-house regional coordinator for case management services.

Are the insurer's operations contained within one state or does it have national capabilities? Because the activities of case managers are largely mandated by both federal and state regulations, it is the case manager's responsibility to know the effect of state regulations on different health insurance benefits. A state might require that x number of mammographies per year be covered for women in a certain age group as part of the regulations companies must follow if they want to write insurance in that state. (Under Employee Retirement Income Security Act [ERISA] guidelines, companies that self-insure are not compelled to hold to those same minimum benefits regulations and provide equivalent benefits. For example, employer groups can choose to limit their fiscal responsibility for HIV-related treatments over a claimant's lifetime.)

In the majority of cases, case managers are employed by the payers, the insurers, and their work is governed by the group, department, or agency carrying the fiduciary responsibility for the benefit plan. This entity defines what will be covered and when coverage will be cut or phased out to ensure that no one person or group of persons makes excessive claims that consume all the benefits dollars in the plan. As the plan or insured group becomes larger, the efforts to provide appropriate, timely, cost-effective care can become convoluted. With numerous layers of fiduciaries, insurers, administrators, and claims adjustors to contact for approval, the patient's experience is often over before a decision is reached.

BASIC INSURANCE AND ADMINISTRATIVE
COMPANY PLAYERS

In traditional insurer-client relationships, a company or individual pays an annual premium to an insurance firm. The cost of any particular benefits plan is determined by the breadth and length of coverage that will be provided; the age, sex, and health of the individual at the time the plan is drawn up; and the statistical likelihood the individual will suffer from a disease or disability. Generally, group plans, in which insurers cover a body of employees or associates in the same industry along with their dependents, are available at a lower premium than plans for single individuals. The entire administration of the benefits plan is managed and handled by the insurance company. For example, when an individual makes a claim against his or her insurance plan, the claims department within the insurance firm processes the paperwork and arranges for full or partial payment or denies payment. Similarly, it is the insurance firm's responsibility to invest and manage the premium dollars it takes in to ensure its ability to pay claims.

In response to rising insurance costs, many businesses have pursued alternative financing methods, such as self-insurance. The switch to self-funding does result in a significant initial reduction in healthcare benefits costs for individual companies. Business executives nationwide find that self-insurance helps streamline company operations and offers better control over where their healthcare dollars were used. Overall, self-insurance has been a consistently growing trend, especially among large employers, which can be seen in the steadily increasing numbers of employer-funded PPOs, indemnity plans, HMOs, and point-of-service (POS) plans. In self-funding, companies assume dollar-for-dollar responsibility for employee healthcare and avoid the spillover of financial responsibility previously included in their premiums to cover other clients an insurer might be carrying. However, self-insured firms run a risk. By narrowing the universe of contributors to their health benefit fund (by eliminating the old insurer's other clients), companies also limit their payout capabilities. Financial liability is spread among a smaller group, often without the application of support systems, such as preadmission authorization, utilization review, claims review, or case management, to help manage the benefit program. A few catastrophic claims, such as for a premature infant, an organ transplant, childhood leukemia, a head trauma, or a burn or cancer patient, can sap a plan's resources and eliminate any bottom-line savings. Another version of self-funding, the consumer-driven healthcare concept, elicits more employee responsibility financially.

With the appearance of self-funded plans, two other types of service companies became more prominent: TPAs and firms offering administrative services-only (ASO) contracts. TPAs and those insurers or companies providing ASO contracts take on the administrative responsibility of handling claims for self-funded groups. They process claims, answer claimant questions, and act as the liaison between the offices and officers of the payer and the healthcare provider groups. There are a number of TPAs and ASO companies that at the request of their self-insured employers have begun to render claims management services (e.g., educating client company employees via wellness programs, assisting with medically fragile cases, tracking high-cost cases, and providing comprehensive cost-control programs). They provide these services by subcontracting with a case management or utilization review firm or by setting up an in-house case management or utilization review group. Some self-funded companies elect to self-administer their plans as well, processing all claims through their own claims group.

To handle an unexpected rise in healthcare costs or a number of catastrophic or chronic claims, self-insured employers often invest in excess or surplus lines of insurance such as reinsurance or stop-loss coverage. It is often purchased in combination with capitated payment arrangements to help protect employers against the fluctuating utilization within their employer groups, as well as those unforeseen, very costly cases. Premiums are paid to a reinsurance firm, establishing a plan that commits the reinsurance firm to step in and cover health benefits payouts in the event that claims should surpass a set dollar limit. "Specific" stop-loss protection becomes activated when an individual's claims reach the deductible level selected by the self-funding group; such protection usually covers up to one million dollars per lifetime per employee. "Aggregate" coverage, which kicks in when a self-insurer's total group health claims outstrip a predetermined level or percent of its annual estimated claims costs, is another form of stop-loss protection that is available.

Minimum premium is another means of financing medical benefits. In this method, an employer pays a segment of the regular premium to an insurer to administer the benefits program and provide specific and aggregate stop-loss insurance. The employer maintains a "bank account" that the insurance company taps for payment of claims. Minimum premium differs from straightforward stop-loss in that the employer maintains the funding source rather than purchasing stop-loss or reinsurance coverage from an insurer. It provides some of the economic benefits and tax advantages of self-funded plans without the deep restrictions that can be associated with fully insured plans.

Too often, employer groups assume that their insurers "know the business" and settle into a false sense of security. Granted, today's insurers are astute in the business of setting premiums and designing benefit plans, but they may not be well-versed in the business of properly managing available healthcare benefit dollars and the broad array of healthcare claims. Regardless of the size of the company and its method of insuring and administering health benefits, it is the case manager's responsibility to know the allowances and restrictions of the benefit plan.

A case manager subcontracting with a TPA might find that of the TPA's eight clients, three are fully insured and the others are self-insured, each with a unique benefits plan design and claims administration package. Although working in-house with a major insurer and responsible for helping to manage the insurer's own employee benefits, a case manager might have to coordinate her work with the TPA overseeing payment of all claims. A large regional firm with thousands of employees and dependents might be self-funded but contract with an insurance firm for the administration of its plan.

In addition to the setup of the plan, a case manager needs to know the relationship of the referring party to the claimant: Was the request for case management the result of a red flag sent up by the stop-loss insurer? Was it made by the utilization review staff within the insurance firm? Or was it the suggestion of a human resources manager within the employer company? The referral source affects how the case can be managed and the amount of autonomy the case manager will have. Being in a position to ask direct approval to change a treatment plan from a corporate CEO is a far cry from taking a call from the claims department at a TPA—already once or twice removed from the benefit plan decision maker—on a case in which the claimant is covered by an insurer who does not offer reimbursement for case management services. Likewise, if a case manager needs allowance to spend a slightly higher portion of benefit dollars now to prevent spending a substantial amount of money for repeat hospitalizations for complications later on, the CEO of a self-insured firm looking at that scenario might be better able to appreciate the case manager's point of view than the three owners of an HMO, who see dollars spent on case management as an expense that directly diminishes profits because of the way the HMO's profit base is structured. The utmost in cost control and practice autonomy occurs in the self-insured, self-administered employer group that has hired its own medical administrator or case manager to track all stages of the health benefit process, from plan design through claims processing.

ADMINISTRATIVE AND CUSTOMIZED SERVICES

Along with claims payouts, many insurers, TPAs, and ASOs serve as "broker/administrators" and provide a broad range of specialized or ancillary administrative services. These may include claims adjustment, claims analysis (medical, dental, and disability), risk control services, design and creation of national and regional networks, utilization review, Pharmacy Benefits Management (PBM), and disease management programs. TPAs can help redesign plan language, communicate to employees the items included in a Summary Plan Description (SPD) and their relevance, assist with COBRA administrations, and craft Medical Savings Accounts (MSAs) and 401Ks. Case managers can contribute effectively to each of these offerings.

Because of their clinical medical experience, case managers can evaluate a claims run, ascertaining those areas in which claims are excessive and perhaps indicating special needs (e.g., the need for an employee wellness program). Case managers can also analyze specific claims for use of services. Risk control requires a system to identify possible high-care, high-cost cases so they may be properly managed each step of the way. Again, case managers have the experience and expertise to review an employer's or insurer's covered lives and establish an appropriate "grading" system—not to pull out individuals for restricted coverage or treatment but to provide early warning so that each case receives the attention it needs.

The same skills make case managers particularly effective when an employer seeks or an insurer designs an HMO, a PPO, or a blend of the two. Using a geographical or medical services-based strategy, a case manager can help develop the provider profile most appropriate for the characteristics of the employer group being covered. Utilization review, rather than the lower service fees typically associated with HMOs and PPOs, is the ingredient that leads to reduced expenditures, although it has come under fire as a "gatekeeper" strategy that can prevent individuals from getting the care they need. In developing a utilization review program, case managers, because of their medical background and their tradition of managing each case individually, are in a position to elucidate the importance of establishing a treatment path for each patient. Putting the individual back into the care picture enhances the benefits of utilization review for both the patient and the payer.

THE CASE MANAGEMENT DELIVERY SYSTEM AND REPORT CARDS

Employer groups are beginning to understand the complexities of the health benefit system, but there is still a need for more comprehensive employer education. The system is undoubtedly complex, and given the expanding numbers of providers and payers, it is not growing any simpler or more streamlined. Education remains an uphill struggle. When they discovered that their health benefit premiums were often higher than the coverage or reimbursement their employees received in return, many employers turned to self-funded plans, and the first- and second-year savings were substantial. On the flip side, any catastrophic case within the employer group became more keenly felt than before.

To control risk, some employers responded proactively by acquiring reinsurance. Those who took the unwise position that the money saved through self-insuring would cover any big cases that came along have learned otherwise.

Employers also had to manage employees' growing sense of entitlement in conjunction with their disconnect regarding risk factors and the true cost of healthcare. To bring employer-sponsored healthcare coverage more in line with reality, companies are beginning to share healthcare risks and costs with employees in the form of consumer-driven health plans, and are educating their covered populations on the importance of wellness.

Report cards were a direct response to employers' frustration with the burden of healthcare expenses. These tools compare health plan performance in key areas of accountability (quality, utilization, administrative responsiveness and performance, consumer satisfaction, cost control) and help answer the question: What are we getting for our money?

Similar concerns about the quality of healthcare prompted the Leapfrog Initiative, sponsored by The Business Roundtable in early 2000. It was formed in response to reports on quality in 1998 and safety in 1999 from the Institute of Medicine (IOM), a congressionally chartered, independent organization that gathers and reports objective information on healthcare. The IOM found that upwards of 98,000 Americans die every year from preventable medical errors experienced during hospital stays (outpatient settings were not included in this study). Not all these mistakes resulted in death; however, other results were similarly tragic—permanent disabilities and the need for additional treatment leading to longer hospital stays and recovery periods. The concept behind the initiative was that a large body of hospital service purchasers would have the clout to initiate improvements in the safety and quality of healthcare by taking its business to providers with proven records of strong performance in both areas, while at the same time educating consumers in making better choices on hospital care.[1]

In a recent study, Health Grades 5th Annual Patient Safety in American Hospitals Study, analyzed 41 million MEDICARE patient records. It determined that patient safety incidents cost the Federal Medicare program 8.8 billion dollars and resulted in 238,337 potentially preventable deaths during 2004 through 2006, quite more work is needed and case managers can be part of initiatives through the system.[2]

A coalition of more than 135 public and private organizations providing healthcare benefits, the Leapfrog Group represents approximately 37 million healthcare consumers in all 50 states. It works with medical experts around the country to identify problems and suggest solutions in hospital systems to avoid preventable errors in patient care.[3] Those in the group, including IBM, PepsiCo, Verizon, Xerox, Empire Blue Cross/Blue Shield, and New York Business Group on Health, base their healthcare purchases on a hospital's progress in adopting three safety measures, or "leaps": computer physician order entry systems, evidence-based hospital referral, and ICU physician staffing. These leaps are considered by the Leapfrog Group to be a starting point toward improving care and will likely be broadened over the years.[4]

Payers want to know how successfully a case might be handled through case management prior to giving the go-ahead for its application. So, current standards lump all cases together. Any patient claim exceeding a specific dollar limit or falling into a specific diagnostic category is earmarked for case management. But what of the situations that lend themselves to case management more readily than the diagnoses would indicate? A pregnancy experienced by a healthy 22-year-old differs from that experienced by a healthy 14-year-old or 45-year-old. Because there is often little leeway in the standards set by payers for case management intervention and there are numerous restrictions on how and when case management can come into play, many opportunities to provide high-quality, cost-effective care are lost.

Case managers have created a win/win scenario; patients and payers are both well-served. Instead of routinely spending $50,000 on a treatment, employers, providers, payers, and case managers manage that money, putting it to its best use. However, case management has a distance to go before it is integrated as a routine element of a benefit plan rather than as an alternative treatment applied to specific cases upon request. Case managers need to expand their communication with employers and decision makers. (For more information on communicating with payer sources, please see Chapter 8.)

Case managers are providing services and working cases in many practice settings. When they are employed directly by an employer group, hospital, or insurance company, case managers have a greater opportunity to review medical care and benefit dollar protection issues thoroughly and to position case management as a solution to escalating healthcare costs. There are case managers holding positions now (registered nurses, occupational health nurses, social workers with teaching backgrounds), but only a few case managers are involved in marketing the service to CEOs and relatively none in the benefit plan design and decision-making loop. The next step in educating insurance providers and administrators is to convince these companies to put case managers in more pivotal positions and make them an integral part of higher-level management, able to report the true benefit of case management, to expand case management services to multiple lines of insurance, and to increase the value, marketability, and awareness of case management.

NOTES

1. "About Us," The Leapfrog Group, http://leapfroggroup.org/about.htm; June 10, 2003 and "BRT-Sponsored Initiative Focuses on Patient Safety," The Business Roundtable, http://brtable.org/press.cfm/375; June 10, 2003.
2. "Medical Errors Cost $8.8 Billion, Result in 238,337 potentially preventable deaths." April 8, 2008 release HEALTH GRADES.
3. The Leapfrog Group home page, http://leapfroggroup.org - October 22, 2008.
4. The Leapfrog Group Fact sheet, http://leapfrog.org - October 22, 2008.

Chapter 4

Insurance Lines and Health Benefit Plans

What is the health benefit plan? And why does it matter? Often, what a case manager can accomplish and the positive impact she can effect upon a patient's outcome are dictated by the terms of the benefit plan under which an individual is covered. It is vital that case managers understand what their role is relative to the type of coverage in question. Some plans contain no provision for case management services, leaving case managers struggling for approval to implement alternative treatment strategies at the eleventh hour—with answers at hand but no means with which to put the care-at-home or subacute care scenario into action. In the optimum situation, case management services are covered by the benefit plan, enabling case managers to make the best use of one of their assets— the ability to respond quickly to complex problems.

Case management, disease management, and utilization review are product lines that may be offered to providers and members within a plan. Indemnity, consumer-driven, disability, and point-of-service are all insurance plans.

In all cases, a case manager must know a policy's caps on dollars or duration, service exclusions, and any specific treatments that may or may not be covered. Basic coverage terms of a plan are available in the Summary Plan Description, an easy reference guide written in lay language that describes the benefits. However, the master contract— called the plan of benefit or the policy of insurance—prevails in any matter. A plan of benefit is a technical and legal contract containing definitions of the terms within the text, all eligibility requirements, and a list of treatments that are not covered.

WORKERS' COMPENSATION

Workers' compensation was one of case management's earliest practice settings. Workers' compensation insurance costs for medical care and cash payments declined in 2005 after a continual rise over the previous years. As of 2005, 4.2 million injuries and illnesses were reported in private industry workplaces. Of them, 2.2 million cases required days off from work or restricted duties, according to the Insurance Information Institute. The total number of reported injuries and illnesses has fallen dramatically over the past two decades, however the length of time away from work has been increasing. As noted in CMSA's National Case Management Week 2003 Media Kit, a 2002 Alexander and Alexander survey of more than 2,000 corporate executives found that 86% of them use case management to help control the upward spiral.

According to Jennifer Christian, M.D. MPH, FACOEM, the President and CMO for Webility Corporation, 2006 may have marked a milestone in the Workers' Compensation long history. She noted in an article in *Case in Point* that stakeholder and industry leaders from around the country have embraced an innovative guideline "Preventing Needless Work Disability by Helping People Stay Employed" put forth last year by the American College of Occupational and Environmental Medicine (ACOEM) that is steadily gaining support. The guideline has 16 main points within four general categories which are:

- Adopt a work disability prevention model.
- Address behavioral and circumstantial realities that create and prolong work disability.
- Acknowledge the contribution of motivation on outcomes and make changes to improve incentive alignment.
- Invest in systems and infrastructure improvements.[1]

The complete guideline is available at www.acoem.org, and Christian describes this as a "commonsense plan . . . a very simple, easy-to-read blueprint for process improvement . . ." Concerning the increasing length of time that injured or disabled employees are away from the workplace, Christian attributes this, at least in part, to the disconnect between employees, payers and medical offices during the medical treatment/RTW process, such as the lack of a shared goal or effective communication.

According to Tom Strickland, CRC, President of Systemedic Corporation and founder of the first case management association, conference, and *The Case Manager* magazine, the birth of modern-day case management can trace its roots back to the workers' compensation market in the early 1970s. A true pioneer in the field, George Welch was the driving force behind an in-house "rehabilitation nurse" program within the Insurance Company of North America (INA), known initially as the MEND program. INA's parent company merged with Connecticut General Corporation (CG Corp.) to become CIGNA. The early success of Welch's initiative evolved into a successful CIGNA subsidiary, International Rehabilitation Associates, still in existence today under the name Intracorp.

Describing the workers' compensation setting of a decade ago, Linda L. Chalmers, RN, CRRN, CCM, WCLA, Early Intervention Nurse Case Manager for Zurich Insurance North America, notes that case management started in the workers' compensation field with major insurance carriers, such as Liberty Mutual and Wausau Insurance, hiring "rehabilitation nurses" to help handle the medical aspects of work-related injury claims for the employees of its policyholders.

In those early days, Chalmers notes, the case managers were all RNs that "worked in the field." The registered nurses would meet with the injured employee, their physician, and the employer. The goal of this contact was to assess the injury, develop the treatment plan, implement the plan, coordinate the identified service needs, monitor the results, and evaluate the outcomes. The field grew tremendously during the early 1980s when carriers and employers realized that they could save dollars and get their employees back to work sooner while reducing their loss costs. The difference between the decades is that today there are many more carriers that have their own established programs with internal staff, or who use the services of a regional or national company offering a full menu of case management and managed care products.

The introduction and growth of the managed care model has impacted workers' compensation in many ways. Chalmers feels the change has been significant, saying,

> As states began to write rehabilitation benefits into their statutes, that actually fueled the need for medical and then vocational services and personnel. While this was happening, the cost of medical care began to rise at an alarming rate. It was thought that a major reason for this was the cost shift that was occurring. The group health carriers were developing products to contain their costs, such as PPO and POS programs, usual and customary bill review, second opinion requirements, utilization review, pharmacy management programs, and more, while the medical providers were shifting their expenses to the

workers' compensation carriers, with extended care, unbundled, or unnecessary care. This was happening, many thought, because the providers viewed a work-injured patient as a blank check; there were no cost or service controls, no bill review, no PPOs, and no utilization or any significant means of cost control. The first effort to control medical costs in the workers' compensation arena was the development and mandate for a workers' compensation fee schedule for physician services in a number of states.

As the cost of medical care continued to escalate, increasing the cost of workers' compensation premiums, many states stepped up their methods to control or at least try to manage the medical costs associated with work-injury care. States and carriers began adopting many of the strategies that were developed and implemented by the group health payers. Providers also began to create products that were specifically designed to meet the special needs of the workers' compensation carriers and their customers. For example, in the '80s, PPOs did not include the specialty care providers, such as orthopedic, occupational health, or physical therapy clinics, that are commonly needed and used by workers' compensation, but were heavily weighted with family practitioners, OB, or pediatric specialists, which were not the practitioners appropriate for the care of a work-related injury. Today's PPO looks entirely different, and offers specialty providers that are commonly utilized by workers' compensation carriers and their customers.

So today, even in a state such as Illinois, where the injured worker has "choice" of their physician, cost management strategies can still be used, such as the provision of a list of PPO providers from which the employee can choose.

Looking at the past decade in workers' compensation, Christopher Wood, PhD, CRC, CDMS, Senior Vice President for Managing Care. Managing Claims (MCMC, LLC) notes the following changes and trends have occurred:

- There has been an increased focus on managing medical care and related medical expense and disability lost time more *proactively*, starting from the initial First Report of Injury. Wood notes that the elements of more *proactive* medical and disability lost time management can include any or all of the following:

- 24/7 injury reporting with availability of telephonic Nurse Case Management
- Use of disability guidelines such as ODG (Official Disability Guidelines) to set expectations for anticipated medical care and lost time from day one
- Immediate direction of care to preferred medical provider networks including physician, diagnostic, therapy, prescription drug, and durable medical equipment providers with an increased focus on "occupational" health
- Tremendous acceptance of and growth in the tiered use of Telephonic Nurse Case Management and Field-Based Nurse Case Management integrated with claims handling and allowing nurse involvement in more cases overall and earlier identification of cases requiring ongoing management. This has lead to the development of formalized case management guidelines concerning what cases can be managed telephonically and what cases require field-based management
- Greater use of Job Analysis concerning physical/functional job demands as well as "Transitional" duty with defined parameters for time of participation and much more active management and utilization of Case Managers
- Increased use of technology including shared data bases that allow for improved communication among claims and clinical managers as well as medical providers

Strickland offers his insights into the transformation of workers' compensation and its effects on case management (and vice versa) and expands upon this in Table 4–1. He believes that there certainly have been a lot of changes in workers' compensation case management in the last 20 to 30 years. However, the philosophical foundation of this specialty remains basically the same—assisting the injured worker in maximum recovery, and cost containment for the carrier and/or employer by helping manage medical treatment, equipment, lost time, employee/employer relations, and more. Something else that has not changed over the years is the dominance of registered nurses in compensation case management. In the late 1970s and early 1980s, vocational rehabilitation counselors swelled the rank of compensation case management, with the increasing focus on return-to-work issues and several states going to mandatory vocational rehabilitation.

Currently, the specialty pendulum has swung substantially toward nurse case managers in workers' compensation, Strickland notes, and he

Table 4–1 Issues Impacting Workers' Compensation and Case Managers

---

There are areas now in workers' compensation that are somewhat new and different from the past, and which will impact the practice of comp case management for several years to come.

1. Work Setting – In the early days of comp case management, you had a relatively small number of case managers working within the insurance industry, but there was a rapidly growing private/for-profit trend which saw a proliferation of private case management companies formed by nurses and vocational counselors, or combinations thereof. Case managers doing primarily workers' compensation now find employment areas in four major categories:

   • Insurance Carriers – The cycle here has been from only a handful of case managers in the earlier days, to a move within the comp insurance industry to rely heavily on company-based case management staff, and now the trend appears more towards contracting out to large or regional case management companies. Many comp carriers have retained a significant number of telephonic case managers, and contract out on only the more complicated or serious injuries.
   • National Case Management Companies – National case management companies, such as Intracorp, Concentra, GENEX, CorVel, etc., retain a large portion of comp case management on the strength of multiple locations, standardized billing, one-stop shopping, etc.
   • Regional Case Management Companies – Usually strong entrepreneurial companies, with a long history of success and expertise in local markets.
   • Solo Practitioners – Individual RN or vocational professionals who usually do work for a smaller customer base of employers or TPAs.

   In all of the above settings, the case manager is generally required to know only the comp laws and regulations of one particular state. However, some comp case managers are called on to travel into adjoining states to provide services and it is critical that they have at least a basic understanding of the state's comp rules and regulations. As has always been the case, the legal and administrative rules of the individual states in comp can directly effect the development of rehabilitation plans and the feasibility of professional recommendations. Issues such as change of physician, impairment ratings, and time limitations on training programs, are examples.

2. Managed Care – Case management was established in workers' compensation well before the introduction of "managed care." The major financial crisis in American healthcare was in the area of *health* claims, and this was where managed care got its hold. After observing some of the successes that managed care brought to reducing health claims costs, the

Table 4–1 continued

workers' comp industry began to adopt, on a state-by-state basis, various methodologies used in managed care. As is common in workers' compensation, the individual state laws and regulations concerning managed care determine to what extent, if any, the case manager's professional practice is impacted. In those states with minimal or no managed care in comp, the case manager's service – especially medical case management – remains essential for managing effective care and providing cost containment.

In those states that have been active in incorporating comp managed care methodologies, the case managers have to adjust and work with these other cost containment programs. This is true of both telephonic and on-site case managers, as well as those working for employers, carriers, or private case management companies.

In states that allow the use of managed care organizations, there are usually several preferred provider organizations that are utilized by the insurance carriers, employers or Third Party Administrators (TPAs). It is essential for the comp case manager to understand the benefits and structures of these networks, as they are directly related to hospital and provider referrals, obtaining equipment discounts, coordinating physician care, etc. In states where inpatient (or outpatient) preauthorization is required, the case manager must understand the players and procedures to arrange for surgeries and other types of medical treatments.

Not working appropriately with these types of managed care programs can result in excessive and unnecessary expenditures by the payer/customer. The effective integration of these various managed care programs with case management can result in excellent outcomes and substantial cost savings. However, the issues of complex regulations, varying claims philosophies and a poor spirit of cooperation by other managed care professionals, can make case management more of a challenge.

3. HIPAA and Confidentiality – Since the beginning of the 21st century, privacy and confidentiality issues in the whole field of medical care have been a hot topic of conversation and legislation. Under the current HIPAA law, the field of workers' compensation has been excluded and the focus is primarily in the health insurance industry. However, this could change at any time, and it is wise for comp case management practitioners and their companies/organizations to have clear policies, in writing, regarding their specific efforts to safeguard the privacy and confidentiality of those with whom they work. Because of potential exposure to HIPAA guidelines outside the realm of workers' compensation, some case

continues

Table 4-1 continued

---

management companies are seriously considering restrictions of their areas of practice (such as group health, liability, etc.) and thereby not fall under the stringent rules and regulations that apply to companies who are a "covered entity" under HIPAA.

Even if your practice is restricted to workers' compensation, you should have in place confidential safeguard policies and abide by them rigorously. Examples of privacy issues in workers' compensation for case managers would be: not releasing any case management reports or medical records to parties outside the payer without obtaining a signed consent form; doing evaluations or discussing medical issues with a client in a public facility – such as a physician's waiting room; keeping case management records in locked file cabinets for non-working hours; file protection while traveling, i.e., keeping files in a secured trunk as opposed to public view and access in an automobile interior; a clear explanation to new clients at the time of the initial contact as to your role as a case manager and privacy rules that you and/ or your company follow.

Source: Courtesy of Tom Strickland, President, Systemedic Corporation.

---

predicts that nurse case managers will continue to be, by far, the specialty that manages a great majority of workers' compensation cases. He believes this is true for at least two major reasons. One is the substantial increase in healthcare and treatment costs in both compensation and health over the last 20 years. As these costs continue to rise, employers and compensation claims adjusters have personally seen the cost-containment impact of proactive medical case management. Vocational case management has also become established as an important resource in workers' compensation. However, the vocational percentage has decreased over the last several years relative to nurse case management.

In the years since the last edition of TCMH-3rd, published in 2004, Strickland's case managers note that they are seeing sicker and older injured workers, as increasing costs and erosion of 401K and pension plans have kept workers employed beyond the age of 65. A good trend his company is seeing however, is the earlier referral of catastrophic injuries. Earlier intervention promotes good acute care, quality provider selection, smooth home transition, DME coordination, prevention of complications and costly readmissions.

Just as technology has improved medical outcomes in work related injuries, this has had a positive impact on vocational outcomes as well. An increasing number of video job analyses to share with treating physicians and therapists helps to create a more realistic treatment plan as well as appropriately timed RTW.

Another reason Strickland sees for the success of RN medical case management has been its ability to consistently deliver the twin benefits of improved medical treatment for injured workers and the savings of claims dollars through a variety of methodologies. Case management (both medical and vocational) was saving money prior to what became the hot trend of "managed care." Case management held its own quite well through the managed care cycle and remains as strong as ever as an effective resource in workers' compensation, whereas many utilization review and discount network programs have come under fire and have diminished or significantly evolved.

According to Strickland, the diminishment of vocational case management in workers' compensation most likely comes from the fact that mandatory vocational rehabilitation services have changed their laws or have modified them to the extent that they are no longer as lucrative for vocational rehabilitation practitioners. In some ways, the success of vocational rehabilitation/return-to-work programs has impacted the demand, at least in the private, for-profit case management industry. Specifically, the trend with many employers toward self-insurance has slowed vocational referrals. This is not because return-to-work services are not effective, it is because many employers have observed the techniques and successes of vocational counselors over the years and have incorporated these techniques internally. Further, they have been much more proactive in bringing employees back to work on their own in modified jobs or transitional employment programs. The ADA has also had a major impact in getting employers to think in terms of "reasonable accommodations" for workers with residual physical limitations.

As previously mentioned, the basic philosophy of workers' compensation case management has not changed significantly over the years. And in reality, the methods and techniques that worked well 30 years ago still essentially work well today. Obviously, there are newer treatment modalities, improved surgeries, better medications, advanced equipment, funding shifts, and changing legal environments. However, success in workers' compensation case management remains firmly rooted in caring and competent case managers who can be sensitive, firm, creative, and frugal. Combine that with a working knowledge of claims/legal issues and written and verbal communication skills, then success in W.C. case management will occur in most cases, comments Strickland.

The 4 C's—Continuous, Communication, Coordination, Creativity—Keys to Success

Chalmers supports Strickland as well as the observations by Dr. Christian noted earlier concerning the disconnects and communication problems so often found with these kinds of cases. In an article she contributed to *Case in Point*, she shared her recollections about her intervention with an injured worker that changed, not only the employer's policies for future injured workers, but helped her to formulate a case management philosophy that would be imprinted on all future cases. Chalmers recalled a conversation she had with an employer concerning one of their employees who had been involved in an explosion that killed a co-worker and caused burns that covered 30 percent of his body. During a visit with the employee in his home, following his discharge for a rehabilitation facility he shared with her: ". . . I have been with the company 25 years, never missed a day of work, and always came in when they called, worked overtime . . . and I didn't even get a Christmas card from them this year . . ." According to the tradition of the company, every employee received a personal Christmas card, and this man had quite clearly become a casualty of the "out of sight, out of mind" syndrome that affects all too many injured or disabled employees. The 4 C's: Continuous, Communication, Coordination and Creativity have become the criteria employed by their case management staff and the critical factors that have resulted in the successful recovery and return to work of an injured worker. Chalmers shared that the continuous contact and communication can:

- Build the injured worker's sense of belonging, self-confidence, and overall well-being through a positive work experience.
- Enhance the employee's physical and psychological recovery while preparing him for a return to productivity.
- Minimize the chances of the worker seeking legal counsel.
- Control medical costs by minimizing "care seeking" by the employee as a response to feeling less valued.
- Facilitate a successful RTW.[2]

Unlike group medical, long-term disability, or short-term disability insurance, in which a master plan is written for a national company and health benefits will be the same whether the employee of a California company lives in California, Minnesota, or New Jersey, workers' compensation falls under the guidelines of the state in which the policy is written. Workers' compensation regulations, therefore, vary from state to state for companies with coast-to-coast operations. Similarly, a case manager's activities will also be dictated by each state's workers' compensation process. The benefits an employee in Arkansas is entitled to will not match those for an employee in Delaware. The percentage granted for wage replacement funds may range, and can vary, within the same workers' compensation plan dependent upon the employee's selection of options for benefits only, benefits plus sick pay, or benefits plus sick and vacation pay. Rates and medical benefit exposure for the employer will differ as well.

The state workers' compensation guidelines also take precedence over the funding source. Employers must provide employees with the level of benefits the state mandates, not the level of benefits they can afford. Regardless of whether a company is self-funded, self-administered, or utilizing a traditional indemnity plan, workers' compensation cases fall under the jurisdiction of the state Workers' Compensation Commission, whose laws and regulations set the limits and extent of coverage. A liaison or intermediary agent between the claimant, employer, insurance carrier, and funder, the state Workers' Compensation Commission acts as an advocate for the claimant. It determines the level of benefits, the obligations of the employer, the responsibilities of the employee, and the level of capability and performance that constitutes "rehabilitation." In some states, the Workers' Compensation Board may list those doctors individuals may utilize.

Among the greatest challenges case managers face when working across state lines, according to Linda Chalmers, is keeping up with the regulations. One way that her company, Zurich Insurance, addresses this is by making sure that there are designated staff who are licensed to work cases in a particular state. They also assign designated teams to specific jurisdictions. This enables the RN to become a "specialist" for particular areas. The RNs have access to current information and jurisdictional requirements via Internet sites such as Workers' Comp Connection (http://workerscompensation.com), and are provided in-service training regarding the changes occurring in the industry and regions.

Another challenge has been the need to adhere to URAC standards in order to become and remain accredited, notes Chalmers. The workers' compensation carriers are now held to a much higher standard than in days past. Most recently, they have been required to develop programs and educate not only the healthcare professionals they employ but also claims personnel about the Health Insurance Portability and Accountability Act (HIPAA), and the importance of maintaining the confidentiality of the medical information that they handle.

Bound by a greater degree of legislation than group medical coverage, workers' compensation cases tend to be more legally involved and litigious than group medical cases. In order to sell group medical insurance, an insurance company must include certain benefits and coverage as designated by the state. Under ERISA guidelines, self-funded companies are exempt from meeting those same mandates for levels and provisions required of insurance firms covering companies paying premiums for benefits. This is what allows for the elimination of medical benefits or top-dollar caps on medical treatment for AIDS or psychological problems in some employers' group health plans. But workers' compensation cases are different. If state guidelines require that an out-of-work person be reimbursed for medical expenses at 100% of cost and for lost wages at 80% or two-thirds of pre-injury salary, even self-funded employer groups must provide that level of benefits.

Case managers are also regulated much more by legislation in state-by-state workers' compensation cases than in group medical cases. For a time, South Carolina offered employers the option to leave the system but revised its law in 1996, mandating that employers return to the system by July 1, 1997.[3] Workers' compensation has always been elective in Texas for nongovernmental employers, but those who opt out expose themselves to tort law liability.[4] For certain industries, the state does provide for mandatory workers' compensation coverage, like that under Title 25 of State statutes regarding rules and regulations for "Carriers" (Article 911-A, Sec II, Motor Bus Transportation and Regulations by the Railroad Commission). In New Jersey, the complex workers' compensation law allows coverage to be terminated by either party upon 60 days notice in writing prior to any accident. Under Rhode Island's Department of Labor and Training Division of Workers' Compensation, employees are permitted to claim common-law rights and opt out of the workers' compensation system. (Another example illustrating state-to-state variations in insurance is a New Jersey statute allowing 10 or more employers licensed by the state as hospitals to group self-insure.[5])

Further, states are trying to control workers' compensation costs by limiting options for claimants in filing claims, qualifying for benefits, or attempting to change a negative compensation board decision. Arkansas has required workers to identify the day and time of an injury, rather than simply describing it in general terms. This straightforward measure has reduced fraudulent claims. Connecticut stopped awarding disability benefits for mental or psychological disorders unless they were caused by an injury. In Texas, restrictions were placed on legal appeals by workers on rulings by compensation boards. California established a fund, paid for by employers, that finances special teams to go after fraud.[6]

Those who have only worked group medical insurance cases need to be aware that in workers' compensation, most insurance companies and employers face a double exposure. Although states have varying levels of benefits, insurers and employer groups are mandated to reimburse both medical costs and lost wages. Therefore, a carrier is not only interested in optimizing the results from medical care, but also wants the patient back to work as soon as possible. As a result, case management professionals may find themselves asked to achieve inconsistent goals—medical health vs. a timely return to the workforce. It pays to be aware that an employer's first and only concern might be the return-to-work time frame because the replacement of salary is a greater expense than the actual medical care.

For example, imagine a case involving a back injury. The employee might see a doctor once every few weeks without undergoing any major surgical procedure or complex medical care, such as a laminectomy or extensive physical therapy. Nevertheless, the employer is getting hit and hit heavily by salary replacement benefits. In a group medical case, an employee either has sick leave or disability leave, but the employer is not paying a salary indefinitely. In most workers' compensation cases, the employer is required to keep the job open. Added to the employer's constraints is the fact that in workers' compensation cases, employees are more inclined to hire attorneys if they feel they are not getting the benefits to which they are entitled. The involvement of an attorney is sometimes perceived by a claims examiner or an employer as a roadblock: "Well, this guy has an attorney, so why bother with case management now?" However, this might be the juncture at which case management is most needed. In fact, when a case manager can convince a doubting group of liability examiners as to the value of their services, she might have a group that is dedicated to the use of case management for the enhanced ability to evaluate and control the damages associated with liability claims.

Recapping, the payer's exposure in a workers' compensation case can be much greater than in a group medical case, even though the illness or injury is less severe, and the involvement of attorneys sometimes complicates the situation. Complying with the regulations of different states compounds the difficulty for case management professionals, especially those working for a nationwide insurer. Other variables contribute to the challenge. In mandated rehabilitation states, patient report formats must follow stringent guidelines; case managers must also file specific forms for billing. Further, there are more players in workers' compensation cases. In addition to the claims department and medical rehabilitation professionals, there are administrative law judges, vocational counselors, and vocational rehabilitation boards. Working on such cases can be a nightmare for independent case management companies as they try to keep abreast of changes in workers' compensation regulations in all the states they serve.

On the other hand, there have been changes in the workers' compensation industry over the past decade that benefit case managers in their efforts to guide patients toward the best outcomes, while assisting employers with their staffing and disability pay issues as outlined by Chalmers (see Table 4–2).

A single group medical plan or MCO may offer the same benefits from state to state; however, these benefits will be supplied by different providers from state to state. Coordinating and assessing care and services remains a challenge. An independent case management company with licensed nurses in multiple states can work group medical cases in

Table 4–2 Improvements for Case Managers in the Workers' Comp Industry

---

Among the more significant improvements in workers' compensation case management according to Linda Chalmers are the following:

1. Employers are much more proactive and offer modified duty programs for early return to work for their employees. In the 1970s, the common reply I received from an employer was, "The employee must be 100%, or we don't want him/her back." Today, I see iron and construction workers returned to modified duty.

2. Employers finally understand the value of Early Return To Work programs and have developed plans and special handling protocols for carriers to help them implement those programs for their injured employees.

3. There is a greater acceptance and understanding of how an RN case manager assists the claims handler/adjuster with managing the medical aspect of claims. In the '70s and early '80s it was commonplace to get a case assignment months following an injury when it was nearly unsalvageable and the adjuster was asking for a "miracle recovery." Now, carriers are likely to offer Early Intervention services. The medical case manager will "triage" the case within 24 hours of the accident, assess its severity, and assist the claims professional with the medical management of the injury. This helps to ensure appropriate care and coordinate a return-to-work plan with the physician, employee, and employer. It is a win-win situation for the employer, injured employee, and carrier.

Source: Courtesy of Linda Chalmers, RN, CRRN, CCM, WCLA.

---

several states relatively easily. To be effective, case managers have to decide beforehand whether to tackle the workers' compensation arena or stick with group medical.

AUTO INSURANCE

Like workers' compensation regulations, auto insurance policy regulations vary from state to state in terms of medical coverage limits and lost-wage replacement. Some states pay medical costs from the day of the accident. In auto policies, this is called PIP (personal injury protection) or "no-fault" coverage. Whereas New Jersey might offer medical coverage up to $250,000, New York policies may generally cover individuals for $50,000. In North Dakota, PIP of at least $30,000 per person is required. There are states with very low caps, in which auto policies have perhaps $5,000 maximum medical exposure. Where does an individual go when that $5,000 is exhausted? To a group medical plan. Those states with generous medical coverage sometimes provide minimal salary replacement coverage. Because these variations can create incentives or disincentives for individuals to get medical problems resolved quickly and return to work, case managers need to be aware of the fine points of auto insurance coverage. There are states where, as long as an employee can demonstrate some level of impairment, he or she can continue to remain off the job. This type of provision leads people to tend toward prolonging the recovery process.

Every case manager needs to know the terms of coverage for the line of insurance, the state regulations, and any other plans covering an individual to make the best use of time and dollars. As discussed previously, workers' compensation and no-fault auto insurance policies vary from state to state, but they also differ in structure. In a given policy, does the term "state" refer to the location where the accident occurred, or where the employee resides, or where the corporation has its headquarters office? For example, I have had case managers working a case in Arkansas under New York state regulations. A truck driver from Arkansas was injured in an accident in New York, where his company has its headquarters. The driver recuperated in Arkansas, but the case was treated as a New York workers' compensation case, not as an Arkansas resident compensation case.

INDEMNITY PLANS

The meaning of *indemnity* is determined by its usage. In general, *indemnity* refers to a traditional insurance plan in which reimbursement or compensation for loss or personal injury is provided via a contract. A company or individual pays premiums for a policy that outlines a contract of benefits and entitlements. The formation of HMOs, PPOs, and the applications of self-funded plans were responses to the escalating costs of traditional indemnity plans. Interestingly, we have returned to the same double-digit increases that led to the evolution of managed care as we know it today. *Indemnity* can also be used to describe legal exemption from liabilities—the "hold-harmless" clause.

GROUP MEDICAL PLANS

Whereas workers' compensation plans use terms such as *degree of disability* and *causally related,* and auto policies refer to PIP portions, group medical policies contain a different terminology: *caps, limitations, co-payments, coinsurance, preexisting, exclusions.* Aside from knowing the exact meaning of these terms, a case manager needs to be apprised of the source of funding that backs a group medical policy. If it is a fully insured plan, the plan may have to meet certain conditions on a state-by-state basis. Is it a premium-rated plan or is it self-funded, PPO backed, or HMO backed? Because employees are able to choose the plan they want to belong to, one employer group can refer to a case manager individuals in any number of plans: fully insured plans, HMOs, PPOs, and so on. Some of these plans will have case management provisions written in; some might not utilize case management.

The business of healthcare has become so convoluted, created with such complexities, that business owners feel hard-pressed to point out the exact source of the problem. They no longer have long-term relationships with their providers or payers; often, they have a variety of providers and payers from state to state. It appears inevitable: healthcare rates continue to rise.

Case managers can break this pattern and mind-set. By working with patients, employers, providers, and payers across the continuum of care, case managers can demonstrate that there is not one source of high costs but rather a series of checks and balances along the way in which a case can fall through the cracks and spiral out of control. Case managers help to keep all parties informed and that patient at the appropriate level of care.

In my experience, employers tend to be less involved and less interested in the administration of fully insured plans. Some employers continue to pay the premiums and consider themselves done, paying little attention to the potential benefits of case management programs, wellness programs, cost containment, and management of claims. For these reasons, a case manager might find less flexibility for alternative care arrangements when working within a fully insured plan. On the other hand, I believe case managers will be utilized more and more in the self-funded and risk-bearing managed care entities. A case manager will often find a greater degree of flexibility within a self-funded plan, with its increased or direct contact with the employer chief executive officer, chief financial officer, and the human resources manager.

Case managers should be aware that the group medical benefit structure often changes as an individual moves from one level of employment to another. Is the patient an active or retired employee? A retired employee who has COBRA coverage and is now at the age of Medicare eligibility? On disability and moving into retirement? Adjustments may be triggered by the employee's age as well. A case manager working with a 63-year-old active employee who suddenly retires must have an answer to the question, "How does retirement change the patient's coverage?"

For example, under COBRA, the employer must offer terminated employees an 18-month continuation of benefits under the plan the employee had been covered by during tenure with the company. Coverage extends for 36 months to a spouse and all dependents on the policy at the time of termination. If the employee was disabled at the time of termination—an unlikely scenario—coverage continues for 29 months. The employee is responsible for meeting the premiums.

The extent of medical benefits, in terms of length of time, is subject to the determination of the employer group or union contract. Some companies only provide coverage to their active employees. Others offer benefits to retired employees for a specified period, or design plans with less generous benefits over a longer period of time; if an individual had been with the company for 5 to 10 years of continued service, he or she might receive an additional 3 years on the medical plan. The larger the firm, the more likely it is that retirees will leave with their benefits intact—because of management loyalty to senior staff. For those hired at a later date, and therefore younger, the benefits structure might have been revised to meet the expense constraints of the times.

DISABILITY PLANS

Disability plans can be very specifically worded according to the desire of the employer group or single employer. Self-employed individuals can hold disability policies on themselves. Short-term disability (STD) plans can transition into long-term disability (LTD) plans carrying a different level of provisions. Varying in terms—the policy definition of short-term, long-term, and total disability; the portion of salary replaced; the number of months or years covered—disability plans require individual review by a case manager.

Within an LTD policy, there are two major distinguishing provisions: HISOCC ("his occupation") and ANYOCC ("any occupation"). Under HISOCC, a person must be totally disabled from performing any and all aspects of his or her job. Even if the person can perform three out of four job functions, that one missing function entitles him or her to the replacement of salary. HISOCC usually carries specified time limitations, ranging from 1 to 5 years. In general, a HISOCC plan might state that a person totally disabled from performing any and all aspects of his or her job is entitled to receive a specified amount of dollars for no more than 5 years but no less than 1 year. LTD plans may also be group specific. Physicians and other professionals, for example, tend to establish well-worded policies and often "layer" their coverage, purchasing several policies to provide the salary protection necessary should illness limit their earning power. These multiple disability policies are designed to take effect as claims escalate, and because some higher socioeconomic groups readily pay the more expensive premiums necessary to fund such coverage, the entitlements are generally more generous than other ANYOCC or HISOCC plans.

The other portion of an LTD plan, the ANYOCC clause, is where the rubber hits the road. Under ANYOCC, an individual may not be able to perform all aspects of his or her previous job but may well be able to perform the tasks required in other occupations. Most LTD policies cover individuals up to age 65 totally disabled from performing any and all aspects of their jobs and provide perhaps two thirds of their salary. These policies are expensive, and employer groups are trusting the law of averages and an actuary that while all employee premiums are paying into the LTD plan, only a small percentage of the employees will require coverage under it. Therefore, when a patient has improved to the point of moving from HISOCC status to ANYOCC, LTD carriers get very aggressive. Often, case managers are not involved in any type of intervention until the end of the HISOCC stage, when a carrier feels, "Okay, it's been a year now" (or 3 years or 5 years) and takes a closer look at the particular circumstances of the case.

The trust in the law of averages when writing HISOCC policies has proven to be misplaced. Companies often believe they will collect many more premiums than the benefits they will have to pay out. Insurers thought HISOCC policies would be big moneymakers because of the large population of well-paid professionals who would be interested in the income protection and who could afford the premiums. Indeed, many people did invest in them. However, there are now a large number of policyholders claiming benefits, and insurers have to pay each individual until he or she is 65 years old, unless the patient moves from HISOCC to ANYOCC status.

We were called in by a payer to assess a 41-year-old emergency room (ER) nurse for a return-to-work status for her ER job. At the time of her ER injury, she was working 23 hours a week. The question is not, "Can the job be modified or can the hours be restricted?" Even if we could help her return to work in another capacity at the hospital, she would still receive her benefit from the payer (which is, of course, where the payer's interest is focused in this case) as long as she continues to be disabled for her ER job (HISOCC status). This means she will collect from that policy, receiving $2,000 a month, until she is 65 years old, even though she may be gainfully employed someplace else. Unless her physician releases her for the job description of an ER nurse, the payer is obligated to pay $24,000 a year for 24 more years. For this reason, some companies no longer write HISOCC policies that are open-ended until age 65.

Case managers, rehabilitation managers, and anyone else competent to intervene should know that sometimes STD and LTD policies are strictly wage-replacement plans and lack provisions for medical services. Obviously, it is much more difficult to work cases without that medical arm to put to good use. Despite knowing medical treatment could improve a patient's situation, a case manager might be stymied because medical benefits have been terminated or used up and the patient continues to linger on LTD. To cut short theft losses, other LTD carriers are much more willing to be creative and bend the rules. Such carriers, looking at risk management as well, will buy the motorized wheelchair or electrify the employee's van in order to move toward a solution. Carriers concentrating on vocational rehabilitation are more likely to pursue these alternatives.

As an example, when working with a major corporation that had self-funded all its lines of insurance for employees, I could call the benefits manager directly to arrange funding for medical treatment on behalf of an LTD employee. The benefits manager and upper management were familiar with case management and could see that such medical support would make sense.

In contrast, a fully insured employer might have Prudential as its LTD carrier while buying its major medical coverage from Blue Cross/Blue Shield or Aetna. Coordinating two different carriers adds levels of approval and discussion that hinder the case management-medical intervention process. I could get an LTD case and know exactly what needs to be done medically, but if the medical plan does not cover the intervention and the LTD claims examiner cannot see the need for it, I must make a very convincing argument for a medical course. This is where the financial planning capability of case managers comes into play. Depending on a carrier's exposure—the amount of money it is responsible to reimburse under the plan—the carrier can be willing to stretch provision boundaries to include medical treatment when a case manager can demonstrate that once x dollars are spent on medical treatment, an employee could be off LTD and back to work. Carriers are especially willing to look at a creative case manager's ideas when the employee is a heavy-hitting professional with LTD receipts ranging in the thousands of dollars per month.

David Hubbard, RN, a Disability Case Manager with Fort Dearborn Life Insurance Company in Dallas, TX and a member of the Editorial Advisory Board of *Case in Point* offered that he and his company are seeing ". . . a great deal of behavioral health claims and comorbidities that cause somebody not to be able to work . . ." Hubbard asserts that if case managers believe that they are *not* seeing much behavioral health claims ". . . they are simply not paying attention . . ."

As claims for disability are submitted, Hubbard looks to see if the diagnosis provided is even an accurate one. Interestingly, ". . . in a study of 100 claims for a diagnosis of LBP (low back pain) with radiculopathy, the only finding was a disc bulge but with no evidence of stenosis, nerve root encroachment or frank herniation . . . only 15% had physical or electrodiagnostic findings consistent with the diagnosis; in another study of 100 claimed pre-term pregnancies, only 19% had findings on exam consistent with the potential for high risk or pre-term birth . . ."

As a result of increased economic instability, there willl likely be an increase in the submission of disability claims and a need for case management for the most appropriate resolution and/or settlement of the claim.

POINT-OF-SERVICE PLANS

Originating in 1988, POS managed care plans include a range of customized care plans most often offered by larger companies. They evolved from PPO plans as companies sought to combine employee choice, cost reduction, and efficient utilization. The most successful POS arrangements are characterized by effective providers, limited network size, and provisions requiring healthcare providers to share a portion of the payer's risk, making for a more realistic plan design. These plans run the spectrum from open-access HMO plans to gatekeeper PPOs. HMOs with open access tend to incorporate smaller network panels and to be more rigid in their procedures. Consequently, employee resentment is more likely to occur when an employer moves from a traditional insurance plan to an HMO-based plan. POS networks based on gatekeeper PPO models generally include broader network panels, impose fewer restrictions on patients and providers, and allow more range in plan design. Responsibility for overseeing a POS plan falls to a network manager within the company. The key feature differentiating POS plans from PPO arrangements is that a higher level of benefits can only be accessed if care is provided through a primary care provider, such as a pediatrician, an internist, or a family practitioner. (OB-GYNs are the exception to the rule.)

Case managers working cases that fall into the POS category need to ascertain the type of POS the employee is enrolled in—open-access HMO, gatekeeper PPO, or a hybrid falling between the two. To be in a better position to make a case in favor of an alternative treatment, a case manager should also be aware of which party within the network is responsible for what portion of the risk. Is the employer, provider, or payer most exposed to financial risk? The group with the highest exposure to financial risk is the group most likely to benefit from and be interested in case management services.

There is a growing attention being paid to coinsurance rather than co-payment, whether it takes form within indemnity or consumer-driven plans. This emerging option will be interesting to watch.

CONSUMER-DRIVEN HEALTHCARE PLANS

The convergence of several technological, financial, and administrative and provider trends has led to the growth of a new frontier in healthcare management: consumer-driven healthcare (CDH) plans. Born from consumers' ready access to Internet-based health information, employers' need to reign in steadily increasing healthcare costs, the cold reception to medical savings accounts and warm reception to health reimbursement arrangements, and restrictive plan language, consumer-driven healthcare plans are giving individuals greater choice, responsibility, control, and difficult decisions to make. These and other self-directed plans fall under the defined care or defined-contribution healthcare model. Essentially, CDHs allow (or require, depending upon individual reaction to the idea) consumers to decide how they want their available pool of healthcare dollars spent. In this way, the incentive to purchase wisely and limit unnecessary expenditures falls to the employee rather than to the employer.

To be successful, individuals who have no clear idea of the cost of medical care have to become educated consumers and smart shoppers. This is an issue I have addressed throughout my career (some would say, "yes, continually, from a soapbox"). We can recite from memory the price of a loaf of bread, a cell phone with camera capability, a new refrigerator, or a Lexus. How many of us can offer up the price of an MRI, heart bypass surgery, or anesthesia and the technician to provide it?

Early entrants into the CDH plan provider market include Aetna Inc., The Choice Care Card, Definity Health, Destiny Health, Flexible Benefit Service Corp., HealthAllies Inc., HealthMarket, Humana Inc., Lumenos, MyHealthBank Inc., Self Insured Plans Inc., Vivius, and a number of Blue Cross/Blue Shield plans (Blues).

In general, consumer-driven health plans have high deductibles that assign the first several thousand dollars in medical expenses to employees, combined with an employer-funded health spending account. Each employee might receive an annual tax-exempt fund of $500 or $1,000 that he is free to spend on any medical expenses he elects provided by any physician or alternative provider, from dental work and cardiology to massage therapy. The employee may take any money left in this personal account and roll it over into next year's account, with no penalty.

When medical expenses top $1,000, the employee pays the deductible, approximately $500. When expenses reach $1,500, the employer coverage takes over, with 80% of costs being paid by the employer and the remaining 20% charged to the employee.

There are several variations on the basic plan. Flexible plans allow employees to earmark a portion of their pretax paycheck dollars for medical expenses that don't generally fall under traditional insurance, such as dental or vision care. In flexible plans, unused dollars must be forfeited at the end of the year.

Using another type of CDH, workers can personalize their coverage by selecting benefits from an on-line menu of coverage offerings. They balance deductibles, premiums, and co-payments to suit their individual needs.

Another plan variation offers a CDH tier inserted into a more traditional insurance policy. This type is favored by some Blues. The variables might include drug formularies, hospital networks, and benefit choice. Premiums are set according to the benefits an employee selects, and workers take on the financial risk for their choices when costs overrun the fixed contribution of the employer.[7]

At this time, providers and consumer groups alike are split on their response to CDH plans. Interest is widespread, although actual enrollment remains low. Cautioning voices cite high administrative costs, the possible loss of tax advantages and provider network negotiated savings, potential rising costs with broader enrollment, and the fact that employer savings are not ensured.[8] Although momentum seems to be building, the next 5 to 10 years will tell us whether this new product is here to stay.

DIAGNOSIS-SPECIFIC BENEFITS

There are conditions and diagnoses that may allow for additional funding through federal, state, and local programs. The availability of programs varies from state to state. A premature baby with developmental delays, such as those caused by cystic fibrosis, may be eligible for state early-intervention programs. Coverage varies from state to state. This can be checked through your state's health department, and other programs such as Children with Special Health Needs (formerly Crippled Children's Services and often called Children's Medical Services) and the state-administered cash grant program, Aid to Families with Dependent Children. Medicare automatically becomes the primary funding source for patients with end-stage renal disease, even those who are active employees, after 18 months of dialysis treatment, but only for services related to the renal condition.

For those with physical limitations or disabilities, such as the legally blind, there are also federal and state programs that help stretch funding dollars. Easter Seals aids those with muscular dystrophy; the Shriner's have funds available for burn victims. As citizens and taxpayers, patients are entitled to the offerings of these and other programs. (Unfortunately, most case managers do not take as much advantage of these alternative sources as they could. This is an area in which case managers need to expand their activity.)

Admittedly, utilizing these funds is not always easy or straightforward. Working with state or federal funding sources is often more difficult for case managers because of the bureaucratic layering. In any state-operated or federally funded program, the rules are sometimes so stringent that they allow for no flexibility at all, even when it would seem that a more cost-effective solution is available. For example, some regulations force case managers to spend more money. Case managers are mandated to use only Medicare-certified agencies in some state Care at Home program cases despite the fact that such agencies may be as much as 50 to 100% more expensive than another home care agency. In its effort to protect both those people who might not be able to fend for themselves and the taxpayers, Medicare has adopted rules that are not always in anyone's interest.

Further, case managers will find that government billing and report formats are entirely different from those used in the private sector. Case managers with a high overhead might not be able to afford to handle mostly Medicare cases because of the significantly lower profit margins. In addition to generating an increased number of diverse reports and tracking down agencies that are delinquent in payments, case managers will have to contend with a high turnover rate among government staff (necessitating reintroductions to case management), regulatory changes, and midstream program cuts.

TRADITIONAL INSURANCE VERSUS SELF-FUNDED PLANS

In working with a number of major insurance companies that provide traditional insurance (a.k.a. indemnity plans and premium-based plans), I have found that there appears to be less willingness to be flexible with benefit alternatives. This may be because the premiums have been set based on known experience (the history of health benefit usage for that type and number of employees) and an anticipated projected cost for that employee group over time. The insurer has been investing or managing the premium income to make certain there will be enough funds to cover employee claims. A change in the benefit payout—even if it lessens the payout—is perceived as a disruption to the system. There also seem to be rigid constraints on adopting options that, even at first and second glance, appear sound from a business-management perspective. When case management might result in an extra expense or administrative cost that the insurer will have to absorb at the year's end, a traditional insurance company almost requires a guarantee of projected savings neatly spelled out, which is brought back to the employee group for review at a multitude of levels prior to taking action.

With one major insurer, I had to complete a cost-benefit analysis immediately following my initial evaluation before the insurer could determine whether it felt case management would be viable in each particular case. Instead of being able to blend our experiences, pulling on the volumes of past history, I had to justify case management again and again. While the reams of documentation were prepared for the claims managers and everyone else in the approval process, we were missing opportunities to help the patient and save benefit dollars. During the 3 to 4 weeks it took for all levels to decide that case management might indeed be a good idea, we missed more opportunities. I have no problem with the demand for a round-figure estimate of potential cost savings, but in these instances it seemed that the carrier was asking case managers to become actuaries.

The approval process itself is too convoluted, too enormous to be successful, fraught with so many players and layers, and "we-have-to-talk-with-legal" situations that case management options become too big a "problem" to be resolved. The "problem" is twofold: getting to the decision maker and presenting the information.

If case managers could go directly to the group paying the premiums and tell them their options and alternatives, they could snap the trap and get their jobs done. But case managers dealing with traditional insurance most often talk first to agents, then brokers, and case management reports are finally presented by marketing managers or claims managers instead of the case managers, who are of course closest to the issues. There seems to be insufficient education and preparation by case managers as to what case management can accomplish and an inability on the part of large insurers to take a successful pilot case management project and make the transition to a successful corporate-wide program.

For example, suppose a case manager is assigned a case by a large carrier, a case that had been directed to the carrier by its preadmission/concurrent review contractor. By the time the case has come to the attention of the insurer and has been determined to be appropriate for case management, several days have passed. The patient has cancer and is in the hospital now. The insurance contract has an absolute limit on home health benefits, no more than 30 visits per calendar year, but unlimited dollars can be spent in hospital care. Other than a hospital, it seems there are very few places where this patient could be cared for—at a skilled facility or perhaps at home with multiple support services. The indicators seem to dictate that the person remain in the hospital.

After seeing the patient on-site, the case manager follows up her visit with a verbal report to the insurer's in-house case management contact. The patient wants to go home, and the case manager wants to move him out of the hospital as soon as possible. Such a move will not threaten his current medical status or recovery. The insurance contact has to discuss the plan with her manager, then bring it to the service representative who reviews it with the service manager to determine whether a plan exception can be made. The service manager wants to speak with legal counsel, and then there is the meeting of the trustees next week, where they will see if they can do something about it. Meanwhile, alternative care is in place, the patient is poised to go home, but the contract does not allow it.

The case manager needs an exception but cannot get a decision, and the hospital charges are adding up.

Now consider the same basic scenario with the insurance provided by a self-funded employer group that has a TPA administering its claims. The benefit plan contains the same language limiting home health visits to 30 per calendar year and providing unlimited hospital benefits. Through the same process of identification—via a preadmission/concurrent review contractor—the case is red-flagged in the claims department of the TPA. Knowledgeable about case management, the claims adjuster contacts the TPA's case management contractor. Returning from her on-site visit, the case manager talks directly with the employer's service representative and the claims department within the TPA, outlining the alternatives for the patient, who requires support services and really wants to go home or at least into a less intensive care setting. With case management, a program can be constructed that results in the best care for the patient and saves the plan substantial benefit dollars.

The TPA's service representative contacts the fiduciary or controller of the benefit plan, who sees the economic sense of adopting the use of case management. (Fiduciary responsibility obliges the controller not only to meet the needs of the individual but to safeguard dollars for the needs of the entire benefit group.) By deciding for case management in this instance, the controller creates a win-win scenario—quality of care is increased and cost is decreased. The recommendation and decision take a few hours, as opposed to the days needed in a large insurance firm.

This is not to say all TPAs have seen the light and welcome case management with open arms. The issue really centers on a level of sophistication and the willingness to make decisions and assume a controlled risk regardless of the insurance benefit system. In general, the larger the organization, the more tortuous the decision.

Previously, TPAs tended to be small and local, whereas insurance companies tended to be larger and operate nationally from a central location. Through more recent mergers and acquisitions, there are now larger regional and national TPAs, although this in itself is not a guarantee of more seamless operations. A national TPA with a certain level of sophistication might contain its own case management group, contract with several case management companies across the country, or find a case management provider with nationwide capability. The role of case management within the TPA world is as variable as the TPAs and the organizations that employ them.

I believe my frustration with the convoluted decision-making process within some larger insurance firms remains an industry-wide frustration.

When I have the opportunity to work one-on-one with an employer group or a small group of payers, whether within a claims department or a TPA—or when I speak with CMs in a large company—and show them what a smaller firm has been able to achieve for patients and payers, their eyes light up. If we can restrict the players in traditional-insurance decision making to the key people, we have a chance at success. The difficulty of working with a larger complex bureaucracy provides a strong argument for becoming self-funded—it is the control of decisions and dollars that makes case management programs work. Case managers need to spend more time bringing their successful scenarios and pilot projects to the marketplace. Education and proof of case management's viability will make case management a more readily used medical- and business-management tool.

STOP-LOSS INSURANCE PLANS

Because of their position in the insurance industry, stop-loss insurance carriers (reinsurance carriers) are of special interest to case managers. They can see more clearly the positive effects of case management. Many employer groups, whether utilizing traditional premium-based insurance or a self-funded plan, set a threshold over which the financial responsibility for health benefits will be borne by a stop-loss carrier. Handling only the big-cost cases, stop-loss carriers absolutely see the benefits of case management. Customarily, a reinsurer requests a specific limit report— notification when a claim reaches 50 or 75% of the set threshold. At that point, the carrier might intercede and put case management in place or have written into the stop-loss agreement that a case manager be automatically assigned by the company when a claim hits its specific limit. In fact, many stop-loss insurers mandate cost-containment measures, agreeing to write reinsurance only if the company puts preadmission review, case management, and other managed care strategies in place.

Reinsurers are looking closely at how they can best protect their layer of coverage from exposure to financial catastrophe. A company might have healthcare benefits of a million dollars per covered life, with a threshold set at $100,000 with a reinsurer. This means there is coverage for patients for claims of $150,000 or $250,000, but the company only pays the first $100,000 out of its group coverage and is reimbursed dollar-for-dollar by the stop-loss carrier for any costs over the threshold up to $1 million. Therefore, reinsurers are very interested in using case management to keep benefit payouts beneath the level of stop-loss. If a case manager can help manage healthcare and costs, keeping benefits payouts from moving upward into the stop-loss range, the firm saves not only in its fiscal year but also in the next year, because premiums are based on claims experience. Just as the stop-loss carrier uses case management to protect it from high dollar losses, the employer group itself should be seeking the same protection.

Using this information, case managers can create opportunities by "creating the need" for case management (i.e., identifying the need and demonstrating it). When I talk to employers, I tell them that for many organizations, stop-loss coverage can be hard to obtain. The premiums can become so costly that company managers are forced to raise the group's threshold—the amount of money the company is responsible for—higher than the firm can actually carry. However, if an employer group can tell a reinsurer that it already has case management and other cost-containment strategies (preadmission review, concurrent review) in place in the first layer of coverage, the reinsurer might be more inclined to write coverage for the group, more assured that high numbers of catastrophic cases will not reach the stop-loss layer.

MULTIPLE-EMPLOYER BENEFIT PLANS AND TRUSTS

Prior to the passage of the Taft-Hartley Act in the 1950s, there was no mandated healthcare coverage for individuals who worked for multiple employers during the course of the year. Unlike the office workers employed year-round by a single firm, the organized laborers employed annually by various contractors (carpenters or painters who worked out of a union hall) had no single organization sponsoring a health benefit plan. The Taft-Hartley federal labor law included a number of citations, among them a provision allowing for the establishment of multiemployer benefit trusts (a.k.a. welfare funds). Funded by multiple employers, a trust of this type is regulated by a board of trustees (with union and employer positions equally represented), which determines the operative and administrative rules. As in a pension fund, the monies are gathered and placed in a trust overseen by a welfare plan administrator. The manager at ABC Building Co. will send in a monthly statement listing the individuals employed by ABC, the hours worked, and the amount ABC owes to the fund on the workers' behalf. There is then a pool, the "Carpenters Health and Welfare Plan" pool, for instance, from which health benefits can be drawn.

Unions and associations, such as the local truck drivers or Writers Guild of America also offers benefits to members. These groups are able to purchase services at discounted group rates.

Case managers with patients who are covered by a multiemployer trust should ascertain the name of the welfare plan administrator (or health and welfare officer) for assistance in clarifying benefits. Eligibility for these trusts is complex and can fluctuate from quarter to quarter. The hours a carpenter works in the first quarter will be applied to his or her coverage for the second quarter. If the carpenter does not have the required hours of employment to cover plan participation, he or she might have to self-pay for a quarter to maintain eligibility.

It is illegal to form a union for the sole purpose of providing or obtaining insurance benefits. Case managers can be involved unwittingly in a welfare fund or trust that is not sound. After negotiating a discount in good faith for prompt payment, and putting one's reputation on the line with a provider, it is a shock to find that there is no money to pay claims. It might be that the fund monies were poorly administered, or dollars fell short as unmanaged cases drove up costs and drained the fund. It is always wise for case managers to know as much as possible about the type and health of the welfare fund payer.

VIATICAL SETTLEMENTS

Originated in the late 1980s and very popular in the late 1990s, viatical settlements enable someone facing a terminal illness to utilize the present-day value of their life insurance policy to ease financial burdens. They are arranged when companies purchase life insurance policies from people with limited life expectancies (less than 8 years), offering the *viator* (the owner and potential seller of the life insurance policy) a cash settlement based on the policy's value and the viator's life expectancy, generally ranging from 40 to 80 cents on the dollar. Viators may also elect to collect an accelerated death benefit in cash and viadicate the remainder of the policy. Shorter life expectancies generally translate to larger viatical settlements.

A viator with 6 months to live might be offered 80% of the policy's face value, whereas a person who is expected to live for 36 months might receive only half of the policy's face value. This is because ownership of the policy and beneficiary rights transfers to the viatical company, which continues to pay the premiums. When the viator dies, the viatical company cashes in the policy for its full face value. Its strategy is to make a profit by reaping a higher return from the policy's face value than it paid out in premiums or to the viator. Although certain viatical companies will purchase insurance policies from people with life expectancies of more than 4 years, some only buy from viators with less than a 6 months' prognosis. If a viator lives longer than anticipated, the viatical company's profits diminish due to increased premium payments.

Viatical settlements offer viators—people with terminal illnesses who often are unable to continue working and are, therefore, financially squeezed—the funds to pay for food, rent, medical bills, unreimbursed medical expenses, the mortgage, or a vacation. Policy owners, rather than beneficiaries, benefit from the settlement, as is appropriate; a mentally competent person has a right to decide how and when to use his or her assets.

A person can decide to sell only a portion of his insurance policy value to the viatical provider and leave the remainder of its assets to beneficiaries. Using some or all of an insurance policy's worth can enable a person/family to keep a house, property, or an heirloom chest of drawers, rather than having to put them on the market to raise funds for healthcare, food, and the electric bill.[9]

Initially a response to the financial needs of people with AIDS, the viatical industry now is a resource for any terminally ill patient. As protease inhibitors and pharmaceutical cocktails have proven more effective in treating AIDS, fewer viatical companies are purchasing policies from people with AIDS, and some have stopped altogether. Those utilizing the settlements might have cancer, Alzheimer's, or other conditions.

Any individual, family, or group of friends coping with a terminal illness is obviously in a stressful and sometimes heartrending situation. When case managers are working with a client considering arranging a viatical settlement, they can assist by helping them obtain accurate information. Areas to cover include:

- Tax ramifications and the settlement's effect on other benefits, such as Social Security or Medicaid
- Alternatives, such as a personal loan, cash advance on credit cards, or liquidating other assets
- The viatication of a portion of the value of the life insurance policy according to the viator's needs
- A review of licensed viatical companies (some "companies" are merely brokers who connect a self-funded group of investors with an interested viator)
- A contract containing a reclusion clause of 15 to 30 days, which allows the viator to void the contract
- The assistance of a knowledgeable financial adviser
- The assistance of AIDS service organizations to identify reputable viatical companies
- Negotiations with at least four viatical companies

Resources for information on viatical settlements include the Viatical Association of America, National Consumers Helpline, National Viatical Association, viaticaladvocate.com, idealsettlements.com, and viatical-expert.net, listed in the book's Appendices A and C.

Similarly, life settlements create cash from a non- or underperforming asset, allowing policy owners to cash out of unwanted, unaffordable, or obsolete life insurance policies. Senior settlements and lifetime settlements are two forms of lifetime settlements that have become tools in the estate planning for seniors.

NONTRADITIONAL POLICIES

There are also a number of nontraditional supplemental policies currently available that, although not necessarily recommended for purchase, are often selected by individuals seeking more comprehensive coverage.

Disease Insurance Policies

While most insurance plans cover the typical conditions, some of these present extraordinary financial burdens to patients. There are two main types of disease insurance: specific-disease and critical illness. Specified-disease is a policy for a particular condition such as cancer, heart attack or stroke; critical illness policies are more broad-based and may cover up to 24 ailments. These policies provide lump-sum payments that individuals may use as they wish. Instead of payments to providers, these policies can reimburse non-medical costs such as transportation, meals and lodging . . . or even spousal reimbursement for care provided. Case managers should explore the existence of this kind of coverage and assist families in the best use of these funds.

While these policies may seem attractive to some, many consumer-advocacy groups advise that individuals would be better served by expanding their health and disability insurance plans.[10]

Cancer Policies

While working on behalf of one patient, I discovered he had paid for a cancer insurance policy due to the high incidence of cancer in his family. This policy allowed for greater benefits than his health plan or an LTD policy would have provided. To receive the entitlements of a cancer policy, an individual must have a confirmed diagnosis of cancer as described in his or her policy. Although a broad number of cancer policies have been purchased, they are not recommended to the general public because of the limitation of the coverage. People are usually encouraged to put the money they might spend on a cancer policy toward expanded health plan coverage instead.

Alzheimer's Policies

These are seen as very limited and costly policies. The stated qualifications for nursing home coverage—a key issue with this type of policy—generally preclude any history of Alzheimer's within a family, eliminating the patient group most likely to benefit.

Occupation-Specific Policies

AIDS and HIV policies are sold to law enforcement officers and fire fighters, who, because of their occupation, are at a high risk of exposure to HIV infection through lifesaving efforts, resuscitation procedures, or hostile bites.

Care Settings: Long-Term Care, Home Care, and Nursing Home Policies

Long-term care plans (a.k.a. home-care policies) are now being perceived as an insurance vehicle that everyone in our society needs to look at and consider for themselves. We are now seeing high numbers of these policies, and will continue to see them as people age and face financial liabilities that could be devastating. Meant to meet the bulk of expenses for unexpected catastrophic events, such as a head injury, long-term care policies fill the gaps in a plan that might not cover custodial care or other treatments no longer considered part of a traditional healthcare plan. As employers look for ways to protect themselves from long-term health-care responsibilities, medical policies—whether traditional indemnity plans or ERISA (self-funded) plans—are becoming more stringently worded. As an example, a group medical plan might cover 30 days of inpatient rehabilitation. However, if someone claims that this amount of rehabilitation is not sufficient to restore a patient to his or her prior degree of function or capability, the group medical response will likely be, "That's not restorative you're requesting, that's long-term custodial care, and we don't pay for that."

The long-term care policies being offered by some employer groups to employees and their immediate family or dependents do respond to a tremendous need in the healthcare marketplace. Unfortunately, even these policies are so narrowly written, restrictive, have many exclusions, and/or are expensive that they bar a great number of people from access to care or limit the actual length of care to be covered. The industry is just now seeing a gradual move toward more consumer-friendly long-term care policies.

Medigap Policies

Similar to long-term care policies, Medigap plans were devised as a safety net for those areas of coverage where Medicare stopped short. A Medigap policy is an independent policy purchased by individuals through an insurance agency to augment Medicare coverage. Launched in the marketplace with a great deal of hype, some Medigap policies are actually less than they appear. Guidelines on items that should be included in every Medigap plan can be obtained from the federal Department of Aging or the Department of Health and Human Services.

Dental Insurance

Dental insurance policies are currently popular in the marketplace. Further developments in this product line include a shift toward dental managed care networks, PPO networks, and POS arrangements as alternatives to "indemnity" dental plans.

RIDERS TO LIFE INSURANCE POLICIES

Individuals may also purchase additional coverage through a rider, material or paragraphs added to an existing life insurance policy.

Accelerated Benefits

Additional funds for terminal illness care may be obtained through a rider to a life insurance policy. Should a policyholder develop a terminal illness (as validated by a physician statement that the person is likely to die within a year), the person can gain access to approximately one half of the life insurance policy's benefits.

Accidental Dismemberment Clause

Also written as a rider to a life insurance policy, this clause has not come into common use. It provides for a flat dollar amount to be paid, regardless of the medical care delivered and its cost, if a person loses an arm, a leg, his or her vision, or suffers multiple losses.

COORDINATION OF BENEFITS

When there are two or more coverages on a claim—perhaps a wife and husband both work and are covered by their employers, a no-fault auto policy, or Medicare—there are rules governing which of the plans is primary and pays first and which pays second. In an "intact" family, an employee's plan pays first on that employee. When the claim is for a child covered by both parents' plans, the "birthday" rule comes into play. The plan of the parent with the earlier birthday, by month and day, not year, is utilized. If Mom's birthday is April 12 and Dad's birthday is August 20, Mom's plan is primary. (In the past, Dad's plan was always primary; some plans still hold the male parent as primary.)

Medicare is primary if a person retires on pension and his or her spouse is not an active employee with coverage as an active employee. However, an employer group health plan is always primary vis-a-vis Medicare. A 74-year-old active employee is entitled to Medicare, but his employer plan is primary. That same plan also is primary for his 69-year-old spouse named on the plan. If an employee is disabled but still covered by an employee group plan, Medicare is the secondary payer.

To clear up any unknowns and prevent future confusion, a case manager should always ask about all insurance in effect during an initial visit or telephone call. The source referring the case might not have all pertinent information on file. All findings regarding multiple coverage, coverage origin, plan sponsor, and who is insured under each plan should be recorded. In divorced families and step families, coordination of benefits becomes more intricate, as custody and court-order issues may be involved.

Coordination of benefits is always specific to the types of plan involved in a case, and a coordination of benefits statement is customarily included in each plan.

NOTES

1. CIP Staff, "A New Model – Workers' Compensation Awaits an Overhaul," *Case in Point,* October/November 2007, pp. 23–25.
2. Chalmers L, "Marooned" – *Case in Point,* Dec/Jan 2009.
3. Bradford M, "Texas Employers Defend Workers Comp Opt Out," *Business Insurance* 31, no. 7 (1997): 18.
4. Conerly WB, "Is Workers' Compensation a Model for Unemployment Insurance?" *National Center for Policy Analysis Brief Analysis no. 435* (2003): http://www.ncpa.org/pub/ba/ba435.

5. Department of Labor, *State Workers' Compensation Statutes,* "Table 1. Type of Law and Insurance Requirements for Private Employment," John Burton's Workers' Compensation Resources (2003): http://www.workerscompresources.com/.

6. Quint M, "Crackdown on Job-Injury Costs," *The New York Times,* CXLIV, no. 50,002 (1995): D1, D7, D9.

7. Benko LB, "Jury Still Out on Consumer-Driven HealthCare Plans," *Business Insurance* 37, no. 11 (2003): 16.

8. Kaplan E, "Early Results Mixed for Consumer-Centric Plans," *Employee Benefit News,* (2003): 11.

9. Petrie D, "Are Viatical Settlements Appropriate for Your Patients?" *The Case Manager* 14, no. 4 (2003): 48.

10. Duffett C, " Disease Insurance Gets Money to the Customer," *Central New York Business Journal,* Aug 12, 2005.

Chapter 5

Legal Responsibilities of the Case Management Profession

LICENSURE AND LIABILITY

An important issue surrounding the practice of case management is that involving the licensure of the professionals providing these services. While case management is an intradisciplinary profession, nursing constitutes the majority number. There is an evolving number of practice settings for nurses, and technology has made it "possible" for us to work globally, but our licensing restrictions have not given us "permission". Corporations that employ these nurses as case managers, health coaches, health and wellness consultants, utilization reviewers, call-center nurses etc. also have their business across the country and their nurses have caseloads not just in one state but in multiple ones. Unfortunately, little has been done to address this situation of nurses working with patients in states other than the one in which they are licensed. In conversations that I have had with colleagues over the last several years, I realized that many are blissfully unaware of the potential liability they are facing, and many others didn't even realize that this was an issue at all! Why would we not see this as a problem, what are the consequences and what can we do about it?

Some case managers believed that what they were doing in this "non-hands on" or non-traditional setting for nurses, and didn't involve the actual administration of medications, treatments etc., that, well somehow, maybe it wasn't ". . . real nursing . . ." In fact in some of my interviews with Medical Directors in managed care, some of these physicians had the same opinion. Those nurse case managers that did believe (and rightfully so) that what they did was most definitely within the scope of nursing, believed that if their employers weren't getting them licenses, or requiring that they pursue licensing in other states, then it must be OK. Because many nurses are assured by their employers that the organization carries its own malpractice insurance and that as employees they are covered under that policy, they too were not concerned. Providers of malpractice and liability insurance, if they knew, would not provide coverage to organizations or individuals that were engaged in illegal activities . . . and practicing without a license is in fact, illegal. As I began having more in-depth conversations with senior management in several of the employer groups, they shared that this would be a very expensive and labor-intensive process and perceived that it was possibly the nurses' problem rather than the organizations'. Obviously, this was a problem for both.

Nurse licensure is regulated on a state-by-state basis, through the successful passing of the NCLEX (National Council Licensure Exam–RN) exam with state boards of nursing requiring nurses to be licensed within the states where patients reside whenever telephonic or on-site intervention occurs. If a nurse practices *without* a license-to-practice in the state where the *patient* lives, he or she is violating the law. The violation is punishable with penalties of up to $1000, permanent loss of licensure, and up to one year in jail. Obviously if there is a harm-causing event to the patient (malpractice) the consequences can be devastating both professionally and financially.

Recognizing that the practice of nursing is changing, the National Council of State Boards of Nursing (www.NCSBN.org) began exploring several different licensing models in the late 1990's that would simplify government processes and remove some of the regulatory barriers, while increasing the access to safe nursing care. This could be compared to the process used to grant and regulate a state driver's license, i.e., the candidate passes the exam, is given a license and is allowed to drive . . . infractions are handled in the state where the offense occurs. The nurse, after passing the licensing exam, would be allowed to practice across state lines (only in the states that are participating in the Nurse Licensure Compact (NLC) . . . there are, as of July 2008, 23 states—(Figure 5–1) whether physical or electronic, as long as she acknowledges that she is subject to each state's practice laws and discipline.

Additional resources to assist with licensing issues are available at each state's professional licensing board, the CMSA website www.cmsa.org (there is a template of support letters that case managers can use to encourage one's own state to join the compact—Figure 5–2), and Center for Telemedicine Law (www.CTel.org) and www.telehealthlawcenter.org.

Figure 5–1 Nurse Licensure Compact (NLC) States

Last Updated: [July 2008]
Nurse Licensure Compact (NLC) States

COMPACT STATES	IMPLEMENTATION DATE
Arizona	7/1/2002
Arkansas	7/1/2000
Colorado	10/1/2007
Delaware	7/1/2000
Idaho	7/1/2001
Iowa	7/1/2000
Kentucky	6/1/2007
Maine	7/1/2001
Maryland	7/1/1999
Mississippi	7/1/2001
Nebraska	1/1/2001
New Hampshire	1/1/2006
New Mexico	1/1/2004
North Carolina	7/1/2000
North Dakota	1/1/2004
Rhode Island	7/1/2008
South Carolina	2/1/2006
South Dakota	1/1/2001
Tennessee	7/1/2003
Texas	1/1/2000
Utah	1/1/2000
Virginia	1/1/2005
Wisconsin	1/1/2000

If you have questions regarding NLC licensure, please contact your state board of nursing in your primary state of residence for specific requirements. For state board of nursing contact information, please click here.

States Pending NLC Implementation (these dates could be subject to change).

PENDING COMPACT STATES	STATUS
Currently no states are pending NLC implementation	

Source: printed with permission of National Council State Boards of Nursing (NCSBN) http:// www.NCSBN.org.

Figure 5–2 Template for Your Organizations to Support the Nurse Licensure Compact

---

Template for Your Organizations to Support the Nurse Licensure Compact

(these are suggestions only, please feel free to modify as you see fit)
DATE
Kathy Apple, RN, MSN, CAE
Executive Director
National Council of State Boards of Nursing, Inc.
676 North St. Clair Street
Suite 550
Chicago, IL 60611-2921
Dear Ms. Apple:
On behalf of the more than XXXX members of the XXXX, which represents XXXX, I would like to state our unqualified support of the Nurse Licensure Compact (NLC). XXXX supports the individual efforts at the state level to enact model legislation, currently in 19 states, providing for participation in the NLC.

XXXX, whose members XXXXX, recognizes the importance of the NLC as legislation to enhance the public's protection by simplifying governmental processes and removing regulatory barriers to increase access to safe nursing care. In today's fast paced healthcare environment of new technology and practice modalities, it is critical that nurses are able to comply with state licensure laws that cross state lines. These types of situations occur with increasing regularity in areas such as nurse advice lines, tele-nursing, home health, long distance monitoring of patients, hospital follow-up care, mobilization in times of disaster, and the increased mobility of the nursing workforce across state lines. New threats of bioterrorism and the role of nursing as part of rapid response teams place an increased urgency on the implementation of the NLC.

XXXX and its nationwide network of XXXX (local/state chapters) are happy to support NCSBN's efforts to bring more states under the NLC. Please contact XXXX at XXX with any questions.
Sincerely,

        XXXX
        XXXX
        cc: Kristin Hellquist, NCSBN Director of Policy and
                  Government Relations
           Members of the Nurse Licensure Compact
                  Administrators (NLCA)

Donna Dorsey, NCSBN President

Source: permission granted by Case Management Society of America.

Other Legal Issues

To serve as an advocate for individuals in today's massive, intricate healthcare delivery system, a case manager needs to know the laws governing patient rights and entitlements as well as the criteria determining "fair treatment" under the law. This does not mean that case managers must have each minute detail of workers' compensation legislation committed to memory, but they do need to understand policies to know when it is appropriate to file for COBRA coverage or set an appeals process in motion. For self-protection and protection of her employer, a case manager must also be aware of any recognized standard of practice by which her work will be judged. Like nurses, physicians, social workers, and physical therapists, case managers now have protocols (practice guidelines) that are becoming the established benchmarks for appropriate case management services.

PATIENT BILL OF RIGHTS AND PATIENT CONFIDENTIALITY

Every hospital has a patient bill of rights that outlines the individual's prerogatives regarding care, including the right to emergency aid, the right to diagnosis and prognosis information, the right to unbiased treatment, and the right to voice grievances. Prominent among the items covered are the right to privacy and the right to confidentiality of all patient records. (Table 5–1 is a sample patient bill of rights from the New York State Department of Health Web site (www.health.state.ny.us/nysdoh), Table 5–2 is another sample patient bill of rights created by the American Hospital Association, and Table 5–3 is a patient bill of responsibilities, a list of corresponding duties a patient is expected to fulfill.)

In its *Accreditation Manual for Hospitals*, The Joint Commission identified privacy and confidentiality as two patient rights, entitling a patient to the following:

- To refuse to talk with or see anyone not officially connected with the hospital, including visitors, or persons officially connected with the hospital but not directly involved in the patient's care
- To wear appropriate personal clothing and religious or other symbolic items, as long as they do not interfere with diagnostic procedures or treatments
- To be interviewed and examined in surroundings designed to ensure reasonable visual and auditory privacy

Table 5–1 Patients' Bill of Rights

As a patient in a hospital in New York State, you have the right, consistent with law, to:

1. Understand and use these rights. If for any reason you do not understand or you need help, the hospital must provide assistance, including an interpreter.
2. Receive treatment without discrimination as to race, color, religion, sex, national origin, disability, sexual orientation or source of payment.
3. Receive considerate and respectful care in a clean and safe environment free of unnecessary restraints.
4. Receive emergency care if you need it.
5. Be informed of the name and position of the doctor who will be in charge of your care in the hospital.
6. Know the names, positions and functions of any hospital staff involved in your care and refuse their treatment, examination or observation.
7. A no smoking room.
8. Receive complete information about your diagnosis, treatment and prognosis.
9. Receive all information that you need to give informed consent for any proposed procedure or treatment. This information shall include the possible risks and benefits of the procedure or treatment.
10. Receive all the information you need to give informed consent for an order not to resuscitate. You also have the right to designate an individual to give this consent for you if you are too ill to do so. If you would like additional information, please ask for a copy of the pamphlet "Do Not Resuscitate Orders—A Guide for Patients and Families."
11. Refuse treatment and be told what effect this may have on your health.
12. Refuse to take part in research. In deciding whether or not to participate, you have the right to a full explanation.
13. Privacy while in the hospital and confidentiality of all information and records regarding your care.
14. Participate in all decisions about your treatment and discharge from the hospital. The hospital must provide you with a written discharge plan and written description of how you can appeal your discharge.
15. Review your medical record without charge. Obtain a copy of your medical record for which the hospital can charge a reasonable fee. You cannot be denied a copy solely because you cannot afford to pay.
16. Receive an itemized bill and explanation of all charges.
17. Complain without fear of reprisals about the care and services you are receiving and to have the hospital respond to you and if you request it,

Table 5–1 continued

a written response. If you are not satisfied with the hospital's response, you can complain to the New York State Health Department. The hospital must provide you with the Health Department telephone number.
18. Authorize those family members and other adults who will be given priority to visit consistent with your ability to receive visitors.
19. Make known your wishes in regard to anatomical gifts. You may document your wishes in your healthcare proxy or on a donor card, available from the hospital.

Source: Courtesy of the New York State Department of Health, 2003, Albany, New York.

Table 5–2 The Patient Care Partnership: Understanding Expectations, Rights, and Responsibilities

These rights can be exercised on the patient's behalf by a designated surrogate or proxy decision maker if the patient lacks decision-making capacity, is legally incompetent, or is a minor.

1. The patient has the right to considerate and respectful care.
2. The patient has the right to and is encouraged to obtain from physicians and other direct caregivers relevant, current, and understandable information concerning diagnosis, treatment, and prognosis.

   Except in emergencies when the patient lacks decision-making capacity and the need for treatment is urgent, the patient is entitled to the opportunity to discuss and request information related to the specific procedures and/or treatments, the risks involved, the possible length of recuperation, and the medically reasonable alternatives and their accompanying risks and benefits.

   Patients have the right to know the identity of physicians, nurses, and others involved in their care, as well as when those involved are students, residents, or other trainees. The patient also has the right to know the immediate and long-term financial implications of treatment choices, in sofar as they are known.
3. The patient has the right to make decisions about the plan of care prior to and during the course of treatment and to refuse a recommended treatment or plan of care to the extent permitted by law and hospital policy and to be informed of the medical consequences of this action. In

continues

Table 5-2 continued

---

case of such refusal, the patient is entitled to other appropriate care and services that the hospital provides or transfer to another hospital. The hospital should notify patients of any policy that might affect patient choice within the institution.

4. The patient has the right to have an advance directive (such as a living will, healthcare proxy, or durable power of attorney for healthcare) concerning treatment or designating a surrogate decision maker with the expectation that the hospital will honor the intent of that directive to the extent permitted by law and hospital policy.

    Healthcare institutions must advise patients of their rights under state law and hospital policy to make informed medical choices, ask if the patient has an advance directive, and include that information in patient records. The patient has the right to timely information about hospital policy that may limit its ability to implement fully a legally valid advance directive.

5. The patient has the right to every consideration of privacy. Case discussion, consultation, examination, and treatment should be conducted so as to protect each patient's privacy.

6. The patient has the right to expect that all communications and records pertaining to his/her care will be treated as confidential by the hospital, except in cases such as suspected abuse and public health hazards when reporting is permitted or required by law. The patient has the right to expect that the hospital will emphasize the confidentiality of this information when it releases it to any other parties entitled to review information in these records.

7. The patient has the right to review the records pertaining to his/her medical care and to have the information explained or interpreted as necessary, except when restricted by law.

8. The patient has the right to expect that, within its capacity and policies, a hospital will make reasonable response to the request of a patient for appropriate and medically indicated care and services. The hospital must provide evaluation, service, and/or referral as indicated by the urgency of the case. When medically appropriate and legally permissible, or when a patient has so requested, a patient may be transferred to another facility. The institution to which the patient is to be transferred must first have accepted the patient for transfer. The patient must also have the benefit of complete information and explanation concerning the need for, risks, benefits, and alternatives to such a transfer.

9. The patient has the right to ask and be informed of the existence of business relationships among the hospital, educational institutions, other healthcare providers, or payers that may influence the patient's treatment and care.

Table 5–2 continued

10. The patient has the right to consent to or decline to participate in proposed research studies or human experimentation affecting care and treatment or requiring direct patient involvement, and to have those studies fully explained prior to consent. A patient who declines to participate in research or experimentation is entitled to the most effective care that the hospital can otherwise provide.
11. The patient has the right to expect reasonable continuity of care when appropriate and to be informed by physicians and other caregivers of available and realistic patient care options when hospital care is no longer appropriate.
12. The patient has the right to be informed of hospital policies and practices that relate to patient care, treatment, and responsibilities. The patient has the right to be informed of available resources for resolving disputes, grievances, and conflicts, such as ethics committees, patient representatives, or other mechanisms available in the institution. The patient has the right to be informed of the hospital's charges for services and available payment methods.

Source: Reprinted with permission of the American Hospital Association, © 2003. This document has been superseded by The Patient Care Partnership, available at http://www.hospitalconnect.com:80/aha/ptcommunication/index.html

Table 5–3 Patients' Bill of Responsibilities

The Nassau County Medical Center recognizes the primary role its patients play with regard to their care, their safety and the safety of others, and the safeguarding of the rights of other patients and staff.

A bill of patient responsibilities describing this role is set forth below in the interest of promoting a safe, comfortable environment in which the best possible care may be rendered.

Patient Responsibilities:
NCMC patients shall be responsible:

1. To provide, to the best of his/her knowledge, accurate and complete information about present complaints, past illnesses, hospitalizations, medication and other matters relating to his/her health.
2. To report unexpected changes in his/her condition to the responsible practitioner, as soon as possible.
3. To make it known whether he/she understands a contemplated course of action and what is expected of him/her.

continues

Table 5–3 continued

4. For following to the best of his/her ability the plan for medical care as recommended by the physician primarily responsible for his/her care.
5. To keep appointments and when unable to do so, to notify the hospital with sufficient time to reschedule.
6. For his/her actions if he/she refuses treatment or does not follow the practitioner's instructions.
7. For assuring that the financial obligations of his/her healthcare are fulfilled as promptly as possible.
8. For following hospital rules and regulations regarding patient care and conduct.
9. For assisting in the control of noise and the number of visitors.
10. To comply with the No Smoking Policy as posted and assist Medical Center staff in their efforts to provide a smoke free environment for all.
11. For being respectful of the property of other persons and of the hospital.
12. For being considerate of the rights of others.
13. To fill out the patient evaluation form to provide feedback to the hospital.

Source: Courtesy of Nassau County Medical Center, East Meadow, New York.

- To expect that any discussion or consultation involving the patient will be conducted discreetly and that individuals not directly involved in the patient's care will not be present without the permission of the patient
- To have the medical record read only by individuals directly involved in the patient's treatment or in the monitoring of its quality, and by other individuals only with the patient's written authorization or that of a legally authorized representative
- To expect all communications and other records pertaining to the patient's care, including the source of payment for treatment, to be treated as confidential
- To request a transfer to another room if another patient or visitor in the room is unreasonable, disturbing the patient by smoking or other actions
- To be placed in protective privacy when considered necessary for personal safety[1]

(In 1995, the Joint Commission adopted new accreditation standards that addressed the ethical practices of healthcare organizations and implemented a code of behavior regarding marketing, admission, transfer, discharge, and billing practices, as well as the relationship of the organization and its staff to other healthcare providers, educational institutions, and payers.)

The American Hospital Association has adopted a Patient's Bill of Rights that encourages healthcare institutions to use a template, revise it for their patient community and populations, and simplify or translate language as needed to make it of best use to patients and their families.

As healthcare professionals, case managers are ethically charged to maintain the maximum amount of confidentiality possible on matters of health and finances on behalf of patients. Confidentiality touches on a number of issues and relationships. Regardless of the health plan and their health status, patients are equal. The getting of information is not an arbitrary and capricious procedure. It can be argued that providers, payers, case managers, and patients all have rights, and in fact they do, but in particular cases the rights of one group will override those of another. Each member of a health plan enjoys the same right to know about his or her condition, and the same protection must be given to the privacy of any member. A cancer or HIV-positive patient has the right to keep his or her health status from being known by anyone else; an employer requesting such particular information from a case manager is out of line.

However, some patients need to be educated on how far they can push their right to confidentiality. A case manager cannot forge a document or fudge a claims report, altering the diagnosis, treatment, or medication, for example, to cloud facts about an illness because it might be a tip-off to the patient's condition. Although claims forms generally include a patient's name, social security number, age, and illness, patient codes are utilized to help protect the patient's identity on reports that might be sent to a corporate office, such as cost-benefit analysis reports.

Jeanne Boling, a previous executive director of the Case Management Society of America (CMSA), assembled information on confidentiality issues that case managers typically must face. The material was adapted from "Confidentiality: An Issue CMs Must Understand," conference hand-outs developed by Susan Scheutzow. Case managers will ask themselves two very basic questions to clarify confidentiality concerns: When must information be disclosed? When must information not be disclosed?[2]

Following the principle that the sensitivities of patients must be respected while facilitating the truthful and complete disclosure of information necessary for proper healthcare determinations, Scheutzow says that information must be disclosed when a patient requests it (as qualified by state law). Many states have statutes requiring that any patient be given access to his or her medical records except when the content might be damaging to the patient. In the absence of statutes, courts generally hold that patients must be allowed to see their medical records.

Varying from state to state, statutes may require that the following events be reported: births; deaths; child or elder abuse and neglect; violent injuries; animal bites; contagious, infectious, and occupational diseases; certain conditions of newborns; abortions; impaired healthcare professionals; and breath, blood, and urine testing for alcohol and drugs. Federal law mandates the reporting of certain adverse transfusion reactions, certain misadministration of radioactive materials, and certain medical device defects and failures. According to Scheutzow, case managers have a duty to warn authorities in cases of communicable diseases or violent inclinations of the mentally ill. They are also compelled to respond to subpoenas and court orders; if information is privileged, a case manager should request a signed consent from the patient and consult a lawyer.

When can't case managers share information? When it comes from a drug or alcohol abuse treatment provider or a patient's mental health records or when it concerns AIDS or a sexually transmitted disease. As an example of why case managers should consult legal counsel, the list of confidential matters includes cases of abortion, in direct contrast to state statutes that might require disclosure of abortion. To help clarify such issues, Scheutzow recommends that case managers have a strict, well-defined confidentiality policy, operate with the informed consent of patients, and get adequate and valid releases or consent authorization forms for all disclosures of confidential information.

Confidentiality, privacy, and access to information are issues of concern at hospitals, within managed care organizations, and on Capitol Hill. Key pieces of confidentiality legislation were debated in 1996 and 1997, with elements of the Health Insurance Portability and Accountability Act and the Patient Right to Know Act opening up debate on how to prevent breaches of privacy. The overarching legislation now in effect is HIPAA, which calls for full disclosure to patients regarding how their healthcare information will be used and who might see it (see Chapter 7). It has been the position of the National Coalition for Patient Rights to point out that everyone wins in a system that improves health and prevents illness at the lowest cost. However, if employees and patients feel the healthcare system leaks personal information, they will begin to withhold that information, lying about their lifestyle and concealing their genetic background, resulting in delayed treatment, and, coincidentally, outcomes data based on erroneous input.

CONSENT/DISCLOSURE AND CONSENT AUTHORIZATION FORMS

Empowerment derives in part from awareness. Therefore, a case manager, as patient advocate, must have the utmost respect for a patient's right to knowledge. During a well-conducted assessment, the case manager will discover just how much the patient understands about his or her condition and prognosis. In most instances, not enough background has been provided to enable the patient to safely manage his or her illness or injury. The wife or husband or eldest child perhaps knows a few more details, but the patient remains in the dark. There must be a free disclosure of information so that an informed decision may be made.

When a case manager begins working with a patient, she should have in hand a consent authorization form (Table 5–4), signed by the patient or the person authorized to act on the patient's behalf, whenever arranging for an alternative care location or provider, considering an optional medical procedure, or developing a case management plan. This document provides for the release of information to the case manager and certifies the patient's permission to review case information with the treating physician, other healthcare providers, the payer, the employer group, and so on, when some data must be shared to further the case. It also incorporates permission for the provision of case management services. In a group medical plan, consent forms are not strictly required, although certainly recommended and increasingly a standard of practice. They are a necessity in a workers' compensation or no-fault case, especially in situations more prone to litigation than others. A consent form can

Table 5–4 Consent Authorization Form

CONSENT
Date:

To assure appropriate medical case management services, I, _____, authorize any physician, hospital, or other professional involved in my treatment to disclose medical, hospital, vocational, or related information. I authorize that the information may be shared with other professionals, agencies, or insurance companies who may be involved in the provision or payment of necessary services.
A copy of this authorization may be accepted, if necessary.

     Signed
     Guardian
     Witness

   Source: Courtesy of Options Unlimited, Case Management Services Division, Huntington, New York.

---

be written very specifically or broad-based to cover a number of medical situations, but it should authorize access to information for the duration of the case. A copy of the consent form is kept on file and accompanies all case management reports sent to a physician, lawyer, claims examiner, and so on. For long-term cases, a consent form should be signed annually.

A case manager might think, "John is in the hospital and I need to see him." So off she goes, driving 45 minutes to the hospital. But John feels that case management intervention is not necessary and certainly does not want to sign any consent form. There is no other family member present. The case manager has now trekked to the hospital and gotten nowhere because she was not prepared. It would have been better to have moved a little more slowly, but thoroughly, through the case management process. Perhaps the case manager is planning on seeing a man who is on life support; she needs to review his hospital records. The man's wife, authorized to sign for him, cannot meet the case manager at the hospital. The case manager may send the consent authorization form by mail, e-mail, or fax and have a signed copy with her when she visits the hospital. In essence, it safeguards the patient–case manager relationship, noting who the case manager is, those people she will need to speak with, and the records that will be discussed.

Perhaps the patient is in an intensive care unit (ICU). The case manager has spoken with the doctor and the family; both parties think case management is a great idea. She arrives at the ICU and a family member says, "Oh, we have an attorney. You'll have to show this to him." Unable to speak to the patient without the counsel's permission, the case manager is back to square one. To prevent this, the case manager will want to ascertain whether the patient is represented by an attorney. However, she will want to be careful not to put herself in the position of inadvertently "suggesting" that the patient needs an attorney. Instead of saying, "Do you have an attorney? I need to know because I will need his or her authorization as well," the case manager can call, explain her role, mention the use of a consent authorization that will enable her to speak to the doctor, and ask as an "afterthought" if there is anyone else who the patient thinks she might need to contact. The patient may respond, "Well, my lawyer already told me that I can't sign anything, so you'll have to talk to her." In this way, without asking directly, the case manager finds out an attorney is involved.

In some cases, a consent form is not critical but is used to give the patient confidence. When a case manager gets a referral from an employer group or an insurance carrier and the patient's diagnosis is a psychiatric disability, cancer, a degenerative disease such as ALS, or AIDS, a consent form offers the patient an assurance of confidentiality. (There is extra anxiety in the case of an AIDS diagnosis, and justifiably so, because insurers and companies have been known to cut benefits or employment for individuals with AIDS.) In response to this growing concern, some states have imposed additional mandates to ensure the confidentiality of HIV/AIDS status. I send a consent form with a brochure on my services and a note requesting the patient's signature so I can speak to the doctor, the therapist, and others, to help them work with the patient. With such a form, there is a record that a case manager is working in tandem with the patient and the doctor and that sensitive patient information will not be disclosed to a boss or an insurance representative.

Many case managers have difficulty with consent forms, feeling that as soon as they have to ask for a signature, the patient will respond negatively. It is true that many people are intimidated by anything requiring their signature. What I basically do is follow rules of full disclosure, explaining the authorization and telling the patient that it is good for his or her protection and for my protection. Often, case managers must call a doctor on the telephone for details of a treatment plan. Sometimes, broader background must be gleaned from patient records, or assistance is needed on an emergency basis. How can a case move forward if the patient must be contacted for each and every release? I tell each patient that the document is a simple statement showing that he or she is aware of what is going on, that it is similar to the form signed upon entering the hospital or when a doctor wants to forward patient records to someone else for review. I also explain that my ability to help might be severely compromised without the authorization. When the patient understands all this, consent is customarily given readily.

In her comments regarding consent and disclosure issues, Scheutzow outlines the process of informed consent:

- Give the information verbally and in writing.
- Offer an opportunity for questions and answers to clarify patient understanding.
- Witness the signing of the consent form and retain the current consent in case management records.
- Recognize the two legal standards for disclosure: Disclose the information that a reasonable medical practitioner would disclose under the same or similar circumstances, and disclose all the background needed to make the decision-making process meaningful.

When there is a question of a patient's competency (legal judgment rendered by a court after hearing evidence) or capacity (the patient's functional ability to understand the diagnosis, treatment, risks, and alternatives), the case manager should involve family members in the case management plan and also recommend that they seek legal help for purposes of establishing power of attorney, durable power of attorney, or guardianship.

MEDICAL RECORDS

Case management files are considered medical records and, consequently, must be retained for the period of time mandated by state and federal statutes. In most states, this period is 5 years or the period of time in which lawsuits may be filed, whichever is longer. Children's medical records must be kept until the children reach legal age, as defined by the state.

THE RIGHT TO KNOW VERSUS THE NEED TO KNOW

When case managers work directly with employer groups, especially self-funded employer groups, the issue of an employer's right to know (as opposed to need to know) comes to the forefront. Involved with the bigger, more expensive cases, charged with tracking a company's stop-loss ceiling, or facing an employer who can—if dedicated to the search and wishes to illegally sort through computer files or paperwork—identify a particular employee by matching a benefit claim to the corporate checkbook register or social security number, case managers find that their fiduciary relationship with patients can be compromised. (A fiduciary relationship is the legal relationship of confidentiality that exists when one person relies on another, as in the case manager–patient relationship.)

Despite the risks of a lawsuit, some employers might ask for specific information on a patient. Citing pending layoff, promotion, or management decisions that need to be made or the responsibility to protect dollars now that it self-funds and administers its health package, the employer might assert that it has the right to know which employee is costing the most. A CEO might say, "Before I can approve that home care alternative, I need to know who we're talking about here."

It is true that the boss does need to have a broad perspective on employee problems, but the "who" must be protected to the greatest extent possible. Without naming an employee or dependent, the case manager can respond in generalities. Cost-benefit analyses and other reports can give credible but not identifiable narrative data. John, the

45-year-old drill bit specialist who works in the machine shop, becomes a "middle-aged man." Further, the case manager can explain to the employer that it is in the employer's best interests *not* to know exactly who John is in the event of an unlawful discharge or workers' compensation lawsuit.

DISCLOSURE ISSUES

Issues of disclosure and confidentiality are not as clear-cut as they once were. Susan O. Scheutzow noted how changes in the ways in which society, the government, and the courts perceive these issues impact a case manager's responsibilities and liabilities. At her session, "Confidentiality: How a Case Manager Can Protect It," given at the Medical Case Management Conference V, she included these comments in her materials:

> The issue of disclosure of information includes mandatory reporting of information to the government, disclosure of information to protect third parties such as when there is a duty to warn third parties about the illness of a patient, and disclosure of information pursuant to judicial or quasi-judicial process. Information may be required to be released in these instances even if there is otherwise a general legal requirement to keep information confidential.

> Generally there has been a trend to increase mandatory disclosure of information. The physician–patient privilege, which generally came into being in many states over 100 years ago and protected confidential communications from release pursuant to judicial process, is largely inadequate today. The physician–patient privilege generally is limited to communications made to physicians. With the proliferation of licensed healthcare professionals rendering care in today's healthcare system the physician–patient privilege is inadequate to protect healthcare communications.

> The laws requiring confidentiality and requiring disclosure of medical records are on a collision course for healthcare providers as providers are increasingly required to release information to comply with the law yet are subject to liability for errors in making such disclosure.[3]

Given this environment, it is still the case manager's responsibility to protect the rights of the patients she is working with by keeping medical (as well as financial and emotional) information confidential unless required by law to disclose it. In questionable instances, case managers should consult legal counsel for advice.

ADEQUATE INFORMATION

Because they may be held legally responsible for their decisions, it is important that case managers make certain the information they use is accurate and adequate. Secondhand information, unless it comes from a reliable source, might not be good enough. Long-distance telephonic case management, conducted without on-site or in-person visits, can be dangerous if an element of the treatment plan is overlooked. In all cases, the case manager should document decisions, medical sources, transitions from one care facility to another, and so on, to support the selected case management plan.

CONTRACTS AND LETTERS OF AGREEMENT

Case managers working in-house for insurance carriers, HMOs, TPAs, and so on, will not have to consider this question, but those working independently as case management consultants should review the use of case management service contracts. As Thomas K. Hyatt pointed out in a presentation titled "Contracting for Case Management Services," the decision to utilize a formal business contract must be based on legal and practical considerations and the case manager's working relationship with the client. How frequently does this payer or client refer cases? What is the range of services the client is expecting and how much responsibility will the case manager have?

If a written contract or letter of agreement is used, Hyatt recommends that it include the following:

- A "due diligence" section. Basically, this section includes the practices, conduct norms, documentation, and so on, that both parties can reasonably expect from each other. As an example, the payer will expect the case manager to document his or her credentials and qualifications. The case manager will expect to receive the benefit plan (Summary Plan Description) and all amendments applicable to the beneficiary. The case manager should review the insurance contract for a statement giving the insurer the authority to perform case management and to delegate this function to an outside entity.

- Evidence of the payer's professional liability insurance. Does the insurance cover case management services and, if so, for how much?
- Specific terms, if any, between the payer and a TPA or any TPA terms for case management intervention
- Written releases allowing the case manager access to confidential medical information
- Any applicable medical protocols
- The payment structure
- A clear delineation of the duties of the payer and the case manager
- Confidentiality protection
- Physician and patient consent
- Professional liability insurance protection
- Compliance with laws

A case manager's ability to negotiate with a large payer might depend on her specialty, the needs of the payer, and a host of business circumstances, Hyatt suggests. In my mind, the most important requisite for negotiating is that the case manager adopts the firm position that she is a healthcare professional working to achieve a positive outcome for all parties. This stance enables the case manager to pursue the contract she deserves and to turn away contracts that are inadequate.

Hyatt also notes that case managers should read carefully any prepared written agreements presented by a payer and should not sign anything they do not fully understand. It is appropriate to line through any provisions that are unacceptable even if the agreement is subsequently signed and returned to the payer. If a payer rejects the need for a written agreement, Hyatt says, the case manager should consider developing a letter stating her understanding of the business terms and the case manager–payer relationship, including the case manager's duties, the payer's duties, compensation (per hour, per day), payment schedule (payment within 30 days of receipt of the case manager's invoice), insurance coverage and indemnification (e.g., a "hold harmless" clause to protect the case manager from claims, liabilities, damages, etc.), and the length of the term for case management services (for one particular case, a group of cases for 5 years, etc.).[4] See Appendix 5 at the end of the chapter for Hyatt's sample written agreement.

LEGAL ISSUES IN CASE MANAGEMENT

Noted speaker Alice G. Gosfield, Esq., said, "Case managers are at the fulcrum of where the care management aspect of the healthcare delivery system currently is focused, and a great deal of what you do is going to get much more scrutiny as years go by. The concept of liability and accountability for the outcomes of care is not just going to be competitive but is increasingly going to be based on whether patients are harmed as a result of the choices that are made in this changing system." This means that case managers will not only need to document "controlled costs with appropriate outcomes demonstrated on the basis of data," but also that a case manager's recommendations for care might have to stand up in court.

Following is an overview of case management and the law. The basis of this section is a reference document compiled by Jeanne Boling titled "Legal Issues in Case Management." In her brief, Boling succinctly captured the range of diverse elements that may legally impact on a case manager's practice. (A section of this document appears as Appendix 5–B.)

The first focus is on a case manager's competence, noting that it must be and will be measured against accepted standards of care in the industry. Among the existing formal standards of care pertinent to case managers are those developed by the CMSA, URAC, the Association of Rehabilitation Nurses, the National Association for Social Work, the National Association of Rehabilitation Professionals in the Private Sector, The National Association of Geriatric Care Managers, the National Institute on Community-Based Long-Term Care, and the American Nurses Association, as well as nurse practice acts and standards of care developed by individual hospitals or practice-based protocols, as well as the Department of Human Services or Department of Health in individual states. Corporate, organizational, and facility standards of care and protocol are other resources, including those from the NCQA referenced earlier and the HEDIS performance measures. Also appropriate are the Guidelines for Health Benefits Administration (a joint effort of the American Hospital Association, American Medical Association, American Managed Care and Review Association, Blue Cross and Blue Shield Association, and Health Insurance Association of America), the series of 19 Clinical Practice Guidelines created by the former Agency for Health Care Policy and Research and released from 1992 to 1996 (see the Agency for Healthcare Research and Quality), and the HEDIS performance measures and NCQA protocols noted in Chapter 2. The National Guideline Clearinghouse is a public resource for evidence-based clinical practice guidelines located on the Internet. Currently relevant certifications available to case managers are discussed in Chapter 7.

Beyond these protocols and certifications are the basic educational curricula and degrees for the various healthcare professions, continuing education credits, and the more informal standards of care "set" by peers in case management practice and other healthcare professionals. Taken together, such standards will be used as criteria to ascertain whether a case manager has the background and experience to practice case management.

From a legal standpoint, what are the questions of liability that may arise? Attorney Lynn S. Muller succinctly addresses the basics in "Legal Issues: An Ethical Dilemma" (Table 5–5).

Table 5–5 Legal Issues: An Ethical Dilemma

Legal Basics

By what standard would a nurse case manager be judged? In the absence of new case law, we must rely on history, as the law is based on what came before. Res Judicata is a fancy legal term for the idea that the thing has already been decided.

Professional Negligence arises out of Tort Law. Negligence is a tort, a civil wrong. This is distinguished from crimes.

Negligence is the conduct that falls below a standard of care required by the law for the protection of persons . . . from foreseeable harm. Negligence may result from an act or omission.

The Standard of Care applied to a tort suit is not normally derived from an external authority, such as a government standard. In the developing Case Management Field, as with other professionals, standards develop in a complicated way through interaction with leaders of the profession, professional journals and meetings and networks with colleagues. Over time, hundreds of separate statements and comments become the "Standard Practice." Eddy, Clinical Policies and the Quality of Clinical Practice, 307 *New Eng. J. Med.* 343 (1982).

Proving Plaintiff's Case: Standard or customary practice by those in a specialty area is normally established through the testimony of experts. The purpose of the expert is to assist the trier of fact (usually a jury . . .). Such experts base their testimony on their knowledge, education, and experience. Fed. R. Evid. 703, 704, N.J.S.A. 2A:84A-2, et seq.

The Plaintiff must offer proof that the Defendant Physician (includes peer review), Nurse (including case managers, UR, QA, Discharge Planners, etc.), and Therapists (including all licensed therapists) acted contrary to the accepted standards of practice in the area.

Where do you fit into this picture?

Source: Reprinted with permission from L. S. Muller, Legal Issues in Case Management Practice, An Ethical and Legal Roundtable, Questions and Quandaries in Case Management: Quest for Resolutions, p. 44, 1996, Case Management Society of America.

Case managers may be held liable for negligence in the form of malpractice, bad faith actions, or for the actions of a certain provider or staff member, in the sense that the case manager was not sufficiently careful or knowledgeable about the selection of a provider or the competence of staff. Charges of negligence look at an individual's conduct, rather than state of mind or intent. Malpractice is seen as the negligent conduct of professionals, such as case managers, nurses, physicians, and others.[5] Malpractice includes any professional person's wrongful conduct, improper discharge of professional duties, or failure to meet standards of care that results in harm or undue costs to another person. Bad faith actions involve a breach of implied duty conducted in good faith and fair dealing as part of providing managed care services. There are a few relevant cases that help illustrate the implications for case managers regarding liability and malpractice. A number of cases that have passed through the courts focus on a payer's denial of claims, or the size of damage payments. Although a case might not include a case manager on the stand, case managers will want to be aware of trial process and outcomes.

Discharge

The first four cases reviewed here concern issues that arise with regard to patient discharge. The first, *Wickline v. State of California* (1986, 1987), is one of the more widely known cases with elements pertinent to case management practice. Alice Gosfield summarized the basic message of the *Wickline* decision as follows: Anyone can be held liable for damages or harm to a patient when (1) services being provided in the utilization management environment are not in accordance with standards of care, (2) the attending physicians disagree with the utilization management function, or (3) appeals on a medical decision are not pursued or are arbitrarily ignored or denied.[6] For case managers in particular, these implications follow:

- Case management is a reasonable activity.
- Case managers can be held accountable when something bad happens to the patient.
- Case managers must meet a reasonable standard of care.
- Case managers must not conduct their activities in a way that corrupts medical judgment.
- Case managers must act within the scope of their licensure and their own competence and education.

- The case manager's role is as a consultant to clients and physicians (who make the final medical decision).
- Case managers should not practice medicine and should not interfere with the doctor–patient relationship.
- Alternative treatment plans should be placed in writing as much as possible and be signed by the physician.

In the light of legal ramifications and consequences, case managers must act on complete information. If contradictory information exists, it is the case manager's responsibility to determine what is true. The case manager should consider carefully whether sufficient information can be gathered over the phone or whether an in-person meeting is necessary. At a minimum, the case manager should work from a claims history and all available medical records, and the case management plan should be based on data that a competent professional in the case management role would deem sufficient for clinical decision-making purposes.

At the end of the day, the court decision placed responsibility for the *Wickline* discharge solely on the shoulders of the physician. However, because they may be held responsible for the patient's care, case managers should not comply with unreasonable third-party payer limits without written protest. Case managers are patient advocates foremost, and the courts demand that a patient's interests come first. Also, if employees make treatment decisions based on payment mechanisms or a fear of denial rather than on what is appropriate for the patient, the company may not be protected.

Protection against liability claims when dissent from a treatment plan exists requires that the case management review process be conducted by adequately qualified reviewers using valid medical criteria and include a thorough review of medical records and a discussion with the treatment team. If discharge is called for, the review should incorporate an assessment of the risk of discharge.

The second case with discharge issues at its center is *Wilson v. Blue Cross of Southern California and Blue Cross/Blue Shield of Alabama and Western Medical Review* (1990). This case involved the premature discharge of a patient from a psychiatric hospital. At the time of discharge, the physician had written in his notes that the patient was discharged on the recommendation of the utilization review company. The patient went home and committed suicide. The family did not sue the physician or the hospital; they sued the insurer and the utilization review company that had suggested the discharge. In court, the insurer and utilization review firm held that they were not responsible for the decision to discharge the patient and that the attending physician was responsible for making his own decisions and, if at all concerned, should have appealed the decision for discharge. The jury felt that the insurer violated three of the four elements of the case, and only held back on finding the insurer guilty of a "bad faith denial of claims." Because all four elements against the insurer did not hold up in court, the insurer was not held liable in this particular case. (Alice Gosfield commented, "Some in the industry now say, 'Oh good, we can't be held liable.' My view is that this was a squeaker and somebody better start paying attention to the processes by which these judgments are going to be made."[7])

As for the implications for case managers, there are two. First, case managers should check benefit plan contract language. Does it include coverage for case management? Has the insured authorized case management? If not, the case management entity can be charged with interfering with the insured's insurance contract and perhaps with liability for any harm resulting from that interference. Second, it is critical that a case manager's treatment plan have the approval of the treating physician and the patient or family.

Two additional cases of record with lessons for case managers are *Hughes v. Blue Cross of Northern California* (1989) and *Linthicum v. Nationwide Life Insurance Company* (1986). In *Hughes,* as noted by Marilou M. King, an appeals court upheld a trial court's award of $700,000 in damages, finding that there was a "defective determination of medical necessity because only a part of the beneficiary's medical records were reviewed by the utilization reviewer." This case also contained some "bad faith" implications for case managers. When a case management plan denies a patient access to the benefits of an insurance contract, it is usually the result of intentional and outrageous conduct, but to avoid any problem in this area, a case manager should thoroughly review and/or discuss contractual obligations with the insurer, should formulate a recovery plan or plan of care in concert with the treating physician and patient, and should ensure that it is satisfactory to them.

In *Linthicum,* the insurer was held liable for failing to consult the treating physician. The implications for case managers are as follows: All medical records must be reviewed and reflected in case management reports and recommendations, and a case manager must consult the treating physician. Consult the treating physician? Sounds like very basic advice, but someone somewhere along the line at Nationwide forgot and was held accountable.

These cases underscore the importance of one's ethical and clinical responsibilities, whether fulfilling the role of case manager, social worker, home healthcare nurse, discharge planner, or "other" in the discharge planning process. Over and over, I see case managers neglecting to cover the bases, not sweating the details. There are principles and guidelines that exist to help define the criteria for appropriate activities in discharge planning. (See Appendix 5–C for the "Evidence-based Principles of Discharge and Discharge Criteria" developed by the American Medical Association.)

Negligent Referral

The next legal area to be considered is negligent referral. When referring a patient to a facility or provider, case managers have a responsibility to act in good faith in the best interest of the patient, investigate the competency and qualifications of the facility or provider, and use reasonable care in making the referral. The more choices a case manager offers the patient or physician, the less her risk of being held liable for that referral.

When considering a practitioner or facility for referral, a case manager should examine current licensure and accreditation, the outcomes of cases similar to the one under consideration for referral, billing practices, insurance coverage, and the records of any previous pertinent malpractice judgments. The National Practitioner Data Bank, www.npdb-hidb.com, retains information on all malpractice judgments and settlements, catalogued by practitioner and institution. Although there is a recommendation currently under consideration to open these records to all inquiries, only those nurses and physicians with cases on file and hospitals can retrieve their own data. Thus, an independent case manager would have trouble checking a physician's record through the data bank.

The National Practitioner Data Bank (NPDB), the Healthcare Integrity and Protection Data Bank (HIPDB), and the Federal Credentialing Program (FCP) are managed by the Division of Practitioner Data Banks, a division of the Bureau of Health Professions (BHPr) within the Health Resources and Services Administration (HRSA).

Case managers should document their continuous inquiry into the credentials and performance of the practitioners and facilities to which they refer patients, offer the patients and families a choice of practitioners and facilities, and always follow up with patients who are referred to review their status and response. Further, a case manager should disclose any problems to the patient and physician for their informed consent and obtain the patient's and physician's consent in writing, keeping it on file in a case management report.

Relevant case law citations include the nationally publicized case of *Bergalis v. CIGNA Dental Health Plan* (1991). Kimberly Bergalis of Florida sued her dentist for allegedly infecting her with the AIDS virus and also sued CIGNA for $20 million on the basis of a negligent referral to this particular dentist. According to Marilou King, "The claim is not that CIGNA knew the dentist had AIDS but that CIGNA should have undertaken a reasonable investigation to discover if the dentist to whom CIGNA referred patients had a disease that could be communicated like AIDS."[8]

Another case, *Moshe v. Rush-Presbyterian St. Luke's Hospital* (1990), alerts case managers to the fact that utilization review (UR) and case management activities may be interpreted as inhibiting the ability of physicians to render care. Therefore, in making a referral, a case manager must use a reasonable process for determining that the referral is in the patient's best interest, give complete referral instructions, and, if the agency or facility is providing questionable levels of care, take corrective action immediately.

This issue of access to care is also seen in *Nazay v. Miller,* a 1991 Pennsylvania case, in which the original court ruling supported a retiree who did not comply with PreCert/UR requirements and was subsequently penalized for noncompliance by the plan. A subsequent ruling reversed that decision. Even in a cost-containment environment, denial of access to care is a very sensitive issue. A case management plan should always be proactive and in the patient's best interests.

Bad Faith Actions

One of the tenets of ethical practice is veracity, telling the truth. A case manager preparing marketing materials should avoid overemphasizing capabilities or guaranteed results. In *Warne v. Lincoln National Administrative Services Corp.*, a jury awarded Warne $26.8 million for his school district's plan because it did not cover his liver transplant. The benefit plan language clearly stated that this surgery was not covered; however, the plan's benefit brochure included organ transplants as a covered procedure. The jury felt the plan's denial of payment was a bad faith action.[9]

Emerging Case Law

Lawyer Stephen J. Schantz has noted cases that fall short of what he calls "black letter law" but offer guidance and fuel for thought for case managers. In *California v. State Care Health Plan,* a husband and wife, members of a managed care plan, found through a series of referrals that their daughter had Wilm's tumor, which can be a problematic, dangerous diagnosis. Surgery was recommended. After many conversations with physicians, the plan, and various providers, the family found a multidisciplinary medical team that followed protocol developed by a prominent national body to treat Wilm's tumor. The family wanted the plan to approve surgery by this team. The plan had approved another surgeon, at the same hospital, even though the individual lacked the depth of experience or the exact same credentials. Timing became critical. There were discussions, appeals, and allegations that the evening before surgery, the healthcare plan called the parents to request their presence at a meeting. Bedside with their daughter, the parents declined. The family went ahead with the team, following its protocol. Afterwards, payment was denied because the procedure was not completed by a preapproved provider.

In California, the California Department of Corporations is the regulatory entity overseeing HMOs and managed care entities. It sought to institute a fine against the HMO for $500,000 on the premise that, if you say you are an HMO, you must have the ability to give ready referrals in a variety of specialties. That fine was appealed and upheld, based on extensive review of the referral process, expertise available, and who did what and when, indicating that, in California at least, the right to provide managed care services is predicated on the ability to fulfill the "care" element.

Another class action filed in federal court, *Drolet v. Healthsource,* includes a number of allegations, one holding that the physician–patient relationship is compromised by the various financial incentives the provider company provides to participating physicians to reduce specialty care expenditures and referrals. There is a growing concern that financial incentives within some managed care organizations almost serve as disincentives for referral care, diagnostics, and services. This area is ripe for litigation and bears watching.[10]

Providers are beginning to turn to the courts for protection against liability or claims that go unpaid. In a 2001 case, *Rogers v. Cigna Health-Care,* a group of physicians in Texas alleged that Cigna had evaded paying for medical services that had been provided. In a similar vein, the Maryland Insurance Commissioner in 2001 declared $1.4 million in administrative penalties plus disciplinary action to five health plans for allegedly neglecting to reimburse claims within the 30-day time frame allotted, and failing to comply fully with state insurance law.[11]

LEGISLATION

In addition to tracking case management protocols and practice guide-lines, case managers need to monitor local and national legislative and regulatory changes and statutes to make certain their practice is in line with current regulations. This task can appear daunting. Major pieces of pertinent legislation include the following:

- The Employee Retirement Income Security Act (ERISA) of 1974 governs the majority of nongovernmental employee benefit plans. It exempts companies that self-insure from meeting the same mini-mum benefit regulations that govern insurance companies.
- The Tax Equity and Fiscal Responsibility Act (TEFRA) of 1982 amended the Social Security Act and made Medicare secondary to employer group health plans for active employees 65 to 69 years old and their spouses in the same age group. It also revised the Age Discrimination in Employment Act (ADEA) of 1967 by requir-ing employers to offer active employees age 65 to 69 and their spouses the same health benefits as those made available to younger employees.
- As a result of the Social Security Amendments of 1983 (Title IX), Medicare reimbursement shifted from reasonable costs to diagnosis-related groups (DRGs). The amendments also clarified professional review organization (PRO) functions.
- The Consolidated Omnibus Budget Reconciliation Act (COBRA) of 1986 eliminated the age cap of 70; made the employer's plan the primary payer for all active, Medicare-eligible employees and their spouses regardless of age; mandated the extension of medical plans after termination from a job and after a person becomes ineligible under medical coverage; required employers with healthcare plans to provide healthcare coverage to former employees, divorced or widowed spouses of employees, and for-mer dependent children of employees at group rates over a fixed amount of time.
- The Omnibus Budget Reconciliation Act (OBRA or *oh boy, regula-tions again,* with a nod to Alice Gosfield) of 1986 made private employer health plans primary and Medicare secondary for claimants who were permanently disabled and were covered depen-dents under a working spouse's health plan or for claimants who returned to active employment.
- The Health Care Quality Improvement Act (HCQIA) of 1986 estab-lished the National Practitioner Data Bank mentioned earlier.

- The short-lived Medicare Catastrophic Coverage Act (MCCA) of 1988, which was repealed in 1989, mandated the largest expansion of Medicare since its introduction in 1965: a cap of $1,370 for personal expenses for physicians' services; elimination of all cost sharing for inpatient hospital care after the deductible; and revisions in skilled nursing, home health, and respite care benefits.
- AIDS-related legislation passed in 1988 by Congress provided funds for research, education, HIV testing, and home health demonstration projects.
- Ryan White Comprehensive AIDS Resources Emergency Act of 1990—provides emergency financial assistance to communities that are disproportionately affected by the AIDS epidemic. These communities are allowed monies to provide whatever essential services are necessary to maintain the patient. Case managers unfamiliar with this act can contact their state's Health and Human Services department for information on the available resources and the process for accessing services for their patients.
- The Omnibus Budget Reconciliation Act (OBRA) of 1989 and 1990 included updates to HCQIA and required states to extend Medicaid coverage to all pregnant women and children up to age 6 with family incomes less than 133% of the federal poverty level.
- The Agency for Health Care Policy and Research (AHCPR) was created as a result of OBRA of 1989. The agency has developed the Office for Forum on Quality and Effectiveness to publish and disseminate national clinical practice guidelines. It is now called the Agency for Healthcare Research and Quality (AHRQ).
- The Civilian Health and Medical Program of the Uniformed Services (CHAMPUS) gives all active and retired military personnel and dependents access to treatment at any Department of Defense medical facility. Retired military personnel, their dependents, and dependents of deceased personnel are compensated by CHAMPUS if they are not eligible for Medicare.
- The Federal Employees Health Benefits Program (FEHBP) provides health insurance coverage for federal government employees. The coverage is voluntary and includes variable benefit and premium levels and a choice of competing health plans.
- The Federal Patient Self-Determination Act of 1990 required that adult patients be given written information about the state's policy regarding advance directives, living wills, and durable powers of attorney. The AHA Patient's Bill of Rights noted earlier in this chapter was an outgrowth of this bill.

- The Americans with Disabilities Act (ADA) of 1990 (federally enforced beginning in 1992) required that employers not prevent employees from returning to work even if they can no longer perform 100% of their jobs. In her presentation "Case Management & Alphabet Soup: Understanding FMLA, ADA, OSHA & DOT" at the CMSA's 1997 national conference, Deborah DiBenedetto noted that the ADA prohibits discrimination against "qualified individuals with disabilities," regarded as having an impairment and/or a record (or history) of impairment, and seeks to balance reasonable accommodation and undue hardship.
- The Family and Medical Leave Act (FMLA) of 1993 applies to companies and public agencies employing at least 50 people and enables covered employees to apply for 12 weeks of unpaid time off in each 12-month period, taken intermittently or in a block. This short-term leave is set aside for the care of themselves (in the case of illness or injury); a sick spouse, child, or infant; or for the birth of a child. During the leave, the employer must maintain health benefits as the worker desires. In a 1997 article, *Business Insurance* noted the interrelationship between FMLA, the ADA, and workers' compensation benefits. Citing expert advice from speakers at the Risk & Insurance Management Society, Inc. conference in April 1997, the piece states that benefits from other sources, such as short- or long-term disability and workers' compensation, may be used toward the 12-week FMLA limit. According to government rules, "workers' comp leave can count against the 12-week FMLA allowance if the absence is due to a qualifying illness or injury and the employee is properly notified in writing that the leave will count as FMLA leave." Also, "the employer is not required to pay health benefits beyond the 12 weeks if the worker cannot return to his or her job; in that case, COBRA benefits should be assigned."[12]
- The Health Insurance Portability and Accountability Act (HIPAA) of 1996 (first known as the Kassebaum-Kennedy Act) curbs employers' ability to deny health benefit coverage to employees with preexisting medical conditions and allows Medical Savings Accounts (MSAs) on a trial basis for employers with fewer than 50 employees. It also included amendments that set a timetable for putting in place privacy regulations and electronic standards for medical record keeping, as well as penalties for breaking them. These went into effect mid-year 2003.
- The Health Centers Consolidation Act of 1996 included a definition of "required primary health services," incorporating patient case management.

- In 1996, more than a dozen states enacted legislation requiring health plans to provide inpatient coverage for at least 48 hours following normal childbirth and 96 hours following a caesarean section. Among these states were Alaska, Connecticut, Georgia, Illinois, Maine, Maryland, Minnesota, Oklahoma, Pennsylvania, South Carolina (72 hours for C-sections), South Dakota, and Washington.
- Federal legislation requiring health plans to provide at least 48 hours of inpatient coverage following a normal birth and 96 hours of coverage following a caesarean was enacted at the federal level in 1996, as well, as the Newborns' and Mothers' Health Protection Act. Federal regulations issued in late 1998, and put into effect January 1, 1999, provided guidance to employers on how to comply with the law. Approximately six states either passed or were considering bills to give managed care enrollees direct access to certain specialists, customarily obstetricians and gynecologists, without first having to see a primary care physician.
- Other federal legislation that would have impacted case management included the Comprehensive Long-Term Care Act of 1997, which would require case management plans under Medicare long-term care and permit a Medicare beneficiary to request case management assessment regarding one's status as a "dependent individual," and the Medicare Patient Choice and Access Act of 1997, which would require direct access to specialists as determined by the case manager and provider, and allow a specialist to serve as a case manager regarding chronic conditions, were actively debated with portions of each folded into the Balanced Budget Act of 1997.
- The Balanced Budget Act of 1997 established the State Children's Health Insurance Program (SCHIP), Medicare+ Choice plans, provider-sponsored organizations (PSOs), TEFRA limits, and other education programs, payment schedules, etc. It also mandated a demonstration of coordinated care in the fee-for-service Medicare program, the impetus for the Medicare Coordinated Care Demonstration Project.
- The Patient Protection Act of 1997 defined utilization review broadly, requires health plans to have utilization review programs that meet standards or are state certified, mandates provider credentialing, [13] and established The Health Care Consumer Advisory Board.
- The Children's Health Insurance Program, legislation dubbed "Kid Care," was passed by Congress in mid-1997 providing federal funding to the states to build programs offering healthcare coverage to children in low-income families who are uninsured and to those

whose parents' employer plans don't offer family coverage. From 1998 to 2000, $3.2 billion in federal funds was left unspent, eliciting George Bush's proposal that states have until 2006 to use the money, before it's returned to the treasury. (Some states deliberately under-used the fund to maintain their eligibility for other programs, as well.) Case managers will have to track their state's utilization of its portion of the $24 billion in block grants to ascertain how this safety net can be best used by their clients.

- In late 1997, President Clinton presented his healthcare agenda, out-lining legislation he planned to pursue, including a ban on so-called drive-through mastectomies, when coverage is denied for an overnight hospital stay following a mastectomy. Clinton called on Congress to enact legislation for mastectomy coverage similar to the mandated 48 hours of inpatient/normal birth and 96 hours of cae-sarean coverage. In 1997 and 1998, several states (Connecticut, Okla-homa, Rhode Island) adopted Breast Cancer Patient Protection Acts requiring insurers to cover a minimum of 48 hours of hospitaliza-tion for mastectomies and 24 hours for lymph node excision. Intro-duced to the 106th Congress as part of H.R. 383 in 1999, the concept was referred to the Committees on Commerce, Education and the Workforce, and Ways and Means. Mastectomy length of stay was reintroduced in the 107th Congress and designated The Breast Can-cer Patient Protection Act, H.R. 536. Let's fast forward. In 2003, leg-islation requiring a minimum hospital stay for mastectomies and lymph node dissections was introduced to the 108th Congress in H.R. 1886.IH (Breast Cancer Patient Protection Act of 2003) and H.R. 1448.IH (Women's Cancer Recovery Act of 2003), and to the Senate as S. 10 (Health Care Coverage Expansion and Quality Improvement Act of 2003). Let's see what happens next. In addition, Clinton also called for a ban on gag rules, a clause that was included also in the Patient Right To Know Act. He cited as problems the lack of early retiree healthcare coverage for those not yet eligible for Medicare and the need for subsidized healthcare coverage for the unemployed.

- In December 2000, President Clinton announced Patient Privacy regulations, issued under the authority of the bipartisan Health Insurance Portability and Accountability Act (HIPAA). President Bush authorized these early in 2001, with full compliance required by April 2003. Under the regulations, patients gained the right to see their own medical records and to limit what information doctors can give to insurance companies, rights that had been limited in some states.

- The Mental Health Parity Act of 1996 expired in October 2001. Lawmakers have extended it each year since then, and did so again in December 2002. The act calls for health plans to set mental health services reimbursement limits that are at least equal to those for medical and surgical care. As studies prove that mental diseases such as depression can be linked directly to genetic makeup, the call for mental health parity is becoming stronger.

- In mid-2003, President Bush's first proposal to give seniors a drug benefit by forcing them to move into managed care was dropped, following its poor reception. House and Senate representatives then passed bills for two different pieces of $400 billion legislation to add a prescription drug benefit to Medicare, the biggest expansion of the program since its inception in 1965, intended to take effect in 2006. Both bills included private, stand-alone insurance policies for drug coverage and similar deductibles. Lawmakers working to reconcile the two bills have hit a sticking point: finding a compromise for the way each bill provides extra assistance to low-income elderly or disabled. (In July 2003, the House voted to guarantee that Congress and civilian federal workers would be able to hold onto their prescription drug benefits when they retire, even if the final Medicare drug bill provides significantly lower benefits. In essence, they are working to pass a bill they hope never applies to them.)

- Medical Malpractice/Tort Reform was hotly debated in 2003, especially on the state level. Physicians in West Virginia reported a 150% increase in their medical liability insurance rates in 18 months and reacted by planning early retirement, moving to other states, and requesting state legislation to control escalating costs. In Pennsylvania, a general surgeon pays twice what his fellow surgeon in New Jersey pays in malpractice insurance premiums. Recruiting new doctors to the state has become a problem. Several states are pursuing tort reform as a solution, and setting caps on noneconomic (pain and suffering) damages in medical malpractice cases. We will be hearing more on this subject.

- Also in the pipeline are several bills concerning coverage for veterans: H.R. 533, the Agent Orange Veterans' Disabled Children's

Benefits Act of 2003, H.R. 1048, the Disabled Veterans Adaptive Benefits Improvement Act of 2003, and H.R. 966, the Disabled Veterans' Return-to-Work Act of 2003.

DAY-TO-DAY PRACTICES

There are a number of areas in case management practice in which common sense and thinking ahead helps case managers prepare for liability claims (see also Appendix 5–B). As mentioned throughout this handbook, discussions and decisions regarding the case management treatment plan should be documented. If a patient, family member, or physician resents or is unhappy with case management intervention, this too should be documented, along with memos on steps taken to resolve any concerns or problems. Routine patient and provider satisfaction surveys will help monitor quality assurance and serve as an indicator of responsiveness to patient needs (see Chapter 12).

In practice, follow the agreed treatment plan. Noncompliance with the plan can be construed as mismanagement. In any publicity or marketing efforts, avoid puffery or claims that case management guarantees better outcomes or cost containment. In contract making, be very cautious of any type of incentive compensation arrangement with a payer or provider. Again, remember that case management is customarily administrative in nature. However, in rural areas and certain situations, a nurse case manager might provide hands-on care. Consequently, case managers should not insinuate that they are in any way determining the medical treatment plan.

Case managers should keep suspicions, conjectures, and allegations out of their correspondence and reports; these documents can be subpoenaed. A situation can be objectively covered in a report without accusation and without giving legal weight to either side in court. It is enough to record a patient's verbalized wish to return to work and the missed job interviews as well, letting the judge decide the motivations behind the actions. Similarly, a case management report can mention that a patient has stated his or her benefit payments have been significantly delayed, causing hardship; that the patient has been directed to contact a claims examiner; and that the case manager has undertaken to relay this information to the claims examiner—end of story. Case managers should consider what might happen if "the other side" sees the report.

Individuals and payers increasingly are suing plans for adverse decisions. Some UR nurses and individuals called case managers simply shorten length of stay (LOS) and deny benefits, which can be perceived (as well it might be) as harmless by patients, increasing the number of suits naming case managers.

Further, case managers may be requested by either party in a court case to appear as witnesses. (Although nurses are rarely called, the tide may be turning; certified rehabilitation counselors and vocational counselors can and do serve as witnesses in court.) If requested to appear in court, a case manager should consult with the client and a lawyer.

To defend her own interests, a case manager needs to remain involved in a case. If taken off a case ("We don't need you now; the home health company will take care of it"), the case manager should document the situation in an accurate and objective manner. The report might include language such as this: "Despite our suggestions that we continue to monitor this case actively and despite our concern for the patient, which was communicated to our client, the client has decided to end case management involvement in this case." Further, the case manager should file copies of the written notices to the patient, the medical provider, and all other members of the treatment team informing them that she is no longer involved at the client's request, not because the case manager thinks there is no need. The case manager should also make certain the patient knows whom to contact: the physician, therapist, claims examiner, and so on if a problem arises.

GETTING LEGAL INFORMATION

No case manager has to be a lawyer, but it is important to be current regarding case management professional guidelines. There are conferences specifically for case managers, training seminars, a host of national conferences relevant to case management, and magazine coverage of pertinent issues. *The Case Manager,* for instance, included a regular feature called "Laws, Liabilities & Legislation." Other publications, such as the *Case Management Advisor, Inside Case Management, Remington Report, Managed Care Interface, Care Management, Journal of Case Management, NARPPS Journal, Journal of the American Medical Association, Journal of Clinical Ethics, Continuing Care, Wall Street Journal, Rehabilitation Nursing Journal,* and the *American Journal of Nursing* also carry articles on medicolegal issues.

Unfortunately, much of the law that will eventually affect case management practice is currently in the process of creation. While clear codes of conduct are being formulated, case managers should do the following:

- Work within the guidelines that already govern case management practice settings.
- Develop a risk-management mentality. ("How do I protect myself, my company, and my patients against lack of knowledge?")
- Act according to their best judgment and keep apprised of changes in the profession. ("Is this how another prudent person in this profession would act in similar circumstances?")
- Use common sense and instinct. If something does not feel right, it probably is not. Network and ask questions of peers.
- Get a lawyer who is knowledgeable about case management.
- Document case management activities and decisions in an objective manner.
- Purchase professional liability insurance in the form of a personal or corporate policy.

NOTES

1. Boling J, "Legal Issues in Case Management," in *Managing Case Management Seminar Manual* (Little Rock, AR: Individual Case Management Association, 1991), 183.
2. Boling J, "Legal Issues in Case Management," prepared for the Individual Case Management Association, January 1994. (The material was adapted from "Confidentiality: An Issue CMs Must Understand," handouts developed by Susan Scheutzow for the Medical Case Management Conference IV in Orlando, 1992.)
3. Scheutzow S, "Confidentiality: How a Case Manager Can Protect It," in *Medical Case Management Conference V Manual* (Little Rock, AR: Individual Case Management Association, 1993), 323.
4. Hyatt T, "Contracting for Case Management Services," in *Medical Case Management Conference V Manual* (Little Rock, AR: Individual Case Management Association, 1993), 395–398.
5. Carneal G and Caprio L, ed., *Case Management Trends: An Overview of Recent Industry and Regulatory Developments* (Washington, D.C.: URAC, 2002).
6. Gosfield A, "Clinical Practice Guidelines and Managed Competition: Legal Implications for Case Managers," session audio tape recorded at the Medical Case Management Conference V, Orlando, Florida, September 1993.
7. Gosfield A, "Clinical Practice Guidelines."
8. King M, "Liability for Negligence," *Legal and Risk Management Issues in Case Management Seminar Manual* (Little Rock, AR: Individual Case Management Association, 1991), 87.
9. Kongstvedt PR, *The Managed Healthcare Handbook*, 4th ed. Gaithersburg, MD: Aspen Publishers Inc., 2001: 1227.

10. Schantz S, "Legal and Legislative Aspects of Case Management," presented at Upward Bound, CMSA 7th Annual Conference and Educational Forum, Boston, MA, June 1997.

11. Hendricks AG and Cesar WJ, "How Prepared are You?" *The Case Manager* 14, no. 3 (2003): 58.

12. Kazel R, "Leave Act Shouldn't Scare Employers," *Business Insurance* 31, no. 17 (1997): 39.

13. Schantz S, "Legal and Legislative Aspects of Case Management," 320–321.

APPENDIX 5–A

Written Agreement: Some Typical Provisions

Caveat: While these provisions have been prepared by a professional attorney, they should not be used as a substitute for legal counseling in specific situations. Readers should not act upon the information contained herein without professional guidance.

1. Recitals.

This Agreement is entered into by and between _____ (Payer), a _____ corporation and _____ (Case Manager), an individual residing in _____.

Whereas Payer has entered into an agreement with one or more employee health benefit plans (the Plan) and thereunder has agreed to provide case management services to beneficiaries of those plans; and

Whereas Case Manager is a registered nurse licensed in _____ and certified by _____, who desires to perform case management services to beneficiaries of the Plan, as appropriate;

Now, therefore, for adequate consideration, the receipt and sufficiency of which are hereby acknowledged, the parties agree as follows:

2. Duties of Payer.

(a) Payer authorizes Case Manager to perform services defined in Section 3 for beneficiaries referred by Payer to Case Manager pursuant to _____.

(b) Payer shall provide to Case Manager current, accurate and complete benefit plan information pertinent to beneficiary and shall cooperate with Case Manager in explaining terms of such benefit plans and in supplying Case Manager with any information.

(c) Payer shall provide to Case Manager all necessary waivers of confidentiality for release of medical information, which it warrants, are valid for beneficiary.

(d) Payer represents and warrants that plan documents are sufficient to authorize the performance of the case management services to be performed by Case Manager pursuant to this Agreement.

(e) Payer represents and warrants that it shall maintain professional and general liability insurance coverage in the amount of _____, which shall provide primary coverage for any claims arising from the acts of Payer pursuant to its agreement with the Plan and this Agreement.

(f) Payer represents and warrants that it shall make and communicate to beneficiary all benefit determinations regarding beneficiary's health insurance coverage and that Case Manager's reports and recommendations shall be advisory to Payer and may form the basis, in whole or in part, of Payer's benefit determinations. Case Manager shall have no responsibility to make or communicate benefit determinations.

(g) Payer represents and warrants that as part of its benefit determination program it has in place an appeals process that complies with the Guidelines for Health Benefits Administration published by _____ _____.

3. Duties of Case Manager.

(a) Case Manager shall receive referral of beneficiary by Payer pursuant to _____.

(b) Case Manager will review beneficiary's coverage as supplied by Payer and necessary waivers of confidentiality. If this information is incomplete or inadequate, Case Manager shall contact Payer and shall not take any further actions until such information is complete and adequate.

(c) Case Manager will obtain pertinent medical information from beneficiary, facility or primary or admitting physician(s) as necessary and shall devise an alternative plan of treatment for beneficiary. Case Manager shall provide beneficiary and physician(s) with alternative plan of treatment and thoroughly discuss plan with same. If physician(s) and beneficiary competently agree with the alternative plan of treatment, Case Manager will obtain their written consent thereto. Thereafter, Case Manager will contact providers of such alternative treatment and secure rates.

(d) If agreeable to beneficiary and physician(s), Case Manager shall facilitate beneficiary's access to alternative treatment. Case Manager shall report in writing to Payer within _____ business days its recommendations and outcome with originals of all written consents by beneficiary and physician(s).

(e) If not agreeable to beneficiary and physician(s), Case Manager shall report in writing within _____ business days to Payer its recommendations and outcome. Thereafter Case Manager's responsibilities with regard to said beneficiary shall end.

(f) Case Manager represents and warrants that it shall maintain professional liability insurance coverage in the amount of _____, which shall provide primary coverage for any claims arising from the acts of Case Manager pursuant to this Agreement.

4. Compensation.

For the duties performed by Case Manager under this Agreement,

(a) Payer agrees to compensate Case Manager at a rate of $_____ per hour, which shall include travel time as necessary.

(b) Payer shall pay Case Manager within thirty (30) days of its receipt of invoice from Case Manager.

(c) [Penalty for late payment.]

(d) [Additional fees for expenses of Case Manager such as supplies and Xeroxing.]

5. Relationship of Parties.

Payer and Case Manager mutually agree that there shall be no relationship between them other than an independent contractor relationship, and nothing herein shall be construed to create a principal-agent, employment or partnership relationship. Payer shall neither have nor exercise any control or direction over the methods by which Case Manager performs its duties under this Agreement. Case Manager recognizes that Payer shall not pay or withhold on behalf of Case Manager any sums for income tax, unemployment insurance, social security or any other withholding requirement of any law.

6. Indemnification.

(a) Payer agrees to indemnify Case Manager and hold it harmless from and against any and all claims, losses, liabilities, suits, damages and expenses incurred by Case Manager, including court costs and attorney's fees, to the extent such claims, losses, liabilities, suits, damages, and expenses arise out of any acts or omissions of Payer, its officers, agents or employees, or arising from any breach or default on the part of Payer in the performance of its duties under this Agreement or under the Plan.

(b) [Only if Case Manager has to, insert corresponding indemnification of Payer by Case Manager.]

7. Term and Termination.

This Agreement shall commence on _____ and continue for a term of one year. Thereafter, this Agreement shall automatically renew each year for successive one-year terms. Either party may terminate this Agreement without cause upon _____ days prior written notice to the other. In the event Case Manager is in the process of performing services hereunder for referred beneficiaries at the time of termination, Case Manager shall complete such performance even if to do so extends past the date of termination. The right of Case Manager to be paid for services already performed hereunder shall continue past the date of termination of this Agreement.

8. Miscellaneous.

(a) Choice of law/venue;

(b) Assignment;

(c) Compliance with applicable laws;

(d) Entire agreement/amendment; and

(e) Other.

In witness whereof, the parties hereto have caused this Agreement to be executed on _____, 20_____.

Payer	Case Manager
Name:	Name:
Title:	Title:
Date:	Date:

Source: Reprinted from *Medical Case Management Conference V Manual,* pp. 399–404, with permission of ICMA and Thomas K. Hyatt, Esq., © 1993.

APPENDIX 5–B

Legal Issues in Case Management Checklist

COMPETENCE OF THE CM

1. Are you properly trained and licensed? Have all qualifications been checked and documented?
2. Are you working toward the highest appropriate credential license or certification? Are you maintaining appropriate continuing education units to support the existing credential/license?
3. Are you first a client (claimant) advocate? Does your CM practice reflect this standard?
4. Are your case management plans created in concert with treating physician and client?
5. Are you familiar with your company's Job Description and Organization Chart and Policies and Procedures?
6. Is there anything in your current operations that seems inconsistent with existing formal standards for CM? (If so, discuss with your supervisor and/or legal counsel to resolve.)

CONSENT/DISCLOSURE

1. What consent form and written materials explaining case management services are you using? What is required? (Discuss any concerns about appropriate procedure or materials with supervisor and/or legal counsel.)
2. How do you explain CM services?
    —by phone?
    —by brochure?
3. Is your explanation consistent with staff, appropriate, and accurate?

CHANGE OF PROVIDER

1. Is your CM role empowering/facilitating to physicians and clients? Are you directing care or transfer without physician and/or client agreement? (If so, stop. Rethink and revise your role.)

2. Are you always acting within the scope of your licensure, your own competence and education? (If not, focus your CM practice on your area of competence and/or obtain additional supervision, education or experience to support you in an expanded role.)

In reviewing referral policy procedures

3. How are practitioners/agencies/facilities evaluated?
4. Is a continuous inquiry into credentials and practice of the above documented?
5. Is patient/family offered a choice? Are pros and cons reviewed with family appropriately? Is referral in patient's best interest?
6. Have you followed up after referral to assure good care?
7. Are referrals with knowledge of benefit/funding structure?

CONFIDENTIALITY

1. Do you know state legislation relating to confidentiality and reporting concerns, which apply to your CM practice?

    Check Areas of Applicable Legislation

    Patient right of access to medical information
    Abuse/Neglect—Child and Elder
    Contagious/Occupational Disease
    Alcohol Treatment
    Chemical Abuse Treatment
    Mental Health Treatment
    AIDS/Sexually Related Disease
    Abortion

2. Do you know and/or have you reviewed and are you complying with your company's confidentiality policy? (Review and revise if necessary with legal counsel.)
3. Are you clear about the appropriate path of medical information in your office to assure confidentiality is protected?
4. Are discarded medical records shredded?
5. Are faxed medical records handled so they are only seen by appropriate people?
6. If CMs have field files away from office, are they locked at all times in car or home? Are they safe? Who might have access?
7. If electronic records, are they accessed only by appropriate people?
8. If information returns to employer, is it "sanitized" so individuals cannot be identified? Who sees this information?

9. Are CM files retained according to state law then destroyed as medical records? (Adults 5–7 years; Children, to age of majority)
10. Is documentation concise yet complete for CM assessment, plan, implementation, follow-up, and outcome?
11. Do you know clearly how to handle medical information with employers, self-insureds, families of competent clients, others requesting access to your files?

CONTRACTING

1. Are contracts or letters of agreement (LOA) in place for all major referring accounts?
2. Are these contracts or LOA reviewed by legal counsel before signing?
3. Do contracts clearly define
   - your duties?
   - payer's duties?
   - your compensation and time of compensation?
   - insurance coverage and identification?
   - term for performance?
4. Do agreements/contracts avoid incentive compensation (or waste) arrangements? (May cause appearance of overemphasis on financial arrangements corrupting judgment regarding your primary responsibility of client advocacy.)
5. Do the entities referring cases to you have the authority to authorize you to perform CM services? Do they warrant that fact?
6. Do you understand the benefits and restrictions of different payer/reimbursement systems? (i.e., group health, indemnity HMO, PPO, reinsurance, COBRA, work comp, liability, Medicaid, Medicare, CHAMPUS, military, etc.)

CLIENT CARE NEGOTIATION

1. Does state insurance law allow you to proceed with quality and cost negotiation for client care and services?
2. Do quality issues always supersede cost issues?
3. Are you operating in concert with the primary physician and client? With their understanding and support?
4. On major decisions, do you have client and physician written consent?

5. Have you documented referral data on all options being considered?
6. Is there a direct contract in place, which establishes a rate? Is this nonnegotiable?
7. How and to whom will the agreed upon quality and cost of care be documented? Monitored? Concluded?

CUSTOMER SERVICE/RISK MANAGEMENT

1. What's your company's Incident Occurrence Reporting System?
2. What is your CM quality assurance program? Do you keep routine patient satisfaction surveys as a quality assurance monitor?
3. Are all advertising/marketing materials and procedures fair and appropriate? (not overstated)
4. Is staff consistent in offering information describing CM services and CM company?
5. Are written materials and policy reviewed by legal counsel?
6. Who communicates benefits decisions? (Never communicate a payer benefits decision unless the payer indemnifies you for it.)
7. What are your corporate, personal liability, medical malpractice, and errors and omission policies? Do you review them regularly with the carriers?
8. Do you keep current by
   • reading journals, medical, and general literature?
   • attending seminars, conferences in your area of practice?
   • networking with peers on local, regional, and national level?
9. Are potential clients transported by CM? (Be sure liability insurance is in place to support.)
10. Is there a policy regarding staff protection when there is possible exposure to violent and high-risk neighborhoods?

Source: Developed by Jeanne Boling, MSN, CCRN, CDMS, CCM for the "Case Management Practice" Seminar. Used with permission of the Foundation for Rehabilitation Certification, Education and Research, © 1994.

APPENDIX 5–C

AMA Evidence-Based Principles of Discharge and Discharge Criteria

H-160.942 EVIDENCE-BASED PRINCIPLES OF DISCHARGE AND DISCHARGE CRITERIA

1. The AMA defines discharge criteria as organized, evidence-based guidelines that protect patients' interests in the discharge process by following the principle that the needs of patients must be matched to settings with the ability to meet those needs.
2. The AMA calls on physicians, specialty societies, insurers, and other involved parties to join in developing, promoting, and using evidence-based discharge criteria that are sensitive to the physiological, psychological, social, and functional needs of patients and that are flexible to meet advances in medical and surgical therapies and adapt to local and regional variations in healthcare settings and services.
3. The AMA encourages incorporation of discharge criteria into practice parameters, clinical guidelines, and critical pathways that involve hospitalization.
4. The AMA promotes the local development, adaptation and implementation of discharge criteria.
5. The AMA promotes training in the use of discharge criteria to assist in planning for patient care at all levels of medical education. Use of discharge criteria will improve understanding of the pathophysiology of disease processes, the continuum of care and therapeutic interventions, the use of healthcare resources and alternative sites of care, the importance of patient education, safety, outcomes measurements, and collaboration with allied health professionals.
6. The AMA encourages research in the following areas: clinical outcomes after care in different healthcare settings; the utilization of resources in different care settings; the actual costs of care from onset of illness to recovery; and reliable and valid ways of assessing the discharge needs of patients.
7. The AMA endorses the following principles in the development of evidence-based discharge criteria and an organized discharge

process: (a) As tools for planning patients' transition from one care setting to another and for determining whether patients are ready for the transition, discharge criteria are intended to match patients' care needs to the setting in which their needs can best be met. (b) Discharge criteria consist of, but are not limited to: (i) Objective and subjective assessments of physiologic and symptomatic stability that are matched to the ability of the discharge setting to monitor and provide care. (ii) The patient's care needs that are matched with the patient's, family's, or caregiving staff's independent understanding, willingness, and demonstrated performance prior to discharge of processes and procedures of self care, patient care, or care of dependents. (iii) The patient's functional status and impairments that are matched with the ability of the care givers and setting to adequately supplement the patients' function. (iv) The needs for medical follow-up that are matched with the likelihood that the patient will participate in the follow-up. Follow-up is time-, setting-, and service-dependent. Special considerations must be taken to ensure follow-up in vulnerable populations whose access to healthcare is limited. (c) The discharge process includes, but is not limited to: (i) Planning: Planning for transition/discharge must be based on a comprehensive assessment of the patient's physiological, psychological, social, and functional needs. The discharge planning process should begin early in the course of treatment for illness or injury (prehospitalization for elective cases) with involvement of patient, family and physician from the beginning. (ii) Teamwork: Discharge planning can best be done with a team consisting of the patient, the family, the physician with primary responsibility for continuing care of the patient, and other appropriate healthcare professionals as needed. (iii) Contingency Plans/Access to Medical Care: Contingency plans for unexpected adverse events must be in place before transition to settings with more limited resources. Patients and caregivers must be aware of signs and symptoms to report and have a clearly defined pathway to get information directly to the physician, and to receive instructions from the physician in a timely fashion. (iv) Responsibility/Accountability: Responsibility/accountability for an appropriate transition from one setting to another rests with the attending physician. If that physician will not be following the patient in the new setting, he or she is responsible for contacting the physician who will be accepting the care of the patient before transfer and ensuring that the new physician is fully informed about the patient's illness, course, prognosis, and needs for continuing care. If there is no physician able and willing to care for the patient in the new setting, the patient should not be discharged. Notwithstanding the attending physician's responsibility for continuity of patient care, the healthcare setting in which the patient is receiving care is also responsible for evaluating the patient's needs and assuring that those needs can be met in the setting to which the patient is to be transferred. (v) Communication: Transfer of all pertinent information about the patient (such as the history and physical, record of course of treatment in hospital, laboratory tests, medication lists, advanced directives, functional, psychological, social, and other assessments), and the discharge summary should be completed before or at the time of transfer of the patient to another setting. Patients should not be accepted by the new setting without a copy of this patient information and complete instructions for continued care.

8. The AMA supports the position that the care of the patient treated and discharged from a treating facility is done through mutual consent of the patient and the physician; and

9. Policy programs by Congress regarding patient discharge timing for specific types of treatment or procedures be discouraged. (CSA Rep. 4, A-96; Reaffirmation I-96; Modified by Res. 216, A-97)

Source: Council on Scientific Affairs Report 4. Evidence-Based Principles of Discharge and Discharge Criteria. American Medical Association, Annual Meeting, Chicago, IL; June 1996. Available at http:www.ama-assn.org/ama/pub/article/2036-2459.html. Accessed: July 18, 2003.

Chapter 6

Ethical Responsibilities of the Case Management Profession

Closely connected with questions of legality are questions of ethics or morality. In any healthcare delivery system, our primary motivation should be the health, welfare, respect, and dignity of the individual. The moral principles and ethical values attached to this . . . autonomy, beneficence, fidelity, justice, nonmalfience, and veracity . . . are at the core of patients' rights and case managers' responsibilities.[1]

Autonomy is a respect for the patient's right to self-determination; that is, we ought to respect his right, as much as possible, to make his own decisions about his care. Beneficence is our charge to promote and act for the patient's good, to further a person's legitimate interests, and to actively prevent or remove him from harm. Fidelity involves faithfulness, trustworthiness, and duty; keep your promises. Justice is the maintenance of what is right and fair, nonmalfeasance means to do no harm (and as ethicist Mark Meaney points out, repair harm caused), and veracity requires that we tell the truth.

It is not illegal for a case manager to accept a finder's fee from a durable medical equipment supplier, but neither is it ethical. There is no law prohibiting a case manager from taking the season football ticket from a rehabilitation center contact, but it does cloud the objectivity of the relationship. Whether self-employed or working in a healthcare setting or insurance firm, case managers have to make clear decisions regarding their ethical standing.

Money is shifting to case management. Providers understand the purchase power case managers wield and their ability to refer to one facility over another. It has been an accepted marketing strategy in the medical industry for providers and pharmaceutical houses to wine and dine physicians and others who might recommend their institutions or products. Given the relative newness of case management and its professionals (e.g., nurses just entering the field from hospital settings), such perks are unexpected and they look very good. To avoid the criticism that case managers have become just another part of the "fat" medical bureaucracy (and, even more important, to avoid the possibility of litigation), case managers must rely on their inner conscience to remain free from associations in which objectivity could be questioned.

As a stronger incentive, association directives and legislation are putting handcuffs on any type of overemphasis on a certain drug when the pharmaceutical company making the drug is sponsoring the conference on the condition the medication is used to treat. The Pharmaceutical Research and Manufacturers of America (PhRMA) adopted a voluntary code on Interactions with Healthcare Professionals in 2002 which was subsequently revised and is effective January 2009. This code includes comprehensive guidelines limiting offers of scholarships and educational funds, practice-related items, gifts (stethoscopes versus golf balls, for example), travel, lodging, use of a corporate box at a football game, and more.

There are ethical dilemmas on the patient side of case management as well. John appears fit, is begging to return to work, and has mentioned his readiness to his employer, who is eager to have him back in the machine shop at his old station . . . the only job that is available to him at this time. However, John has not been able to control a hand tremor completely, which will jeopardize his safety at the drill. Does the case manager fudge her report on his capabilities and release him to work?

Jane, while recuperating from a skin graft, has returned to a drug habit she had kicked 3 years ago. Her employer and family are unaware of the problem. Does the case manager keep this "secret" to herself or take steps to enroll Jane in a drug rehabilitation program?

Mary has made it clear to her family and the case manager that she does not want her life prolonged by any artificial means under any circumstances. The treating physician has authorized the insertion of a feeding tube and family members are reluctant to challenge the doctor's authority. Does the case manager raise the issue or let it pass?

Three cases that involved ethical and/or moral concerns are included in Tables 6–1, 6–2, and 6–3. In each case example, we address the choices made to resolve the challenges we faced.

PATIENT RIGHTS AND CASE MANAGER RESPONSIBILITIES

Case managers have access to a great deal of information. What will the decision be regarding the disclosure of someone's substance abuse or HIV

Table 6–1 Ethics Case Study 1

The case of a 29-year-old female with an extremely communicable disease was reported to Options Unlimited by the acute care treating facility, 1 day after admission. In speaking with the patient directly, we learned that she had recently been overseas, visiting her native country. She is married and has two very young children. One week after her return to the United States and her employment (through the client group with which we are affiliated), the patient demonstrated symptoms of her illness and shortly thereafter, was admitted to the hospital.

During her course of treatment (while inpatient), questions arose at Options:

1) Was the case, with this diagnosis, reported to the Centers for Disease Control (CDC)?
2) What risk factors pertain to her immediate family and to her coworkers with whom the patient was in contact after her return to work?
3) Should measures be taken (and if so, what/how; with/to/for whom) regarding notification to the employer in order to prevent exposure to other employees, the patient's coworkers?
   a) How will this affect confidentiality issues with/for the patient?
   b) Specifically, what are Options Unlimited's responsibilities in this matter?
4) What, if any, responsibility does Options Unlimited have with regard to protection of the patient's immediate family (spouse and two very young children, ages 1 and 3)?

What we did:

1) Verified that the CDC was provided with appropriate, reported information;
2) Discussed with CDC and treating physicians and researched (from our end) the necessary precautions that must be taken by the patient, her family, her employer, and her coworkers to prevent spread of the disease;
3) Educated the patient and her family regarding the necessary precautions to take; verified understanding and willingness to comply/adhere to the necessary precautions;
4) Asked the patient whether she had discussed her illness with her employer/coworkers;
   a) We found that she had, in fact, discussed her condition with her HR Department and coworkers. (This fact opened the door for us to then intervene in that regard.)
5) Spoke with HR Department at the patient's job (with the patient's permission);
   a) Verified the necessary precautions/measures needed/taken to prevent contamination/spread of the disease.

continues

Table 6–1 continued

Thought-provoking concerns/dilemmas:

1) What was the responsibility to patient versus responsibility to employer and/or coworkers had the patient not previously discussed her condition with them?
2) What should/could have been done with that scenario?
3) Did Options perform actions appropriately in this case as noted?
4) Is there something else which should/could have been done?

Source: Courtesy of Options Unlimited, Case Management Services Division, Huntington, New York.

Table 6–2 Ethics Case Study 2

A 50-year-old female was admitted to acute care for treatment of substance abuse, opioid dependence. During the course of her treatment in acute care, Options Unlimited learned of her history of drug use/abuse, which she advised began after a motor vehicle accident many, many years ago. Her "neck problems" continue, she is "in constant pain," and needs further care and treatment of her cervical disc situation. The MD who prescribed all of her addicting drugs was (per the patient) "recently brought up on charges for issuing too many prescriptions for drugs." We also learned that she was molested as a child, and that she is currently employed as an individual who works with mentally handicapped, young adults.

Concerns/questions that arose:

1) Ability of patient to perform her job requirements
2) Concern of abuse for those committed to her care:
   a) Neglect due to her drug use
   b) Possible physical abuse to those in her care due to her own history of abuse
   c) What, if any, responsibility/obligation belongs to Options in this matter?
3) Need to determine (or rule out) actual medical/surgical concerns that need to be addressed in addition to her substance abuse and psychological issues
4) Do we have any obligation with regard to the report about the physician who ordered the numerous addictive drugs?

Dilemma:

1) What are our responsibilities to the patient versus responsibility to her employer and the young adults in her care (as far as disclosure of our information obtained and the concerns that followed)?

Table 6–2 continued

---

2) What are the legal ramifications of any actions taken on the part of Options Unlimited in all regards?

What we did:

1) Consulted with psychiatrists and medical doctors to rule out any physical conditions that would/should be monitored/addressed
2) Followed case through discharge from acute care
3) Set her up with outpatient care for follow-up treatment regarding psych/substance abuse issues, and continued treatment of same
4) Negotiated fees for care and treatment by nonparticipating providers
5) Monitored monies used due to a limited dollar benefit in order to maximize her care and treatment
6) Reported the patient's information with regard to her past history (social and medical), job function(s) and her statement regarding her physician being brought up on charges to the benefit plan to note their system of same. We also encouraged the Plan to have this physician removed from preferred provider listings.

What we wanted to do but did not (because of concerns over breach of confidentiality and legalities):

1) Report our findings about the patient's job functions and our noted concerns regarding same to the employer/HR department
   a) No evidence of abuse toward those in her care was found, therefore, tying our hands in this matter. We understand that without reported misconduct or question of abuse, there is no action possible.

Outstanding questions:

1) Should we/could we have intervened further; if so, in what regard and to what degree?

Source: Courtesy of Options Unlimited, Case Management Services Division, Huntington, New York.

Table 6–3 Ethics Case Study 3

A 33-year-old pregnant female is deemed to be high risk for preterm labor/delivery, and is placed into case management to monitor and assist in coordinating care and treatment to prevent threat of complications, early birth of infant, etc. During our initial interview with the patient, we are advised that she is unmarried, but lives with the father of the child. She is HIV+, which she contracted from her deceased husband, who acquired the disease from a blood transfusion after injuries sustained in an MVA many

continues

Table 6–3 continued

years prior. The father of the child she is currently carrying (her significant other) is aware of all facts. The rest of the patient's family are aware of the pregnancy, but none are aware of the positive HIV status; that's the way the patient wants it.

As far as the patient's job function(s), she reported that she is employed in a manufacturing plant and works on a line in which small pieces of glass and/or metal frequently "fly off" and hit her in the legs, causing bleeding and the necessity for her to "pick out the pieces with tweezers." She states that she has "never put anyone at the job in risk." She adamantly wants any/all information related to her HIV status to be kept from her employer and especially the occupational health (OH) nurse in the plant, who is described as "too nosey."

Within a very short time of obtaining the noted information, the patient (unfortunately) informed our case manager that she did not want to continue with our intervention, as she had others (social workers, physician's nurses, supportive boyfriend, etc.) following up with her frequently.

We believe (but cannot confirm) that she became "skittish" over the fact that we were affiliated with the benefit plan whose client is her employer. We asked if that concerned her, but she denied same, and simply wanted her case closed.

We did so, reluctantly.

What we did:

1) Discussed the possibility of her transitioning into another job function, which would not expose her to flying debris; advised that in following that recommendation she could state that her request was due to her pregnancy status, to make it less taxing on herself by coming off the line, thus accomplishing that issue while also preventing any coworker, the OH nurse, or employer from becoming suspicious as to her HIV+ status

2) Role-played with the patient to empower her to have the confidence needed to have such a conversation with her employer/superior

3) Offered the possibility for psychological treatment intervention (to assist the patient in dealing with her family and their lack of knowledge of her condition, also to assist in her fears of OH nurse/employer finding out about her status)

4) Notified the benefit plan of the patient's status and job function

5) Notified the benefit plan and the physician of case closure per the patient's request

Table 6–3 continued

Dilemma/frustrations/concerns:

1) We believe that our first and foremost concern/responsibility is that the patient's confidentiality issues not be breached regarding her HIV. However, we are also very concerned over the risk of exposure to her coworkers. Are we appropriately prioritizing?
2) Is there a way of decreasing the risk of exposure to the patient's coworkers without breaching the patient's confidentiality? If so, how/what could we have done?
3) Is there anything else we should have done in this case?

Source: Courtesy of Options Unlimited, Case Management Services Division, Huntington, New York.

---

status when the choice involves either compromising one's principles or losing a client? When the choice involves telling the patient's wife or not?

When I talk to case managers across the country about the push and pull of ethical issues, for instance, autonomy versus beneficence, sometimes the patient's right to autonomy is in direct conflict with some of the other principles. The individual has the right to make his own decisions about treatment, the right to refusal, the right to information, all rights we want to safeguard. Although that is true, questions arise with regard to beneficence, doing no harm, or promoting good. Does the patient have the right to select treatment even if it is going to drive up the cost? Does he have the right to continue poor health habits? In patient advocacy versus resource control, a case manager will advocate for the patient and protect his rights. How can one protect the life of a one-pound baby and still strike a balance vis-à-vis plan resource control? Questions arise regarding end-of-life issues: Does the 80-year-old person requesting an organ transplant have fewer rights than a 5-year-old child? How can one make those decisions?

It is a difficult, introspective challenge. You must know what your values are, and respect the rights and values of the individuals upon whose behalf you are working. Ethical matters do not have easy answers, and the continuing emphasis on cost containment and our improving technical abilities contributes to the rising concerns of healthcare professionals. We have not anticipated the horrible outcomes that people live with as a result of some of the wonderful advances. To save that one-pound baby who then becomes dependent on his family for every activity of daily living may be acceptable for the family during the initial stages when the family unit can care for the infant. However, when the baby becomes a young adult and then a full-grown adult, the family and society shoulder a huge burden in caring for this individual. Technology creates both wonders and nightmares.

Many hospital networks today are very competitively pursuing profit margins, perhaps by discharging patients in a timely fashion so they may capture more of the resources, especially in capitated contracts. The hospital-based case manager or social worker involved in discharge planning may not feel comfortable sending a person home, yet there is a push on the utilization review (UR) team to free the bed, or there is a productivity level to be met (a certain number of cases to be carried). When does our professional concern for that patient outweigh the financial motivations and concerns of the institute that employs us? On one hand, the case manager's role and responsibilities have been defined by her employer; on the other hand, she knows how complex some of these issues are. When does she say, enough is enough? Not only is this not fair, it puts the patient, the hospital, and me at risk.

With home care contracts designed for the patient and family to become their own care providers, some case managers in home care agencies are being pushed to transfer patients to less supervised home care far earlier than we would normally deem wise. I think there are many home care case managers with very mixed feelings about the capabilities of patients and families to take on the care programs.

A case manager in a rehabilitation facility may find herself in a different situation. She may know that a person might well go home, deriving more use of the benefit dollars if discharged. Perhaps there are only $50,000 lifetime benefits in terms of rehabilitation needs. Yet the rehabilitation facility that employs her has a need to keep the beds filled as long as possible. Job viability and security might depend on it.

In fact to illustrate just how realistic this "push-pull" dynamic is in place, allow me to share something that occurred during our "Best in Class Case Management" seminar in the summer of 2008 in New York City. There were several hospital case managers in the audience and I was attempting to have them consider that providing case management/discharge planning only up through the day of discharge was inadvisable and quite possibly resulting in many needless readmissions. I suggested that in order to more clearly demonstrate that case management could be effective and realize savings to the bottom line, I proposed that they take a look at the kinds of patients that were most frequently readmitted shortly after discharge, e.g., patients with congestive heart failure. I proposed that they develop a pilot program that would identify these patients and then proactively follow them for those critical days, possibly weeks post discharge. Encouraging them further, I recommended that they specifically look at patients that had this same diagnosis for the previous six months, look at the rate of readmissions, the length of stay etc. . . . and then *compare* those in the pilot case management program. I assured them that they would absolutely see a marked decrease in readmissions. Feeling quite confident with this suggestion, especially when seeing some in the audience nodding in enthusiastic agreement, I then saw a few with raised hands. Indicating that I welcomed the questions, one of the attendees said: ". . . Well, that *sounds* good, but that's not going to help my facility . . . we'll be losing revenue if we don't have those readmissions! . . ." Regrettably, there were several others who nodded in agreement. Concerned, I challenged them: . . . but is this the *right* thing for the patient? Is it right to have him readmitted so your facility can increase its revenue? Is it *right* to subject the patient to the risks and discomfort of another hospital admission, when we *could* have and possibly *should* have done something to keep him safely in his home? This situation, and there are so many others, have no easy answer for case managers . . . but these questions and issues need to be raised.

In a managed care organization, a case manager might find herself participating in a bonus arrangement for most number of days saved or highest dollar amount saved. With this incentive to cut days for a personal or team award, she might do something that is, if not illegal, certainly ethically questionable. At the very least, the bonus system creates competition rather than coordination among departments.

We were never divided in quite this way. Under the traditional healthcare system, there was no question that our role was as an advocate for the patient. I am not sure that nurses or employers (or patients) still wholeheartedly believe that we serve solely in the patient's best interests, especially for those employed by managed care organizations.

Many of these issues are money-driven. I believe most case managers feel the ethical pull now because of finances. As nurses and social workers, we never really had to be involved with money matters, never had to make those kinds of decisions, and were not directed to push patients out of hospitals. There was no reason for it. They remained in hospital care until they were well enough to go home. We did not have the technology to enable them to survive, so it was not an issue, and no one lived long enough to use a million dollars worth of benefits. Money is certainly driving many of the healthcare decisions being made, who gets it, for how much, and for how long. Healthcare professionals, physicians, social workers, nurses, and therapists now are all involved in these financial issues and are no longer so well-guided by the standards of practice and codes of conduct that gave us answers earlier in our more traditional settings.

Case management was a direct response to both technological advances and the monetary constraints and issues, but because we sit squarely in the middle of the healthcare process, we must deal with these ethical problems. Because health care is now managed like a business, healthcare professionals often find themselves reporting to business managers who might not understand or be sympathetic to the ethical dilemmas. We are working in buildings that look the same but are run quite differently. To survive, we must respond in kind. We need to know more about the financial issues of health care. Just as we want the CEO, hospital director, or medical director to understand our role, we have to comprehend their need to balance the budget. They face the same ethical dilemmas and are as unequipped as we are to address them. Whereas earlier we experienced overutilization of services, possibly driving costs up, now we have underutilization as an area for fraud and abuse because patients are not being given access to services. Futility of treatment is another issue. Are we being empathetic professionals? Is this patient really suffering, or are our actions really driven by another motive . . . profit?

More dialogue needs to take place between healthcare managers, financial managers, and case managers. Certainly, when dialogue happens, some of the issues are so confrontational and confusing that we need ethicists and legal professionals to assist us in the decision-making process. Are the treatment paths we are considering legal? What is the appropriate ethical choice? I believe our healthcare colleagues feel they are swimming in the same deep waters we are trying to navigate. On Long Island, New York, the Stony Brook University Hospital formed the nonprofit Long Island Center for Ethics, designed to increase the practical application of ethics in the academic, medical, and business worlds.

Groundwork is being laid to bring outdated codes of conduct into line with the realities of the healthcare industry's day-to-day practices. The American Academy of Physical Medicine and Rehabilitation Code of Conduct includes sections on ethics relating to the patient and patient's family, the practitioner's relationship with members of the rehabilitation team, physician-to-physician relationships, relationships with the community and government, and research and scholarly activity (www.aapmr.org).

The ethical challenges and responsibilities we face heighten in direct proportion to a patient's degree of impairment; when a patient cannot be a partner in care due to cognitive or speech difficulties, acting out, or inappropriate or impulsive behaviors, a case manager's ethical responsibilities increase. When cost-control issues are involved, ethical dilemmas multiply as well. If an insurance company initially refuses to pay for medically indicated treatment, is it ethical for a primary care doctor to lie to get the coverage for a patient? Should a doctor deceive an insurance company to gain coverage for bypass surgery for a patient with severe angina or chronic atherosclerosis? How many case managers might misrepresent a condition to get the coverage a patient desperately needs?

Our industry is focusing on these ethical dilemmas. John Banja, PhD, Assistant Director for Health Sciences and Clinical Ethics, Center for Ethics, and Associate Professor of Clinical Ethics at Emory University, speaks and writes on the ethical accountabilities of case management and the medical industry in general. During one intense session, topics under discussion included futility of treatment, continuation versus withholding of treatment, the "injury of continued existence," and "distributed justice." The concept . . . that we, as case managers, take or do not take action based on our professional interpretation of ethical conduct . . . led to some passionate exchanges.

At issue was the case of a 4-year-old, unconscious and in a persistent vegetative state since age 2, loved by his family and fully treated as a family member, who develops frequent respiratory infections that require ventilatory support and occasional pediatric intensive care support. Further, the child is developing contractures that interfere with his home care and that physicians believe will require surgical intervention.

The child's physician is under pressure to de-escalate the child's treatment. Given the prognosis, the hospital staff questions the clinical appropriateness of continued ventilatory support and future surgery. Other physicians in the pediatrics group wonder about spending significant resources on a child who will not improve and whose care might have adverse repercussions on accessing care for other children in the plan. The HMO considers the proposed surgery to be heroic, whereas the family insists that everything possible be done.[2]

Selected responses from panel and audience members portray the multiple considerations that constitute an ethical dilemma and decision:

> It is true that case managers are often caught in the middle, and I guess that's where I think they ought to be. What I would like to suggest is that the case manager is going to have an increasingly important role as a mediator. You advocate for the patient, yet you also balance cost and quality. In the process of mediation, there is a lot of emotion. It is very important to provide a forum where we can vent these emotions and patients can voice their concerns.
>
> ~Mark Meaney, Executive Director, Institute for Clinical and Corporate Ethics[3]

This case is fairly typical of cases that we as case managers find ourselves in. In the previous fee-for-service system with unlimited funding available for care, anything that was clinically possible was considered clinically appropriate and necessary treatment. Now, we are hearing more discussion about whether or not care is futile, or inappropriate.
~Author as a panel member[3]

The whole idea of futility is important to look at, but I'd like to address two issues that relate to the family and the child. Is this child any longer a person? I would like to suggest that there is a philosophical difference between having a life and being biologically alive. Also, it is not necessarily the responsibility of society to give that family everything it wants for this child. The family can elect to act with their own discretionary resources. It is a harsh view, but we must also consider the obligations to the other siblings in the family. And, what happens to other members of the health plan if the resources are spent on this child? It is possible for people, such as these parents, to make themselves moral heroes at the expense of others.
~M. Jan Keffer, assistant professor of family health nursing, Indiana University School of Nursing in Indianapolis[3]

When case management is done well, it is pursuing at least two moral goods. One moral good is patient advocacy and the other is proper use of resources. The key issue is distributive justice. Whenever case managers are faced with a managed care case where the health plan is pushing for conservative care, they should ask the following questions before jumping to any conclusions: What is going to happen to the money and resources saved by our not doing this? Who said that doing everything possible for the patient is in the patient's best interests? Until we start making decisions about what constitutes good managed care and unethical managed care, and what constitutes good case management and unethical case management, any situation involving a health plan denying payment will be greeted by cries of "rationing" and I think that's bunk.
~Emily Friedman, adjunct assistant professor, Boston University School of Public Health[3]

There is suffering on the part of the family caregivers; there is suffering on the part of the professional caregivers, and there

certainly seems to be suffering on the part of the child. There is a concept called "the injury of continued existence." Is there a point at which being dead is better than being alive?
~Keffer[3]

A couple of years ago I went back and looked at what my nursing license says I can do. All it says I can do is teach and advocate. That's all; teach and advocate.
~audience member[4]

How do we measure the worth of this little child against someone who may grow up to be 16, 17, 18, and who becomes sexually promiscuous, on drugs, and we're spending a lot for that as opposed to this?
~audience member[5]

There isn't one option; there are many options. Parents may opt for everything, but they need to know the consequences of what that everything may be. Frequently they do not because no one has taken the time to explain it to them. Ethics panels help bring to the forefront all of those issues in making sure that everyone understands fully not only the rights and responsibilities, but the possible consequences as well.
~Author, during the keynote[6]

I also voiced my concern that many case managers seem reluctant to enter the ethical arena, to speak up, take a stand as the patient advocate, or blow the whistle on unbundled billing practices, upcoding, or Medicare fraud. We are waiting for a committee to be formed. We are waiting for someone else to take the first step. I would like to see a heightened empowerment of case managers, with an understanding that being a patient advocate is not something we do in name only. We must be willing to confront employers, confront physician groups, and confront plan administrators.

Ethics and Medical Errors

There is another issue often left unsaid but gaining importance. We live in the days of swift technological advances that can sustain life longer than was ever possible. We also live in the age of increasing medical errors. Who pays for the surgery that included a gross medical error—the insurance company, or is a bill ever sent back to the provider? In a pilot program, does a full-disclosure report go back to the insurer?

Case managers sometimes stumble across legal or ethical problems. Among those issues a case manager has an ethical responsibility to report are patients who are potentially or habitually dependent on their medication, who are overmedicated or overtreated by multiple physicians, or who are lying to their physicians regarding compliance. If a patient has not been receiving the treatment that claims are filed for, if an occupational therapist is treating a patient outside practice guidelines, or if a physician inappropriately refers a patient to a center he or she has a financial interest in, the circumstances should be reported to the plan administrator, the treating physician, or a peer review organization. A case manager must develop knowledge of professional ethics, standards of practice, and the appropriate code of behavior, and must report through proper channels whatever is intolerable, fraudulent, or abusive in hospital or private practice.

In another CMSA conference in 2004, there was a session moderated once again by John Banja, PhD that addressed medical errors. (Banja had been working on his book dealing with medical errors, mentioned in the "Resource" section at the end of this chapter.) His presentation focused on the moral, ethical and legal issues surrounding the increasing numbers of medical errors occurring in health care, but with increasing frequency in our hospitals, and the possible role that case managers and other healthcare professionals could have. At the end of his formal presentation, he introduced members of a panel which represented a Medical Error Response team in a large hospital. Panel members described in good detail how they had developed a strategy that would proactively respond when errors were discovered. They developed a team who would promptly review the particulars of the error, and then go directly to the patient and advise him what had occurred. They would then offer the sincere apology, and provide additional information as to what steps would be taken to insure that this wouldn't happen again to other patients. While it has long been a practice in healthcare settings for an incident report to be completed by the employee who committed the error, and an internal process to review the matter and determine what education and/or disciplinary action would be needed, in the majority of cases, the error was rarely, if ever, disclosed to the patient. In its white paper in 1999, the Institutes of Medicine acknowledged that health care in the US was not as safe as it should be and defined medical error as: ". . . the failure of a planned action to be completed as intended . . ."[7] In 2001 the Joint Commission on Accreditation of Health Care Organizations issued the first nationwide disclosure standard that required that patients be informed about medical errors. In 2005, 69 percent of healthcare organizations had established disclosure policies, which ranged from simple statements to detailed disclosure statements.[8] While, once again, this matter of disclosure is not necessarily a legal matter, it most certainly is an ethical one.

Banja in a series of articles he contributed to *The Case Manager* acknowledged that the disclosure of an error is easier said than done. He believes: ". . . that many remain undisclosed for two primary reasons. One is the fear of inviting a lawsuit from disclosure; the other is the embarrassment and assault on the professional's ego that such a conversation poses . . ."[9] Banja acknowledges that when the case manager is employed by the organization, the inclination to protect the organization which is the same one that provides one's salary, benefits etc., may challenge the case manager's ethical obligations. He cautions that regardless of whether they are internal or external case managers, one must not allow the advocacy for the patient to diminish and notes: ". . . as painful as they are to confront, harm-causing errors demand deep ethical commitment and moral courage from everyone in the healthcare industry."[10]

In another article in the same edition of *The Case Manager*, Banja proposed some specific recommendations regarding the disclosure of harm-causing medical errors and suggested:

- the causal connection between the error and the harm that the patient experienced should be reasonably established.
- there should be a conversation with the patient (and as appropriate, the family as well) that specifically addresses the nature of the error, that problems from that have already occurred or are likely to occur (and explanation of these should also be given), and that these may require additional treatment (and again, explanation of what this treatment may include should be provided).
- that there should be the development of an organizational policy to clearly delineate the disclosure process. (Banja advised that this responsibility should not be defaulted to the case manager.)[11]

CODES OF ETHICAL CONDUCT

To assist case managers in their day-to-day practice, our industry (as well as others) has responded with standards of practice and codes of conduct. The CMSA issued the CMSA Statement Regarding Ethical Case Management Practice (Appendix 6–A) to "provide guidance to the individual case manager in the development and maintenance of an environment in which case management practice is conducted ethically." The CCMC adopted its Code of Professional Conduct for Case Managers with Disciplinary Rules, Procedures, and Penalties, initially in 1996 incorporating three kinds of standards (Principles, Rules of Conduct, and Guidelines for Professional Conduct), along with guidelines and procedures for processing complaints and possible sanctions. It was completely revised for a third time in 2004. The complete and current version of the Code is available on the CCMC website (www.ccmcertification.org). In its preamble, it is stated that the Code was designed to achieve goals that include the following: CCM certificants accept the responsibility that their actions or inactions can aid or hinder clients in achieving their objectives; that they provide services in a manner consistent with their education, formal training, and work experience; and that they demonstrate their adherence to certain standards. CCMC in its Code, provides the definitions of case management as developed by CMSA and CCMC (Figure 6–1), the Principles of the Code of Professional Conduct for Case Managers (Figure 6–2), the Rules of Conduct

Figure 6–1 Example Definitions of Case Management.

CMSA:	A collaborative process of assessment, planning, facilitation and advocacy for options and services to meet an individual's health needs through communication and available resources to promote quality cost effective outcomes (CMSA, 2002).
CCMC:	A collaborative process that assesses, plans, implements, coordinates, monitors, and evaluates the options and services required to meet the client's health and human services needs. It is characterized by advocacy, communication, and resource management and promoted quality and cost-effective interventions and outcomes (CCMC, 2005).

Source: Reprinted with permission from the Commission for Case Manager Certification.

Figure 6–2 Principles of the Code of Professional Conduct for Case Managers.

Principle 1:	Certificants will place the public interest above their own at all times.
Principle 2:	Certificants will respect the rights and inherent dignity of all of their clients.
Principle 3:	Certificants will always maintain objectivity in their relationships with clients.
Principle 4:	Certificants will act with integrity in dealing with other professionals to facilitate their clients' achieving maximum benefits.
Principle 5:	Certificants will keep their competency at a level that ensures each of their clients will receive the benefit of services that are appropriate and consistent for the clients' conditions and circumstances.
Principle 6:	Certificants will honor the integrity and respect the limitations placed on the use of the CCM designation.
Principle 7:	Certificants will obey all laws and regulations [relevant to case management practice].
Principle 8:	Certificants will help maintain the integrity of the Code.

Source: Reprinted with permission from the Commission for Case Manager Certification.

Figure 6–3 Rules of Conduct.

Rule 1:	A certificant will not intentionally falsify an application or other documents.
Rule 2:	A certificant will not be convicted of a felony.
Rule 3:	A certificant will not violate the code of ethics governing the profession upon which the individual's eligibility for the CCM designation is based.
Rule 4:	A certificant will not lose the primary professional credential (or licensure) upon which the eligibility of CCM designation is based.
Rule 5:	A certificant will not violate or breach the Standards for Professional Conduct (i.e., professional misconduct).
Rule 6:	A certificant will not fail to pay required fees to CCMC.
Rule 7:	A certificant will not violate the rules and regulations governing the taking of the certification examination.

Source: Reprinted with permission from the Commission for Case Manager Certification.

Figure 6–4 Standards for Professional Conduct—Six Areas of Practice.

Standards	Areas of Practice
Advocacy	Acting on behalf of clients and ensuring that a comprehensive assessment identifies the client's needs. Options for necessary services are provided to clients. Clients are provided with access to resources to meet individual needs.
Professional Responsibility	Representation of practice, competence, representation of qualifications, legal and benefit system requirements, use of CCM designation, conflict of interest, reporting misconduct, and compliance with proceedings.
Case Manager/Client Relationships	Description of services, relationships with clients, termination of services, and objectivity.
Confidentiality, Privacy and Recordkeeping	Legal compliance, disclosure, client identity, medical records, electronic recording, reports, and records maintenance/storage and disposal.
Professional Relationships	Testimony (judicial or non-judicial forum), dual relationships, unprofessional behaviors, fees, and advertising and solicitation.
Research	Legal compliance and client privacy.

Source: Reprinted with permission from the Commission for Case Manager Certification.

(Figure 6–3) and the Standards for Professional Conduct—Six Areas of Practice (Figure 6–4).

In addition, CMSA's Standards of Practice for Case Management, revised in 2002, and *Case Management Practice Guidelines*, discussed further in Chapter 9, offer guidance to direct case management practice.

What I have yet to see is the real use of these documents to empower the case management community. I think if more case managers were to use these documents as they define roles and responsibilities within their departments and make them active, working documents, it would help eliminate some of the problems they are having. It would give them recourse when faced with a choice, presented by an employer, that they feel is unethical.

In early 1997, I developed, along with Mark Meaney, a survey instrument to solicit from case managers in a range of practice settings the scope and type of ethical issues by which they feel challenged on a daily basis. The purpose of the survey (Appendix 6–B), which was subsequently followed up by intensive one-on-one interviews with case managers of various expertise levels, was to establish a field-tested consensus on ethical dilemmas, enabling the CMSA to prepare training tools (a manual, video tapes, training guides) to address those most pressing issues and assist in the education of case managers toward more ethical practice. It might be useful in your own practice setting to utilize this instrument or a modified version of it to conduct a bit of introspective analysis of you and your colleagues . . . to explore your feelings; examine your actions; consider the potential for conflicts and develop a strategic plan to address them.

Objectivity and Common Sense

As a commissioner for six years on the Commission for Case Manager Certification (CCMC), and member of its Ethics Committee, John Banja, PhD gained additional perspective on the ethical challenges that case managers face. Case managers who are charged with ethics violations can face a reprimand, suspension from CCM certification or revocation of the CCM credential and he and members of the committee review each of the cases. In an interview with the *Case Management Advisor*, Banja shared that the vast majority of case managers do not commit ethics violations but added: ". . . Overwhelmingly, case managers are good-hearted, well-educated professionals who advocate intensively for their patients, but there are about 100,000 people out there who call themselves case managers and not all of them are that careful, professional and discreet . . ."[12]

In some instances, we may allow our personal feelings to dictate the way we manage a case; other times we become frustrated and discouraged and this may be apparent in the wording of our reports or documentation in our records. Banja cited a few examples: " the injured worker was clearly exaggerating his pain . . ."; ". . . the client's wife is argumentative and obnoxious . . ."[13] He advises case managers that ethics violations occur when we overstep our limits or make determinations outside our scope of practice and provided examples of this as well: ". . . I will not authorize this MRI; the client doesn't need one . . ." or ". . . physical therapy is not indicated after this procedure . . ." While, based upon our many years of experience these assumptions or judgments may indeed be accurate, however, determining the medical need for something is clearly within the scope of practice of a physician, and not a case manager's. Banja offers this "No-Brainer Test of Ethical Behavior" and recommends:

Ask yourself three questions:

1. Is it legal?
2. Would my mother approve?
3. What if my behavior was described on the front page of tomorrow's New York Times?[14]

LOOK TO YOUR RESOURCES

I have encouraged every managed care organization and every case management department to create an ethics panel or review board to help mediate some of these problematic cases. I do not think any single case manager should have to face alone the kinds of issues touched upon in this chapter. Mediation, collaboration, and input from other professional disciplines will assist in some of these tough calls. A case manager needs a network of people to bounce around ideas about ethical challenges. Perhaps there is an ethicist at a local college or other case managers not in direct competition who can act as sounding boards. The unexpected case will arrive, and case managers need resources for ethical counseling.

Additionally, case managers have an obligation to be as knowledgeable as possible in order to promote the best outcomes for our patients and have a professional as well as an ethical obligation to pursue continuing education. Thankfully, our professional associations include sessions that address not only the most current treatment guidelines for the conditions we help to manage but those that help to provide us with guidelines for "best practices," which of course would include and encompass our standards of practice and codes of professional conduct. CCMC also has on its website (www.ccmcertification.org) an ethics educational module which will be revised as appropriate to remain current with the Code.

Because not every case manager would be able to attend conferences, books such as Kenneth Blanchard and Norman Vincent Peale's *The Power of Ethical Management*, and magazine and newspaper columns that address the issues of professional ethics are valuable resources. Look for a 2004 book titled *Medical Error and Medical Narcissism: Bioethical Explorations* (working title) by medical ethicist John D. Banja, PhD, an associate professor of clinical ethics education at Emory University Hospital, on the ethical issues that arise from medical errors. Ethics issues are also addressed consistently in *Case in Point* (Contexo Media), *Professional Case Management* (Lippincott) and *Case Management Advisor* (AHC Media).

Books that are helpful in exploring ethical issues include *The Elderly: Legal and Ethical Issues in Health Care Policy* (M. L. Levine, ed., Ashgate Publishing Company, 2004); *Clinical Ethics: A Practical Approach to Decisions in Clinical Medicine*, 5th edition (A. R. Jonsen, M. Siegler, and W. J. Winslade, McGraw-Hill/Appleton & Lange, 2002); *Managed Care: Financial, Legal, and Ethical Issues* (D. A. Bennahum, Pilgrim Press, 2000); *Ethical and Legal Issues in Home Health and Long-Term Care: Challenges and Solutions* (D. A. Robbins, Aspen Publishers, 1996); *Ethical Decision Making in Nursing* (G. L. Husted and J. L. Husted, Mosby, 1995); *The Ethics of Health Care: A Guide for Clinical Practice* (R. Edge and J. R. Groves, Delmar Publishers, 1994); *Ethics on Call* (N. Dubler and D. Nimmons, Vintage, 1992); *Principles of Biomedical Ethics*, 5th edition (T. Beauchamp and J. Childress, Oxford University Press, 2001); *Clinical Ethics*, 3rd edition (Jonsen, Siegler, and Winslade, McGraw Hill, 1992); and *The Crisis in Health Care: Ethical Issues* (edited by N. F. McKenzie, Meridian, 1990).

NOTES

1. Mullahy CM, "Satisfaction of Persons Served," in *Ethical Dimensions of the CARF Standards,* ed. J. D. Banja (Tucson, AZ: Commission on Accreditation of Rehabilitation Facilities, 1997).
2. Hoffman LF, "Ethics Helps CMs Handle Difficult Cases," *Case Management Advisor* (8, no. 8, 1997): 138 (for more information, please call 800-688-2421), and J. Banja, E. Friedman, J. Keffer, M. Meaney, C. M. Mullahy, "Ethical Accountabilities of Case Management," *Journal of Care Management* 3, no. 4 (1997): 4, 12.
3. Hoffman LF, "Ethics Helps CMs Handle Difficult Cases," 138.
4. Banja J, Friedman E, Keffer J, Meaney M, Mullahy CM, "Ethical Accountabilities," 24.
5. Banja J, Friedman E, Keffer J, Meaney M, Mullahy CM, "Ethical Accountabilities," 16.

6. Banja J, Friedman E, Keffer J, Meaney M, Mullahy CM, "Ethical Accountabilities," 17.

7. Wilson J, McCaffrey R, "Disclosure of Medical Errors to Patients" *MedSurg Nursing* October 2005.

8. http://AHRO.org.

9. Banja J, "Medical Errors 101: A Primer," *The Case Manager,* Volume 16, May/June 2005 pp. 57–59.

10. Ibid.

11. Banja J, "Ethically Speaking: The Case Manager's Response to Harm-Causing Error," *The Case Manager,* Vol. 16, May/June 2005, pp. 60–64.

12. Banja J, "Avoid Common Ethics Violations While Keeping Patients," "Best Interests In Mind," *The Case Management Advisor,* Vol. 19, No. 1.

13. Ibid.

14. Ibid.

APPENDIX 6–A

CCMC RULES OF CONDUCT

Violation of any of these rules may result in disciplinary action by the Commission up to and including revocation of the individual's certification.

Rule 1: A Certificant will not intentionally falsify an application or other documents.

Rule 2: A Certificant will not be convicted of a felony.

Rule 3: A Certificant will not violate the code of ethics governing the profession upon which the individual's eligibility for the CCM designation is based.

Rule 4: A Certificant will not lose the primary professional credential (or licensure) upon which eligibility for the CCM designation is based.

Rule 5: A Certificant will not violate or breach the Standards for Professional Conduct (i.e. professional misconduct).

Rule 6: A Certificant will not fail to pay required fees to CCMC.

Rule 7: A Certificant will not violate the rules and regulations governing the taking of the certification examination.

SCOPE OF PRACTICE FORF CASE MANAGERS

I. Assumptions

- Case management is not a profession but rather a collaborative and trans-disciplinary practice.
- Certification indicates that the case manager possesses the education, skills, moral character, licensing and experience required to render appropriate services based on sound principles of practice.
- Certificants will practice only within the boundaries of their competence, based on their education, training, appropriate professional experience, and other professional credentials. They will not misrepresent their role or competence to clients. They will not represent the possession of the CCM credential to imply a depth of knowledge, skills, and professional capabilities greater than those demonstrated by achievement of certification.

II. Underlying Values

- Belief that case management is a means for improving client health, wellness and autonomy through advocacy, communication, education, identification of service resources, and service facilitation.
- Recognition of the dignity, worth and rights of all people.
- Understanding and commitment to quality outcomes for clients, appropriate use of resources, and the empowerment of clients in a manner that is supportive and objective.
- Belief in the underlying premise that when the individual(s) reaches the optimum level of wellness and functional capability, everyone benefits: the individual(s) served, their support systems, the health care delivery systems and the various reimbursement systems.
- Recognition that case management is guided by the principles of autonomy, beneficence, nonmaleficence, and justice.

III. Definition of Case Management

Case management is a collaborative process that assesses, plans, implements, coordinates, monitors, and evaluates the options and services required to meet an individual's health needs. It uses communication and available resources to promote quality, cost-effective outcomes.

IV. Ethical Issues

Because case management exists in an environment that may look to it to solve or resolve various problems in the health care delivery and payor systems, case managers may often confront ethical dilemmas.

Case managers must abide by the Code as well as by the professional code of ethics for their specific profession for guidance and support in the resolution of these conflicts.

SELECTED DEFINITIONS

Advocacy – a process that promotes beneficence, justice and autonomy for clients. Advocacy especially aims to foster the client's independence. It also involves educating clients about their rights, healthcare and human services, resources, and benefits, and facilitating appropriate and informed decision making, and includes considerations for the client's values, beliefs and interests.

Assessment – The process of collecting in-depth information about a person's situation and functioning to identify individual needs in order to develop a comprehensive case management plan that will address those needs. In addition to direct client contact, information should be gathered from other relevant sources (patient/client, professional caregivers, nonprofessional caregivers, employers, health records, educational/military records, etc.).

Autonomy – A form of personal liberty whereby the individual possesses sufficient mental capacity to determine his or her course of action in accordance with a plan chosen and developed by himself or herself.

Beneficence – The obligation or duty to promote good, to further another's legitimate interests, and to actively prevent harm or diminish its impact as much as possible.

Client – the individual to whom a Certified Case Manager provides services for or on behalf of.

Code – The CCMC Code of Professional Conduct for Case Managers.

Commission or CCMC – The Commission for Case Manager Certification.

Coordination – The process of organizing, securing, integrating, and modifying the resources necessary to accomplish the goals set forth in the case management plan.

Evaluation – The process, repeated at appropriate intervals, of determining the case management plan's effectiveness in reaching desired outcomes and goals. This might lead to a modification or change in the case management plan in its entirety or in any of its component parts.

Implementation – The process of executing specific case management activities and/or interventions that will lead to accomplishing the goals set forth in the case management plan.

Justice – Achieving a fair distribution of benefits and burdens.

Monitoring – The ongoing process of gathering sufficient information from all relevant sources about the case management plan and its activities and/or services to enable the case manager to determine the plan's effectiveness.

Nonmaleficence – Refraining from harming others or, if harm is inevitable, insuring that as little harm occurs as possible.

Planning – The process of determining specific objectives, goals, and actions designed to meet the client's needs as identified through the assessment process. The plan should be action-oriented and time-specific.

Veracity – Truth telling.

STANDARDS FOR PROFESSIONAL CONDUCT

Section 1—Advocacy

S 1—The Advocate

Certified case managers will serve as advocates for their clients and ensure that:

a) a comprehensive assessment will identify the client's needs.
b) options for necessary services will be provided to the client.
c) clients are provided with access to resources to meet individual needs.

Section 2 – Professional Responsibility

S 2—Representation of Practice

Certificants will practice only within the boundaries of their competence, based on their education, training, professional experience, and other professional credentials. They will not misrepresent their role or competence to clients.

S 3—Competence

Certificants will not:

a) handle or neglect a case in such a manner that falls below the Certificant's reasonable obligations and responsibilities.
b) exert undue influence that adversely affects the outcome of case management services to the client.
c) exhibit a pattern of negligence or neglect in the handling of the Certificant's obligations or responsibilities.

S 4—Representation of Qualifications

Certificants will not represent the certification designation to imply a depth of knowledge, skills, and professional capabilities greater than those reasonably demonstrated by achievement of certification. Certificants will take the necessary steps to correct a misstatement made by a third party with respect to the Certificant's qualifications.

S 5—Legal and Benefit System Requirements

Certificants will obey state and federal laws and the unique requirements of the various reimbursement systems by which clients are covered.

S 6—Use of CCM Designation

The designation of Certified Case Manager and the initials "CCM" may only be used by individuals currently certified by the Commission for Case Manager Certification. The Certificant will not utilize the designation or initials as part of a company, partnership, or corporate name, trademark, or logo.

S 7—Conflict of Interest

Certificants will fully disclose any conflict of interest to all affected parties. If, after full disclosure, an objection is made by any affected party, the Certificant will withdraw from further participation in the case.

S 8—Reporting Misconduct

Certificants possessing knowledge, not otherwise protected as a confidence by this Code, that another Certificant has committed a violation of any provision of this Code will promptly report such knowledge to CCMC and to such other authority as may be empowered to investigate or to act upon such actions or violations. Certificants will not initiate, participate in, or encourage the filing of complaints that are malicious, unwarranted, or without a basis in fact.

S 9—Compliance with Proceedings

Certificants will assist in the process of enforcing the Code by cooperating with investigations, participating in proceedings, and complying with the directives of the Committee on Ethics and Professional Conduct.

Section 3—Case Manager/Client Relationships

S 10—Description of Services

Certificants will provide information to the extent reasonably necessary to permit clients to make informed decisions. At a minimum, information provided by Certificants to clients about case management services will include a description of the services, possible benefits, significant risks, alternatives and the right to refuse services. Where applicable, Certificants will also provide the client with information about the cost of case management services prior to initiation of services.

S 11—Relationships with Clients

Certificants will not enter into any relationship with any client (business, personal or otherwise) that will interfere with the Certificant's professional objectivity.

S 12—Termination of Services

Prior to the discontinuation of case management services, Certificants will provide written notification of that discontinuation to all relevant parties consistent with applicable statutes and regulations.

S 13—Objectivity

Certificants will maintain objectivity in their professional relationships and will not impose their values on their clients.

Section 4—Confidentiality, Privacy and Recordkeeping

S 14—Legal Compliance

Certificants will be knowledgeable about and act in accordance with federal, state, and local laws and procedures related to the scope of their practices regarding client consent, confidentiality, and the release of information.

S 15—Disclosure

At the outset of the Certificant-client relationship, Certificants will inform the client that any information obtained through the relationship may be disclosed to third parties. Disclosure of information will be made only to clients, payors, service providers, and governmental authorities and limited to what is necessary and relevant, except that the Certificant must reveal information to appropriate authorities, as soon as and to the extent that the Certificant reasonably believes necessary, to prevent the client from: a) committing acts likely to result in bodily harm or imminent danger to the client or others; and b) committing criminal, illegal, or fraudulent acts.

S 16—Client Identity

As required by law, Certificants will hold as confidential and private the client's identity, especially when using data for training, research, publication, and/or marketing unless a lawful, written release regarding this use is obtained from the client.

S 17—Records

Certificants will maintain client records, whether written, taped, computerized, or stored in any other medium, in a manner designed to ensure confidentiality.

S 18—Electronic Recording

Certificants will not electronically record communications with clients without first obtaining the client's written permission.

S 19—REPORTS

Certificants will be accurate, honest, and unbiased in reporting the results of their professional activities to appropriate third parties, to avoid exerting undue influence upon the decision making process.

S 20—Records: Maintenance/Storage and Disposal

Certificants will maintain records necessary for rendering professional services to their clients and as required by applicable laws, regulations, or agency/institution procedures. Subsequent to file closure, records will be maintained for the number of years consistent with jurisdictional requirements or for a longer period during which maintenance of such records is necessary or helpful to provide reasonably anticipated future services to the client. After that time, records will be destroyed in a manner assuring preservation of confidentiality.

Section 5—Professional Relationships

S 21—Testimony

Certificants, when providing testimony in a judicial or non-judicial forum, will be impartial and limit testimony to their specific fields of expertise.

S 22—Dual Relationships

Certificants who provide services at the request of a third-party payor will disclose the nature of their dual relationship at the outset of the Certificant/client relationship by describing their role and responsibilities to parties who have the right to know. Dual relationships, other than payor/client, include, but are not limited to, Certificants working with clients who are the Certificants' employer, employee, friend, relative, and/or research subject, and must also be disclosed.

S 23—Unprofessional Behavior

It is unprofessional behavior if the Certificant:

a) commits a criminal act;
b) engages in conduct involving dishonesty, fraud, deceit, or misrepresentation;
c) engages in conduct involving discrimination against a client because of race, color, religion, age, gender, sexual orientation, national origin, marital status, or disability/handicap;
d) engages in sexually intimate behavior with a client; or accepts as a client an individual with whom the Certificant has been sexually intimate.

S 24—Fees

Certificants will advise the referral source/payor of their fee structure in advance of the rendering of any services and will also furnish, upon request, detailed, accurate time and expense records. No fee arrangements will be made that could compromise health care for the client.

S 25—Advertising

Certificants who describe/advertise services will do so in a manner that accurately informs the public of the services, expertise, and techniques being offered. Descriptions/advertisements by a Certificant will not contain false, inaccurate, misleading, out-of-context, or otherwise deceptive material or statements. If statements from former clients are to be used, the Certificant will have a written, signed, and dated release from the former clients. All advertising will be factually accurate and will not contain exaggerated claims as to costs and/or results.

S 26—Solicitation

Certificants will not reward, pay, or compensate any individual, company, or entity for directing or referring clients to the Certificant. Nothing contained herein will preclude Certificants from making reasonable expenditures in entertaining individuals who have referred or may in the future refer clients to the Certificant or from giving gifts of minimal value to such individuals.

Section 6—Research

S 27—Research: Legal Compliance

Certificants will plan, design, conduct, and report research in a manner consistent with ethical principles and federal and state laws and regulations, including those governing research with human subjects.

S 28—Research: Subject Privacy

Certificants who supply data, aid in the research of another person, report research results, or make original data available will protect the identity of the respective subjects unless an appropriate authorization from the subjects has been obtained or as required by law.

Source: Reprinted with permission from Case Management Society of America, © 1996.

APPENDIX 6–B

Excerpts from the CCMC Code of Professional Conduct for Case Managers

PREAMBLE

Throughout this document and for the purposes of this document, "client" is used to refer to the individual for whom a CCM certificant provides services; likewise, "payer" is used to refer to the CCM certificant's customer.

CCM certificants recognize that their actions or inactions can either aid or hinder clients in achieving their objectives, and they accept this responsibility as part of their professional obligation. CCM certificants may be called upon to provide a variety of services and they are obligated to do so in a manner that is consistent with their education, formal training, and work experience. In providing services, CCM certificants must demonstrate their adherence to the Committee on Ethics and Professional Conduct.

The basic objective of the Code is to protect the public interest. Accordingly, the Code consists of Principles, Rules of Conduct, and Guidelines for Professional Conduct, as well as the CCMC Procedures for Processing Complaints.

The Principles are fundamental assumptions to guide professional conduct and are advisory in nature. The Rules of Conduct and the Guidelines for Professional Conduct prescribe the level of conduct required of every certificant. Compliance with these levels of conduct is mandatory and will be enforced through the CCMC Procedures for Processing Complaints.

PRINCIPLES

Principle 1: Certificants shall endeavor to place the public interest above their own at all times.

Principle 2: Certificants shall respect the integrity and protect the welfare of those persons or groups with whom they are working.

Principle 3: Certificants shall always maintain objectivity in their relationships with clients.

Principle 4: Certificants shall act with integrity in dealing with other professionals so as to facilitate their contributions with respect to achieving maximum benefits for the client.

Principle 5: Certificants shall keep their technical competency at a level which ensures their clients will receive the benefit of the highest quality of service their profession can offer that is consistent with the client's conditions and circumstances.

Principle 6: Certificants shall honor the integrity and respect the limitations placed on the use of the CCM designation.

Principle 7: Certificants shall obey all laws and regulations, avoiding any conduct or activity that could harm others.

Principle 8: Certificants shall help maintain the integrity of the Committee on Ethics and Professional Conduct for Case Managers.

CCMC RULES OF CONDUCT

Violation of any of these requirements may result in denial or sanctions on the part of the Commission up to and including revocation of the individual's certification.

Rule 1: Intentionally falsifying an application or other documents.

Rule 2: Conviction of a felony that involves moral turpitude.

Rule 3: Violation of the code of ethics governing the profession upon which the individual's primary professional credential upon which eligibility for the CCM designation is based.

Rule 4: Loss of the primary professional credential upon which eligibility for the CCM designation is based.

Rule 5: Violation or breach of the guidelines for professional conduct (i.e., professional misconduct).

Rule 6: Failure to maintain eligibility requirements once certified.

Rule 7: Failure to pay required fees to CCMC.

Rule 8: Violation of the rules and regulations governing the taking of the certification examination.

SCOPE OF PRACTICE FOR CASE MANAGERS

I. Assumptions

- Case management is not a profession in itself but rather an area of practice within one's profession. It is collaborative and trans-disciplinary in nature.
- Certification determines that the case manager possesses the education, skills, moral character, licensing and experience required to render appropriate services based on sound principles of practice.

- Certificants shall practice only within the boundaries of their competence, based on their education, training, appropriate professional experience, and other professional credentials. They shall not misrepresent their role or competence to clients. They shall not attribute the possession of the certification designation to a depth of knowledge, skills, and professional capabilities greater than those demonstrated by achievement of certification.

II. Underlying Values

- Belief that case management is a means for achieving client wellness and autonomy through advocacy, communication, education, identification of service resources, and service facilitation.
- Recognition of the dignity, worth and rights of all people.
- Understanding and commitment to quality outcomes for clients, appropriate use of resources, and the empowerment of clients in a manner that is supportive and objective.
- Belief in the underlying premise that when the individual reaches the optimum level of wellness and functional capability, everyone benefits: the individuals being served, their support systems, the health care delivery systems and the various reimbursement systems.
- Recognition that case management is guided by the principles of autonomy, beneficence, nonmaleficence, justice, veracity and distributive justice.

III. Definition of Case Management

Case management is a collaborative process that assesses, plans, implements coordinates, monitors, and evaluates the options and services required to meet an individual's health needs, using communication and available resources to promote quality, cost-effective outcomes.

IV. Ethical Issues

Because case management exists in an environment that looks to it as a solution for many of the problems in the health care delivery and payer systems, case managers frequently find themselves in ethical dilemmas.

Each case manager must abide by the Committee on Ethics and Professional Conduct for Case Managers as well as by the professional code of ethics of their specific profession for guidance and support in the resolution of these conflicts.

GUIDELINES FOR PROFESSIONAL CONDUCT

G 1—Representation of Practice

Certificants shall practice only within the boundaries of their competence, based on their education, training, appropriate professional experience, and other professional credentials. They shall not misrepresent their role or competence to clients. They shall not attribute the possession of the certification designation to a depth of knowledge, skills, and professional capabilities greater than those demonstrated by achievement of certification.

G 2—Competence

Certificants shall not:

a) handle or neglect a case in such a manner that the certificant's conduct constitutes gross negligence (which for the purposes of this guideline shall mean willful, wanton or reckless disregard of the certificant's obligations and responsibilities).

b) exhibit a pattern of negligence or neglect in the handling of the certificant's obligations or responsibilities.

G 3—Representation of Qualifications

Certificants shall take the necessary steps to represent their qualifications and to correct a misstatement made by a third party with respect to the certificant's qualifications.

G 4—Legal and Benefit System Requirements

Certificants shall work in accordance with applicable state and federal laws and the unique requirements of the various reimbursement systems involved.

G 5—Testimony

Certificants, when providing testimony in a judicial or non-judicial forum, shall be impartial and limit testimony to their specific fields of expertise.

G 6—Dual Relationships

Certificants who provide services at the request of a third-party payer shall disclose the nature of their dual relationship at the outset of the certificant/client relationship by describing their role and responsibilities to parties who have the right to know. Dual relationships, other than payer/client, include, but are not limited to, certificants working with clients who are the certificants' employer, employee, friend, relative, and/or research subject, and must also be disclosed.

G 7—Description of Services

Certificants shall explain services to be provided to the extent reasonably necessary to permit the client to make informed decisions, understand the purpose, techniques, roles, procedures, expected outcomes, billing arrangements, and limitations of the services rendered and identify to whom and for what purpose the results of the services will be communicated.

G 8—Objectivity

Certificants shall maintain objectivity in their professional relationships and shall not impose their values on their clients.

G 9—Relationships with Clients

Certificants shall not enter into any relationship with any client, business, personal or otherwise, that will interfere with the certificant's professional objectivity.

G 10—Confidentiality: Legal Compliance

Certificants shall be knowledgeable about and act in accordance with federal, state, and local laws and procedures related to the scope of their practices regarding client consent, confidentiality, and the release of information.

G 11—Confidentiality: Disclosure

Certificants shall inform the client, at the outset of the certificant-client relationship, that any information obtained through the relationship may be disclosed to third parties. Disclosure of information shall be made only to clients, payers, service providers, and governmental authorities and limited to what is necessary and relevant, except that the certificant must reveal information to appropriate authorities, as soon as and to the extent that the certificant reasonably believes necessary, to prevent the client from: a) committing acts likely to result in bodily harm or imminent danger to the client or others; and b) committing criminal, illegal, or fraudulent acts.

G 12—Confidentiality: Client Identity

Certificants shall maintain the confidentiality of the identity of the client when using data for training, research, publication, and/or marketing unless a written release is obtained from the client.

G 13—Confidentiality: Records

Certificants shall maintain client records, whether written, taped, computerized, or stored in any other medium, in a manner designed to ensure confidentiality.

G 14—Electronic Recording

Certificants shall not electronically record communications with clients without first obtaining the client's written permission.

G 15—Reports

Certificants shall be accurate, honest, and unbiased in reporting the results of their professional activities to appropriate third parties, to avoid exerting undue influence upon the decision-making process.

G 16—Records: Maintenance/Storage and Disposal

Certificants shall maintain records necessary for rendering professional services to their clients and as required by applicable laws, regulations, or agency/institution procedures. Subsequent to file closure, records shall be maintained for the number of years consistent with jurisdictional requirements or for a longer period during which maintenance of such records is necessary or helpful to provide reasonably anticipated future services to the client. After that time, records shall be destroyed in a manner assuring preservation of confidentiality.

G 17—Use of CCM Designation

The designation of Certified Case Manager and the initials "CCM" may only be used by individuals currently certified by the Commission for Case Manager Certification. The certificant shall not utilize the designation or initials as part of a company, partnership, or corporate name, trademark, or logo.

G 18—Research: Legal Compliance

Certificants shall plan, design, conduct, and report research in a manner consistent with ethical principles and federal and state laws and regulations, including those governing research with human subjects.

G 19—Research: Subject Confidentiality

Certificants who supply data, aid in the research of another person, report research results, or make original data available shall maintain the confidentiality of the identity of the respective subjects unless an appropriate authorization from the subjects has been obtained.

G 20—Unprofessional Behavior

It is unprofessional behavior if the certificant:

a) commits a criminal act that reflects adversely on the certificant's honesty or trustworthiness;
b) engages in conduct involving dishonesty, fraud, deceit, or misrepresentation;
c) engages in conduct involving discrimination against a client because of race, color, religion, age, gender, sexual orientation, national origin, marital status, or disability/handicap;
d) engages in sexually intimate behavior with a client; or
e) accepts as a client an individual with whom the certificant has been sexually intimate.

G 21—Conflict of Interest

Certificants shall fully disclose an actual or potential conflict of interest to all affected parties. If, after full disclosure, an objection is made by any affected party, the certificant shall withdraw from further participation in the case.

G 22—Termination of Services

Certificants shall recommend the termination of case activity when the certificant reasonably believes that the client is no longer benefiting or when services are no longer required.

G 23—Fees

Certificants shall advise the referral source/payer of their fee structure in advance of the rendering of any services and shall also furnish, upon request, detailed, accurate time and expense records. No fee arrangements shall be made that would reduce the quality of care.

G 24—Advertising

Certificants who describe/advertise services shall do so in a manner that accurately informs the public of the services, expertise, and techniques being offered. Descriptions/advertisements by a certificant shall not contain false, inaccurate, misleading, out-of-context, or otherwise deceptive material or statements. If statements from former clients are to be used, the certificant shall have a written, signed, and dated release from the former clients. All advertising shall be factually accurate and shall not contain exaggerated claims as to costs and/or results.

G 25—Solicitation

Certificants shall not reward, pay, or compensate any individual, company, or entity for directing or referring clients to the certificant. Nothing contained herein shall preclude certificants from making reasonable expenditures in entertaining individuals who have referred or may in the future refer clients to the certificant or from giving gifts of minimal value to such individuals.

G 26—Reporting Misconduct

Certificants possessing knowledge, not otherwise protected as confidence by this Code, that another certificant has committed a violation of any provisions of this code shall promptly report such knowledge to CCMC and to such other authority as may be empowered to investigate or to act upon such actions or violations. Certificants shall not initiate, participate in, or encourage the filing of complaints that are malicious, unwarranted, or without a basis in fact.

G 27—Compliance with Proceedings

Certificants shall assist in the process of enforcing the Committee on Ethics and Professional Conduct for Case Managers by cooperating with investigations, participating in proceedings, and complying with the directives of the Committee on Ethics and Professional Conduct.

Source: Reprinted with permission from Code of Professional Conduct for Case Managers with Disciplinary Rules, Procedures, and Penalties, © 2001, Commission for Case Manager Certification.

APPENDIX 6–C

CMSA Ethics Survey

I. Your Practice Setting and Discipline

I am a:

❑ Nurse
❑ Social Worker
❑ Therapist
❑ Other _____

Employment Setting:

❑ Independent
❑ Facility-Based
❑ Home Care
❑ HMO/PPO
❑ Insurance Carrier/TPA
❑ Employer Group
❑ Other

My contact with patients/claimants is:

❑ Telephone only
❑ By telephone and on-site, as needed
❑ None, but I know of their status through physicians, providers

As a decision maker:

❑ I can assess, plan, recommend, implement and change services, levels of care for patients in conjunction with the physicians.
❑ I can monitor services, but others do the above.

II. Metaethical Analysis (what is important)

When you conduct yourself as an ethical and moral professional, rank your goals in order of importance (1 being MOST important, 5 being LEAST important):

___ patient outcome   ___ professional reputation and success
___ quality of life   ___ appropriateness of care
___ cost savings   ___ advocacy of patient

III. Descriptive Analysis (how they work)

Which character traits are essential for ethical case management? List as many as you feel are appropriate.

_____

_____

_____

_____

To whom is a case manager responsible?

Assign to each: (1) important, (2) somewhat important, or (3) least important

   ___ Patient   ___ Family of Patient
   ___ Self   ___ Employer
   ___ Payer   ___ Society

Decisions that case managers are asked to make frequently present ethical challenges. The following represent some of them. Please note your response when confronted with the situations below by writing in an a, b, or c:

a) I make the decision comfortably and unassisted.
b) I frequently consult with others.
c) I make the decision, but often or occasionally wonder if it was the right one.

Rank, a, b, or c:

_____1. When I have to provide a referral to providers about whom I know little

_____2. Referral to in-network providers (physicians, hospitals, home care, etc.) about whom I have reservations, but not doing so results in:
      increased costs to my patients _____
      employment problem for me _____

_____3. Family members ask me not to discuss the seriousness of a condition with the patient

_____4. Patients ask me to withhold information from their family members or employers

_____5. Called upon to manage cases beyond my comfort level or knowledge

_____6. When quality of care, poor outcomes or safety of patient is in serious jeopardy but confronting the provider or informing the patient/family of the situation can jeopardize my relationship with the patient or threaten my employment

_____7. When I have to balance quality of care with the need to demonstrate savings

_____8. Respecting patient autonomy when his/her choices may result in further deterioration and increased costs

_____9. Intervening on a patient's behalf whenever a physician continues aggressive treatment despite expressed wishes of the patient

IV. Normative Ethical Analysis (how we do things around here)

Have you ever:

- been offered bonuses directly tied to the amount of savings you or your department achieved?

  ❏ yes   ❏ no   ❏ not applicable

- been offered gifts, finder fees or other incentives for referrals to certain facilities, providers or dealers?

  ❏ yes   ❏ no   ❏ not applicable

- been asked to change contents of a report or other documentation to obscure facts or to remove "damaging" information?

  ❏ yes   ❏ no   ❏ not applicable

- been asked to report outcomes or cost savings that were greater than you felt you obtained?

  ❏ yes   ❏ no   ❏ not applicable

- Are there other ethical issues or dilemmas that you face that were NOT addressed in this survey?

  ❏ yes   ❏ no   ❏ not applicable

If your answer was yes, would you please describe in the space provided.

_____
_____
_____

I would be willing to be contacted for an interview or discussion or to assist as a member of the Ethics Committee:

  ❏ yes   ❏ no

Optional:
Signature: _____
Name: _____
Address/City/State/Zip:_____
Phone: _____

Are you a current CMSA Member?   ❏ yes   ❏ no

Source: Reprinted with permission from Case Management Society of America, © 1997.

Chapter 7

Case Manager Credentialing

CERTIFIED CASE MANAGER (CCM)

The Certification of Insurance Rehabilitation Specialists Commission (CIRSC) in Rolling Meadows, Illinois, was the credentialing agency selected by the National Case Management Task Force in February 1992 to develop the case management certification process. This group defined case management and announced the first credentialing process for case managers in September 1992. The report drafted at CIRSC offices and published in 1992 became the basis for the *CCM Certification Guide*, published in 1993 and updated regularly, including basic information regarding application for the Certified Case Manager (CCM) certification. (In 1995, the Interim Commission was incorporated as an independent credentialing body and renamed the Commission for Case Manager Certification [CCMC]. CIRSC is now known as the Certification of Disability Management Specialists Commission [CDMSC]. CCMC continues to publish the *CCM Certification Guide*, revised to meet the changing roles of case managers in numerous practice settings within the evolving managed care industry.) The CCM credential brought into existence a nationally accepted standard for case management practitioners. As of 2009, there are approximately 28,000 professionals who have obtained the CCM certification. This research-based, peer-reviewed process has been awarded accreditation by the National Commission for Certifying Agencies. In a 2008 Salary and Trends Survey conducted by *Case in Point*, 81% of the respondents had the CCM credential, so it continues to attain recognition as the gold standard in certification.

THE CCM EXAM

The CCM exam and certification process are administered by the Commission for Case Manager Certification (CCMC). In the fall of 2008, the CCM examination migrated to computer-based testing, and in fact the application, renewal, and continuing education unit (CEU) tracking is available online. Currently, the CCM exam is made up of questions across six knowledge domains, further defined into subdomains in the *CCM Certification Guide*. These domains include Case Management Concepts, Case Management Principles and Strategies, Healthcare Management and Delivery, Healthcare Reimbursement, Vocational Concepts and Strategies, and Psychosocial and Support Systems. Although it certainly tests clinical knowledge, the exam is intended to be a tool for the evaluation of the skills necessary for the practice of case management. Factual knowledge is tested, as is the practical application of such knowledge. By having to answer situational test questions, candidates cannot merely memorize facts, laws, formulas, and so on, but must demonstrate that they have actually engaged in case management activities. Currently, the exam contains 180 multiple-choice questions, and applicants have $3\frac{1}{2}$ hours to complete the exam. The fee for application and the exam is $290.

Obviously, those currently in practice will be more comfortable with many of the "hands-on" type of questions, such as the following:

A worker with a reported back injury is referred by his physician for noninvasive diagnostic testing. Which of the following procedures will most likely be performed?

   a. Angiogram
   b. Myelogram
   c. Ultrasound
   d. Computerized Axial Tomography

Due to nutritional deficiencies, the chronic alcoholic may develop peripheral neuropathy. This disorder is best described as:

   a. A progressive deterioration of sensory and motor functions at the lower extremities which can be reversed if treated early.
   b. A disease of the spinal nerves that causes immediate and permanent damage and results in paralysis.
   c. Affecting only the most severe, long-term alcoholics who have extensive liver damage.
   d. A rapidly progressive loss of sensation and function of the facial and neck muscles.[1]

The correct answers are *d* and *a*.

Are there ways to prepare for this examination? There are several conferences, both local and national, that are useful in obtaining the kind of information and insight required to pass the CCM exam. These include the national conferences sponsored by CMSA, National Association of Rehabilitation Professionals in the Private Sector (NARPPS), and other organizations. Presenters at such conferences are often case management professionals, lawyers, physicians, and others who can share their expertise and the kind of hands-on knowledge that is invaluable to prospective test takers.

Currently, there is no official study guide for the exam, but several of the works listed in Appendix A at the end of the book will be of help. The CCMC also includes a reading list on its web site. The information covered in the exam is always contained in published, readily accessible sources.

Although attending seminars and reading are beneficial, several hours or days of study will not by itself result in a passing grade. Actual working experience and competence are being tested, as well as theory, and although the exam is for entry-level practitioners, it is interesting to note that most case managers have more than 20 years experience in the healthcare field.[2]

Because there are many clinical areas involved in the practice of case management, individuals who have experience in only one specialty area (for example, neonatology or AIDS) may struggle with certain aspects of the exam. So, too, may allied professionals other than nurses who perform some but not all case management activities or who are members of a case management team but do not have all of the responsibilities. For these individuals, additional preparation may be necessary to round out their knowledge.

BEFORE CCM, TO THE WIDE ARRAY OF CREDENTIALS

Other applicable certification designations, which were in place prior to CCM, are Certified Rehabilitation Registered Nurse (CRRN) from the Rehabilitation Nursing Certification Board and Certified Occupational Health Nurse (COHN) from the American Association of Occupational Health Nurses.

In early 2002, CMSA surveyed a cross section of case management professionals from a wide array of backgrounds. Results showed that the vast majority of case managers that are certified hold the CCM. The second largest group of case managers, approximately half the number of those who have earned the CCM, have some "other" certification. These are followed, from most to least, by case managers with the Certified

Disability Management Specialist (CDMS), the Certified Case Manager (CM) credential from American Nurses Credentialing Center, Certified Occupational Health Nurse (COHN), Certified Rehabilitation Counselor (CRC), Continuity of Care Certification, Advanced (A-CCC), and the Case Manager, Certified (CMC).[3]

A number of new case manager credentialing bodies and credentialing opportunities have been developed, and others increasingly are being applied by case manager professionals. Each of these was designed to meet the needs of case managers in certain settings, and candidates may find it helpful to examine each offering prior to sitting for an exam. Some of the most recognized are included in the following pages, drawn from web sites, articles and papers published in *The Case Manager, Case Management Advisor*, and *Case Management Trends: An Overview of Recent Industry and Regulatory Developments*, published by URAC.[4] The credentialing groups for these programs are included in Appendix A at the end of the book.

CERTIFIED DISABILITY MANAGEMENT SPECIALIST (CDMS)

In place for a number of years as the CIRS credential, the CDMS has six eligibility categories. Each category is specific in its requirements, and it is suggested that interested candidates call the Certification of Disability Specialists Commission to request written materials outlining the categories. Briefly stated, they include a valid registered nurse or certified rehabilitation counselor certification/license plus a minimum of 2 or 3 years, respectively, of acceptable supervised experience; a master's degree in rehabilitation counseling with hours and certified supervision requirements; a bachelor's degree and license or certification, plus a minimum of 2 years acceptable, full-time employment with 1 year under the supervision of a CMS, CCM, or CRC; or a bachelor's, master's, or doctorate degree in any discipline, plus a minimum of 5 years of acceptable, full-time employment under the supervision of a CDMS, CCM, or CRC.

The half-day computerized exam includes 175 multiple-choice questions covering disability case management, psychosocial intervention, vocational aspects of disability, managed care and disability management concepts, and business knowledge related to disability management. Application and examination fees are $385. Recertification must occur 5 years after the certification is awarded. The candidate must show completion of 80 hours of approved continuing education and pay a $160 fee.

CERTIFIED OCCUPATIONAL HEALTH NURSE (COHN)

One of three credentials offered by the American Board for Occupational Health Nurses, Inc. (ABOHN), the certifying body for occupational health nurses in the United States, the Certified Occupational Health Nurse (COHN) is offered to registered nurses. Its exam no longer requires a degree, due to a change in requirements of the ABOHN. Its core focus is on the nurse as a clinician, advisor, and coordinator. Any graduate study in occupational health or completion of a baccalaureate program, after basic nursing preparation, can be used toward the experience or education requirement for taking the exam. These options are covered in detail in the application form.

CERTIFIED OCCUPATIONAL HEALTH
NURSE–SPECIALIST (COHN-S)

The Certified Occupational Health Nurse–Specialist (COHN-S) credential, also from the ABOHN, reflects the nurse's role in direct care, management, education, and consulting. An applicant must have registered nurse (RN) licensure and a bachelor's degree. It does not require a bachelor of science in nursing. To sit for the COHN-S, an individual must have earned the COHN.

Eligibility criteria for the COHN and the COHN-S require active licensure as a registered nurse or its international equivalent, as well as 4,000 hours experience (or a minimum of 2 years of full-time employment) in occupational health nursing and 50 documented contact hours earned within a 5-year period prior to the application deadline. The continuing education credits that comprise those contact hours must be related to occupational health. An applicant may use professional presentations, nursing leadership, and publications toward meeting this.

CERTIFIED OCCUPATIONAL HEALTH NURSE/CASE
MANAGER–COHN/CM AND CERTIFIED OCCUPATIONAL
HEALTH NURSE–SPECIALIST/CASE MANAGER (COHN-S/CM)

The Certified Occupational Health Nurse/Case Manager (COHN/CM) and Certified Occupational Health Nurse–Specialist/Case Manager (COHN-S/CM) are both specialty credentials in case management offered by the ABOHN. These case management credentials require current, active status as a COHN or COHN-S, current licensure as an RN or its international equivalent, and 10 documented hours of case management continuing education in the 5 years before the application is submitted.

Recertification for ABOHN credentials is required every 5 years. Available from ABOHN, a candidate handbook covers in depth a variety of topics related to its credentials.

CERTIFIED REHABILITATION COUNSELOR (CRC)

Offered by the Commission on Rehabilitation Counselor Certification (CRCC), the Certified Rehabilitation Counselor (CRC) is designed for rehabilitation professionals practicing rehabilitation counseling, a specialty within the rehabilitation profession, which assists those with physical, mental, developmental, cognitive, and emotional disabilities. There are several rehabilitation disciplines and related processes integral to this credential, including vocational evaluation, job development and job placement, work adjustment, and case management. Created with a number of eligibility levels to sit for the exam, the CRC, its certification standards, a Code of Professional Ethics, its certification guide, and application can be viewed on its web site, www.crccertification.com.

CONTINUITY OF CARE CERTIFICATION, ADVANCED (A-CCC)

Available from the National Board for Certification in Continuity of Care, the Continuity of Care Certification, Advanced (A-CCC) is open to multiple disciplines, including nurses, social workers, therapists, dietitians, and physicians. It can be achieved by those with a baccalaureate degree or higher, licensure in your discipline, and 2 years of full-time experience in continuity of care within the last 5 years prior to sitting for the exam. Candidates without a baccalaureate degree need to verify 8 years of full-time experience in continuity of care within the last 12 years. Documentation of employment, proof that the applicant's job responsibilities include continuity of care functions, and a copy of her current job description must be submitted with her application. Included in the exam content is the continuity of care process, healthcare delivery systems, professional issues, standards, reimbursement, legal issues, and clinical issues. The certification is valid for 5 years.

CASE MANAGER, CERTIFIED (CMC)

The American Institute of Outcomes Case Management (AIOCM), a membership organization, offers the Case Manager, Certified (CMC) credential. Applicants must be members of the institute who have attained a certain number of points based on education and experience. The AIOCM has established two certification processes: a standard process and a portfolio review process. Using the standard certification process, applicants must meet general education, professional experience, outcomes care, education, and ethical requirements, and pass the 2-hour exam. The portfolio review procedure, by which candidates who do not meet the standard criteria can apply, requires submission of a portfolio of one's education, training, and experience for evaluation by the AIOCM. Only applicants with more than 10 years of related professional experience may utilize the portfolio review application process.

The AIOCM also offers the Advanced Utilization Managers (UMC-A), Clinical Chart Auditing Professionals (CAPC), and Case Manager Associates (CMC-A, described later in this chapter) credentials.

CARE MANAGER CERTIFIED (CMC)

Case managers and case manager candidates should take note that there are two CMC credentials. Care Manager Certified (CMC), from the National Academy of Certified Care Managers (not to be confused with the Case Manager, Certified, also abbreviated CMC, from the AIOCM), requires that applicants meet one of three criteria. They must have a minimum of 2 years of supervised, paid, full-time care management experience that includes face-to-face interviews, assessment, care planning, problem solving, and follow-up. The experience must be subsequent to obtaining a master's degree in a field related to case management, such as social work, nursing, counseling, gerontology, or psychology.

The second criterion is a minimum of 4 years of paid, full-time direct experience with people in fields such as social work, nursing, mental health, counseling, or care management, 2 years of which must be supervised, paid, full-time care management experience that includes face-to-face interaction as described previously. A bachelor's degree in a field related to care management (social work, nursing, counseling, mental health, psychology, or gerontology) is required.

Third, a candidate can sit for the exam if she holds a high school diploma or any degree unrelated to the field of case management and a minimum of 6 years paid, full-time, direct experience with clients in areas such as social work, nursing, mental health, counseling, or care management. Two years of this work must have been supervised, paid, full-time care management experience as noted in the second criterion listing.

CMC certification must be renewed every 3 years.[5]

REGISTERED NURSE-NURSE CASE MANAGER (RN-NCM)

The Registered Nurse-Nurse Case Manager (RN-NCM) credential is administered by the American Nurses' Association through its subsidiary, the American Nurses Credentialing Center. Candidates must hold an active RN license in the United States or its territories, a bachelor's degree, and another ANA certification. They must document a current, nationally recognized core nursing specialty certification, and have worked within the scope of practice for a minimum of 2,000 hours within the 2 years prior to their application for the exam. The RN-NCM certification is valid for 5 years.[6]

CERTIFIED PROFESSIONAL IN HEALTHCARE QUALITY (CPHQ)

Effective January 1, 2004, the Healthcare Quality Certification Board of the National Association for Healthcare Quality voted to eliminate the education and experience criteria that had been required to sit for the Certified Professional in HealthCare Quality (CPHQ). The Board suggests that candidates assess their readiness to apply to take the CPHQ exam.[7]

CASE MANAGEMENT ADMINISTRATOR, CERTIFIED (CMAC)

To sit for the Case Management Administrator, Certified (CMAC) exam, sponsored by The Center for Case Management, applicants must meet one of five eligibility requirements. They must hold a master's degree and have 1 year experience in case management administration; a master's degree and 3 years experience as a case manager; a bachelor's degree and 3 years experience in case management administration; a bachelor's degree and 5 years experience as a case manager; or hold one of the following active case manager certifications as entry into the CMAC examination: A-CCC, CRRN, CCM, Certified Social Work Case Manager (C-SWCM), Certified Advanced Social Work Case Manager (C-ASWCM) or CDMS.

This certification is valid for 5 years.[8]

CERTIFIED REHABILITATION REGISTERED NURSE (CRRN)

The Certified Rehabilitation Registered Nurse (CRRN) credential, administered by the Rehabilitation Nursing Certification Board, requires that candidates have a current, unrestricted RN license and have completed within the 5 years preceding the examination: 2 years of practice as a registered professional nurse in rehabilitation nursing, or 1 year of practice as a registered professional nurse in rehabilitation nursing, plus 1 year of advanced study (beyond a baccalaureate) in nursing.

The certification is valid for 5 years providing that the individual maintains an unrestricted RN license, has at least 2 years rehabilitation nursing experience within the previous 5 years and 60 acceptable CEs as defined by the organization. For additional information, contact the organization's website at: http://www.rehabnurse.org.[9]

CERTIFIED SOCIAL WORK CASE MANAGER (C-SWCM)

Applicants for the Certified Social Work Case Manager (C-SWCM) credential from the National Association of Social Workers (NASW) must hold active NASW membership in good standing; hold a bachelor's in social work (BSW) degree from a Council on Social Work Education accredited institution, and 1-year (1,500 hours) paid, post-BSW, supervised work experience. (These hours must be accumulated in more than 1 year and less than 5 years.)

Further eligibility criteria include adherence to the NASW Code of Ethics, the NASW Standards for Social Work Case Management, and the NASW Standards for Continuing Professional Education; an NASW Academy of Certified Baccalaureate Social Workers (ACBSW) credential, a current state BSW-level licensure, if applicable, or a passing score on the American Association of State Social Work Boards basic exam; a reference from a BSW- or MSW-level colleague, and an evaluation from an approved supervisor.

The C-SWCM must be renewed every 2 years.[10]

The NASW also offers the Certified Advanced Social Work Case Manager (C-ASWCM) credential for MSW social workers.

CERTIFIED MANAGED CARE NURSE (CMCN)

Certified Managed Care Nurse (CMCN) is offered by the American Board of Managed Care Nursing, an association dedicated to providing training and educational services to nurses in managed care. Eligibility criteria for the CMCN is a Registered Nurse license, Licensed Practical Nurse (LPN) license, or a current license to practice nursing in any American state, territory, or protectorate. The written, 150 multiple-choice question exam is based on the home study course made available by Thomson Prometric. Applicants must qualify under one of four employment experiences listed at "Eligibility Requirements," www.abmcn.org.[11]

CASE MANAGER ASSOCIATE (CMC-A)

The Case Manager Associate (CMC-A) credential from the American Institute of Outcomes Case Management is under development.

OTHER CREDENTIALS AND CREDENTIALING GROUPS

In the late 1990s, the American Nurses Credentialing Center (ANCC), a subsidiary of the American Nurses Association, held its first exam for a case management credential specific to the discipline of nursing, with its primary focus on nurse case management, the Cm. Later this became the Certified Nursing Case Manager (RN,Cm). Now, it is a module called the RN,C or Registered Nurse, Certified.

I am concerned about the number of credentials that have emerged for case managers and the divisiveness they seem to contribute to our industry. Because of interest in case management and its nature as a cross-disciplinary practice, a number of credentials will, of course, evolve. As more companies specify a credential in their employment ads for case managers, and as more case managers enter the field, it will be interesting to note those credentials that move to the top as the most desirable and are recognized as indicators of established professionals. One needs to be informed as to which credential will meet one's needs and serve the industry and our patients well.

In summary, attaining a case management credential should be the goal of each case management professional, and once it is attained, each professional needs to maintain both competency and the credential. Taking the time to get the credential demonstrates both a professional and personal commitment to the case management process and serves to validate its importance for ensuring quality outcomes and the preservation of healthcare resources. If there are over 23,000 CCMs today, how powerful will our voices be when these numbers continue to expand? We will be firmly positioned for the future, helping our patients, their families, the payers, and the providers. As case managers, we know how valuable our work can be, and the CCM credential will underscore and further promote our contributions.

NOTES

1. Commission for Case Manager Certification, *CCM Certification Guide* (Rolling Meadows, IL: CCMC, 2003).
2. Boling J and Carneal G, "Case Management Trends," in *Case Management Trends: An overview of Recent Industry and Regulatory Developments* (Washington, D.C.: URAC, 2002).
3. Boling J and Carneal G, "Case Management Trends," 12.
4. Hoffmann L F, "Directory of the Top 12 CM Credentials," supplement to *Case Management Advisor* 11, no. 11 (2000): 1 (for more information, please call 800-688-2421); Boling J and Carneal G, "Case Management Trends"; and Stolte C M, "The Commission for Case Manager Certification Widens Eligibility Criteria," *The Case Manager* 13, no. 5 (2002): 50.
5. Hoffmann L F, "Directory of the Top 12 CM Credentials," 7.
6. Stolte C M, "The Commission for Case Manager Certification Widens Eligibility Criteria," 53; and C. M. Hoffmann, "Directory of the Top 12 CM Credentials," 1–2.
7. Healthcare Quality Certification Board, "2004 Candidate Handbook," pp. 2–3.
8. Hoffmann L F, "Directory of the Top 12 CM Credentials," 3–4.
9. Association of Rehabilitation Nurses, "CRRN Certification," http://www.rehabnurse.org/certification/.
10. National Association of Social Workers, "Credentials and Specialty Certifications: Certified Social Work Case Manager (C-SWCM)," http://www.socialworkers.org/credentials/specialty/c-swcm.asp.
11. American Board of Managed Care Nursing, home page, http://www.abmcn.org; Stolte C M, "Commission for Case Manager Certification Widens Eligibility Criteria," 53.

REFERENCES

American Board of Managed Care Nursing. "What Is the American Board of Managed Care Nursing?" http://www.abmcn.org.

American Board for Occupational Health Nurses. Certification Information Kit. http://www.abohn.org.

American Institute of Outcomes Care Management. Web site. http://www.aiocm.com.

American Nurses Credentialing Center. Web site. http://www.ana.org/ancc/.

Case Management Society of America. "Certification—Primary Case Management Certification Options." FAXT Sheet. 2003. http://www.cmsa.org.

Central Connecticut State University. "Social Work Program." http://www.sociology.ccsu.edu/SocialWork/NASWbrochure.htm.

Center for Case Management. *Certification Examination for Case Management Administrators Handbook for Candidates.* Information kit.

Certification of Disability Management Specialists. "Why CDMSC." http://www.cdms.org.

Commission on Rehabilitation Counselor Certification. Web site. http://www.crccertifi cation.com.

Healthcare Quality Certification Board. "Welcome to the Web site for the Certified Professional in Healthcare Quality (CPHQ) Program." http://www.cphq.org/.

Hoffmann LF, "Directory of the Top 12 CM Credentials." Supplement to *Case Management Advisor* 11, no. 11 (2000): 1–8.

National Board for Certification in Continuity of Care. Web site. http://www.nbccc.org.

Stolte CM, "The Commission for Case Manager Certification Widens Eligibility Criteria." *The Case Manager* 13, no. 5 (2002): 50–54.

U.S. Department of Justice. Web site. http://www.usdoj.gov.

Part II

Case Management Process

Chapter **8**

Communications

Because case management has become an integral part of the medical mainstream, it is essential that new dialogues and heightened levels of communication be maintained. Case management is a person-to-person service, and open pathways must be laid for good interaction. More focused and conscious communication is needed between case managers and physicians, patients, families, payer sources, and related legal entities. To communicate effectively with each of these groups, case managers must recognize the obstacles to communication and strive to overcome them.

I think it is also important for case managers to make their letters, phone calls, and reports useful to the people they are addressing. It sounds simplistic, but it is appalling how many case managers totally ignore this basic rule of communication. Case management nurses in particular, more than rehab professionals or vocational counselors, tend to offer explicit, medically oriented information to individuals who have not the foggiest idea of what the terms mean, that this blood gas is saturated or unsaturated, elevated or unelevated. The data may be of some use to another nurse or physician, but they are of no help to an adult child of a patient or to a claims examiner. This does not mean that a case manager should never attempt to produce a professional-looking report or should never use medical terminology when speaking with a claims examiner, but I suggest reinforcing the medical terminology with remarks to further educate the referral source or recipient.

COMMUNICATING WITH PHYSICIANS

Working against positive communication between case managers and physicians are stereotypical judgments long held by each group about the other. In many ways, the stereotypes derive from the personality traits that cause an individual to become a physician or a case manager in the first place. Physicians tend to be results oriented, trained to "diagnose and treat," with only episodic patient involvement. Case managers, who usually come from traditional caretaker professions such as nursing and social work, maintain ongoing patient contact to perform their functions. Therefore, from the onset, case managers tend to view physicians as being less interested in their patients, whereas physicians tend to regard case managers as being overly involved or downright obstructionist.

In addition, there are gender-related disparities that contribute additional communication challenges. The now commonly heard expression, "he said, she said," has particular significance in the case manager–physician dialogue.

Another obstacle to case manager–physician communication is the healthcare system itself. Churning with change, it is unwittingly pitting healthcare professional against healthcare professional. Despite a common cause (the well-being of patients), physicians and case managers are becoming adversaries in an eroding system in which territorial struggles run rampant. With the bureaucracy collapsing around them, physicians view case managers with a wary eye, wondering, "Are they going to take my patients away?" or "Are they going to try to tell me how to treat my patient?"

In addition to issues of care control, there are issues of cost control. Misperceptions and misunderstandings stem from the emergence in the 1980s of cost containment as a factor influencing healthcare delivery. Necessitated by advancing medical technologies with advancing price tags, a longer-lived population requiring care, and a shrinking pool of dollars funding both general and high-tech treatment, managed care practices have placed case managers and physicians in "uncharted territory." Neither group of professionals is accustomed to considering, much less negotiating, the cost of care.

Mistrusting them as "claims police" who deny patient access to needed care (and confusing them with "gatekeepers" who sometimes deny care based on computer software programs), some physicians perceive case managers as a threat to their medical judgment and their income. For example, when RNs began assuming clinician roles, establishing clinics in rural areas or in disciplines less attractive to MDs, the traditional physician–nurse relationship remained unchallenged. Nurses were making medical decisions and advising patients on their treatment plans, but there were no physicians in the picture. When case managers, on the other hand, began to be accepted by corporations, insurers, and the public and play an active and high-profile role in devising care plans, some MDs felt their medical opinions were being second-guessed. It does not help either when some case managers mistakenly believe they must assume a militant or overly aggressive stance when communicating with physicians. Worse yet, some may attempt to wield control by using the "purse strings" of benefit dollars in cases where primary insurance is the payer, *and* the employer of the case manager!

Placing additional stress on the case manager–physician relationship are patients who, in today's more consumer-driven healthcare environment, are beginning to assert themselves. Armed with more information, accessible in real-time via the Internet, on a multitude of diagnostic conditions, treatment alternatives, and the ratings of providers, they are unknowingly challenging the physician's traditional place as the absolute decision maker regarding patient treatment plans.[1]

Case managers can address both the stereotypes and the stresses of a shifting healthcare system by opening up positive dialogues with physicians. With a new case comes both the responsibility and opportunity to take a proactive stance and begin promoting better case manager–physician relations. The initial phone call is an example. It is important to communicate the purpose of that call—concern for the patient. Certain cases, by nature of their circumstances, may automatically cause a physician to be on guard regarding the case manager's intent. For example, a case manager may be called upon to intervene on behalf of a patient who has been in an acute care setting for 3 weeks and for whom new healthcare settings are being explored. The case manager needs to relay that there is a concern over the patient's limited policy and that she wants to work with the physician to make better use of the patient's benefit dollars so that funds will be available for a longer period of time. The communication is upfront and professional, and the case manager's role is clearly defined.

This kind of direct communication should not be confused with taking a militant or overly aggressive attitude. Too often, case managers starting out mistakenly believe that in speaking with physicians they need to validate their role—by emphasizing they are representatives of a large insurance company, for instance. However, they soon learn that, instead of causing physicians to acquiesce, this approach alienates them. The more secure case managers are in their role, whether speaking with physicians, hospital discharge planners, social workers, or patients, the better able they are to convey their objectives and all necessary information.

Because of the changing working relationship between case managers (nurses, social workers, and counselors) and physicians, the transition to full collaboration is often awkward. Involved are differences in orientation, training, spheres of influence, and recognition of each group's expertise. Generally, society conceives of physicians as being at the apex of medicine. Buying into this mythical pyramid, nurses, along with other healthcare professionals, have failed to recognize their own contributions to the system. Caught in their traditional roles by their own and others' perceptions, case managers are sometimes seen as "simply" nurses or assistants. As a result, case managers may not be confident in dealing with physicians and have difficulty assuming anything more than a secondary or tertiary function. Also hindering the establishment of a collaborative alliance with physicians is the so-called sacred physician–patient relationship and physicians' perceptions of their legal responsibility to protect confidentiality. This impediment can also be hurdled by empowering case managers to recognize the value of their role and to understand what their abilities have brought and can continue to bring to healthcare management.

Case managers who master the art of communicating with physicians can then use their skills to train and empower their patients to also enhance their discussions with their providers. In effect, case managers should strive to broaden the circle of communications to also include patients and their families. They should share with these individuals helpful tips on how to convey their concerns and feelings, and how to resolve their issues. Equally important, case managers should teach their patients and patients' family members how to carefully *listen* to what their doctors are saying. Additionally, there are nuances in communicating with each physician, and case managers should share those nuances. For example, some physicians are somewhat controlling and don't appreciate being "challenged" (*their* perception); others are very willing to listen to every detail, even encouraging questions and additional discussion.[2]

STEREOTYPES BECOME REALITY

Physicians and case managers (regardless of their professional discipline) may share mutual goals of wanting the best outcomes for patients and delivering high-quality care. However, their approaches and philosophies are different and not always compatible. Additionally, although the healthcare delivery system has been changing around us, we often are unwilling to change the way we think or operate, believing that because what we did in the past worked there is no reason to change it. Physicians, who, for the most part, have been educated and trained to diagnose and treat, tend to be results oriented and generally have limited or episodic involvement with patients. It is relatively safe to say that the topic of communication skills is not something that gets a lot of time in medical school. And while we're on the subject of stereotypes, the majority of physicians in years past were men, and even today, this remains true. Gender disparities do influence people's perceptions, even though it may go against the reality of the situation. Studies continue to bear out what we have instinctively known: women are more effective communicators than are men. Because women comprise the majority of professionals engaged in case management, one can readily appreciate how the differences in styles of communication, or even an ability to communicate at all, would become evident as we attempt to establish effective relationships.[3]

CREATING COLLABORATION

Case managers have the kind of knowledge and insight into patients' needs that derives from a tradition of 24-hour patient attendance. Most also come with strong medical credentials and experience. Taking on a role that MDs were less inclined or less able to assume due to time constraints, case managers honed their skill in locating and recommending alternative treatment facilities and suggesting options for the provision of care via community services and resources. Some now feel their income and status as professionals are being jeopardized by MDs who are challenging their role in healthcare delivery and by medical directors at insurance companies and HMOs who do not appreciate or fully understand their contribution to care. It is difficult for case managers to have to confront such resistance and to feel they are being denied entrance into the "inner circle" as widely recognized medical professionals.

In working with physicians, case managers need to make it perfectly clear that their first and foremost concern is for the patients, that their interest is in ensuring the highest quality of care and the best possible outcomes. In addition, physicians must be assured that the case managers are not there to control or dictate patient treatment plans. Instead, the communication between the two groups should create an atmosphere of cooperation and collaboration. Case managers, after all, possess a different knowledge base than physicians (e.g., an understanding of the patients' insurance policies as well as information about various community resources that may be accessed to effect better outcomes).

In short, what must be conveyed is, "We are all focused on our patient." This statement not only sets the stage for a unified effort, but also communicates that the case manager will assume an integral role in the care of "our patient."

To facilitate physicians' receptivity to and cooperation with case managers, exchanges should occur in a certain order. First, case managers must clearly state whom they are representing. Because case managers come from diverse practice settings, ranging from within an insurance company to healthcare provider or corporate entity, they must establish whom they represent, the organization's interest, and what can be offered in the way of services. A waiver of confidentiality or consent from the patient or guardian should be presented to permit the physician to legally share the necessary information. This introduction should also include an explanation of the line of insurance involved, which shapes the case manager's objectives.

If the case manager comes from a payer group (e.g., an employer group, a Medicare/Medicaid plan, a company's premium or indemnity plan, or a workers' compensation carrier), it is important that she state, for instance, "I am the case manager representing John's employer group working within his workers' compensation plan. John was injured on the job, and my goal is to help your patient get the best possible results and return to work in the shortest period of time, as medically comfortable as possible. If he can't return to his previous type of work, I want to help him find other suitable employment."

Especially given the current chaos in the healthcare system, including the confusion between case management and managed care, it is critical that this complete introduction and communication of intent is done at the outset. Remember, not every call a physician has received from a case manager has been a positive one. The last "case manager" with whom the physician spoke may in reality have been a clerk in the utilization review department of an insurance carrier. This individual may have called the physician to say that the carrier's software tracking system indicated that her patient's condition should only require a 3-day hospital stay rather than the 5 days the physician authorized. Understandably, the physician may recall the experience with anger. Because of the possibility of this kind of scenario, the case manager may want to try to establish rapport with the physician's nurse or office administrator in order to pave the way for better communication. This person will also be a tremendous resource in maintaining ongoing communication with the physician.

Timing the Initial Physician Contact

The means by which a case manager acquires a case often dictates the order in which the exchanges with a physician will proceed. Some insurance companies do not permit involvement of a case manager until the treating physician has approved case management. This is akin to putting the cart before the horse. It is also unfortunate, because most physicians, once knowledgeable about case management, welcome the case manager's intervention at the earliest possible stage of treatment. In addition, it is probably unethical, because patients, unless incompetent, should be empowered by the case providers to make decisions on their own behalf.

Typically, the case manager first contacts the patient or family, then the treating physician. In making the initial contact with the patient, and hopefully winning over that individual, the case manager can gain valuable information that can later be passed on to the physician. The preliminary contact can also be used to confirm the identity of the patient's physician and determine his or her schedule for visiting the patient. The case manager can enlist the patient to alert the physician to expect her call and to tell the physician, "I think it might be helpful to have you and this case manager working together." This plants the seed with the physician that the patient has accepted the case manager and supports a joint effort.

If a patient is in the hospital setting or critically ill with no family members in attendance, the case manager may need to contact the treating physician first (or concurrently with attempts to reach relatives). The first outreach to the physician should be well-planned and well-executed.

It is important to take into account that, like all professionals, physicians have their own work schedules and daily priorities. A surgeon's day, for example, may consist of morning rounds at a hospital, followed by surgeries, then time spent at the office for patient appointments or paperwork, and finally a return to the hospital for postoperative rounds. The case manager should be cognizant of this regimen and acknowledge it when contacting the physician's office. The case manager might say, "I understand Dr. Jones is very busy and may not have time to meet with me during his office hours. Would it be possible for me to call him after hours? Is there a particular time that is better for him?"

Once someone in the physician's office understands that the case manager is aware of the physician's busy schedule demands and is trying to be accommodating, he or she will usually be helpful in coordinating a meeting or telephone contact.

The information gleaned by the case manager in the initial exchange with the patient also influences how time-sensitive the physician communications must be. The case manager may have uncovered relevant information that the patient neglected to tell the physician and that may alter the treatment plan, but it is essential to use common sense in determining the appropriate urgency of the call. By understanding the importance of effective physician contact and properly timing dialogues, the case manager is more likely to make a real contribution toward a successful outcome for the patient.

Finally, in establishing good communication with physicians, case managers should not agonize over their knowledge of a particular medical specialization. Although some large insurance companies or provider organizations may have case managers who concentrate on pediatric or elder care, oncology or cardiac cases, head injuries, and so on, many very effective case managers are generalists. There is nothing wrong with saying to a physician, "I am really not that familiar with your patient's particular treatment plan. Would you explain it further?"

On the other hand, many nurses have had the opportunity to work with very fine physicians, renowned in their fields, and have in-depth experience in specialized areas. Drawing on these resources to gain better insight into a particular case can only serve to equip case managers for more effective partnerships with physicians.

When I started my case management company, I was asked to handle a case involving an infant with a brain stem aneurysm. He had survived an extremely intricate surgical procedure but was left with multiple problems. His neurosurgeon, highly respected and also a clinical professor in a university hospital, was very much in demand and maintained a full schedule. The family was insistent that the physician be involved in all aspects of their child's care. I realized that to gain their trust, I needed to establish a good relationship with the physician.

In trying to reach him, it seemed I was jumping through one hoop after another and getting nowhere. I eventually ended up calling him at his office on a Saturday morning and arranging to meet him the following week after his office hours.

When we met, he was very relaxed and helpful in providing information. He even took the time to draw medical diagrams to clarify his points. He was also outwardly appreciative of my involvement and admitted he did not really understand case management. In fact, he opened up and expressed some of his own difficulties. He said that he entered neurosurgery because of an infinite fascination with the brain, never considering that some cases would require him to give advice regarding a patient's long-term care. He helped me to see that, like many physicians, he just did not have the time or even the preparation for this type of case, one that called for ongoing participation on a number of levels. I, in turn, proved my value by recommending a state-funded early intervention program for the child. The neurosurgeon and I visited the facility and, along with the pediatrician, attended team meetings together. He soon became convinced that this program, by affording the right care and social interaction for the child while alleviating much of the family's stress, was the best alternative. Ultimately, he helped convince the family, who were initially reluctant to remove their child from a home care setting. In that case and others to follow, the physician became a strong ally. This example underscores how a free-flowing and solid case manager–physician relationship facilitates effective communication between the case manager and the patient or family.

Practical Steps to a Win-Win Relationship Between Case Managers and Physicians

The following list details some practices case managers can put into play to better their working relationships with physicians and improve the standing of the entire case management community. These practices assume an understanding that although case managers have much in common—similar jargon, codes of conduct, standards of practice, and most important, the goal of helping and achieving successful patient outcomes—there are distinct differences.

1. Develop an understanding of the physician's practice setting. When is the physician in OR? When is the best time to call the physician's office? Who is the best contact in the office? Sometimes, a nurse or receptionist can provide a quick answer if you frame a clear question over the phone.
2. Go in as a savvy professional. Send the physician credible information on you and your role. Include your credentials.
3. Use your business card. Giving out your card facilitates Rolodex reference and supports your presentation of yourself as a professional.
4. Assure the physician that you will not be talking to him or her every day about every patient. Present yourself as a collaborative partner, a right-hand associate.
5. Reassure the physician that you will never presume that you can put a better treatment plan into action. You care about license liability and patient outcome as much as he or she does. State that you recognize the need to back up your assessment, and plan to review your findings, concerns, and suggestions with the physician.
6. Never drop in on the physician unannounced. Confirm all your appointments. Emergencies do arise.
7. When you attend a meeting with the physician, state how much you appreciate the time being given. Time is a valued commodity among physicians.

8. Make it easy for the physician to give you the information you need. Often, physicians lack the time to meet in person. Type a question-naire requesting specific information and enclose a self-addressed, stamped envelope for the reply. Include a copy of an appropriate signed release of information from the patient. In preparing your questions, remember that you are trying to avoid responses that will have to be dictated to a receptionist and typed, delaying a prompt response. Do everything you can so all the physician has to do is generate clear answers. Use e-mail as a communications tool, if the doctor prefers it. (See the introductory letter and questionnaire samples in Chapter 9.)

9. Attend the physician's hospital visits. It underscores your dedication and gives you the opportunity to directly ask the physician, "How can I help you?"

10. Let the physician know you are a resource: "I have this brochure with specific and clear information on open-heart surgery. Would you mind if I pass it along to Mr. Jackson?"

11. Express your recognition of excellence and a job well done. A brief note (with copies sent to the insurance carrier and the patient, if appropriate) can make a big impact. Writing such notes tells the physi-cian that you value his expertise and effort and communicates to your client company that you and the physician are working well as a team.

12. Make it clear that you are also a resource for referrals. After a suc-cessful effort on behalf of a patient, let the physician know that you are aware of and value his or her care and concern and that you will certainly make patients in similar straits aware of his or her skill and manner.

13. Get to know the physicians in your community and develop a good relationship with a support person in each office.

14. Do not trust your memory. Maintain a physician database to docu-ment specialty areas, preferred communication patterns, and previ-ous experience.

15. You know how to problem solve with other case managers, so use the same techniques in your associations with physicians. For exam-ple, every case manager and every physician struggles with patient compliance, so let physicians know you will be their eyes and ears to ensure that treatments are carried out. For a broader perspective, attend a physicians' conference or pick up publications written for physicians, such as *Physicians Practice Digest.*

16. Maintain the collaboration. Offer to give the physician an update after your house call or hospital visit.

17. When appropriate, provide the physician with copies of your case management report, enclosing an authorization release. Such updates can be particularly helpful for the physician seeing a patient on a consultation basis.

18. Hone your diplomacy skills and try to handle any problems in an ethically and morally responsible manner. Perhaps you discover a patient is taking medication that has an adverse effect in combination with another pill. He may be using over-the-counter medication or have forgotten to mention a drug he has been on for 10 years. Make it clear that you are interested in the best outcome, not in pointing a finger, when you uncover a bad situation. Document your concern as a partner, without laying blame, unless you are confronted by overt negligence.

19. Do not undermine a physician's position in front of patients. Request a moment in the hall or office afterward.

COMMUNICATIONS WITH PATIENTS AND FAMILIES

Let's agree that patients and their families can be difficult. Many families have unresolved issues, sibling rivalry, disparities relating to inheritances, and/or unequal burdens of responsibility for taking care of a chronically or catastrophically afflicted family member. All of these issues complicate the case manager's communications with patients and families and must be taken into account from the outset.

The timing of a patient's referral to a case manager helps describe how her role should be introduced and explained to the patient or family. For instance, consider this workers' compensation case. The patient has left the hospital, has completed a physical therapy program, and is now involved with various follow-up services. He has not returned to work, prompting the case to be referred to a case manager. Understandably, the patient may view this intervention less than positively. In fact, all parties may have been better served by earlier involvement of the case manager. Helping to educate clients as to the ideal time for case management intervention should be a constant objective of all case managers. However, because case managers cannot always influence when a case is referred, they must learn how to establish good patient communications regardless of the circumstances. Empathy is the key.

Case managers should put themselves in their patients' shoes. For instance, a case may have been referred within 24 hours of a catastrophic event—a massive stroke, an explosion, or the severing of a limb. Or perhaps a patient has just entered a rehabilitation center or experienced a difficult or dangerously premature delivery. To facilitate the best possible exchange, the case manager needs to have as many facts as possible about the patient and the reasons for the referral. The case manager should be aware that the patient and family may be experiencing much more than a medical crisis and should take the time to consider the patient's and family members' feelings. The medical circumstances may have created financial difficulties, marital problems, role reversals, and so on. Knowing this, the case manager should not simply pick up the phone and dial.

The person receiving the call may be waiting for news from the treating physician or the hospital. The case manager may be calling the wife of a patient who was involved in a head-on collision and is in a hospital 300 miles from home. Consider the impact of a call by a case manager who begins by introducing herself as a representative of the insurance company for the driver whose car struck her husband. The case manager must understand that there will probably be negative feelings and low receptivity and try to surmount these obstacles by using good communication skills.

Similarly, if it is a workers' compensation case and a patient was injured on the job, the case manager should recognize that management–employee or management–union relations may affect the patient's response to the case manager. The individual may have been injured in a plant recently cited for hazardous working conditions. If the patient was a new employee, he or she may be somewhat threatened and skeptical of the employer's position, fearful that management is questioning the veracity of his or her accident report. Conversely, a key senior employee of a company may have none of these concerns owing to his or her more secure position and possibly positive experiences relating to past insurance claims.

A simple matter of whether or not a company has sent flowers and cards to an injured worker also can influence how the case manager will be received. Although some organizations act in a humane way toward employees—sending gifts, calling on family members to express their interest, and setting up a "sunshine organization" to help maintain contact—others do not. The case manager should bear this in mind and try to get a sense of the company's corporate culture before calling on an employee. Especially in programs in which the case management service is new, the case manager might want to make a joint contact with the claims department or the employer benefit department to help ease patient concerns.

After introducing herself, the case manager should ask, "Is this a good time to talk?" The case manager must appreciate the suffering going on and offer support by asking how the family is, what information they have been given by the hospital, and so on. It is not a good strategy to assume family members know everything about the case and launch into the specifics of changing the treatment plan before giving them time to accept the involvement of someone new in an emotional and intense family crisis. If the case manager flounders, she can lose the family's good will before she begins her work.

Group medical cases also introduce special challenges to patient communication. Consider a patient who was just diagnosed with brain cancer. He comes from a rural community and was transferred to a major metropolitan hospital for optimum care. His family is distraught, shocked by the news. Family members may be completely out of their element, not knowing what to ask or whether they are making the best decisions. When the case manager comes on the scene, they may believe she is there to control things or keep down the high medical costs. She is looked upon as an unwanted intruder. Particularly in such situations, it is imperative that the case manager make a timely introduction and state something like this: "It may be possible, after we have spent a little more time talking and I've visited with your husband, that my assessment will be that he is receiving the best possible care and we will not be suggesting any changes. My role is to act as a coordinator of medical services and a resource for additional alternatives. Your insurance company (or employer) does not require you to accept case management. It is totally up to you."

Our healthcare system has been a very paternalistic one; we believe we know best what the patient needs. But we assume this without input from the patient. From a patient's perspective, a good scientific outcome may not be relevant. Patients do not have access to clinical research data; they are not familiar with care maps or care pathways. Have we asked: Are you comfortable? Did you understand this recommendation? Do you want to die at home?

A May 2003 Commonwealth Fund/Harvard/Harris Interactive survey of patients with health problems in the United States, Australia, Canada, New Zealand, and the United Kingdom showed poor communication between doctors and patients, high rates of medical errors, lack of coordination in patient care, and barriers when accessing care. The findings, published that same month in Health Affairs and available online at The Commonwealth Fund site (cmwf.org/media/releases/), points out missed opportunities for improving care. The survey report authors suggest that reforms targeted to populations with health problems could reap system-wide improvements in quality of care and potential cost savings (here, case managers around the world are replying, "You rang?").

The report notes that U.S. patients were more likely than those in other countries to mention communication problems with their doctors. "Three of ten respondents in the U.S. (31%) said they left a doctor's office without getting important questions answered." In Australia and New Zealand, the ratio was one in five (21% and 20%, respectively); in the United Kingdom it was 19%; and in Canada, 25%. Fully half of those adults with health problems in the United States, Australia, Canada, and New Zealand, and two-thirds of those in the United Kingdom said their regular physicians do not ask for their ideas and opinions about treatment and care, and one-fifth to one-fourth of physicians did not provide information on their goals via the treatment they recommended. Again, half the survey takers in the United States, Australia, Canada, New Zealand, and two thirds of United Kingdom adults reported that their doctors never discussed the emotional problems associated with their condition.[4] This certainly sounds like a communication breakdown to me.

Such statistics are telling regarding the state of the industry. As healthcare professionals, we really have been functioning all by ourselves. A case manager should interview a patient and family members for their expectations regarding the future: What do you think this rehab program is about? What do you hope to gain from this medical procedure? Patients should be encouraged to participate and collaborate in the process via the use of open-ended questions. Further, open-ended questions can be used to delve deeper than check-off questions, and in some cases, fill-in-the-blank queries.

Then, the case manager can begin providing the family with educational materials that describe this next step in the healing/recovery phase. This grants the patient and family the chance to form realistic expectations. My company worked with a 39-year-old corporate vice president who had a massive stroke. He along with his wife were a career couple. He entered a world-renowned rehabilitation facility and his wife really felt that within the 30-day stay covered by her policy he would improve sufficiently to come home and "be fine." Adequate information regarding his status was not communicated or, if communicated, was not reviewed for perception. In this case, her misguided perception was her version of reality.

I believe that people view acute care hospitals as the dramatic stage of recovery: They have survived. From my conversations, I gather that rehab is seen as fine-tuning. They feel that "when I leave rehab, I'm not going to have my slurred speech anymore, I'm going to have complete mobility, although I may be a little bit slower." These and other care expectations are far off the mark. Case managers need to better understand a patient's perspective and help clarify reasonable goals. Has his experience been either very negative or positive? Are his goals realistic? That's not only the caring thing to do, in fact it's the ethical thing to do, because it gives patients the information they need to know about the decisions that they need to make. Tell them the dollar amount of coverage their policy offers, the length of time provided for rehabilitation facility or nursing home care coverage, what they can reasonably expect medically, and the program's parameters; in a word, assist them with patient goal setting.[5]

The care program coordinated by the case manager may be far off the mark from the patient's perspective. Now is the time to address that. "Okay, John, these are your short-term goals; these are the physician's short-term goals for you—how far apart are you? What do we need to do to bring them back together again? Were they reasonable or not? Let's review long-term goals; are there any shortcomings? How many days does your health benefits plan cover?"

Here is an opportunity to share with the patient. "John, it seems like you are plateauing at the rehab facility. This may be a slow process. Because you only have 2 or 3 weeks of rehab coverage available, maybe it would be better for you to go home for a while and practice on some of these exercises until you reach the next stage. How do you feel about this?" This encourages a more collaborative process with that patient. Patients will see that someone really respects their needs or desires. Perhaps John was in an acute care hospital for 3 or 4 weeks with a horrendous illness. From there, he entered the rehab facility. Now, he is lonely for home and really wants to get back into more normal surroundings.[6]

Communications with a family are as important as those with the patient. There is a saying in case management, "If you lose the family, you lose the patient." It is often a good idea for case managers to give the patients and family members examples of how they have worked with other people in similar circumstances. This helps families perceive case managers as caring human beings and not just additional bureaucrats in the healthcare system.

The Patient Communication Chain of Command

Communications between a case manager and a patient should ideally follow a certain sequence. However, many factors can alter this sequence. Today's society has introduced new family units, including step-, mixed, common-law, gay, and multigenerational family units, creating different hierarchies for patient communications. The case manager needs to remember that communications with the patient and family might affect and be affected by numerous other people. Generally, the patient communication chain of command is as follows:

1. Patient (if of legal age)
2. Spouse (if married)
3. Parent or legal guardian (if patient not of legal age)
4. Oldest child (if patient widowed or divorced)
5. Significant other (if patient has an alternative lifestyle)
6. Individual with power of attorney (if patient is incapacitated)

A caveat exists in regard to the "significant other" category. Although new legislation has begun to clarify the legal rights of close companions, it is important that case managers adhere to what society and the legal community recognize to be the significant other on behalf of a patient. Also, in many workers' compensation or auto cases, although the referral may come from the carrier or the employer group, if an attorney represents the individual, the attorney, not the individual, is contacted first. For legal reasons, the case manager must explain the role of a case manager and obtain the permission of the attorney before contacting the patient.

Elder care cases in which only one sibling is represented or cases involving children whose parents are divorced may also have a skewed communication sequence. The oldest child in a family might not be the most appropriate child to assist a needy parent, being too distant physically or emotionally or being simply unable to take on the responsibility of making a life-and-death decision. At some point, the case manager might want to suggest that the on-site child contact any brothers or sisters for additional support in dealing with a parent who is critically ill.

When the Family Becomes a Patient

Many medical cases, particularly those of a catastrophic nature, will devastate a family. In tough medical situations, all attention is focused on the ill or injured person, even though the caretaker or family member might be hanging from a thread. Case managers must understand that their role includes advocacy for the families. Family members should be encouraged to say what is on their minds and be reminded to ask for help if they need it. Keeping a family intact through a difficult period can ultimately be one of the case manager's greatest achievements in managing a particular case. The case manager should communicate to the family that she is there to assist in any way possible, whether that means helping the family sort through accumulating bills or preparing for the patient's return home by providing information about special equipment or home care services.

Case managers have to meet people where they are. One of my very first cases—and probably one of the biggest challenges to communication that I have had in case management—involved a gentleman who was injured in an automobile accident and rendered a quadriplegic at a C-4 level. He was on a respirator. His daughter, a nurse on a neurosurgical unit in a major metropolitan hospital, worked over 100 miles away. Although she was absolutely devastated by the situation, as the nurse in the family, she had a great deal of responsibility thrown at her. All the relatives were asking her all their questions. She felt that she had to make all the decisions, and she was having tremendous difficulty dealing with the pressure. Although she probably was very capable, she was beset by conflicts. What if she chose wrongly? She remained confident in making determinations for her own patients, but in this case, she was a daughter and not simply a nurse on the case.

Many of the medical professionals supposed that because she was a neurosurgical nurse on a unit, she knew everything she needed to know. They were talking to her not as a family member, but as a peer. I, as the case manager, became the claimant's advocate and his daughter's advocate as well, making it easier for her to be just the daughter in this particular situation. I acknowledged that she had certain expertise, but I did not make further assumptions regarding her knowledge and skills. For example, when we were researching rehabilitation facilities for her father so he could go into a weaning program and eventually get off the respirator, I gave her detailed information. I did not presume that she knew all the various types of mechanical ventilators, or could, in her current state of mind, distinguish the benefits of one rehabilitation program over another. I put myself in her place—and now I've been in that place.

When my mother had a massive coronary and was rushed to the hospital at 3 A.M., the family looked to me to make all the decisions, especially because I had worked as a nurse in a coronary care unit. I had not been as intimately involved with the intricacies of coronary care for a while, and I would have liked to have had someone who could reassure me. Yet my family said, "You're the expert. Tell us what's going on." I was panicked, I was panicked to death. Some case managers might assume that they can take less of a role in such situations because of a family member's medical background, but I would alert them to the possible need for more tailored assurance and support.

With the C-4 case, I spoke to the physicians involved and reminded them that this nurse was a daughter first, that she had doubts and questions and required shoring up. This intervention was effective and in fact became very important because this was a liability case. A municipal vehicle that was being used for something other than official town business had struck the father. I was referred by the insurance carrier that represented the town, so I was on the absolute opposite side, giving the daughter and her family a reason to doubt my intentions. But because I was able to work nurse to nurse and person to person, I helped her see that I really was not there just for the town, just to cut dollars; I was interested in maximizing the auto policy resources. There was a limit to certain benefit dollars, but there was also a huge lawsuit involved. While communicating with both parties and both parties' attorneys, I kept myself from taking a side. It was a difficult situation, but if case managers keep their goals straight and remember exactly what they are contributing, they can handle such challenging cases successfully.

The Question of Confidentiality and the Question of Cost

In their communications, case managers must assure patients and families that their discussions will be held in confidence. Certain diagnoses (substance abuse-related illnesses, cancer, AIDS, depression, etc.) in particular cause patients to worry about others' knowledge of their condition. Although case managers must tell patients whom they represent (an employer's group medical plan, workers' compensation, etc.), they must also make it clear that certain information will not be communicated to employers or supervisors.

Along with issues of privacy, there may also be worries about the cost of the case manager's involvement: "I don't have the money for this. Who's going to pay for this help?" The case manager should explain how the intervention is being funded and indicate that it does not represent another bill to the patient or family. In most lines of insurance, case management is a claims administration expense and the cost is not deducted from the patient's benefits. Regardless of how the service is being funded, some patients consider it unnecessary. They may also sense that the case manager's involvement reflects another agenda (that of the insurance carrier, workers' compensation plan, etc.) and be wary.

Some referrals may in reality be thinly disguised requests for case managers to serve as medical investigators. Soul-searching is in order here. Case managers have to decide whether these assignments are really the ones they want to take on and recognize the consequences of their decision. Particularly in smaller communities, where everyone knows everyone else, being regarded as the individual who interrogated the local grocer about his back injury can definitely cause future patients to become close-mouthed, preventing effective communication and case management. It is appropriate to tell a potential client that claims investigation is not a case management role.

Documenting the Patient Contact

Case managers should document all of their patient communications, whether in-person or telephonic, regardless of the patient's acceptance or refusal of services. Beyond chronicling a case manager–patient exchange, correspondence can be used to reinforce important messages. For instance, the document may highlight certain aspects of the conversation, such as the statement that the services will not cost the patient anything, thereby offering reassurance to the patient and family.

Communication should flow between case managers and patients and families whenever appropriate: at the time of referral, after the referral, and when new information becomes available. Case managers should write to keep lines of communication open, to reassure an invalid parent's adult child who wants to remain in the loop, or to document a change in treating facilities. Sometimes, a case manager needs merely to send a simple reminder, "I'm writing to confirm that I will accompany you when you go to therapy next week." Letters can help establish consensus among those involved in caring for a patient and create the impression that the case manager, far from being an intruder, is one of the team.

Form letters can be used, but they should be personalized. Easily produced using word processing programs, the customized letter projects a personal interest rather than one governed by routine. The case manager might include words that focus on the patient or family: "I hope your husband is recovering comfortably from his back injury by the time you receive this letter." Or, "I just wanted to elaborate on our discussion. I know we covered a lot of information about burns in a short period of time. I thought this might be helpful." Throughout their communication with patients and families, case managers should strive to position case management as apart from the medical bureaucracy.

The case manager–patient correspondence should document the patient's acceptance or refusal of case management services. In the case of refusal, it should note patient and family concerns and their reasons for declining the service, address them, and leave the door open for future dialogue and possible reconsideration.

The correspondence should reinforce and redefine the role of the case manager. It should explain who is being represented and how the services will be paid for, and it should underscore the point that the purpose of case management is to facilitate a positive outcome for the patient. The case manager might well include some promotional material that is user-friendly and helps the patient better understand case management's role and objectives. The initial letter might close with a statement such as this: "I am sending you this letter and brochure to better acquaint you with our services. I will call you in a few days when, hopefully, we can further discuss some of your concerns." Or: "I look forward to seeing you again at the hospital with Dr. Johnson and your husband. In the meantime, one of our brochures is enclosed to give you a better idea of our services." The letter should indicate that the referral source has been provided with a copy. (Sample patient letters appear in Chapters 9 and 10.)

COMMUNICATIONS WITH PAYER SOURCES

Each payer source or line of insurance (whatever entity is referring the case for case management) places certain restrictions or obligations on the case manager. For instance, workers' compensation in one state may mandate that a case manager perform stipulated duties in a set time period, use specific forms, apply stated criteria in an evaluation, and charge only a fixed amount. In other cases, the case manager has to listen very closely to what the payer is requesting and not begin a program that she considers ideal. Specifically, what does the payer expect? What are they asking for? The semantics of the communication must be clarified at the outset.

Following referral, a group medical carrier usually wants to know how big the case is going to be. Is this long-term, or is this short-term? If it is a plan with stop-loss insurance, another umbrella of insurance coverage, is it likely to reach the stop-loss threshold? If so, maybe the group medical carrier is required by the nature of the policy to advise the stop-loss carrier when the accumulated benefits reach 50% of the threshold figure. Part of the case manager's responsibility might be to predict when that will occur.

For each of the various lines of insurance, the case manager needs to be able to help the referral source to know which are going to be the big cases in terms of time and dollars and what case management can do to improve the situation. Can the case manager get John out of the hospital sooner, move him into a more aggressive rehabilitation program, or work with his employer to modify his job site according to his needs?

In their communications, case managers need to make the effort to tell the whole story and illuminate the issues that do not come across on a piece of paper or a claims form. I think case managers too often report major problems and think the job is done. They say, "Oh, this is horrible," without saying, "Listen, you have a problem case here, but I really think we can make this a better scenario" or "I've found the patient is giving us more to work with than we might have thought initially."

For example, if a patient is getting reimbursement for disability care or income replacement, the physician might not distinguish in his or her reports between stages of disability. My office handled a disability case in which the individual had a diagnosis of postmeningitis syndrome. Month after month, the doctor continued to rubber stamp "totally disabled" on the claims form. Well, the guy was totally disabled for his job at the time, but he was absolutely desperate to go to work again. Nobody knew that, nobody took the time to make a telephone call, and when our case manager went out and saw how motivated this guy was and how hard he was trying, we got him into a computer training program. He made arrangements for his own transportation and attended classes like clockwork. All we needed to do was to get out there and see him and bring back the unknown information. Prior to that, the diagnosis was that his disability was forever, based on the lack of knowledge within the claims department. He had gotten lost in the system, he was labeled "postmeningitis" and "neurological disorder" and everyone assumed his condition was permanent.

Group medical cases are the same. It may well be a horrible situation, but the family members are very supportive, they really want the patient home, services can be put in place, and some serious cost containment and positive results can be achieved simultaneously. Again, case managers must realize they are problem solvers. They must not cut short their communications with payer sources by saying, "Just let me know what you want." They do a disservice to the patient, the payer, themselves, and the case management industry.

The following list describes typical challenges for case managers in communicating with payer sources:

- Because of prior experience with case management services, a payer might have assumptions about what case management can and cannot do.
- Lack of medical knowledge within a claims department can slow a case manager's progress. This is where the role of educator is vital.
- The line of insurance might present problems. A fully insured plan can be more difficult to work with than a self-funded plan, due to

restrictions prohibiting some of the more creative interactions between the referral source and the case manager.

- Sometimes, the size of the company can be a hindrance. I often find the bigger companies are not willing to explore the what-ifs of case management, to take a risk. They say, "We've always done it this way and that's it."

Case managers can clarify a number of issues for employers to keep them better informed regarding case management and its benefits. Employer groups have become increasingly concerned about their possible liability when another individual, such as a case manager, becomes involved and perhaps "interferes" in the patient–physician relationship. To address this, case managers would do well to position themselves as a solution within the complex and complicated system. They should stress their advocacy role—that in general they do not provide "hands-on" care—and that only a very small percentage of employees within a given group require the services of a case manager. Those selected are exactly those who an employer would want to receive special attention: the sick, absentee employee (or dependent) who has multiple problems and whose family is suffering because of it.

It is very difficult for the average case manager to have a conversation with an employer group, especially within large managed care organizations, because there are so many layers of administration between the on-line case manager, the one who develops a working relationship with the employee or a family member, and the actual employer. There are account coordinators, marketing people, sales representatives, and chains of people on both the employer group and the managed care side. Case managers could break through this communication barrier if they were more actively involved in the marketing and account coordination meetings between the managed care company and the employer group. The director of a case management department can speak to the issues of case management at a board meeting or annual review and open a different dialogue with CEOs and CFOs, enabling them to better understand the role and process of case management.

One way to delineate the benefits of case management to employers is to highlight its risk management contributions. Every organization today is familiar with the principles of risk management and with reviewing its overall exposure to prevent occurrences and contain loss. The case manager needs to walk in the employer's shoes and use a comparative example to make her point. How does the employer protect itself against disaster or risk? A manufacturing company executive uses risk management tools such as routine safety inspections, employee instructions on driver and/or plant safety, and procedures to prevent injuries and fires or to maintain OSHA compliance. In the same way, healthcare management includes risk management strategies used to maintain and grow an industry, minimizing loss and damage to your resources, and your employees. Case management is one such strategy.

Case managers can ask questions at that board meeting. What presents the biggest risk to your health plan or the greatest use of your valuable healthcare dollars? Here is what we can do to maximize the use of your dollars and minimize the spiraling costs. An integrated multilevel case management program will manage that small portion of people who present the biggest exposure to your plan and who are driving up costs. As the group entrusted with the fiduciary responsibility of administering your plan and safeguarding your benefits, we target these populations and manage them.

Employers and payers at this meeting should be asking the case manager, managed care organization, or TPA the following questions: What strategies do you have in place to identify these cases? When you identify them, what do you do? Are they selected by a computer system? Do people call them on the phone? What red flags do you use to apply industry standards to an employee group to protect my plan assets from known problems? How do you practice case management? The director of a case management program can explain to an employer how an out-of-work employee with multiple diagnostic conditions moves through the managed care system.

For many companies, the first results of switching to managed care were strong and satisfactory. Large savings were realized as healthy people and young people moved into managed care, drawn by the options and benefits, including mammography, new baby care, wellness programs, and prenatal coverage. The sick tended to stay in traditional plans. Now that HMOs and PPOs have had several years' experience *and* are picking up the Medicaid and high-risk Medicare population group, they are experiencing much more dramatically the effects of adverse selection, and they face what insurance plans did years ago. The catastrophically and chronically sick are using up the greater portion of benefit dollars. A database or outcomes profile will not help deal with these people. We still have to work on our delivery system and use the tools, such as case management, that have proven effective in managing high-cost patient populations.

Case management needs a more widespread and ongoing voice in the boardrooms, managed care businesses, and homes as the personalized, proactive benefit that it is. Too often, people first hear of case management when they or a family member are in critical care. Case managers can take advantage of company newsletters and brochures reviewing benefit plan provisions to introduce case management in a consumer-friendly vein. When case examples are communicated on a regular basis, the real work and role of case management are evident.

The value and benefit of case management also needs to be communicated to the employee. As an example, our company routinely sends out patient satisfaction questionnaires. A local union we were working with sent out its own participant survey on its provider groups. A board of trustees member responded to both questionnaires, and his quotes were used in a report to members emphasizing the case management element of the union's healthcare network.

COMMUNICATIONS WITH LEGAL PROFESSIONALS

Attorneys are rarely called on for case-managed group medical claims, with the exception of certain HIV cases, but are frequently contacted in workers' compensation and short- and long-term disability cases and sometimes contacted in auto liability cases. Above all, a clear explanation of the case manager's intent and role, along with an honest and straight-forward manner, goes a long way toward overcoming an attorney's concern regarding case management intervention. Anticipating questions, all communications should underscore the case manager's proactive involvement in a complex delivery system.

During the early years of case management, case managers allowed attorneys to state the case for case management to clients. Intimidated by attorneys (as some still are), case managers had no comfort level for butting heads with a lawyer who portrayed case managers as out to find fault. When legal counsel said no to case management, there was little further discussion. Today, case managers are more apt to use a negative response as an opportunity to begin a brief public relations campaign. "Why are you denying case management on behalf of your client? I'm really surprised. Most attorneys I know have no problem with the service."

The reasons behind a refusal might have merit. Perhaps the carrier has acted in bad faith; perhaps the client's lost-wages payments or a physician's invoices are being held up unreasonably. If the case manager can resolve the problem, she should do so, thereby demonstrating to the attorney that case management can be a catalyst for positive change.

When an attorney refuses to allow case manager–client conversation, we want to know why. Sometimes it is helpful to write a letter to the attorney, with a copy to the patient/client, to again explain as a matter of record the benefits of case management services, the intended proactive role of the case manager. This letter calls the patient's attention to the attorney's denial of services, should he not already be aware.

There are some attorneys who do not understand case management or who are aggressive and challenging. Case managers have to be articulate and assertive in return. The more comfortable they are with their role, the better job they can do as case managers. If they do not challenge a refusal and transform it into an assent, they are walking away from work and very possibly from a career.

There are stereotypical judgments on both sides. Some lawyers think case managers are claims investigators in disguise, and some case managers see lawyers as litigation hounds. And of course there *are* both case managers and lawyers who are less than professional. On the other hand, there are law firms that are interested in case management and how it can benefit their clients. We need to move past the us-versus-them mind-set. Attorneys want patients to get the best from the healthcare system, and this is what case managers want, too. They want patients to be able to go back to productive lives; so do case managers.

In some instances, the time frame in which a case manager is contacted can confuse communications. When a case manager is brought to a case early on, patients and lawyers alike tend to view case management intervention as more beneficial, and some of the long letters of introduction and initial lawyer–case manager meetings can be avoided. If an insurance carrier refers a case 1 year after the fact because the individual is still not at work and the care costs are piling up, a case manager might have more difficulty portraying the payer as truly concerned and herself as an objective advocate. The claimant is likely to ask, "Where were you 6 months ago?" and an attorney would be smart to ask, "Why weren't you offering help when John had his accident?" A more wary lawyer might question the case manager's intent: Is it advocacy or investigation? Case managers must be aware of politics; the carrier might well intend to tap her for information—for example, What is the HIV status of the ill employee? Is she an alcoholic? Is this a case the case manager wants to take? Can she be credible when the payer's motives are so suspect?

In another scenario, an attorney, unbeknownst to the carrier, might become involved several weeks after an accident. The case manager should obtain the attorney's written permission to work with the patient before continuing on the case.

Case managers will want to maintain ongoing communications with attorneys involved in their cases. Especially when a case manager has a particular concern about a claimant, an attorney can be quite helpful (by obtaining, for example, better cooperation from a patient who insists on drinking or smoking in direct opposition to the doctor's recommendation). By sharing information with and giving credit to attorneys, case managers make them a part of the care team.

As with contracted medical services, the case manager should track whether the claimant is well served by his or her attorney. Many attorneys are cooperative and interested, whereas others are aloof and detached. If the claimant voices a concern regarding the attorney's representation, the case manager can suggest that there are alternatives but should stop short of recommending specific replacements, just as she should not name a certain physician as the best choice.

COMMUNICATION SUBTLETIES

Not everything a case manager communicates is verbal or written. The case manager's overall demeanor projects a message to patients, physicians, and social workers. For instance, many nurses in the habit of wearing comfortable clothing in the hospital environment adhere to the same dress code in their role as case managers. They might wear a skirt and blouse with sneakers rather than pumps. Or, they might go to the extreme of wearing a warm-up suit. At the other end of the spectrum are case managers who don the complete "corporate look" (tailored suit and briefcase) without considering that it could intimidate a patient. Minor modifications, such as not wearing the jacket and walking in with an envelope rather than a briefcase, can soften the image and signal a more approachable person.

Case managers also need to know their audience. When visiting a patient whose home is in a low-income neighborhood, it is preferable not to march in dressed to the hilt in designer labels and expensive jewelry. For appointments with physicians or corporate representatives, the power look not only is appropriate, but also places the case manager on a par with other professionals, affording greater credibility.

Demeanor also extends to behavior. Upon entering a patient's home, a case manager should remember that he or she is a guest. Extending courtesies such as complimenting the decor, taking note of photographs, or kneeling down to greet a young child communicates a genuine interest. Commenting on a patient's new level of skill (such as moving from wheelchair to walker) further assists in projecting the image of a caring professional. When meeting a physician or human resources manager, it is a good idea to express awareness of how busy the office seems to be or to request literature regarding the practice or company.

THE RIGHT MIND-SET

A positive attitude and confidence in one's role are essential for good communication. Case managers who are motivated and even proud of their role as catalysts for change convey the value of case management. Those who chose the profession merely to escape a battered existence in another healthcare role are likely to suffer from low self-esteem and be ill-equipped to meet the challenges that case management presents.

The case manager's role can be extremely difficult and, depending on the motives of others involved, quite disheartening. In fact, certain lines of insurance will present case management assignments that may be layered with bureaucracy and rifts between medical personnel, payer groups, and legal entities. Such cases cause some case managers to be timid and even apologetic. Case managers who feel powerless may resort to an opposite tactic. Rather than withdrawing and becoming subservient, they ride roughshod over patients or others, drawing their "authority" from what they perceive to be the powerful "big business" or insurance company. This approach only serves to alienate people, creating barriers to effective communication.

Case managers need to accept the fact that their job will not always give them warm feelings and provide professional satisfaction. They also need, however, to keep feelings of frustration and disappointment in check, particularly when communicating with patients. Usually, the difficulty with making certain calls to patients lessens as a case manager's experience builds. Moreover, if a case manager views each case as a new opportunity to improve a situation, communication can become a more agreeable aspect of providing assistance.

COMMUNICATIONS AND CARING OVERLOAD: BURNOUT

Simply because of the nature of the work, most case managers' caseloads consist of tragic cases. Many are life-and-death situations; the bulk of them have no happy ending. Yes, the high-risk pregnancy often results in the birth of a healthy infant, and getting a partially disabled person well-situated in a new job is especially rewarding, but the balance between success and tragedy that exists in more traditional healthcare delivery roles is not part of case management. Often, case managers deal with people who are angry at the system, at God for allowing this terrible thing to happen, at themselves for not handling it better, or at the patient for getting ill in the first place. Angry patients and families tend to voice their opinions to case managers rather than physicians. Case managers who try to distance themselves emotionally by totally walling themselves off from the pain their clients feel will lose their ability to be effective because they will stop interacting with those clients. They must create for themselves a balance between success and tragedy by finding an appropriate level of involvement.

There is a fine line between "I have a no-hands-on role" and "I am totally responsible for this person," and case managers must be able to walk it by knowing where the function of case management begins and ends. They must take on enough of the responsibility to help fix problems while acknowledging their limitations. In their former roles as practicing nurses, many case managers were able to offer a quick solution to pain; the proper medication "made it better." But case managers cannot deter a terminal illness or make a dying child well; they cannot keep contracted services or equipment from failing; they cannot absorb everyone's woe. Despite the day-to-day challenges, case managers need to maintain their equilibrium and a strong sense of their role; otherwise they will become overwhelmed and burn out.

When a case manager begins to blow up at associates, dreads the next call or any further involvement in a case, is unable to see any positives in her work, and grinds through cases that appear completely hopeless, she needs to step back and get help on the cases that seem overwhelming. Usually, a case manager is burned out on a few cases rather than on the job as a whole, unless she has pushed herself long beyond the point where she needed to take a break.

One way to avoid taking on too much responsibility for a case's progress is to draw on the knowledge and experience of peers, even peers in another state. By calling, putting thoughts and concerns out in the open, knocking ideas around and getting feedback, it becomes easier to see a situation clearly. Perhaps there is a personality clash with the patient, or maybe the case manager has simply run out of ideas for a successful intervention. Sometimes a case has to be given over to an associate or back to a supervisor. How can a case manager turn over a case to someone else and not lose face with the client? Nothing works better than honesty. Some cases benefit greatly by another's expertise in an area; sometimes all that is needed is a better patient–case manager match.

To prevent burnout, a case manager would do well to understand the parameters of the job and not glamorize it. An RN trying a utilization review or case management role needs to prepare for the role's requirements. Many professions have hazards, and recognition of them is three fourths of their solution.

One problem is isolation. Case managers are often on their own, enjoying minimal interaction with other case managers. They are no longer on the nursing team, and they are not physicians, claims adjusters, or rehabilitation specialists. They interact with all these specialists, but their work places them outside the "inner circle" of an office or professional group. This can lead to a lack of input when facing a problem and a lack of recognition for a job well done. There may be few or no peers providing the "safety valve" of shared laughter or griping. Case managers can combat the isolation by creating a case management "team." They can talk to their contacts in the claims department about their lives and interests. They can make an effort to observe and discuss improvements in patient abilities with the family, choosing to dwell on the joy of progress after all the time spent on the tougher aspects of an illness.

Case managers also need to get out of the case management cycle. The job allows for flexibility, and because the job includes great tension and stress, it is vital for a case manager to use some of that flexibility to provide "fueling up" time. Instead of writing all the necessary reports during the 9–5 workday, the case manager might take time off to attend a child's scout meeting, visit a museum or park, water the garden, or exercise, completing the reports in the evening or on a Saturday morning. Regularly going out to lunch, taking no-work-allowed coffee breaks, and attending at least one annual case management conference are the types of activities that can help keep burnout at bay.

NOTES

1. Cathy C, *Care Managers Working with Aging Families* (Sudbury, MA: Jones and Bartlett, 2009).

2. Cress C, *Care Managers Working with Aging Families.*

3. Cress C, *Care Managers Working with Aging Families.*

4. The Commonwealth Fund, "Medical Errors, Lack of Coordination, and Poor Physician–Patient Communication are Pervasive in Health Systems of Five Nations," May 2003, http://www.commonwealthfund.org/newsroom/newsroom_show.htm?doc_id=223545.

5. Mullahy C, "Satisfaction of Person Served," in *The Persons Served: Ethical Perspectives on CARF's Accreditation Standards and Guidelines*, ed. J. Banja (Tucson, AZ: Commission on Accreditation of Rehabilitation Facilities, 1997), 55.

6. Mullahy C, "Satisfaction of Person Served," 55.

9

The Case Management Work Format and Process

When a case manager receives an assignment, she will make a series of contacts, including one with the patient and family, the treating physician(s) and medical facility staff, the employer, and, if the patient is involved in or considering a lawsuit, an attorney. The information gathered is reported in writing, and planning is coordinated with the payer. The process of case management can be broken into categories: case finding and targeting, gathering and assessing information, planning, reporting, obtaining approval, coordination or putting the plan into action, follow-up, and evaluation. Each step of the case management process involves medical, financial, behavioral/motivational, and vocational management activities. It is vital at each phase that case managers analyze and not simply record or report their findings. (See the case management flowchart presented in Figure 9–1.)

Case finding and targeting encompasses the determination of eligibility and the identification of high-risk or high-cost clients. The way in which a case manager approaches a new case is influenced by the referral source (generally the payer) and the line of insurance. The referral source might be an insurance company with clients covered under workers' compensation, auto, or group medical plans, a Third Party Administrator (TPA) that is paying claims for a client company, a hospital discharge planner, a corporate human resources manager, or a home health services agency. It might be a state Medicaid office with case management services within a line of insurance or a population segment, such as high-risk newborns or children who are dependent on technological medical assistance. In today's growing and diversified market, cases may also come directly from consumers. An individual might contract elder care services and request that a case manager evaluate a family member's capabilities and

Figure 9–1 Case Management Work Format Flowchart.

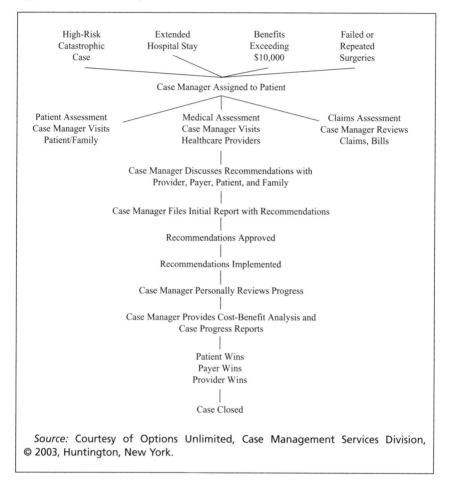

Source: Courtesy of Options Unlimited, Case Management Services Division, © 2003, Huntington, New York.

needs. For the independent case manager, the case might be referred as a "trial run" by a new client she has been soliciting.

Within some larger case management, insurance, TPA, and employer firms, computer software programs are utilized to flag potential cases appropriate for case management intervention. For example, system software can be programmed to pull out every individual with claims totaling over $5,000 or $10,000, each individual with claims bearing the ICD-9 or CPT codes indicating a certain type of illness or condition, or each patient experiencing three or more hospitalizations over a set period of time. (*2003 ICD-9-CM: Professional for Physicians: International Classification of Disease, 9th Edition, Clinical Modification,* one of the ICD-9 code reference books, is published by Medicode Inc. *Current Procedural Terminology CPT 2003* is published by the American Medical Association, which also publishes *ICD-9-CM 2002: International Classification of Diseases, 9th Edition* (Volumes 1 and 2). Medicode publishes *ICD-9-CM Spiral Expert for Physicians, Volumes 1 and 2, 2002, International Classification of Diseases, 9th Revision, Clinical Modification.*)

Other artificial intelligence systems screen cases through a series of reviews. Generally, on the first review level, nurse reviewers might ask 10 standard questions regarding a patient's file. If any of the 10 questions is answered yes, the computer system presents a series of new questions to help single out those cases needing immediate case management attention. The system is making its "decisions" based on data taken from interviews with specialists in various medical fields. The system operator, usually a medical review specialist, answers the computer's questions. Cases are forwarded for case management by the system itself and by the system operator.

There are a range of software programs available, some designating specific illnesses or designed to track progress through a care plan. Computer software can be of significant assistance in finding and targeting cases for case management intervention, but it should not be the sole instrument for reviewing information. It requires the support of a personal interview with the patient, knowledge of the patient's prior history, or an independent professional judgment regarding the data. In other words, the use of computer software should be regularly combined with a case manager's personalized contact.

The variety of referral sources is enormous, as is the variety of backgrounds in case management that referral sources may have. A company recently mandated to offer case management services might be referring its first case and have little or no understanding of case management. A claims examiner might have been told to refer the case and have scant knowledge of what type of report or data to request from a case manager. The source of the case might be another healthcare professional. Large companies and insurance carriers often have in-house medical directors who refer patients for case management. The referral may come from a senior claims person, a physician, or a nurse familiar with case management who coordinates all vended-out services. The source and his or her background will partially determine the information requested, expected, and provided. Case managers must take clues regarding assessment and reporting from the referral source.

GATHERING AND ASSESSING INFORMATION

The accuracy of the entire case management process depends on the information gathered. The process of collecting information might include scheduling a conversation with the referral source (payer), determining policy limits and coverage, interviewing the patient and family, interviewing the physician(s) and the key members of the medical treatment team, reviewing the medical records, holding discussions with employers and attorneys as needed, and determining the availability of community resources.

I always suggest to case managers that they conduct assessments as a reporter first and then as an analyzer of the information. Too many nurses and other case management professionals have functioned like journalists, writing wonderful documentaries about patients but not really telling and selling the role of case management. Because of this, too many client companies and organizations see case managers as observers of care rather than contributors to the care plan. All case managers must be observers, but they must be much more as well. If they never looked beyond "what is wrong with this picture" to "what can I do to improve this," if they never envisioned the contributions they could make—to better the patient's condition, support the family, stretch the dollars, tighten up the treatment plan, coordinate the activities of the providers—then they would be merely a group of reporters who call themselves case managers. With the various functions of case management in mind, case managers should approach each case with an open mind and an eye for problems that must be addressed.

THE R.I.P. METHOD OF CONDUCTING INTERVIEWS

This approach was developed by the Foundation for Rehabilitation Education and Research for a seminar section titled, "Interpersonal Skills for Case Managers."

R is for rapport, the essential connection made by the case manager with the person being interviewed. That connection, which can last 10 seconds or 30 minutes, might take the form of a brief and pleasant introduction, a quick statement of purpose, or a warm comment or observation about the individual, his or her situation, home, or busy schedule.

The *I* in R.I.P. refers to information, the purpose of the communication, be it approval for a previously submitted case management plan, permission for a hospital discharge, or knowledge of the specific medication a patient is receiving. The case manager must focus on the objective of the contact and maintain the contact until she has the background needed to continue the case management process.

Even if the involvement of the interviewed party will be minimal, the conversation should not end before that individual completely understands the next step in the process or the plan *(P)*. The case manager might conclude by saying, "Thank you for letting me visit with you in your home. My report goes to the insurance company shortly, and I'll call you with their comments in 2 weeks." To a physician, she might say, "Thank you for your time (on the phone), Dr. Reynolds. I'll confirm your approval by letter and do everything I can to assist you in making certain John follows his treatment plan."

TALKING WITH THE REFERRAL SOURCE

Prior to beginning an assessment of a case, a case manager (CM) provides a clear definition of assessment and a description of the report she plans to file based on the needs of the referral source (claims examiner, vice president of human resources, corporate CM department head). Not every client wants the same type of initial needs assessment, nor does every client have the same document in mind when an "initial needs assessment" is requested. Because responsibilities for administering claims within an insurance policy are different, client requirements are different. The case manager might work for a company that considers an initial evaluation an on-site personal contact with the claimant, an on-site personal contact with the employer, and an on-site personal contact with the treating physician—a three-point, on-site contact. Another company's "initial evaluation" may be either an extensive phone call or an on-site contact visit with the claimant only.

What is the referral source being asked to do? What is the problem that case management might have a role in solving? Perhaps the case will not merit case management intervention. There is no plain vanilla case management and no plain vanilla initial needs assessment.

Depending on the case manager's type of employment—whether working for an insurance firm, within a TPA, or self-employed as an independent CM, for example—and the kinds of clients served, request-for-service referral forms may be forwarded for completion. Some case managers have developed their own forms, but corporations often have a "Directive for Service" that is mailed to the case manager to utilize at the outset of a case. Perhaps the case manager works in a branch office of a company with national accounts, providing case management services for a large client group. The company might have its own referral intake sheet incorporating very specific data regarding past medicals, file numbers, and so on. A form designed and used by an independent case manager might also function as a marketing tool and include information on the range of services.

Referral form data can be taken in person, by phone, by e-mail, or sent by fax. Again, there are numerous variations that influence how and what information is obtained.

In a workers' compensation case, the payer might ask the following questions: How extensive is this injury? What is my exposure in terms of dollars? How long is this individual likely to be out of work? If the client is paying medical costs and replacement of salary and is also handling liability issues, there may be multiple concerns, with the medical portion being the least important. A case manager accustomed to delivering an intense discourse on clinical aspects of the case will be preparing an initial assessment report that is of little use to this client.

In other situations, the case manager might be called in as an intermediary, perhaps to confirm the status of a case. In an auto liability case, a client might request that the case manager call two doctors or visit the hospital to determine the extent of an injury. If the policy carries $50,000 in benefits and the injury is so severe that the patient will be in an intensive care unit for two months at $3,000 per day, the benefits dollars are already spent. The client may decide that there is no action a case manager could take to save any money at this juncture. In a disability case, the client may have little interest in the course of medical treatment but be especially concerned with whether the disability will be permanent. Therefore, the case manager may be asked to conduct a telephonic assessment rather than make an on-site visit.

Imagine a situation in which a case manager works for a company that has a set policy on procedures and a referral comes in regarding a workers' compensation case:

Case Manager: Kate, you've asked for an initial evaluation of John Jones. Does that mean you want us to visit John, his employer, and his treating physician, or are you just interested in a visit with John?

Payer: We'd like you to conduct a visit with John only.

Case Manager: All right. Are you interested in our customary initial evaluation with a claimant, Kate? It includes a medical history, a current medical status, a vocational history, and a financial profile. It's fairly extensive. I anticipate that it will take me an hour and a half or two hours, and John is an hour away. [If John is represented by an attorney, there is a whole new angle and additional time required for an initial assessment.] Is that what you're interested in?

Payer: No. All I want you to do is go to the hospital and find out what's going on right now. Write it up and get me a report.

Case Manager: OK. Do you have a time limit, Kate, on when this needs to be done, or a specific format for that report? Do you want just a phone report, do you need a letter, or do you want this to be a full report? Do you have any benefit limits? What are you really looking for here? [Again, the case manager needs to find out the desires of the particular client and get as much of the client's agenda on the table as possible. The first case from a referral source is a key case: If the case manager messes it up, she may not get another referral from that payer. If the case manager goes on and on about what "we always do" but the payer has different requirements, the case manager runs the risk of losing the opportunity for future work. She should not make the assumption that she knows what is best for the client; the client is buying her services.]

Case Manager: Does the report need to be completed in 72 hours? Do you have to reserve dollars on this case? Is your home office looking for this information quickly?

Payer: As a matter of fact, I need to get someone out on it right away.

Case Manager: I am sorry, the staff that I have right now that's closest to John already have appointments. If you can wait a little while, I can get one of our other case managers to do it, but it won't be until the end of the week. [A case manager should never, just to get that first case, make a promise that cannot be fulfilled. A broken promise will definitely destroy any hope of future referrals.]

Payer: Well, I am sorry, Jessica. I'll have to get someone else, but we'll give you all another opportunity in the future.

Are there any limits on travel time? The call may come from a regional office in Atlantic City: "I hear you do great work in New Jersey. I need you to send somebody out as soon as possible on this person." Maybe the case manager has a representative in Paterson, New Jersey. She should say, "We can take that, but are you concerned about travel-time expenses? This particular case is 3 hours away from our office. Do you have a problem with that?"

Or, a client may request a particular case manager for the case: "I want Jack to work this case. He did a great job for me on a head injury 3 months ago." The fact that he lives 2 hours away and his travel time will be factored into the case management fee might not matter to the client, but the case manager ought to verify this.

All business details—fees, how much is charged per hour, what service elements are charged (travel, phone, fax, postage), what service elements are not charged (report copies), the length of status reports—need to be clarified. The case manager might give a synopsis: "Our initial evaluation with these parameters probably will take from 6 to 8 hours. Is that in the ballpark of what you would expect?" The payer may feel that is agreeable or excessive. The payer might have been expecting to be charged for 4 to 5 hours tops or might say, "We never pay for travel time" or "We only pay half the rate for travel time." The case manager must then decide whether to work within those guidelines.

It may be that the case manager is busy working a broad client base and may choose not to reduce any of her fees, including those for travel time. It may be that the case management company is big enough, good enough, that it does not need to compromise on prices. The response could be, "Listen, I'm sorry, but our expenses are such . . ." or "In this part of the country, costs are such . . ." The case manager would then close with a request that the payer keep the firm in mind for other cases. On the other hand, the case manager might have been looking for the chance to work with that individual or payer company and say, "Our fees for this are $100 an hour. I understand that seems a little bit high, but I'd like you to see what we do. If you like what we do, maybe we can negotiate a lower cost another time."

Fees can be discussed on a case-by-case basis or can be set, for example, through the establishment of a 2- or 5-year contract. The important thing is to discuss fees openly at the beginning of the relationship and, if rates are raised over the course of the relationship, to communicate that as well.

A case manager should make certain that she is comfortable delivering the type of job a client is requesting. If the case manager feels incapable of completing an accurate and objective assessment of a particular case via the telephone, for example, or thinks there might be liability concerns with a particular assessment issue, the concern must be broached ("I only conduct on-site assessments" or "I've found that all physicians on a case must be consulted for an assessment"). When the criteria are clear, then information gathering may begin.

Prior to beginning an assessment, eligibility for coverage under the specific line of insurance paying for case management should be defined. The case manager needs to discover the client's responsibility on this case, for this individual, under this policy. She needs to have contact information for the employer, the plan administrator, and the stop-loss carrier, if there is one. Often, eligibility has not been ascertained, so the case manager must ask, "What is the line of insurance?" and "Is this individual covered under this policy?" "Is there stop-loss coverage?" (see Figure 9–2.) Suppose the case manager works in the preadmission and concurrent review department of a large company and receives a call that James Jones is in the hospital with multiple injuries. James is named on the policy of his father, employee John Jones, and covered under the company's medical plan. But in talking to John Jones, the case manager finds that James was involved in an auto accident or hurt at work. Therefore, James is not eligible for benefits under his father's group medical plan, because it is an auto insurance or a workers' compensation case.

In the event that a child is covered under a parent's policy, other questions arise. Many insurance policies include a "birthday rule," a clause that states that the insurance of the parent whose birthday falls earliest in the calendar year is considered the primary coverer and the other parent's plan is used as secondary coverage. Perhaps James Jones fell off a ladder while putting up an antenna on the roof of his parents' house. John Jones's birthday is in August and his wife's birthday is in March. In this instance, the wife's coverage is primary and John's is secondary. John's company may have referred James's case to the case manager under the illusion it was the responsible carrier. During a preassessment review, the case manager discovers the correct status and refers the case back to the wife's insurer.

At the outset of a case, the case manager should ask, "How long has the patient been ill?" or "When did the accident or injury occur?" to review the case for the potential of high-risk or long-term cost factors. In general, the more severe the event is in terms of injury, accident, or illness, the more likely the case will be long-term. Rarely does a person in a coma wake up in a day or two and go about the normal business of life. Based on diagnosis alone, a case manager can outline short- and long-term needs. Even if the referral source has little information other than "it's a spinal cord injury" or "it's a traumatic brain injury," the case manager can ascertain that this is a complex case and prepare the referral source for long-term case management involvement. In the meantime, the case manager identifies those actions that can be taken immediately. Then, once the likely scenario becomes clear based on the present state of the individual or illness, the case manager can evaluate the long-term impact of case management on the situation. The line of insurance and the dollars available may determine what can be done. The case manager may devise an appropriate long-term plan but be unable to actualize the plan because of insufficient funds.

Therefore, the next question is, "What dollars are available to this individual within the policy?" For example, an individual holds an auto

Figure 9–2 Employer Group Information Sheet.

OU Group Number: _____   ABR's Group Number: _____

Employer Group Information Sheet

Group Name: _____Effective Date: _____

Subsidiary of/Parent Organization: _____

Main Address: _____

Phone: (800) _____Fax:_____E-mail: _____

Web Site: _____

CEO: _____ CFO: _____

Director of Human Resources (Benefits Manager): _____

Phone:_____ Fax: _____E-mail: _____

Other Location(s) and/or Site Addresses: _____

Contact: _____ Title: _____

Phone: _____Fax:_____ E-mail:_____

Tax ID #: _____ Type of Industry: _____

No. of Employees: _____ No. of Covered Lives: _____

Number of Plans: _____

Type of Coverage:

Hospital (only) _____ Major Medical (only) _____ Comprehensive _____

Short-Term/Long-Term Disability _____ Workers' Compensation _____ Other _____

Funding Category:

Self Funded: _____ Minimum Premium: _____ Fully Insured: _____

Figure 9–2 continued

Bill to #: _____

Health Plan Administrator: _____

Address: _____

Phone: (800) _____ Fax: _____ Web Site: _____

Contact: _____ Title: _____

Phone/Ext: _____ Fax: _____ E-mail: _____

Consultant/Broker: _____ Fax: _____ E-mail: _____

Modem Dial-Up Capability: Yes _____ No _____

Customer Service Line: (800) _____

Billing: _____ Title: _____

Phone/Ext: _____ Fax: _____ E-mail: _____

Case Management: _____ Title: _____

Phone/Ext: _____ Fax: _____ E-mail: _____

Claims: _____ Title: _____

Phone/Ext: _____ Fax: _____ E-mail: _____

COBRA Issues: _____ Title: _____

Phone/Ext: _____Fax: _____ E-mail: _____

Eligibility: _____ Title: _____

Phone/Ext: _____ Fax: _____ E-mail: _____

Prenotification: _____ Title: _____

Phone/Ext: _____ Fax: _____ E-mail: _____

Reports: _____ Title: _____

Phone/Ext: _____ Fax: _____ E-mail: _____

continues

Figure 9–2 continued

Stop-Loss Issues: _____ Title: _____

Phone/Ext: _____ Fax: _____ E-mail: _____

Specific Limit Reports: _____%

Type of Plan:

Indemnity: _____ PPO: _____ EPO: _____ POS: _____ Other: _____

Networks:
Name: _____ Phone: _____ Web Site: _____

Prescription Drug Card: Yes _____ No _____

Name of Plan: _____

Contact: _____ Title: _____

Phone: _____ Fax:_____ E-mail: _____

Mail Order Plan: Yes _____ No _____

Name of Plan: _____

Contact: _____ Title: _____

Phone: _____ Fax: _____ E-mail: _____

STOP-LOSS INSURANCE INFORMATION

Name of Group: _____

Carrier: _____ Policy #: _____

Address: _____

Contact: _____ Title: _____

Phone: _____ Fax: _____ E-mail: _____

Managing General Underwriter (if applicable): _____

Limits: Specific: _____

              Aggregate: _____

Figure 9–2 continued

Does Carrier Require Case Management? Yes _____ No _____
Does Carrier Request Contact from Case Manager? Yes _____ No _____
Does Carrier Request Stop-Loss Advisory: Yes _____ No _____

ATTACHED ARE:

    Plan group number for each division: Requested: _____ Received _____
    SPDs—2 copies (for each plan/division): Requested _____ Received _____
    Cheat Sheets (for each plan/division): Requested _____ Received_____
    Large Claims Info, if available: Requested: _____ Received _____
    Paid Claims History (prior year): Requested _____ Received _____
    VIP List (if applicable): Requested _____ Received _____
    COBRA Enrollees: Requested _____ Received _____

Source: Courtesy of Options Unlimited, Case Management Services Division, © 2003, Huntington, New York.

policy with only a minimal amount of coverage ($25,000). He has multiple injuries and multiple problems and has been in a hospital intensive care unit for 3 days. Would case management be effective in controlling costs? No. The claimant's injuries are severe, he requires high-level care, and all medical treatments being delivered are necessary. The benefit dollars have been spent, but spent wisely.

On the other hand, a group medical plan providing up to $50,000 worth of rehabilitation care may not stipulate that those dollars have to be spent in an inpatient setting. If the claimant has had a stroke, the case manager looks at the available dollars and determines how to maximize benefits while containing costs.

In addition to the dollar amounts, a case manager must ask about limits and restrictions on types of care, care facilities, and lengths of stay. Is there $100,000 or $500,000 for medical coverage? Is coverage limited to 1 year or is it open-ended until a cap of $1 million is reached? Are there restrictions on the number of days the individual will be covered for hospital care? Perhaps the individual is in a coma in an acute care hospital. The case manager should then ask, "Are there any limitations on inpatient rehabilitation? What are the benefits for a skilled nursing facility?" A benefit cap of $1,000,000 may appear adequate to cover all needs, but the policy may dictate very specific ways in which those dollars may be spent.

There are times when case managers can foresee an unsuccessful intervention despite a policy generous in dollars and services. A case manager may not be able to make a meaningful impact because of the limits of a line of insurance; because a number of attorneys have become involved with a case that is in litigation, requiring the case manager to obtain the approval of each lawyer prior to speaking with the patient and in some cases to have the lawyer present for each conversation; or because of a preexisting condition. Case management is undertaken on a voluntary level; a patient pleased with the medical services he or she is receiving may not be interested in any changes. Sometimes, a patient is so heavily invested in a particular team of physicians that he or she discourages or even refuses case management involvement.

Beyond the type of policy, line of insurance, dollars, and limitations, the data that case managers request from referral sources varies slightly depending on the line of insurance. In a workers' compensation case, the case manager needs to know not only the date of the injury, but also the employee's "time and grade," the length of time the individual has been an employee at the company, and his or her position and job responsibilities. How vested is the company in this employee? The founding fathers of a firm may be more likely to make special allowances for a key employee than for a short-term employee with under a year at the company—less is known about him and his contribution.

Salary and the person's status as a union or management employee also become issues in workers' compensation cases, and the case manager needs to be aware of this aspect of finances. Workers' compensation salary replacement regulations vary from state to state. Further, every union negotiates its own salary replacement. A union may dictate that an injured worker receive full salary for a year. This type of financial arrangement impacts a person's motivation and inclination to return to the workplace. Receiving 100% of normal salary can be a strong disincentive, even when the person is well enough to perform a portion of his or her job or work half-days. Lack of income also influences a person's decision to return to work. Perhaps the individual on disability gets full salary for a month and then goes on state disability and receives only two thirds of salary. This may be financially devastating for the family, to the extent that the person might attempt to return to work prematurely. Premature return to a hazardous environment is of as much concern to case managers as individuals who draw benefits for too long. Not everyone reacts the same way to financial stress, and not every family faces the same amount of stress. Some employees are the sole support, and others have partners who work full- or part-time. In the latter case, a role reversal often takes place, and the partner assumes the role of sole support for a time, easing the financial problem.

One question a case manager needs to ask in a workers' compensation case is, "How did the injury happen?" The idea is not to launch an investigation into who was at fault or to elicit background information for use in court but to prevent a recurrence of the incident. Sometimes, an employee will say to a case manager, "I told my boss that this piece of equipment was falling apart" or "I knew the belt on that sander needed to be replaced and I reported it." This may be the third worker injury at that job station in 2 years, causing the case manager to go back to the claims examiner and urge that a risk management team be sent to the job station before another employee is disabled.

There may be litigation pending or in place. If a claimant begins to volunteer information, the case manager must stop him or her from inappropriately discussing the case. The case manager can acknowledge the claimant's anger, state that she cannot get involved in the legal issues, and put the focus back on the case management program. However, certain circumstantial questions may be appropriate. Has the injury impacted the individual's mental comfort level with his or her job? Is the individual concerned about safety back at the sander belt? Seeking answers to these types of inquiries, the case manager can then help put services or worksite modifications in place that will help the patient overcome his or her fear.

Some workers' compensation issues can hinder the case manager's ability to be effective on behalf of the patient and the referral source because they point to hidden agendas being played out. The mentality that leans toward suing and retiring on the proceeds is an obstacle to successful case management intervention, as is a lawsuit involving a piece of equipment or a manufacturer. The case manager might know from the get-go that a company is mistreating its workforce and that the patient's anger is such that the case manager's efforts will be sidetracked. If the role is to minimize the disability and improve the return-to-work outlook, the case manager needs to take an objective look at the situation, realize its lack of potential, and discuss with the referral source whether the continued use of case management is appropriate.

In group medical plan cases, case managers are only responding to medical care issues; there are no return-to-work or lost-earnings-replacement issues. A carrier will not be asking, "When can I expect John back in the office?" Again, key points will be the type of policy, the dollars available, the dollar limitations, the services included in the plan, and the plan's flexibility. Some group medical plans are very, very generous, incorporating provisions for home care, skilled nursing facilities, rehabilitation facilities, and rehabilitation, especially when provided outside of an acute care facility. On the other hand, other policies may include generous benefits for inpatient care and hardly any language supporting an alternative setting. Such limitations may dictate a case manager's degree of success. If the case manager uncovers these limitations as she is collecting information from the referral source and begins to see the intended care plan unraveling, what are the options? Work with half the case management plan? Work the case any way possible? The case manager might go ahead with the full assessment and offer options after ascertaining that there are decision makers who would consider covering benefits that are not outlined in the policy but that are more appropriate to the case and potentially less expensive as well. In group medical plans and fully insured plans, there is often less flexibility, as plan language has been set in stone because it is formulated based on group experience (e.g., premium rates are assigned based on age, sex, and lifestyle). With self-funded or employer-funded plans, even though the plan language may not include provisions for alternative care, there may be more willingness to consider other possibilities.

Like workers' compensation cases, auto insurance and disability insurance cases are governed by state regulations. When taking notes on an auto policy case, a case manager should request information on medical and lost-wages provisions, the amount of dollars available, the covered years, and whether the carrier has direct control of the policy. Is an individual covered for any medical treatment wherever it may be administered? If the auto accident happened out of state, which state's laws take precedence? It may be the state in which the injury occurred, the state in which the policy is written, or the state in which the employer's headquarters office is located. In short- or long-term disability cases, the extent and framework of the policy must be known before the case manager can begin an assessment.

A Wrap-Up of Referral-Source Communication Steps

1. A referral call to the case manager is made.
2. The case manager gets the appropriate business details and confirms the needs of the referral source (e.g., expectations, fees, format, and time frame for reports).
3. The case manager requests case background (e.g., the status of the patient, the diagnosis and prognosis, the type of insurance coverage, the patient's eligibility under the policy, the policy benefit limits, the plan's flexibility, and the restrictions on care).

4. The case manager confirms the initial assessment and report parameters in writing to the referral source and/or payer.
5. The case manager makes a follow-up call to review the confirmation letter.
6. The case manager documents all conversations.

CASE FINDING AND TARGETING

Sometimes, cases are targeted for case management via referral, some are flagged by a software system, and some are spotted by nurse reviewers and case managers during admissions, intake interviews, or initial assessments. To assist our nurse reviewers and case managers, I developed a case management identification worksheet, guidelines, and a "Red Flags" list, which together form an information-gathering tool. Applicable for use in precert departments, managed care organizations, insurance company offices with nurse reviewers, and a variety of other venues in which case management and utilization review/precertification is practiced, the tool's main purpose is to help more selectively identify those cases with the optimum potential for successful case management.

The Case Management Identification Worksheet (Figure 9–3) is used to tally up all our case management indicators; the Case Management Identification "Red Flags" List (Figure 9–4) lists indicators that should "flag" a case for case management review. The Case Management Identification Worksheet Guidelines (Figure 9–5) are exactly that, an explanation of those issues listed under "Reasons for Referral" on the worksheet, such as a request for or need for a service, complications, financial/insurance issues, family/social issues, and paid claims to date.

We have developed advisory forms for case management intervention and stop-loss notification (Figures 9–6 and 9–7). Our nurse reviewers and case managers fill these out when a case is identified for case management services, or when a case needs to be presented to a department manager, claims department, or referral source for approval, prior to initiating case management services. This form includes diagnosis, reasons for referral, type of insurance, our particular case management goals, and whether a claims examiner has been or needs to be notified. The basics of this advisory can easily be reworked to meet the needs of internal or consultant case managers when communicating with internal or client management.

Our Case Management Audit Tool (Figure 9–8) is used as an evaluation tool to track the progress of the patient and our services. The line of

Figure 9–3 Case Management Identification Worksheet.

Date: _____

Nurse reviewer: _____

Patient: _____ D.O.B. (age): _____

Insured: _____ Date of adm.: _____ Date of discharge: _____
                                                              (or unknown)

S.S.#: _____ Admitting diagnosis: _____

Group: _____

  Surgical procedure: _____

  Hospital: _____

  Physician(s)/specialty: _____

Reason for referral for case management—check all that apply

    A ❑ B ❑ C ❑ D ❑ E ❑ F ❑

A. Request or need for: SNF ❑ Rehab ❑   Hospice ❑

            HHC ❑ Infusion ❑ Extended hosp. ❑

           Other ❑

B. Prior admissions & LOS*: _____

C. Complications (existing or potential): _____

D. Financial/insurance issues: _____

E. Family/soc. issues: _____

F. Paid claims to date (if known): _____

     <u>Reviewer</u>   <u>Date</u>

*Attach or refer to system notes _____

* *

<u>Management review:</u>

Accepted ❑

Denied   ❑

  (Reason): _____

Assigned/referred to: _____

Manager: _____ Date: _____

Source: Courtesy of Options Unlimited, Case Management Services Division, © 2003, Huntington, New York.

Figure 9–4 Case Management Identification "Red Flags" List.

Diagnosis or Illness:		
AIDS	End stage or other organ	Neuromuscular diseases
Alcohol and substance	failure/transplant	Parkinson's disease
abuse	Hepatitis C	Psychiatric (anorexia,
Cancer	Head injury	bulimia, substance
Cardiovascular	High-risk infant	abuse, etc.)
Chronic respiratory	High-risk pregnancy	Rheumatoid arthritis
Chronic obstructive	Hip fracture	Severe burns
pulmonary disease	Leukemia	Sickle cell
(COPD)	Liver disease	Spina bifida
Crohn's disease	Lyme disease	Spinal cord injury
Cystic fibrosis	Morbid obesity	Stroke
Diabetes	Multiple trauma	Transplants
		Tuberculosis
Potential Treatment:	Chemotherapy	Monitors (uterine, apnea, etc.)
	Extended ICU	Oxygen (concentrators,
	Home care services	ongoing O_2)
	Hospice care	Pain management programs
	Insulin pump	Rehabilitation (inpatient
	IV antibiotics/IVIG	or day program)
	(other injectables;	TPN/enteral
	Heparin, Lovenox)	Ventilator dependent
Frequent hospitalizations or prolonged confinement:	• Three admits same year for same or related problem • Confinements exceeding 10 days	
Cost of claims:	• Same illness over $25,000 year to date	
Patterns of care:	• Failed or repeated surgeries, hospital-acquired infections, malpractice concerns (quality-of-care issues) • Multiple providers, medications, outpatient surgeries, admissions to a skilled nursing facility	
While patient still hospitalized:	• Consider response to treatment: multiple providers, prior compliance issues, family support, responsibilities issues, complications	
After patient has been discharged:	• Consider patient knowledge of illness, medications and medical directions, involvement of patient/family (have they scheduled follow-up appointments, testing, second opinions, etc.?), satisfaction with medical care —Does patient/family know what to report, to whom, and when?	

continues

Figure 9–4 continued

	—Do they know the treatment plan for the future . . . do they have the ability and inclination to follow it?
Location:	• Complex care delivered in rural setting, small hospital, or facility with poor outcome history
Pharmaceutical profile:	• Multiple providers/drugs, drug interaction potential, abuse patterns, disease management potential

Source: Courtesy of Options Unlimited, Case Management Services Division, © 2003, Huntington, New York.

questioning it presents promotes quality improvement initiatives by helping the case manager think in new ways about the case, in some cases inspiring alternatives if the patient has plateaued or seems stuck. It also helps us monitor the capabilities and development of a new hire.

TALKING WITH THE PATIENT

Following the initial conversation with the referral source, the first person the case manager interviews is the patient. The object is to obtain an overview of the patient's current medical history, the particular individual, and the situation. The case manager must be proactive and non-threatening, perceived as an advocate and viewed as a benefit. The case manager must also encourage the patient to be participatory, which is done by being supportive and not being overly presumptive or controlling. Because the first contact is the key to future success, the case manager must take the time to lay the groundwork. To set up the first meeting or telephone interview with the patient, the case manager should telephone or, in cases where the patient has no phone or contact number, send a letter (see Tables 9–1 to 9–5).

Telephone Call to Patient to Set Up Initial Visit

Case Manager: Ms. Williams, this is Ann Sanders and I am a rehabilitation nurse [medical case manager, nurse case manager, counselor, etc.] here in the Brownsville area. I work with people who have had serious illnesses or injuries. Your workers' compensation carrier [health insurance carrier, etc.] asked me to visit with you to see if I can be of assistance during your recovery. How have you been feeling today?

Figure 9–5 Case Management Identification Worksheet Guidelines.

Instructions for Use

Purpose: The Case Management Identification Worksheet is intended to standardize and ease the process of identifying the most appropriate cases for case management. The upper section of this form has the usual demographic data and needs to be completed by the nurse reviewer.

"Reasons for Referral": This section has a concise "Red Flags" list. Each one of the areas needs to be considered and obviously, if several or all of these are checked off, it is likely to be a serious case, both medically and financially.

A. Request or need for: During the review process, has there been a direct request for any (or several) of these services? Or, does the reviewer anticipate the need for any?

B. Prior admissions and LOS: All prior admissions *and* the length of stay for each should be noted. If there are reference notes or comments, this, too, should be noted, e.g., ". . . see PreCert # 1234 and notes . . . etc."

C. Complications: The presence or potential for complications is always a "red flag" to alert us to quality-of-care issues and/or *other* medical conditions, for example, a post-op wound infection—is it a nursing issue, a compromised immune system, or a matter for an infectious disease specialist? Because case management should be *preventing* complications, we need to be aware of the potential for them, for example, a patient with a stroke returning to a home without other adults *may* be at risk for falls and reinjury. *State the complication.*

D. Financial/insurance issues: Having too little insurance benefits is as much a problem for the case manager as those contracts with very generous benefits and ambiguous language. *State the issue specifically,* for example, traumatic brain injury—only 30 days inpatient rehab *or* 365 hospital days but no subacute hospital benefits.

E. Family/social issues: Patients living alone, patients in rural areas, patients in high-crime, inner city areas, patients with aging spouses, or families in the midst of emotional crises (death, divorce, etc.) are all issues that could signal a need for case management. *State concisely and specifically.*

F. Paid claims to date: When there is access to claims data, it is helpful as a consideration to know how much has already been spent. Enter the dollar amount.

The "Management Review" section is intended to be another screening level to ensure that *appropriate* cases and those with the most opportunity for a successful outcome by a case manager are actually accepted and assigned.

Note: Those cases denied by a member of the management staff need to have the rationale for the denial, for example, family refused.

Source: Courtesy of Options Unlimited, Case Management Services Division, © 2003, Huntington, New York.

Figure 9–6 Advisory: Case Management Intervention.

Options Unlimited, Inc.	ADVISORY	
76 East Main Street		
Huntington, NY 11743	CASE MANAGEMENT INTERVENTION	Advisory Date: ___
Tel: (631) 673-1150		
FAX: (631) 673-8369		O.U. File #: ___

Name:	Title:	S.S. #:

Company Name:	Employer Group:

Address:	Insurance Coverage & State:

City:	State:	Zip:	Tel:	Insured:

Name:	Diagnosis:

Address:	Co-Morbidities:

Tel:	S.S.#:	D.O.B.:

Hospital:	Date of Admission:	Date of Discharge:

Approval for Case Management:

Claimant:	Case Management Approval from other than claimant:
YES: ☐ NO: ☐	Name:
	Relationship:
Potential For Cost Containment:	Tel. No:

Reason for Case Management Intervention: (Please check one or more of the following)

Complex Medical Diagnoses: ☐	3 admissions within year with same diagnosis: ☐
Prolonged Hospitalization: ☐	Transitions to appropriate level of care: ☐
Multiple Treatment Providers: ☐	High Risk/Cost to Plan: ☐

Plan Approval:	Reason for Denial:
Date:	Date:

Notify Plan Via:	Group Renewal Date:
Re-Insurer:	Member Effective Date:

INDIVIDUAL LIMITS:	**AGGREGATE LIMITS:**

Re-Insurer Notified:	Date Notified:

Plan to Contact Re-Insurer:

** IF THIS INTERVENTION DOES NOT MEET WITH YOUR APPROVAL, CONTACT OPTIONS IMMEDIATELY **

Date Received:	Date Assigned:	Assigned To:	Completed By:

Source: Courtesy of Options Unlimited, Case Management Services Division, © 2003, Huntington, New York.

Figure 9–7 Advisory: Stop-Loss Notification.

Options Unlimited, Inc. 76 East Main Street Huntington, NY 11743 Tel: (631) 673-1150 FAX: (631) 673-8369	**ADVISORY** **STOP-LOSS NOTIFICATION**	Advisory Date: _____ O.U. File #:

Name:	Title:	S.S. #:

Company Name:	Employer Group:
Address:	Insurance Coverage & State:

City:	State:	Zip:	Tel:	Insured:

Name:	Diagnosis:
Address:	Co-Morbidities:

Tel:	S.S.#:	D.O.B.:
Hospital:	Date of Admission:	Date of Discharge:

Approval for Case Management:

Claimant: YES: ☐ NO: ☐	Case Management Approval From other than claimant: Name: Relationship:
Potential For Cost Containment:	Tel. No:

Reason for Case Management Intervention: (Please check one or more of the following)

Complex Medical Diagnoses:	☐	3 admissions within year with same diagnosis:	☐
Prolonged Hospitalization:	☐	Transitions to appropriate level of care:	☐
Multiple Treatment Providers:	☐	High Risk/Cost to Plan:	☐

Plan Approval: Date:	Reason for Denial: Date:
Notify Plan Via:	Group Renewal Date:
Re-Insurer:	Member Effective Date:

INDIVIDUAL LIMITS:	**AGGREGATE LIMITS:**
Re-Insurer Notified:	Date Notified:
Plan to Contact Re-Insurer:	

** IF THIS INTERVENTION DOES NOT MEET WITH YOUR APPROVAL, CONTACT OPTIONS IMMEDIATELY **

Date Received:	Date Assigned:	Assigned To:	Completed By:

Source: Courtesy of Options Unlimited, Case Management Services Division, © 2003, Huntington, New York.

Figure 9–8 Case Management Audit Tool.

Options Unlimited
Case Management Audit Tool

Auditor: _____   Case Manager: _____   Pt. Initials: _____
Audit for month of: _____   Date: _____   OU File #: _____

Quality Item	YES	NO	N/A
1. Is the Advisory form current and complete?			
2. Was the case opened in a timely manner, consistent with criteria?			
3. Has the modem sheet been completed, or are the benefits documented in the nurse's notes?			
4. Are all entries in the nurse's notes dated, with billing sheets and noted?			
5. Are patient centered, short- and long-term goals documented?			
6. Documentation of appropriate actions to meet these goals?			
7. Are goals of plan reflected with each patient/family contact?			
8. If a message was left, is there documentation of the nature of the message?			
9. Patient or family contact documented?			
10. Documentation of explanation of CM services?			
11. Documentation of verbal or written permission to initiate case management services?			
12. Documentation that patient information was mailed?			
13. Medical record release of information obtained? (if required)			
14. Is appropriate physician contact documented? (within 72 business hours)			
15. Documentation of diagnosis specific information? i.e., DME, Home Care/Hospice, Physicians, Social Issues			
16. Was contact with the discharge planner/hospital case manager noted? (if appropriate)			
17. Medications noted?			
18. Is there a fax or notation of computer system entry noted within 24-48 hours after receipt of referral?			
19. Were contacts with the frequency appropriate for the level of the case?			
20. Is there documentation regarding whether providers are in-plan?			
21. If providers are not in plan, are there documented attempts at negotiation?			
22. Are fee agreements/alternative treatments present if negotiations were successful (or notation in computer system of same?)			
23. Are fee agreements clear?			
24. Are appropriate records from providers in the record?			
25. If there was drug coverage noted, is there documentation of notification of the needs to use the drug plan coverage?			
26. Is there drug documentation, if appropriate? Re: off-label use of drug, chemotherapeutic agents, atypical treatment, FDA approval.			
27. Is verification of plan language in transplant cases noted?			
28. Re: DME: Is there documentation of provider notification of rental to purchase price only with documentation of both rental and purchase price?			
29. Were outpatient therapy/home care/hospice/SNF/inpatient rehabilitation notes requested and reviewed on a regular basis?			
30. Is there a timely transition to self/family care noted?			
31. Was the initital report done within a month of opening the case?			
32. Were subsequent reports done in a timely manner?			
33. Was a subrogation referral made if potential liability for injuries was involved?			
34. Was the case closed in a timely manner consistent with criteria?			
35. Is there documentation that patient goals have been met?			
36. Re: Case closure: Is there documentation that the appropriate notification was sent to patients/families and clients?			
37. Were case management functions conducted within scope of licensure?			
Comments:			

Figure 9–8 continued

Comments and/or Corrective Action Plan with Timeframes

_____

_____

_____

_____

_____

_____

_____   _____
Case Manager Signature   Date

_____   _____
Director of Case Management Services   Date

COB:ja
Revised 12/2002
MSExcel/P:Reports/URAC file:Case Management Audit.xls

Source: Courtesy of Options Unlimited, Case Management Services Division, © 2003, Huntington, New York.

Table 9–1 Sample Letter to New Client Who Does Not Have a Telephone

Mr. John Williams
132 E. Main Street
Brownsville, TX 84362

Dear Mr. Williams:

I am a rehabilitation nurse [case manager] and I have been asked by your insurance company [name] to meet with you and see if I can provide additional information about or be of assistance in your recovery from your injury [present illness]. In the information that was sent to me, I did not find a telephone number for you. I need to talk with you so that we can arrange a convenient time to meet.

When you receive this letter, would you please call my office collect at (999) 999-9999. If I am not in the office, please leave a message that you called and also a telephone contact number where I may reach you.

I am looking forward to working with you and I hope to hear from you in the next day or two.

Sincerely,

Angie White, R.N.
Medical Case Manager

Source: Courtesy of Options Unlimited, Case Management Services Division, © 2003, Huntington, New York.

Table 9–2 Sample Letter of Introduction to Insured for High-Risk Pregnancy Management

---

Date

Dear Ms. _____:

I enjoyed speaking with you today and, as promised, this letter is to reexplain what my call and our services are all about. As discussed, _____ is a private consulting firm used by *Third Party Administrator* on behalf of your employer group to provide assistance to individuals who may experience difficulties with certain medical conditions.

Diabetes can sometimes make a pregnancy difficult and what we want to ensure is that you and your baby come through it healthy and happy. Our nurse case managers work with patients, their physicians, and families in coordinating the necessary care and services that may be needed both now and in the future months.

This service is at no cost to you and is provided through the benefit plan. It again is not a "hands-on" service, nor is it intended to interrupt or interfere with any care you are now receiving.

In order to determine just how we may be of assistance, one of our nurses would like to meet with you at your home. Because they are often out visiting patients, we ask that you call collect at (999) 999-9999 so that we can put her in touch with you.

Please accept my personal assurance that every effort will be extended on your behalf and our best wishes for a happy, healthy pregnancy and a very healthy, happy baby for you and your husband.

If you have any questions or concerns, please feel free to contact me at any time at the above number.

Warmest regards,

Case Manager

cc: Claims Department

  Source: Courtesy of Options Unlimited, Case Management Services Division, © 2003, Huntington, New York.

Table 9–3 Sample Letter of Introduction for Services Requested for Insured's Child

---

Date

Mr. Thibault Queyroy
13 Bree Lane
Siddleton, New York

Dear Mr. Queyroy:

Please allow this letter to serve as an introduction and explanation of services that have been requested on behalf of your son, Anthony, by _____ Managed Care Services, Group Health Insurance.

Case Management Company is a private consulting firm utilized by Third Party Administrators on behalf of their insureds who may be experiencing difficulties with a variety of medical, psychiatric, and other complicated situations.

These services are provided at no cost to you and are offered to provide assistance and coordination of services that will be necessary both now and in the future. Our role is not intended to interrupt or interfere with any care or therapies that your son is now receiving, nor will our nurse consultants be providing any direct counseling or "hands-on" care. We work with physicians, therapists, the family, and patient, in order that the best outcome is obtained in a manner that is caring, appropriate, and cost-effective.

In order to determine just how we may help, would you please call us collect at _____. One of our consultants would like to arrange an appointment to meet with you, your son, and physician, if available.

Enclosed, please find one of our brochures that describes our services further. Please accept my personal assurance that every effort will be extended on behalf of your son and we look forward to working with you.

Thank you very much for your time and anticipated cooperation.

Very truly yours,

Source: Courtesy of Options Unlimited, Case Management Services Division, © 2003, Huntington, New York.

Table 9–4 Sample Letter of Introduction for a Workers' Compensation Case

---

Date

Dear Mr. _____:

Please allow this letter to serve as an introduction and explanation of services that have been requested on your behalf by _____, the Workers' Compensation Administrator for your employer.

Case Management Company is a private disability management consulting firm that works with individuals such as you who have sustained injuries in the course of employment.

This is not a "hands-on" service, nor is it meant in any way to interrupt or interfere with the care you are currently receiving. The role of our consultant is to work with you, your physicians, therapist, and other health professionals who may be involved to ensure that you derive the best results from these efforts. Our goal is to assist you with a return to a medically stable, comfortable, and productive lifestyle in an employment situation.

In order to determine just how we may be of assistance, one of our consultants, _____, R.N., would like to meet with you at your home. If you have not heard from our consultant, would you please call us collect at _____ in order that we can put her in contact with you.

Enclosed, please find one of our brochures that describes our services. Should you have any questions or concerns, please feel free to contact me directly.

Mr. _____, we look forward to working with you and please accept my personal assurance that every effort will be made on your behalf.

Very truly yours,

Source: Courtesy of Options Unlimited, Case Management Services Division, © 2003, Huntington, New York.

Case Manager: It sounds like you're still having a few problems. I am going to be out in the Hampton area next Tuesday morning. Would 10:00 A.M. be a convenient time for me to drop in and visit with you for a few minutes? [I'm planning to be at the hospital around 9:30 tomorrow and will plan to visit you. As far as you know, will that be a convenient time for you?]

Table 9–5 Sample Letter of Introduction for Services Provided Through a Third Party Administrator

---

Date

Dear _____:

Please allow this letter to serve as an introduction and explanation of services that have been requested on your behalf by _____ of *Third Party Administrator* (TPA), which is the company administrating the health-care benefits on behalf of your employer, _____.

_____ is a private consulting firm utilized by TPA on behalf of their insureds to assist them with the problems resulting from a variety of medical conditions. This service is at no cost to you, and is a benefit provided by the company.

Our nurse consultants work with you, your family, and treating physicians in coordinating whatever care and services are necessary in order that you may receive the best results possible. This intervention is not intended to interrupt or interfere with any care you are currently receiving, nor is this a "hands-on" service.

In order to determine just how we may be of assistance, one of our consultants, _____, would like to meet with you at your home. Because our consultants are frequently out of the office, would you please call us COLLECT at (999) 999-9999 in order that we can put her in touch with you.

Enclosed, please find one of our brochures that further describes our services. Should you have any questions or concerns, please feel free to contact me directly. Please accept my personal assurance that every effort will be extended on your behalf.

Very truly yours,

Case Manager

cc: Claims Department

Source: Courtesy of Options Unlimited, Case Management Services Division, © 2003, Huntington, New York.

If the patient seems hesitant or has questions about what the case manager will be doing in working with her/him, the case manager should briefly explain her role but try to direct the greater portion of her answers to the personal visit. A personal visit, if possible, can help develop good rapport.

Case Manager: OK, fine, I'll plan to see you next Tuesday around 10:00 A.M. Let me give you my telephone number so if your plans change, you can just call me collect at my office. If I don't hear from you, I will look forward to meeting you next Tuesday.

Case Manager: I have your address in my file, but let me get directions to your house. Can you name any landmarks or stores I can note along the way, so I know I'm still going in the right direction?

Case Manager: Those are good directions, thanks. Mary,[1] I've enjoyed talking with you and I'll see you next Tuesday morning.

It is often advisable to send a brief letter, postcard, or handwritten memo to remind the patient of the case manager's pending visit, especially if considerable travel time and mileage are involved.

Initial Evaluation or Assessment

At the initial visit, the case manager's first questions should center on the patient's comprehension of his or her medical condition. What does the patient see as the problem? The patient might say, "My doctor told me I had a heart attack." The case manager can then elicit further information by asking, "What do you think that means? Will it change your lifestyle?" By encouraging the patient to use his or her own words, the case manager can get a reading on the patient's level of understanding and acceptance (or denial) of his or her situation. Perhaps the patient minimizes the illness. The referral source may have told the case manager that the patient has a malignant tumor that has already metastasized to other organs. But the patient says, "Well, I had a growth and the doctor removed it and he said that I should be fine now." It might be that the referral source, the physicians, and the case manager all know the patient's true medical condition but the patient and family do not have a clue. Perhaps the family wants to isolate and protect the patient from knowing his or her true health status. It is the case manager's job to ascertain the reality of the situation by speaking to the treating physician and family members and by getting documentation from the referral source.

A case manager should never assume a patient has the ability to accept a diagnosis. Some of the most brilliant medical professionals are uncomfortable hearing about their own health problems. Patients and their families can block out information or deny the obvious. Case managers must take each person where they are at the time of the assessment and explore his or her view of the situation. Does this particular patient understand that he has had a serious or a minor illness? Does he understand how it is impacting his life now and will impact it in the future? Does he have any knowledge about that part of his body? If surgery was performed, does he understand why? Has his doctor been communicating with him? If he is on medication, does he know what it is for? If he is in the hospital and about to go home, is he knowledgeable about his discharge plan and what he needs to do? What does he need to be watchful for? Does he understand any specific limitations he may have now? Does he accept these? Many patients intellectually grasp such limitations but do not take them in emotionally.

A patient might say, "Yes, I've had a heart attack and I understand that the major wall of my heart was involved." When the case manager asks, "Do you think you can resume all your regular activities?" the response might be, "Oh, yeah, no problem." But the case manager knows that this is not the case. The patient has heard a portion of the doctor's answer, has been selective in listening, and does not have a total grasp of what he or she needs to know to be a cooperative, compliant participant in his or her healthcare plan.

Whereas some patients may be in denial, others are overly dramatic and intent on being a long-term part of the healthcare system. Some patients who have relatively minor problems try to boost them into life-threatening disorders. Having a major illness allows them a respite from life's burdens.

The ideal patient, after having been given good information about his or her condition, accepts that information and is realistic about possible treatments and likely outcomes. Unfortunately, the typical patient in the kind of cases that case managers tend to get may be physically or emotionally overwhelmed as a result of the severity of the condition. The patient might be a poor historian, might be unable to recall information, might be on a life-support system and unable to communicate easily, or might be very young. In a pediatric case, even though family members will be making the "life-and-death" decisions on treatment alternatives and surgical recommendations, the case manager should find out what the child understands. It is part of the case manager's role to make sure every patient has all the information he or she wants and needs about his or her case.

Because past medical history may impact the present, the case manager must also ask leading questions about other medical conditions that might, from a medical management perspective, affect recovery. This is best done by example, as the patient may not perceive how another condition (one that seems minor or that the patient has lived with for years) might influence treatment. For instance, the patient might decide his or her high blood pressure is "nothing" and never mention it. In the case of a patient about to undergo surgery to repair multiple fractures to a leg bone, the case manager might ask, "Have you ever had problems with your circulation, any bone disease or diabetes? Is this a recurrence of an old injury? Have you had prior surgeries or prior hospitalizations?" A person with a healthy, active lifestyle suffering a first injury should be able to recover in a reasonable amount of time given good medical care. An individual who has been through it all before, especially with a knee or back injury, or even one who has suffered similar work-related injuries with the same employer, might experience delays in recovery.

Another important query centers on medications. This area is crucial, and too little attention is paid to it by all members of the medical delivery system, including case managers. A case manager should ask a patient to bring out all the pills and medications being taken, including over-the-counter medications and herbal vitamins, whether or not the patient thinks they factor into his or her condition. There is a gap between what a patient perceives as a problem and what the medical profession knows is a problem.

I was working with a gentleman in New Hampshire who was diagnosed with cellulitis and thrombosis. Recently starting a new job as a security guard, this 275-pound man had been given a brisk physical and had been hired with this preexisting condition because no one really looked at his legs. A member of an HMO plan, he had been seen by a different physician every time he had an appointment, and no one was tracking his needs and care. My role was to evaluate his status as a short-term disability patient.

At my on-site home visit, I found him living alone in a filthy house where he had just shared a can of stew with the cat. One leg was propped up on a chair and the other was on an ottoman. I asked if he had any other medical problems. The answer was no. I then requested that he show me any pills or medications he took.

He pointed to a shoe box filled with bottles, "Well, I've got these water pills here and my sugar pills. . . ."

"What are these for?"

"My diabetes, but that's nothing. I've had it for years." In fact, he also had been diagnosed as having hypertension and emphysema in addition to the diabetes, was supposed to be on a low-sodium diet, and had just consumed a high-sodium lunch.

"And what's this bottle for?"

"I take those when I feel my blood pressure is high."

"How do you know when it's high?"

"Sometimes I get a headache."

It seems that when he was diagnosed as having hypertension, the presenting problem was his headaches. In his mind then, he had high blood pressure on the days he got a headache. In other words, high blood pressure was not a serious condition he felt he had, but a minor problem that might occur on one day or another. We repeated the question-and-answer scenario until we had reviewed all the bottles in the box.

People tend to follow their own rules for taking medications. Case managers need to ask not only "What are you taking for this diagnosis?" but also "Are you taking any other medications?" And as I found from experience, the question needs to be pursued. I might note a medication in the physician's report. When I ask the patient if she's taking it, she will say she is not. Why not? She does not like the way it makes her feel, she doesn't want to become dependent on it, she doesn't want to be taking it forever, or she simply got tired of taking it. Has she told her physician this? No, but she will tell him when she sees him. Her next appointment is scheduled for six months later.

In good situations, the medication manipulation has no unfortunate consequences; however, the ill effects of overmedication or lack of medication can be harrowing. Even if the patient appears to be progressing well, it is important for the case manager, as an individual charged with preventing patients from slipping through the cracks in the medical delivery system, to check this aspect of the care profile.

Another part of a case manager's assessment centers on socioeconomic and psychosocial factors. What are the family dynamics at work? Is the patient a child or an adult, married or single, single and living alone? A person with many contacts, active in the community and church, might have a vast network of coworkers, family, and friends who can become caretakers for a time. A single person new to an area is more isolated and will need, for example, an entirely different medical support system for home care.

What is the patient's vocational status? An active, valued member of a company tends to want to resolve any medical problems as soon as possible. A person recently fired or with a bleak economic outlook reacts to treatment differently. An upbeat, optimistic, well-adjusted patient is more likely to follow a treatment plan. A person whom life has beaten about the head and shoulders could be on disability or workers' compensation for years, electing a "disability mentality" in which the illness becomes his or her job and social life. It is also important to find out about the patient's prior jobs in the event the patient is not able to return to his or her most recent type of employment.

Avocational interests and hobbies also influence a patient's recovery curve. If a patient enjoyed a number of active physical pursuits, such as skiing, golf, and horseback riding, but can no longer engage in them, the case manager should help the patient develop other ways of expressing an interest in those pursuits and remain mentally stimulated during recovery (e.g., an avid golfer might be encouraged to read the biography of a golf pro). Generally, those with the most avocations are more likely to be responsive to treatment. People who are not participatory by nature sometimes have to be encouraged to take charge and fight for their health.

To assist the case managers in my office to conduct effective initial assessment/evaluation interviews, I developed an Initial Evaluation Guidelines and an Initial Evaluation Worksheet (Tables 9–6 and 9–7), which take them through each step of the assessment process, recording the vital medical, socio/environmental, vocational, motivational/behavioral, and financial information needed to create a valid case management plan. The use of this worksheet as a tool for collection of the data also ensures an organized, easily accessible location for referral back to the information. The worksheet coincides with each section of the Initial Evaluation Report Format (see Table 9–20 later in this chapter); therefore, following the worksheet also assists in writing the initial report. I encourage my case managers to review the initial report format before meeting with the patient so that they are familiar with each section of the report and the information to be covered. This preparation helps the initial interview proceed more smoothly, achieving its two main goals of gathering data and establishing a sense of trust and rapport with the patient and family.

Before closing the personal meeting with the patient, the case manager should obtain a signed Medical Authorization Release form (Table 9–8) from the patient or the patient's guardian. Required to review medical records and to share information with the patient's physician(s) and attorney if the case is in litigation, a consent form allows the case manager access to medical data regarding the patient.

TALKING WITH THE FAMILY

After talking with the patient (when possible), the case manager should interview the family for their perception of the situation. Again, it is essential to explain the role of case management, citing examples of

Table 9–6 Initial Evaluation Guidelines

There are several parts to the initial evaluation process.

1. Meeting with the claimant/family.
2. Contact with the primary attending physician.
3. Contact with other key team persons.

There are two basic goals for each of these contacts. First, we need to *gather* as much information as possible from them; second, we need to *establish rapport* with the individuals involved.

The satisfactory meeting of these two goals can be a difficult task, and it requires a combination of empathy and listening skills, adequate preparation, and clear note taking. The difficulty lies in letting the relevant individuals feel important (by the use of eye contact and/or verbal techniques) while obtaining the necessary data. (Remember: the data is indispensable for a valid case management plan, but without the establishment of some degree of trust, it will be very difficult to work with the relevant individuals to actually carry out the plan.)

The Initial Evaluation Worksheet should be utilized as a guideline when meeting with and interviewing the claimant and speaking with other team members. Although certain cases may require additional data collection, obtaining at least the information required by the form guarantees the information needed for the development of a viable plan of action. The use of this worksheet as a tool for collection of the data ensures an organized, easily accessible location for referral back to this information.

The worksheet coincides with each section of the Initial Evaluation Report Format (Table 9–20). Therefore, following the worksheet should make it that much easier to write the initial report. We suggest that the consultant review the Initial Evaluation Report Format prior to meeting with the claimant in order to become familiar with each section and the information required.

In general, the referral of a case entitles us to meet with the claimant and the physician if deemed necessary. Usually, the contact should be made, and a case management plan determined within 2 weeks of receipt of the case. If there is a valid delay in this time line, a *brief* letter should be written to the client (referral source) addressing the reason for the delay.

If the claimant is located farther than 1 to 1.5 hours from your location, the visits to both the claimant and physician should be scheduled to occur in the same trip. The purpose of this is to save the client dollars. This requires appropriate scheduling, with assertive encouragement to busy physicians. Any exception to this should be well-documented and possibly cleared or approved by the client.

continues

Table 9-6 continued

Should the consultant deem that multiple physician visits are a necessity, the consultant should inform the client of the additional visits required to perform an adequate initial assessment.

Source: Courtesy of Options Unlimited, Case Management Services Division, © 2003, Huntington, New York.

activities with other patients in order to help illustrate the case manager's potential contribution.

Due to the stress of an illness or injury, particularly in long-term cases, the family will undergo role changes, dependency shifts, anxiety, anger, and an inability to make decisions. Therefore, the case manager must get a clear picture of the family structure and function prior to and after the illness.

When meeting with a patient and his or her family, it is important to observe the personal dynamics. As an illness progresses, some family members may foster a mentality of dependence on the part of the patient. Although well-intentioned, they are so frightened by what has happened that they become overprotective. They no longer allow the patient to participate in conversation; talk goes on around the patient as if he or she were not even there. "He needs to eat more." "She feels uncomfortable." Sometimes, this is the fault of the healthcare system. Assuming that a patient is too weak or tired or medicated, professionals and family talk about, but not with, him or her. The patient lies in bed and is discussed as if lacking the will or desire to be involved in his or her own care. Such behavior, rather than protecting a loved one, is dehumanizing. If the patient cannot converse, of course, another person becomes the historian, but if the patient can communicate, the case manager really needs to involve and empower him or her. In no way would a case manager want to demean a family member or friend, but it must be remembered that the patient is the patient.

One objective of the initial assessment is to determine how family members perceive their roles. If a case manager sees that one person seems to be taking over the conversation and correcting other family members, some questions must be directed at that person. Perhaps this person has a completely different understanding of the problem than the patient; perhaps the physician has talked at greater length with him or her. If this

Table 9–7 Initial Evaluation Worksheet

DATE:

CLAIMANT:

CASE SUMMARY:

Date of interview:
Place of interview:
Individuals present:
Medical diagnosis/status/reason for case management intervention:

INTRODUCTION

Sex:
Race:
Age/date of birth:
Height:
Weight (prior and current):
Physical appearance (pale, weak, etc.):
Sensorium (alert, confused, cooperative, etc.):
Signed authorization? (if not, reason):

MEDICAL

Recent medical history

Recap of events for this illness only (events leading to point we are at now):

Previous medical care

Prior medical/surgical history including diagnosis, medications, dates, physicians, outcome:

Current medical status and treatment

Current treatment plan, review of medical record (if indicated):

continues

Table 9–7 continued

(What is actually being done medically for claimant at this time, related to current diagnosis):

If appropriate, complete a body system review:

Neurological

Gastrointestinal

Cardiovascular

Urological

Dermatological

Respiratory

Psycho/Social

Orthopedic

Endocrine

Medications

(Types, dosage prescribed, actual dosage taken, reason for medication):

Medical team

(List current treating physicians, addresses, telephone numbers, specialties):

Physician consultation

(Summarize the physician/case manager personal meeting, or telephone consultation):

Date of contact:

Pertinent data:

Physician plan of care:

SOCIO/ENVIRONMENTAL

Family makeup/position in family:

Extended family/friend support:

What is family's apparent understanding and feeling regarding illness and treatment:

Religion notes:

Table 9–7 continued

Cultural/Language notes:

Description of home/neighborhood:

VOCATIONAL

Occupation:

Education:

Impact of illness on work status:

[In Workers' Compensation—Accident and Health and LTD, vocational will be more involved.]

MOTIVATIONAL/BEHAVIORAL

Claimant's apparent behavior:

Understanding/acceptance of current problem:

Claimant statement regarding compliance:

Subjective emotional adjustment data:

Psychological issues:

Substance abuse issues:

FINANCIAL

Apparent financial difficulties?

Retired or active employee?

Medicare eligible?

Disability:

Workers' Comp.:

Multiple insurance policies:

If not a problem, can be stated as such:

SUMMARY/IMPRESSIONS

Subjective data regarding your personal observations regarding the claimant and issues. Put concerns, positive aspects, and case management goals. (If having difficulty creating case management plan, list problems here.)

continues

Table 9–7 continued

RECOMMENDATIONS:

    1.

    2.

    3.

    4.

    5.

ESTIMATED

    Estimated hours plus expenses:

Source: Courtesy of Options Unlimited, Case Management Services Division, © 2003, Huntington, New York.

Table 9–8 Medical Authorization Release

MEDICAL AUTHORIZATION

I, _____ , hereby request and authorize any hospital, physician, or other person who has attended or examined me, or who may hereafter attend or examine me for _____

_____

_____

to disclose any and all information obtained thereby, relative to this injury or illness, to Options Unlimited. I further authorize that this information may be shared with other professionals, agencies, or insurance companies who may be involved in the provision or payment of services that may be necessary.

(Date)   (Signature of Party)

(Date)   (Signature of Guardian)

Witness: _____

Source: Courtesy of Options Unlimited, Case Management Services Division, © 2003, Huntington, New York.

---

person will be the primary caretaker at home, he or she might feel a responsibility to be the spokesperson for the family.

The case manager needs answers to the following questions: What was the primary caretaker's role in the family prior to this illness? Did the primary caretaker run the household? Hold down a job? Does the caretaker still have those responsibilities in addition to caring for the patient? Will the caretaker's job be jeopardized by this illness? How is the caretaker reacting to the illness? Will he or she be a willing participant or be frightened by the disease? What is the caretaker's intellectual and emotional capability? The caretaker might understand the situation intellectually but be emotionally devastated and barely able to cope.

Referral for case management intervention might come 3 months or 3 years after an accident or the onset of an illness, and the case manager might be confronted at the initial assessment with a family member who has been handling stressful physical, emotional, and financial aspects of an illness every day and is now burned out and about to walk out the door. (It is not uncommon for the spouse of a person with multiple sclerosis, after managing the disease for years, to suddenly cave in and leave the marriage.) The family member has used all his or her personal resources and unless someone does something soon, the case manager will no longer have an intact family with which to work.

The case manager needs to look at all the members of the family and determine their physical and emotional health. If children are involved, how has the situation affected them? Is there an older child who is now going to have to assume the responsibilities of one parent, perhaps taking time off from school to help? Are the children really worried because mom or dad may be dying? Is a brother or sister irrevocably injured to the extent of being unable to resume his or her prior place in the family? Depending on their age, children may develop symptoms or illnesses or engage in emotional outbursts as they try to come to terms with the changes in their lives. Even very young children, unable to talk, will sense that some acute changes have occurred and will react in some way.

It is important to ask the family members about their own health as well as the patient's health. Especially if the case manager anticipates that a family member might become the primary care provider at home, even if that possibility has not been discussed, questions regarding this person's medical status are in order. Is the person healthy enough to assist or overwhelmed by his or her own illness? The case manager should also compile a "medical family tree." Are parents and grandparents still alive and well? Do they have medical disorders? In talking to a 42-year-old man recovering from a heart attack who says, "Well, yeah, my father died from heart disease when he was 53," the case manager will know that this individual is not only coping with the fact that he now has a problem, but is also facing his own mortality because of a strong history of cardiac disease in the family.

All these elements—the illness or injury, present condition, medical history, current medications, family dynamics, vocation, and avocation—help point up the pluses and minuses of the treatment plan and help the treating team do their best work on behalf of the patient.

TALKING WITH THE TREATING PHYSICIAN

In 2003, an expert panel of medical directors and directors of case management for leading healthcare organizations across the nation met in a Physician and Case Management Summit, cosponsored by the CMSA and Professional Resources in Management Education, Inc. Dr. David B. Nash, MD, MBA, FACP, of Jefferson Medical College, Thomas Jefferson University and Kathleen Moreo, RN, Cm, BSN, BHSA, CCM, CDMS, of P.R.I.M.E. Inc. cochaired the meeting. The panel had reviewed intellectual and scientific data, and case studies exploring successful collaborations between physicians and case managers. Their goal was to design a framework to establish and improve working relationships between the two groups. The panel identified both facilitators and barriers to effective physician–case manager collaborations. Kathleen Moreo brought their findings together in the "Consensus Paper of the 2003 Physician and Case Management Summit," which appeared in the September/October 2003 issue of *The Case Manager*.

To set the stage for a good working relationship with the treating physician, the case manager should explain the role of case management and communicate a desire to work with the physician to ensure the best outcome for the patient. The physician should be made to realize that help is available for dealing with any problems with the patient that may occur. The more a physician understands about case management, the more collaborative the partnership can be.

One thought toward building better professional relations is to focus on the aspects of the doctor–patient relationship primarily related to healthcare quality. In the paper "Doing Well by Doing Good: Improving the Business Case for Quality," Alice G. Gosfield, JD, and James L. Reinertsen, MD, note that a core activity of physicians is to take healthcare information and transform it into a "higher order of information," to satisfy the fundamental needs of explanation for understanding, prediction of the course of healthcare, and description of needed change. Here is a meeting place for physicians and case managers, a goal they both share.[2]

When I am introducing myself and the case manager's role to physicians, I find it helpful to mention that I have no intention of calling regarding many patients. In general, less than 7% of a patient population needs case management, and that number might be high for some populations. I also note that my job is to support the physician in communications with the patient, to ensure medications, dosages, and the treatment plan is understood and followed. We are patient advocates; at the same time, we assist all members of the care team.

Finding a good time for a personal meeting with the treating physician can be a challenge. A case manager can attempt to reach the physician at the hospital when he or she has just met with the patient or can telephone the physician's office to set up a visit. To smooth the path, it is a good idea to become friendly with a receptionist or nurse in the office.

Initial Phone Contact with Physician's Office to Set Up Personal Consultation

In setting up a consultation with the physician, it is best to address the receptionist or nurse by name if possible:

Case Manager: Good morning. My name is Sandi Miller, and I am a case manager [rehabilitation nurse, rehabilitation specialist, etc.]. I'm calling in reference to Dr. Brown's patient, John Fuller. I've been asked by Mr. Fuller's insurance company, U.S. America, to develop a rehab plan with him. To make sure my plan for him is appropriate, I need to schedule a brief personal meeting with Dr. Brown. [OR: I wonder if you can help me. I'd like to speak with Dr. Brown regarding Mr. Fuller today or tomorrow if at all possible. What would be the best way to contact him?]

[The receptionist or secretary advises that Dr. Brown does not see rehabilitation nurses and she requests that a letter be submitted.]

Case Manager: In some cases, a letter is adequate for a rehabilitation plan. However, in Mr. Fuller's situation, his medical care is very complex, and there are several issues that can't be adequately resolved by letter, because we are coordinating communications with his rehab and physical therapists, as well. I understand that Dr. Brown's time is valuable but it's critical that I have several minutes of his time.

Case Manager: I am willing to flex my schedule as much as possible to get this consultation. Would late afternoon be my best possibility?

Case Manager: Well, because Thursday afternoons are better for you for these kinds of meetings, could I come in about 3:00? I promise I will be brief and to the point.

Case Manager: Fine, I appreciate your help. I will be in next Thursday at 3:00. I'll mail you a confirmation letter with a medical release for Dr. Brown's file. Could you give me your name please in case we need to get back in touch with you?

Case Manager: Jill, thanks again for your help.

Table 9–9 contains a sample conversation of the actual visit to discuss Mr. Fuller's case.

Initial Phone Contact to Schedule Phone Consultation with a Physician

When the case is medically less complex or the physical distance great, a phone conversation with the treating physician is sufficient. Again, it is unusual to reach a physician by phone on the first call, so developing rapport with the office personnel can speed the establishment of a phone consultation date and time.

Case Manager: Good morning, this is Sandi Miller and I am a rehabilitation nurse. I'm calling in reference to Mr. John Fuller, who I believe has been a patient of Dr. Brown's for the past 4 months.

Case Manager: I'm putting together a long-term care management plan for Mr. Fuller, and I have several medical questions I need to discuss with Dr. Brown as soon as possible. Would I be able to speak to Dr. Brown this morning about Mr. Fuller?

Case Manager: Let me check my calendar. I'm going to be out of the office this afternoon after 3:00. If I called around 4:00 tomorrow, would that work?

[Next day]

Case Manager: Yes, Jill, good afternoon. This is Sandi Miller. We spoke yesterday regarding Mr. Fuller, and you asked me to call back at 4:00 for Dr. Brown. Is he available to talk?

Case Manager: Yes, I'll be glad to hold for a minute. I appreciate your time.[3]

What is the physician's orientation to the patient? How long has the physician been treating the patient? Is this a recent illness or has the physician been overseeing the treatment plan for some time? Is

Table 9–9 Sample Doctor Contact Script

INTRODUCTION

"Hello, Dr. Brown." (Shake physician's hand, comment about office.) "I'm the Medical Case Manager working with Mr. Fuller. I saw him for the first time on Tuesday and he seemed to be:

- getting along well."
- having trouble with his medication, his diet, restrictions on his activities . . ."
- anxious to return to his work doing construction, tree trimming, tennis instruction . . ."

If case manager has met with another doctor, briefly review conversation. (Case manager should offer specific information. If possible, offer it in a way that complements the doctor's treatment.) "In order to plan appropriately with you for Mr. Fuller's recovery [return to work, most comfortable and fullest quality of life], I need your direction. I'll be brief; I know you are quite busy. I just have a few questions."

CURRENT MEDICAL STATUS

"How do you see Mr. Fuller's current medical status? Where are we now with him medically?" (Case manager should listen for projected treatment plans and current limitation/abilities, filling in answers to as many questions as possible.)

FUTURE TREATMENT PLANS

"What are your future treatment plans for him [medication, length of treatment, surgery type and timetable, physical limits and duration, etc.]?"

LONG-RANGE PROGNOSIS

"You would anticipate maximum medical recovery when?"

VOCATIONAL ISSUES

"Mr. Fuller's job has been _____. He needs to be able to [case manager describes physical requirements of job]. His employer will let him return with half day/full day/limited activity [describe]. I'd like to set a target date when that might be possible. Would [date] be realistic?"

continues

Table 9–9 continued

RESIDUAL DISABILITY

"At this time, do you anticipate any permanent disability from the injury? If you anticipate permanent disability, what is your estimation of the percentage of this disability after maximum medical recovery?"

LONG-TERM DISABILITY

"I will continue to stay in touch with you through his recovery process."

CLOSING COMMENTS

"That answers all my initial questions. Is there anything else you can think of that I may have overlooked? Is there any way I can be of assistance to you with Mr. Fuller?

"What is the best way for me to contact you [phone, day of week, time of day, through nurse/receptionist]? Thank you for your time."

Source: Reprinted with permission from Interpersonal Skills for Case Managers, *Case Management Practice,* pp. 120-122, © 1993, Foundation for Rehabilitation Education and Research.

---

the physician new to the patient or does he or she have a longstanding relationship as the family practitioner? The physician may have cared for a brother, sister, mother, or father and thus have some insight into the health needs of the patient. Is he someone who is trusted by the family or is he, as in many cases today, a consulting physician who saw the patient for the first time in the hospital and does not yet have a feel for the patient and family? Maybe the physician had an assistant conduct the patient history.

The case manager should hear the patient's status in the physician's own words. I encourage case managers to pursue details by saying, "Doctor, I am going to be asking you some questions that I've already asked your patient. Although you believe you have already done a thorough job of explaining his condition to him, we find that when it all settles in, the information retained is very selective. Patients understand some elements and let others drift away. I need to find out in your words what his problem is. What have you told him? What do you think he understands?"

If I am able to reach the physician prior to speaking to the patient, I explain my reasons for asking about what has been said. "I need to know what you've told your patient for my own information and because, after speaking with you, I plan to talk to your patient and I don't want to tell him anything that you have not. If you feel he has a certain understanding, and when I speak to him I find that it seems to be lacking, I hope you don't mind if I call you. I feel it might be important. Sometimes, we find that patients minimize their disease or choose to 'forget' the parts they can't cope with. This will impact your treatment plan. I want to make sure that we're all speaking the same language—that he has all the information you need him to have to be able to cooperate and follow your care plan for him."

Of course, it is also important to ask the following questions: What is the diagnosis? What is the treatment plan and prognosis? What do you think is going to be the outcome for this individual, both in the short-term and long-term? Do you anticipate any complications? Is there anything you feel you might need assistance with—patient information, lifestyle changes, or diet modifications? The whole physician–case manager introduction process should focus on eliciting and sharing of information and jointly establishing the best way to provide proper care.

The physician also needs to know how the case manager fits into the picture. "I represent the workers' compensation carrier," "I represent the employer group," or "I represent the employer group's insurance carrier for the medical plan, and I wanted you to know that the patient really has limited benefit dollars for inpatient care. Let's make those dollars stretch for the long-term. May I suggest alternatives to you? You may be more comfortable with one rather than the others. Do you have any alternative-care ideas you'd like to suggest?"

When the case manager knows upfront there is a limit on care dollars, he or she has a responsibility to make the physician aware of the limit and share in the goal of using the money in the best way. Although some care options may be ideal, the expenses connected with them make them poor first choices. An alternative plan may not be the ideal, but it will not pose any risk to the patient and may buy care and services over a longer period of time. It also helps to give the physician examples of the kind of work case managers do and to suggest alternatives in a professional but noncombative manner. "These are the kinds of things I have done with other doctors before to help them with patients and they have appreciated it. It is not the patient's fault that there are limits on his benefits dollars. To ignore that reality is to deprive your patient of an alternative that will provide care over the longer term."

Letters of Introduction and Physician Questionnaires

Tables 9–10 to 9–13 consist of sample letters of introduction to a physician, several of which are designed to be sent accompanied by a physician questionnaire, a good tool for obtaining information for an initial needs assessment, as well as for follow-up reports. Table 9–13 includes an attached physician questionnaire, Table 9–14 is a blank physician questionnaire, and Table 9–15 is a completed physician questionnaire with an introductory cover letter.

When there is more than one treating physician, the case manager needs to touch base with all those having an active and ongoing role. The case manager might also discover during the family interview that there was a prior treating physician who may have some very valuable information that even the current medical team does not know.

TELEPHONIC CASE MANAGEMENT

The increasing practice of telephonic case management is not in itself alarming; however, the increasing practice of poor-quality telephonic case management does bother me. I always advocate the in-person visit as an integral element of good case management, yet I understand that in the current managed care environment, such in-person contacts are not always possible. We have case managers overseeing huge caseloads in geographically distant areas; the increasing use of e-mail, facsimiles, and teleconferences; plus the push to manage more cases more cost-effectively, all moving our industry toward the greater application of telephonic case management strategies. I wholeheartedly advocate the telephone as one of the strong and effective tools of our trade. However, my concern is that much can be lost unless the individual practicing telephonic case management is very skilled and devoted to the small particulars of the job.

I believe it is difficult and, in some cases, impossible to provide the tight management required for good basic care unless a case manager is able to meet the patient, see his home environment, and hear how he interacts with his family. But not all of us have the opportunity to manage a case in the best of all possible words. Some view on-site as the most costly case management intervention. They would be correct. An on-site visit can be extremely expensive. However, in the long run, I believe it may be the most effective step to take because the case manager can establish a rapport with the patient and family, and learn much from the interactions (or lack of them) between family members.

Table 9–10 Sample Letter of Introduction to Physician (Neonatal Case)

Date

Dr. _____
Neonatology
17 Smith Street
Morristown, NJ 07960

Re:
Insured:
S.S.#:
Employer Group:

Dear Dr. _____:

As per our previous conversations, I would like to take this opportunity to express my appreciation for your input with regard to the above referenced infant. As you are aware, I am the Nurse Case Manager that was following his mother prior to her delivery. I would further appreciate a few moments of your time to become familiar with Case Management Company.

The services of Case Management Co., a private medical case management firm, were requested by the administration of Mr. _____'s group health policy to assist this family with any problems or needs experienced during the course of this high-risk pregnancy. This benefit also extends to the infant that was delivered as a result, especially in light of his premature birth.

My role as the case manager is not to interfere with but to complement your prescribed plan of care. Having a neonatal nursing background, I can certainly appreciate the complications attendant to a premature birth. By coordinating with you, should the discharge plan include home services of any type, I would be able to arrange for those services while not creating additional stress for the family, and in many cases with minimal out-of-pocket costs to them.

I realize that at this time, it may still be premature to discuss the discharge plan, though a periodic update will enable me to anticipate possible needs and be prepared to implement ways of meeting those needs. As I believe that our mutual goal is to help this family and infant achieve the most optimal level of well-being available, your professional expertise and opinions are greatly appreciated.

continues

Table 9–10 continued

I also realize that your time is at a premium, and am grateful that you have made it possible for me to obtain the updates from your office. It would be very helpful for further communication to occur as discharge becomes imminent so that any posthospitalization care could be put in place in as expedient a fashion as possible.

I thank you for your assistance with this case, and appreciate that you have taken the time to consider the information in this letter. I am enclosing a copy of our brochure to further explain our services, along with my business card. Should you have any questions about this material, or concerns about your patient that you feel we need to discuss, please feel free to contact me at (999) 999-9999.

Very truly yours,

Case Manager

cc: Claims Department

Source: Courtesy of Options Unlimited, Case Management Services Division, © 2003, Huntington, New York.

I understand many case managers are hard-pressed to convince their referral sources that on-site assessment is a necessary element of the case management process. I would ask the bean counters, do you have an idea of how much money your plan pours out each year for noncompliant patients? Other compliance studies show that as many as one half of patients who begin taking antihypertensive medication stop within a year. Twenty-nine percent of people 45 and older stop taking their prescription medication early. Over 10% do not fill their prescription orders, and another 13% receive their prescriptions but do not take them.[4] Such patients' compliance might be better tracked were on-site visits a possibility.

To get the most out of telephonic case management, I encourage my case managers to get behind the "no." If they ask a patient if he experiences any difficulty testing his blood sugar level, and he says no, I have them ask him to give them his readings for the last 2 days. If he cannot provide this, or his response is inappropriate, there is a good chance he is

Table 9–11 Sample Letter of Introduction to Physician to Be Sent with Questionnaire

---

Date

_____, M.D.
_____ Pediatric Association
P.O. Box 5
417 State Street
Oklahoma City, OK 73101

Dear Dr. _____:

Claimant:
Insured:
Employee #:

I have been asked by _____ Companies to provide medical case management services to the above named patient and to assist with any needed medical services. I met with Mrs. _____ and _____ at their home in _____ on July 11th for an initial evaluation.

My business card and brochure describing *Case Management Company* and our services are enclosed, in order to better describe my involvement with the _____. Mrs. _____ referred me to you on details regarding _____ past and present illness, as she was unable to recall specific details.

For your convenience, I have prepared and enclosed a questionnaire that I ask you to complete, along with a stamped and self-addressed envelope. Enclosed, you will find a signed release of medical information form.

Thank you very much for your time and assistance in answering these questions. I look forward to working with you and the _____ and assisting with any needs or services that may become necessary, both now and in the future.

I extend my sincere appreciation for your time and valuable input and I look forward to our future contact. Should you have any questions or concerns, please feel free to contact me at _____.

Very truly yours,

_____, R.N.
Rehabilitation Consultant
RC:co
Enc.

Source: Courtesy of Options Unlimited, Case Management Services Division, © 2003, Huntington, New York.

Table 9–12 Sample Letter of Introduction to Physician to Be Sent with Questionnaire

---

Dr. Timothy James
10 Smith Street
Chicago, IL 60611

Re:
S.S.#:

Dear Dr. James:

Please allow me to introduce myself as the case management consultant, with _____, who is currently following the progress of your patient, _____.

The services of _____, a private medical case management firm, were requested by the administrators of Mr./Mrs. _____'s group health policy, on his/her behalf, to assist him/her with any problems or needs that he/she may experience during the course of his/her illness.

My role as Mr./Mrs. _____'s case manager is not to interfere with but to complement your prescribed plan of care. This is accomplished through my interactions, not only with this patient, but also with you, his/her physician, as well as all other healthcare providers involved with his/her care.

I believe that our mutual goal is to help Mr./Mrs. _____ achieve the most optimal level of well-being available to him/her. To do so, I must anticipate his/her needs based on available medical data and physician input. Your professional expertise and opinions, on behalf of this patient, would be greatly appreciated.

Would you kindly take a few moments of your time to complete the enclosed questionnaire? Please return this to me, at your earliest convenience, to _____, in the enclosed stamped, self-addressed envelope. Also, please find a signed release of medical information.

If you have any questions regarding this matter, please do not hesitate to contact me at _____.

Thank you for your anticipated cooperation.

Very truly yours,

Medical Management Consultant

Source: Courtesy of Options Unlimited, Case Management Services Division, © 2003, Huntington, New York.

Table 9–13 Sample Letter of Introduction to Physician with Specific Questionnaire Attached

---

Date

Dr. Frederick Zimmermann
_____ East 37th Street
New York, NY 10016

Re: Claimant

Dear Dr. Zimmermann:

As I explained to you in an earlier conversation, I am the Nurse Case Manager who is working with _____ at the request of _____, the Third Party Administrator of his healthcare benefits. As his case manager, I have followed him now for approximately 9 months. In that time, I am aware that he has recently had a liver biopsy and is presently awaiting the results. Because of this, and also because he has informed me that his T-Cell count is at 56, I am enclosing a questionnaire that I would like you to complete. I feel that the time for additional intervention may be coming and in order for me to be as effective as possible, it is important that I have some additional information.

Because of the sensitive nature of this diagnosis, I am also including a copy of the authorization that the claimant signed enabling me to obtain such information. You will also note a copy of the _____ brochure, which I hope will help to answer any questions you may have with regard to my role, is also enclosed. Should you have any questions, I would welcome hearing from you.

I thank you very much for your time. I know that your time is a very valuable commodity. I trust that this information will help me in assisting _____. I also hope that this letter will provide an introduction for you so that you will contact me when I can be of assistance to both you and _____.

Should you have any questions or need to reach me with regard to my interventions on behalf of _____, please contact my office at _____ and leave a message. I will contact you as soon as possible.

Very truly yours,

_____

cc: Claims Department

continues

Table 9–13 continued

QUESTIONNAIRE

1. What is Mr./Mrs. _____'s specific medical diagnosis and extent of metastases?
2. In your medical professional opinion, what is the anticipated progression of this cancer?
3. Is his/her condition terminal in nature? As Mr./Mrs. _____'s case manager, I am responsible for providing qualitative yet cost-effective services when needed. This will help to reduce the family's stress levels as well as keep their out-of-pocket expenses to a minimum.
4. What types of therapies are being planned to treat the patient's disease?
5. In your opinion, is Mr./Mrs. _____ a candidate for any home therapy services, i.e., chemotherapy, pain management, hospice care?

Dr. Zimmermann   Date

Source: Courtesy of Options Unlimited, Case Management Services Division, © 2003, Huntington, New York.

Table 9–14 Sample Physician Questionnaire

1. What is the primary diagnosis?
2. Does the patient have any secondary diagnoses?
3. Do you think the patient might benefit from a cardiac rehabilitation program as an outpatient?
4. What are the prescribed medications?
5. What is the specific diet of the patient?
6. What, if any, are the limitations or restrictions?
7. What are your further plans for the patient regarding his rehabilitation period?
8. What is the prognosis?

             Date

Source: Courtesy of Options Unlimited, Case Management Services Division, © 2003, Huntington, New York.

Table 9–15 Sample Letter of Introduction to Physician with Completed Physician Questionnaire

---

A. Edwards, M.D.
808 Olive Avenue
Sand City, CA 91313

Re: S.R.
S.S.#:

Dear Dr. Edwards,

Please allow me to introduce myself as the case management consultant with OPTIONS UNLIMITED who is currently following the progress of your patient, S.R.

The services of OPTIONS UNLIMITED, a private medical case management firm, were requested by the administrators of Mr. R's group health plan, on his behalf, to assist him with any problems or needs that he may experience during the course of his illness.

My role as Mr. R's case manager is not to interfere with, but to complement your prescribed plan of care. This is accomplished through my interactions, not only with this patient, but also with you, his physician, as well as all other healthcare providers involved with his care.

I believe that our mutual goal is to help Mr. R achieve the most optimal level of well-being available to him. To do so, I must anticipate his needs based on available medical data and physician input. Your professional expertise and opinions, on behalf of this patient, would be greatly appreciated.

Would you kindly take a few moments of your time to complete the enclosed questionnaire? Please return this information to me by fax at my office. I have enclosed a copy of the signed authorization for release of medical information for your records. My fax number is (999) 999-9999. Please feel free to call me if you have any questions regarding this letter or my role. I look forward to working with you.

Thank you for your anticipated cooperation.

Very truly yours,

Sandra T., R.N., C.C.M.
Medical Management Consultant

ST:lm
Enc.

continues

Table 9–15 continued

QUESTIONNAIRE

Patient: S.R.

1. What is Mr. R's specific medical diagnosis?
   Papillary thyroid carcinoma metastatic to lung and multiple lymph nodes.
2. Does Mr. R have metastases of his original thyroid cancer?
   Yes.
3. In your professional opinion, what is the anticipated progression of this cancer?
   Sparse data are available; however, disease recurred quickly postoperatively and tumor progressed under treatment. This makes the anticipated progression rapid.
4. Could you please explain the prognosis at this time? As the case manager, I will assist the family with supportive services, when and if the time comes. The information you can supply me can help me with anticipating care needs.
   Have recommended one-on-one counseling for Mr. R, for his wife too, with Liza G., RN, MS Oncology Counseling & "Friend to Friend" Cancer Pt Support Group Program @ Good Samaritan Hospital.
5. What is the current treatment plan?
   Radiation therapy and chemotherapy.

A. Edwards, M.D.   Date

Source: Courtesy of Options Unlimited, Case Management Services Division, © 2003, Huntington, New York.

---

either having difficulty or no longer testing his blood sugar level. In training sessions, I tell case managers to try to avoid asking questions that can be answered by yes or no. Instead of asking, "Are you changing your dressings every day?" ask, "Who is helping you change your dressing every day?" Explore the patient's answer by asking another leading question. Perhaps the patient has said that his rehabilitation experience has been "okay." Ask him, "Are you where you want to be with your new prosthesis? Can you see your level of improvement?" Whatever the response is, you will have more information to work with, and your instincts will pick up on a false answer or potential problem if you are asking thoughtful questions.

The *Case Management Advisor* offered practical tips to help case managers master telephonic case management:

- Be cognizant of how your own experiences and personality affect your impressions of your patient. Have you had a similar experience? How quick are you to make judgments based on your patient's responses? Are you allowing her to speak? Have you made any assumptions about her before placing the call?
- If you are in a hurry, your results will be poor.
- Reschedule the conversation if your patient is under severe stress or in pain.
- Answer her immediate questions before proceeding with other treatment issues.
- If you do not know the answer to a patient question, admit it. Tell her you will get an answer for her, or have another person who knows call her back.[5]

INDEPENDENT MEDICAL AND SECOND OPINION EXAMS

In some cases, an independent medical exam or a second opinion exam is requested. A case manager's involvement is linked to the type of exam performed (see Figure 9–9). An independent medical exam is generally utilized by insurance carriers to determine the diagnosis, the need for continued treatment, the degree of disability (partial or total), the duration of a disability (temporary, long-term, or permanent), and the patient's ability to return to work. Customarily arranged by the carrier (see Table 9–16), it is often seen by the patient as an exam he or she is required to undergo. The physician most often remains in a nontreating role. Depending on the circumstances, a rehabilitation nurse or a case manager may assist in setting up the exam and may accompany the patient, but in most instances, neither the nurse nor the case manager is present at the exam.

When should a case manager expect an independent medical exam to be requested? Such exams are used routinely by some carriers when treatment appears excessive (e.g., prolonged duplication of services, such as physical therapy or chiropractic manipulation), when the recovery time from an accident or injury appears overly extended, or when there is a delay in the patient's return-to-work schedule. They are also employed upon request to authorize surgery, expensive equipment, or unusual diagnostic testing or when there is an increase in the number of treating professionals. Certain diagnostic conditions (e.g., stress disorders) might also signal use of an independent medical exam.

Sometimes, the ordering of an exam results from one of a few administrative practices. Many examiners work selected cases using a "diary" system, in which files are reviewed once monthly. In the third or sixth month, they schedule an independent medical exam if the case is still active. Similarly, if a workers' compensation hearing is scheduled, an independent medical exam is often automatically ordered.

Also used to determine a diagnosis, a second opinion exam is performed to help clarify a complex medical picture or to prepare alternatives to the current or proposed treatment (see Table 9–17). It is typically

Figure 9–9 Comparison of Independent Medical Exams and Second Opinion Exams.

Independent Medical Exams	Second Opinion Exams
Utilized by carriers to determine: 1. Diagnosis 2. Need for continued Rx 3. Degree of disability (total, partial) 4. Permanency of disability (temporary, total) 5. Ability to return to work	Utilized to: 1. Determine diagnosis 2. Clarify a complex medical picture 3. Propose alternatives to current or proposed treatment
Would prefer this physician remain in nontreating state.	Often becomes treating physician.
This physician often becomes involved as an expert witness once litigation occurs—and appears *for* the carrier.	This physician often refuses to do exam if testimony may be requested.
Often viewed as an "ordered" exam by the claimant.	Presented as proactive examination.
Rehab nurse often does not attend (depending on circumstances, however, may assist in arrangements and may accompany claimant). Usually arranged *by* the carrier.	The nurse/case manager usually attends and, in fact, arranges this exam, obviously with carrier approval.

Source: Courtesy of Options Unlimited, Case Management Services Division, © 2003, Huntington, New York.

Table 9–16 Sample Letter to Physician to Arrange an Independent Medical Exam

---

Date

Robert Jones, M.D.
42 Amsterdam Avenue
New York, NY 10002

RE: James Williams
Insured: ABC Woolens
Carrier File #: 110-24
Date of Accident: 2/2

Dear Dr. Jones:

Please allow this letter to serve as confirmation with Jane in your office today regarding the above captioned claimant.

World Insurance Company is the Workers' Compensation Carrier for ABC Woolens where Mr. Williams is employed as an assistant manager in the Shipping Department.

He sustained an injury to his back on 2/2 and has been in treatment with a number of physicians and therapists. Surgery has been performed, followed by a course of physical therapy. For your review, I am enclosing reports from his treating physicians, hospital records, and diagnostic studies. Mr. Williams will also be bringing with him various X-rays and CAT scans pertinent to this event.

We are at this time 1 year postinjury requesting that you examine this claimant and note your findings with specific attention to (1) current status; (2) objective findings; (3) subjective symptoms; and (4) need for continuance of PT and massage therapy and enrollment in a health spa.

You will also find enclosed a copy of a Job Analysis by our medical management consultant. Please note as you review this that the claimant has a mix of sedentary and physical labor, and the owner can accommodate some restrictions in activity. Following your examination of Mr. Williams and review of the Job Analysis, could you comment on his ability to perform in this job? For your convenience, there is enclosed a physical capacities form, which may be useful in your determination of his actual ability to perform the various tasks.

I have advised Mr. Williams of the scheduled date of his appointment, March 30th at 10:00 A.M., and have requested that he confirm this with your office.

continues

Table 9–16 continued

Thank you very much for your assistance and I look forward to receiving your report.

Very truly yours,

Jane Ellis
Workers' Compensation Examiner

Source: Courtesy of Options Unlimited, Case Management Services Division, © 2003, Huntington, New York.

---

presented to the patient as a proactive exam, and the insurance nurse or case manager who arranged for it is usually in attendance. In group medical plans, a second opinion exam is often required prior to certain surgical procedures that the carrier or the latest utilization review statistics show to have a high usage rate (e.g., hysterectomies, hip replacements, cardiac bypass, disc surgery). Often, the physician conducting a second opinion exam will become a treating physician.

A second opinion exam is called for when there is a conflict between potential treatment plans (surgery versus conservative treatment), when the patient requests one, when there is a multilayered medical scenario or a questionable treatment underway, or when the existing treatment plan is not achieving the expected outcome. The diagnosis may call for a second opinion exam, as when the need for a physician with more or different expertise is indicated. Considering the increasing, documented incidences of medical errors, it may be the wise choice to seek a second opinion. In some cases, a second opinion exam is ordered if a treatment is deemed inappropriate or excessive (e.g., when multiple drugs have been prescribed and all of them have the potential for abuse).

To get the most benefits from independent medical and second opinion exams, a case manager should thoroughly understand the purpose of any exam ordered and be specific as to what should be addressed in the physician's report. The physician most appropriate for the diagnosis of the patient should conduct the exam; a general orthopedist is not the most appropriate physician if the claimant is using an acknowledged expert in hip replacement or needs specialized treatment. The examining physician should be provided as much information as possible, including operative reports, diagnostic test reports, X-rays, CAT scans, MRI, treating physician reports, and other independent medical exams, and be given enough time to review all the data prior to the actual exam. When appropriate, the

Table 9–17 Sample Letter to Physician to Arrange Second Opinion Exam

Date

Adam James, M.D.
Director of Orthopedic Surgery
Long Island Central Hospital
New Hyde Park, N.Y. 10021

Re: James Williams
Insured: ABC Woolens
Carrier File #: 110-24
Date of Accident: 2/2

Dear Dr. James:

After discussion with your office today, I am referring Mr. Williams to you for a "second opinion" evaluation and consultation. The appointment is scheduled for June 20th at 1:00 P.M. With your permission and with Mr. Williams' approval, I will attend this appointment.

As a medical management consultant working with this man at the request of World Insurance Company (the Workers' Compensation Carrier for his employer), I am in the process of developing a plan to assist Mr. Williams with a return to a productive and comfortable lifestyle once again.

To date and following an injury to his back on 2/2, he has been receiving treatment and testing from a number of professionals, including an orthopedic surgeon, neurologist, chiropractor, and his family doctor.

He has received conflicting opinions as to the suggested course of treatment, including a recent one for a laminectomy. Mr. Williams has, as would be expected, questions and concerns regarding surgery that he feels were not explained to his satisfaction by his doctor.

As a medical management consultant, it is not our intent to interfere with or interrupt current medical care; however, we do assist individuals in obtaining sufficient information in order for them to make informed decisions about their treatment.

I am enclosing prior to our visit copies of various medical reports and diagnostic tests.

Thank you very much for your kind assistance and I look forward to meeting you.

Very truly yours,

Medical Management Consultant

Source: Courtesy of Options Unlimited, Case Management Services Division, © 2003, Huntington, New York.

case manager should arrange to discuss findings with the physician in person or over the phone following the exam. After reading the physician's report, the case manager should again speak to the physician if the report is not specific and responsive to the initial request for information.

TALKING WITH OTHER PROFESSIONALS

In addition to the treating physician, the case manager may need to contact facility staff nurses, attorneys, therapists, and other professionals involved in the patient's care. If the role of any individual is not understood, the case manager should ask questions. In all cases, the case manager should introduce herself and explain her relationship to the patient.

Initial Phone Contact with Medical Professionals to Set Up Personal Consultation

Case Manager: Phil, my name is Angie and I'm working with your patient [Dr. Smith's patient], Ann Simpson, in developing a rehabilitation [case management] program.

Case Manager: I met with Ann last week and she told me that she was seeing you two times a week for physical therapy [occupational therapy, speech therapy, etc.]. I would like to meet with you briefly to get a better understanding of her current treatment program. Your input is very important in developing a recovery plan.

Case Manager: Ann said it would be fine if I met with you, and I'll have a signed consent form for your file. Would there be any possibility of meeting with you either next Tuesday or Wednesday, preferably sometime in the morning? I only need about 10 minutes of your time and I promise to be very brief.

Case Manager: Next Wednesday at 9:30 is fine. I'll put this time on my calendar and if there is any change, I will let you know. Please do the same.

Case Manager: Thanks again for your time. I'm looking forward to working with you.

After the appointment is set, the case manager might want to compose and send a brief letter, postcard, or handwritten memo as a time-efficient way to reinforce the date of the meeting and help ensure the medical professional will be there.

Part of the case manager's role may involve a review of hospital medical records. To facilitate this, the case manager needs a consent form signed by the patient or the patient's guardian. Next, the case manager must determine the hospital's procedure for medical record review and/or visit. Some hospitals are very formal, requiring that all medical record reviews be completed through the medical records department. Others require a form of photo identification, proof of immunizations, and a signed consent form be presented to the primary nurse, head nurse, or hospital contact. If the case manager meets any challenge to her right to examine the patient's medical records, she should ask to speak with supervisory personnel or the hospital administrator. Case managers do have the privilege of reviewing medical records if they have a signed consent.

In an acute care hospital, the case manager should ask to speak to the primary or head nurse, introduce herself, offer a copy of the signed consent form and her card, and ask about the patient's current condition and any concerns or key issues. The case manager should then request to review the medical records. In a rehabilitation facility, the contact person may be the social worker on the case, a discharge planner, or the primary nurse.

Staff nurses are good sources of information. Physicians have one window; nurses see the patient from a different perspective. They can be good historians. "Yes, we know John says he can test his urine to monitor his sugar level for his diabetes but he really doesn't do it. He's noncompliant. His family brings him treats and we see him sneaking things." Realizing the extensive demands made on hospital RNs, case managers should make it clear to the nursing staff that they are available for use as resources.

Another person to contact is the discharge planning coordinator, who is responsible for posthospital patient services and timely discharge. The case manager should let the discharge planner know that she is involved with the case, will be arranging for the patient's home or rehabilitation facility services, and will get coverage approval from the payer for those services. This frees the discharge planner to devote more time to other cases. Social workers involved with the family can also make a contribution by adding valuable background to the patient profile; they might even have a completed profile already prepared.

In workers' compensation or disability cases, the employer is a chief contact for the case manager. What does the employer know about the patient? How secure is the patient's job? Will the patient have a job to return to? Is the employer willing to modify the work site? Will the employer allow the patient to return on a part-time or reduced-hour basis? What is the employee's value in the eyes of the employer?

To obtain answers to these questions, the case manager should call the employer. If it is fairly clear that the patient's limitations will prevent a return to work, it may not be necessary or appropriate for the case manager to spend time arranging and attending a personal consultation. If the case manager feels that there is a reasonable possibility of a patient taking up a previous or modified job with the employer, a personal visit should be requested. In asking for time to meet with an employer, the case manager should never give the impression that she is coming to try to force an injured worker back to the job.

Initial Phone Contact with an Employer

Case Manager: Mr. White, my name is Cathy Simpson and I have been asked by your health insurance carrier [name of company and/or adjuster] to assist Mr. King in his recovery and then back to work. The records that I have show that Mr. King had been working for you up until March 12th and that he has not returned since his injury. Does this sound about right?

Case Manager: I'm in the process of completing my initial evaluation of Mr. King and I would appreciate having your input on some work-related matters.

[for a personal visit]

Case Manager: I am going to be in the Lakewood area next Tuesday. Could I see you for just a few minutes while I am in town?

Case Manager: OK, what would be a better day? I'll see if I can rearrange my schedule.

Case Manager: I really appreciate your help with this. I'll see you next Wednesday at 1:00 P.M.

An employer can also be part of the treatment plan. The case manager might request the employer's assistance for a patient facing a long recovery process. Fellow workers are usually great at sending flowers and cards at the beginning of an illness; can some contact mechanism be established to help maintain morale over the long haul? Is there an employee newsletter that the patient can receive so he or she will feel involved with the company? Does the company have a sunshine fund, a program that reaches out to injured employees so they do not lose touch with fellow workers?

In some cases, particularly when workers' compensation, disability, or liability claims are at issue, an attorney will also be contacted. (Case managers working a group medical case rarely see an attorney involved in the case before getting in touch with the patient.) In some states and among some employer groups, lawyers are called on regularly for minor cases—a neck sprain or a knee injury and the talk is lawsuit. Some attorneys are very hesitant to allow case management involvement; others approve the service right away. The concern stems from the fact that a case manager representing the employer or insurance carrier might pursue a hidden agenda and quiz or interrogate the client regarding his or her accident or illness.

Lawyers can deny a case manager the opportunity to work on a case, approve the case manager's involvement but refuse personal access to the patient, or allow access but deny full cooperation, setting strict stipulations for case management intervention: "You may only talk to him about medical issues, and you may not discuss his job." Or, "Every time you make a phone call, you must call me and get my permission first." Or, "Every time you have a meeting, I'm going to be there and we're going to tape it."

Obviously, the case manager's contact with attorneys is critical. Regardless of the injury, any time there is an attorney of record on a case, the case manager must contact that attorney and state very clearly who she is, whom she represents, and the purpose of her involvement. It is very important to position case management as a proactive service and to make it clear that the case manager's role is not to investigate the accident, not to find out who is at fault, nor to discuss the circumstances and details of the accident with the patient. (Obviously, it follows that during an assessment the case manager will steer clear of questions regarding the circumstances and events leading up to an accident and avoid trying to establish who was at fault.) The object of case management is to assist with the patient's recovery and eventual return to a productive lifestyle. It is often helpful, prior to calling the attorney to answer any questions he or she might have, to send a letter clearly stating the case manager's role (she is not a claims investigator or a hands-on provider of services), along with a brochure describing case management services and a copy of the authorization the patient will be asked to sign.

Initial Phone Contact with an Attorney

Case Manager: Mr. Anderson, my name is Sarah Craig and I am a case manager [rehabilitation nurse, rehabilitation counselor] with Professional Case Management. I'm calling regarding your client, John Roberts. I have been asked by American Insurance Company, the company carrying his workers' compensation [or auto insurance], to visit with Mr. Roberts to see if I can be of assistance to him in his recovery. I'm calling to ask your permission to contact him and proceed with an assessment of his condition.

Attorney: What's the purpose of your service? What do you plan to do to help John?

Case Manager: My meeting with him and my initial assessment would be to determine if his recovery is proceeding well, if there are any additional medical services which may be of benefit, or if we can provide for his needs in a more efficient manner. I'm not really able to tell you anything specific at this point as I have not had a chance to meet with him and discuss his current medical status. Hopefully, after I talk with him and review the various medical reports that I have, I will be in a better position to determine what services he might need to maximize his recovery. I know you also share this goal.

Attorney: I don't see why his doctor can't handle his medical treatment.

Case Manager: His physician is certainly the one in charge of his treatment plan. However, because I work in his community, I can assist the doctor and help him to fully understand Mr. Roberts' special areas of need in regard to follow-up treatment, his home environment, the type of work he's done, his family support system, and things of that nature. I am part of the physician's team, and we all work to provide the best recovery possible.

Attorney: I want a copy of every report you make.

Case Manager: That's fine. I'd like you to be aware of my work with your client. I'll be glad to check with the insurance company; it's not usually a problem to copy a patient's attorney on our reports.[6]

Sometimes, attorneys request copies of a case manager's reports to the referral source before they will approve case management involvement. When this happens to me, I tell the attorneys that the reports belong to the referral source. If that company or insurer allows reports to go out, I ask them to forward a copy of the report or I send a copy from my office given the go-ahead. However, I suggest that case management companies or departments working with lawyers always first give the report to the client (i.e., the carrier group or the employer) and let the client review it before making the final decision on whether to send it to the lawyers. This is because there might be something in the report that is not as objectively stated as it might have been or that perhaps compromises the client's position. Attorneys should never automatically receive a copy of a case manager's reports; they should be forwarded only with the client's approval. Case managers practicing in states with mandatory rehabilitation programs may have to follow specific requirements in reporting to attorneys.

An attorney may ask a case manager to sign a statement that the case management reports will not be used against the client in a court of law. Such stipulations should be referred to the carrier. It is the carrier's role to agree or disagree with the attorney's terms before case management involvement continues.

If an attorney questions a case manager's qualifications, the case manager should respond to this issue and perhaps ask for a brief personal visit to discuss the role of case management. There are some attorneys who really have not heard of case management before, have no idea what case managers do, and need an overview of the profession. The case manager should outline her experience and education, provide examples of case management work with other attorneys, offer to send literature on case management along with a personal résumé, inform the attorney that a refusal of services is very unusual, and address any objections.

The case manager might ask if the attorney would like to be present at the initial meeting of the case manager and the claimant; sometimes this allays fears that the case manager has an unwritten agenda as an investigator. When an attorney insists on being present at any case management meeting, the attorney's office can be used as the meeting place unless the patient is confined to a hospital or another care facility, is homebound, or needs to be seen by the case manager in his or her work environment. If a meeting time and place can be agreed upon, the case manager should let the attorney know that the initial interview may require up to 2 hours. The attorney may demand that he or she be present at every single meeting. This may not be possible given the case manager's schedule, nor be conducive to the most honest exchanges with the claimant.

In one case I had, the first such meeting was not very productive. The attorney stopped the patient every time I asked a question. The second meeting was a repetition of the first. At the third meeting, the lawyer had a tape recorder running with a microphone attachment. He continually interrupted my conversation with the patient. When I asked how the patient was feeling, the lawyer said, "Don't answer that!" I knew that we were getting nowhere. Because the atmosphere, due to the attorney's level of involvement, was no longer supportive of an effective case management intervention, I suggested to the referral source that we close the file. I believe case managers can meet lawyers more than halfway, but they cannot work around the obstruction created when patients are being coached on their answers.

If an attorney denies case management services, the case manager should try to find out the specific reasons behind the decision and address them. If further consideration is refused, the case manager should thank the attorney for his or her time and close the conversation. Some law firms have a reputation for sending patients to certain physicians and therapists, allowing no other involvement.

To keep all lines of communication and participation clear in a legal case, the case manager should document any acceptance or denial of service in a brief but specific letter to the insurance carrier or payer and the employer group. In addition, the attorney should be sent a letter either acknowledging appreciation for his or her approval of case management involvement or noting his or her refusal. In the instance of a denial, the case manager should document for the record that the attempt to institute case management was a good-faith gesture on the part of the employer or carrier. This demonstrates that help was offered, and it also may alert the Workers' Compensation Board that they may be dealing with an uncooperative attorney.

In my letters, I begin by reiterating the lawyer's refusal of case management services, along with the reasons given, noting that of course I will abide by the decision (see Table 9–18). To make a point, I include direct quotations: "You said you 'believe our involvement will jeopardize a fair hearing,'" or "I never work with case managers." I'm not courting a lawsuit myself, so I am careful in my use of quotation and synopses. If someone slams down the phone in my ear, I may write, "You abruptly terminated our conversation despite the fact that I assured you that I was contributing medical expertise to the case and was not a claims examiner." I also include an example of how I have worked successfully with an attorney in the past.

I have also started sending the claimant copies of letters of approval or denial that go directly to the attorney in workers' compensation, auto, or other liability cases. Several times, once an attorney's concerns or agendas were addressed (or the attorney was no longer on the case) and I was able to speak to the claimant, the claimant asked, "Well, where were you when I needed you 2 months ago?" I was there 2 months ago, trying to get in touch with him or her, but the claimant never knew because the attorney did not relay the information. Not every attorney shares everything with his or her clients. I feel that if it is the client's insurance policy, he or she has a right to know that case management is being offered; the client deserves access to information that can directly impact on his or her physical well-being. The attorney should be sent copies as well, giving him or her an opportunity to clarify any misunderstanding regarding the refusal of case management services on behalf of his or her client.

When an attorney denies case management intervention in a particular case, this does not close the door on an association with a case manager in another case. Case managers are wise to inform attorneys about the range of their work. For example, case managers with expertise in life-care planning are often sought by attorneys looking to settle a claim on behalf of a catastrophically injured child. A life-care plan developed by a

Table 9–18 Letter to an Attorney Who Has Denied Case Management Services

---

Mr. John Smith, Esq.
456 Main Street
Buffalo Grove, IL 34678

Re: William Jones

Dear Mr. Smith:

Please allow this letter to serve as a confirmation of our telephone conversation today and your declination of services that have been requested on your client's behalf by Jane Brown of ABC Insurance Company. You have indicated that you "... never allow companies such as ours to work with your clients. ..."

As you may recall, OPTIONS UNLIMITED is a private consulting firm utilized by ABC Insurance Company and other companies to assist individuals with the problems that may occur following accidents, injuries, or illnesses.

Our goal is to ensure that your client receives the best results possible from the services that are available and is able to return to a medically stable, comfortable, and, hopefully, active lifestyle once again.

Ms. Brown had requested that one of our nurse consultants meet with your client in order to determine how he is recovering from his accident and if he would benefit from our intervention.

Our role is not intended to interrupt or interfere with any care or services he is currently receiving, nor do we provide any "hands-on" services. We, hopefully, serve as a resource for your client and his family in resolving and preventing any further difficulties.

Because our services are at no cost to your client, and can only serve to enhance his recovery process, we were hopeful of obtaining your approval; however, we will abide by your refusal.

continues

Table 9–18 continued

Should you wish to reconsider or if I can answer questions or concerns you may have, please feel free to call me. Also enclosed is one of our brochures, which explains our services further.

Thank you once again for your time.

Very truly yours,

Catherine M. Mullahy
President

CMM:lm
Enc.
cc: William Jones

Source: Courtesy of Options Unlimited, Case Management Services Division, © 2003, Huntington, New York.

---

case manager includes the probable costs of supporting that child throughout his or her predicted life span (medical services, care providers, improving technologies, and inflation costs are all figured in).

The time taken to perform an assessment depends on the needs of the patient and the severity of the injury or illness. A half hour might be required to speak to the recovering patient before preparing a 2-month postoperative update; a half hour might be all the time allowable for an easily tired patient in an acute care setting or all the time appropriate for a patient in the last stages of a terminal illness. To conduct a more comprehensive assessment (e.g., for a patient 3 months into a head injury rehabilitation program following a horrific accident), at least 1.5 to 2 hours should be allotted, especially if the evaluation will include a facility walk-through with a discharge planner. The more providers involved, the more time-consuming the assessment will be. Similarly, more recent injuries and singular injuries often require less time than recurring or multiple illnesses. The case manager needs to review the history involved with events in the patient's care plan, because that information impacts the scenario faced today and the plan for tomorrow. From a liability standpoint, the case manager needs to gather sufficient background for a responsible assessment, uncovering everything that will affect her ability to plan intelligently and completely for a patient's anticipated problems and the attainment of the treatment goals.

Factors to consider in estimating the time necessary for an assessment include the line of insurance, the state of health of the patient (a complex medical chart takes time to digest), the site where the interview will take place, and the number of people involved (e.g., the patient, family members needing support, discharge planner, physicians, nurses in the unit). After a case manager determines the amount of time needed, it is important to inform the referral source.

PLANNING

Case management is a process of identifying and solving problems. The first and key issue is whether the treatment is appropriate and being provided in the best possible setting. Given the patient's diagnosis, current medical status, and prior medical history, is the treatment plan attaining the most desirable results? Does it appear that it will lead to an eventual recovery or have there already been too many complications?

Is the treatment plan sound? Is it appropriate, reasonable, and really necessary for this patient? Is it forcing the patient into any undue hardship or discomfort? Case managers might come across situations in which treatment may be deemed questionable based on their experience or knowledge. Some cases may be outside the limits of their expertise. In medicine today, there are numerous breaking technological advances, therapies, and medications. If the disease is an unfamiliar one, the case manager has a responsibility to become knowledgeable about it. When things look questionable, when results are uncertain, it is appropriate to ask the treating physician or to acknowledge a need for more information. It is also the case manager's responsibility to comment on treatments that, based on her experience, may seem unusual or strange. Of course, tone is vital; no one should blurt out an accusation of mismanagement. The case manager might say, "Listen, I'm familiar with this, this, and this, but I've never heard of this. Is this something new? Is this something that you've had good results with? Why is this patient being referred for this particular therapy? I've seen more situations in which patients are treated with another therapy."

If a case manager notes that a patient is in a poor system of care—the physician is not communicating, the patient is having multiple complications, the therapists are unapproachable—part of the case management role is to serve as a patient advocate. The patient's interests definitely should come first. If the patient is not being well-served, the case manager can help create a better system of care. Patients do not always have the information they need to see their position clearly. They often are not even aware of what constitutes proper care. They might not know that they can access a second opinion, that they do not have to stay in a hospital where the ministrations are miserable, that they do not have to put up with what is going on. A key tactic is to present information to a patient in a way that does not overtly interfere with the patient–physician relationship but allows the patient to understand that this is not the only "game in town." I have had patients who really did not know that their care was horrible. I have posed questions to lead them to acknowledge that, although perhaps the physician was doing fine, two heads are better than one and they might want to talk to another physician. For example, I might ask, "Don't you feel that maybe you should be getting better by now? Are you concerned?"

When it comes to making recommendations to patients, case managers must protect themselves against the liability that could result from steering them toward particular choices. I caution case managers not to make direct endorsements but instead to present numerous alternatives to patients. "You have these kinds of facilities to select from; these are physicians who are board-certified; these are home health agencies that can provide the type of care you need." Obviously, if a case manager knows a particular physician in the community is absolutely wonderful, there is nothing wrong with saying, "I hear this physician is excellent. Here are two others as well. You are free to select anyone you want." Even though the choice ultimately needs to be the patient's, I try to select from physicians that I feel are the most qualified. Knowing people's inclination to grab on to the first name suggested, I might tend to arrange the order in which I present the three options, but I never commend one practitioner to the exclusion of all others.

Is the patient in the most appropriate setting for his or her problem? If, for instance, the patient has a rare or difficult disease and is in a small, local hospital picked by the patient for its proximity to home, could he or she be better treated in a university hospital that perhaps has an entire department dedicated to that disease? Maybe the patient's treatment would be more medically effective (and more cost-effective as well) if provided by healthcare professionals who are more knowledgeable about the patient's condition. Is the care setting the most appropriate and most cost effective? Could care be given anyplace else? John is in the hospital, his surgery has been completed, and now he is being observed and receiving medication, pain or infusion care services, or physical therapy. Does he have to be in a hospital? Could the case manager arrange for the same kind of services in a less costly and even more appropriate setting? In some cases, a patient may recuperate well at home through the use of support services at far less cost and with better results both emotionally and physically for the patient and with less stress on the family.

It may be that during the acute phase of his illness, John was absolutely in the best possible place, but now he needs rehabilitation and that particular acute care hospital may not be the best for rehab. This is especially true for some traumatic brain injury patients, for spinal cord injury patients, some amputees, and some burn center cases. When the acute phase is over and a patient needs focused rehabilitation, he or she is probably best served in an area or center that has personnel trained and equipment designed to deal with the specific disorder. Acute care hospitals are geared to address the acute phase of a range of conditions, medical problems occurring in episodic fashion. They are not well-suited for individual, long-term care. Individuals may go from the emergency room to an intensive care unit. After they achieve stability in intensive care, they belong on a medical or surgical floor. At the earliest opportunity, once they can be effectively managed without all the expensive support services of a hospital, they should be moved to a more appropriate and less costly arena for care—the home or another setting.

How motivated are the care provider and the patient in the current setting? Is the provider looking after the interests of the patient or trying to keep beds filled and services going?

During an assessment, a case manager should also be evaluating the money available and the exposure faced. Whose pocket is it and how large is it? Is there a pile of money, or are there piles and piles of money? If unlimited dollars are available, should they be spent whatever way the providers want regardless of necessity? Sometimes that attitude does prevail. People will say, "I have $2 million worth of coverage" or "I called my insurance company and they said I have lots of insurance dollars and I don't have to worry." In my mind, it is not responsible in the healthcare delivery system today to spend money just because it exists or just to line the pockets of providers. I look for the "value-locked dollar" for a demonstration that the treatment is necessary, reasonable, and will achieve good results and that the treatment plan is the most cost-effective way to provide the requisite care.

What impact will the costs of medical equipment, supplies, and therapies have? During an assessment, one indicator of greater exposure is any ongoing condition requiring home care services, infusion care services, total parenteral nutrition (TPN, which can run from $165 to $450 per day depending on the provider), pain control medication (for cancer or chronic pain patients), inpatient or outpatient rehabilitation services, or any other intervention that lasts more than a few episodes. Case managers ought to pay particular attention during an assessment in which such services are involved because their price, quality, and delivery sites vary so greatly. For example, the intensity and frequency of activity multiplies when a patient is moved from the hospital to a home or alternative care setting. This is because the case manager must contract for bits and pieces of services as well as rent or purchase equipment. The case manager must examine what is already in place, look at ultimate costs, and evaluate where and how her time can be best spent. Can the cost of the facility, of equipment, or of drugs be negotiated or bid to bring it down? The expense in time and energy, however, might make haggling a $100 item down to $75 virtually wasted effort. (Note that case management should never be driven solely by costs. If a case manager starts operating with the mind-set that everything is too expensive and that the role of case management is just to save money, then she is laying the groundwork for potential legal action.)

In some cases, cost is not the determining factor. For a patient with a brain injury, an acute care hospital may be the best setting for the first several days or weeks of care. Then, the patient needs to be placed in a traumatic brain injury or coma stimulation recovery program. This might not be less costly and, in some cases, is even more expensive. The case manager must look at the patient's needs and how they can be best met in terms of quality and cost. One factor should never drive the others; there must be an equilibrium among the three. If John is going to be at risk as a result of moving him out of a hospital and bringing him home, with services, obviously the move home is not an acceptable alternative. If he can be moved to a less costly setting where the same results can be achieved in a more cost-effective manner, the case manager should try to get the patient and treating physician to agree to that move.

What is going to happen to the patient and how much is this case going to cost the payer or employer if there is no case management intervention? Is it a good case for such intervention? What can the case manager bring to the table? Is the patient's condition and the patient–family support system going to improve with case management, or will case management be just another layer of expense? The system of care already set in place might be good, medically sound, and conservative in its use of care dollars; the patient may be willing and able to follow care instructions, complications may be minimal at present, and the family may be aware of who to call for help. What more could case management offer? In these instances, a case manager must be honest and admit case management has no real role to play.

Sometimes, however, case management, although having no current value, could offer support down the road when the patient's condition is likely to deteriorate. The medical care required will become more complex, and additional services will need to be coordinated. In the meantime, the case manager does not want to drive up costs by going out to visit the patient every month, but neither does she want to totally pull back and be out of communication, waiting for complications to occur. The lost connection could mean less effective management. In such a situation, the case manager might suggest maintaining contact through regular semimonthly, monthly, or bimonthly phone calls.

In light of the information gleaned through conversations with the patient, family, and members of the care team, what is the most reasonable approach to each problem or issue? What are the alternatives to the current care plan? What are the options for future care? How much will the current or alternative plans cost?

Sometimes there are so many problems that a case manager hardly knows where to begin. Often, newer case managers become overwhelmed, thinking they have to identify every single complication or need and come up with all the recommendations for treatment forever. In reality, a case manager simply must show that there are going to be some long-term problems that eventually need to be dealt with by the case management plan and that there are short-term needs that can be addressed immediately and resolved. Long-term plans for chronic cases include short-term goals and long-term vision. The case manager's job is to know where everyone wants to go and then, in measurable steps, follow the procedures necessary to ensure that the ultimate goals are attainable.

REPORTING

As mentioned previously, the nature of the referral source or payer subtly affects communications from the initial assessment through the reporting stage. The focus should be on client needs at all times, and the information must be balanced to present an accurate picture. A report back to the client should include those things the client is most concerned about. In a disability case in which the client is the employer and the case manager goes on and on about the patient's medical condition but ignores return-to-work issues, the case manager has not really met the client's needs. However, when reporting to a claims supervisor or a workers' compensation examiner, a case manager should include specific medical information in the form of parenthetical explanations to help the readers properly interpret the medical terms they will see in other case reports regarding the diagnosis or prognosis. Even if a case manager is not obligated to send out a report (less and less likely, as outcomes management is an important part of healthcare delivery and our role in the system), such documentation is required for internal accountability.

A case manager in a case management company will probably get referrals from different lines of insurance. If the case manager works in an insurance company and the insurance is basically group medical, she will address medical issues for the most part. However, occasionally the case manager might be required to handle a case referred for workers' compensation evaluation or long-term disability evaluation in which the focus is not necessarily strictly medical.

In workers' compensation cases, carriers are responsible for both medical costs and lost earnings. There usually is "reserving of dollars," in which money is put aside to pay for long-term expenses incurred in big cases. Most workers' compensation administrators or claims departments want to know the extent of medical involvement, the severity of injury, the likelihood that there will be some permanent incapacitation, the potential for a full recovery, the length of medical treatment (episodic or continuous), and the need for long-term or enduring medical services.

The first question might be, will the person be able to go back to his or her prior job? If so, at what point is that likely to occur? If John cannot go back immediately, will he be able to go back at some point? In the meantime, can he return to a modified version of his job, perhaps part-time (reduced hours or reduced number of days per week)? Maybe he could work full-time but with one aspect or task taken away? If he cannot go back to the same employer in a modified job (likely in the case of catastrophic injuries), what past vocational and current avocational capabilities does he possess? What is the likelihood that some kind of employment will be possible for him? Did he only possess specific physical skills? Can he use his work knowledge in some other kind of job? Some people lack transferable skills, have only minimal skills, or have transferable skills but no job site in their part of the country where they can be applied. Then, the case manager needs to look at other alternatives. Past skills or hobbies often have the potential to be developed into viable job skills.

In long-term disability cases, the payer is mainly concerned with disability issues. Many policies have HISOCC (how long he will continue to be disabled for his own job) or ANYOCC (how long he will continue to be unable to work in any job) provisions. (For a more extensive discussion of HISOCC and ANYOCC, please see Chapter 4.) These issues are critical because, unlike workers' compensation, a long-term disability carrier does not pay for medical expenses. Disability insurance replaces lost wages, period. Therefore, the payer is less concerned with the intricacies of medical problems, even though the medical condition is often at the base of any disability. While focusing on work-related issues, case managers also need to keep long-term disability carriers aware of unresolved medical issues because managing those often brings a speedier resolution to the lost-wages situation.

Conversely, group medical payers are not particularly interested in return-to-work or socioenvironmental issues. However, from a case management perspective, these issues impact an individual's recovery ability. A group medical carrier may not require a great deal of information but should get some basics (e.g., the injury occurred at work, the claimant is a valued member of the workforce, she is going to be able to go back, her employer has already told her there is a job for her). These things make a big difference in how a person views him- or herself and are absolutely integrated with recovery from injury or illness.

The frequency and length of case management reports should be confirmed with the referral sources. The nature of the reports is an area of concern for many payers today because of their cost and perceived usefulness.

There are some case management companies specializing in workers' compensation that have a report format that everyone uses for workers' compensation cases. When a group medical case comes in, however, the same report format is used. This format might include a vocational assessment section that calls for a lengthy discussion of work site, transferable skills, return-to-work potential, and so on. As a result, a report on an employee's wife, for example, might include a description of transferable skills and her ability to push and pull and bend. Who cares? Return-to-work issues have no relevance. Someone was on automatic pilot, and the group medical payer has been charged for wasted case management assessment time and report-writing time. Case managers must concentrate on the particular situation, the particular line of insurance, the payer, and the particular needs of the patient. There is no all-purpose case management report.

In my opinion, reports should be written at least once a month. All pertinent case activity should be recorded in a specific, regular format. Clients should not be punished with months' worth of case work attached to a large invoice. Most of the discussion will be old news. By reporting in manageable increments of 3 weeks or a month, case managers gain better control of client files and their cash flow. Significant activity or events requiring clarification should be reported in a timely fashion, first by phone and subsequently through written documentation (within a few days). For example, a case manager who has visited a patient ready for discharge from the hospital and noted that everything is in place at his home does not need to generate another lengthy report on the patient's status. An addendum to a previous report will suffice. This type of reporting should continue for the length of the case and be modified according to the level of involvement.

How extensive should reports be? Some payer organizations have very specific guidelines, limiting initial report writing time to 2 hours or even half an hour. Others request a verbal report, asking that the case manager not take the time to send a document, even an e-mail or fax. In this type of situation, the case manager has to educate the referral source. Case management reports have value as documents chronicling case management activity. I know some of our client companies do not read our every report, but the reports do become a matter of record.

Suppose the case manager, during a phone conversation, reports to the payer a previously undocumented call to the patient or the physician. Will either of them remember this exchange of information? What if the case moves into litigation? What if the patient takes a turn for the worse? Especially when planning services, negotiating services, or putting alternate plans in place, case managers need to document decisions and their implementation. This is just good case management administration.

I confronted the issue of reporting in conversation with a client, a Third Party Administrator, who was seeking to cut administrative costs across the board. I used an example from his office to make a point. Most claims departments will pay for a surgery. But if a claim comes in for $10,000, it goes unpaid unless that surgical bill is accompanied by an operative report. The claims adjuster does not necessarily understand the medical jargon, but the report is requisite and accepted as documentation for a surgical procedure. I reminded the Third Party Administrator that he was paying for those operative reports that no one in his office read, yet they were considered a part of good claims administration. I then noted that case managers had procedural guidelines as well.

Just like physicians (who keep notes and dictate reports) or corporations (which maintain minutes of board of directors meetings), case managers need to document their work. Not everyone will read case management reports, but the medicolegal environment surrounding case management and the high cost and high risk associated with typical cases requires case managers to report their activities carefully and comprehensively.

I believe case managers need to explain our position and insist on providing full documentation because it helps validate and legitimize case management intervention. Case management is being requested by payers, and this is key. Case managers, to justify their involvement and demonstrate their contributions, need to be able to document what they did and how it affected treatment outcomes. Simply stated, case managers might be doing important work, but if they do not record it, it did not happen. Reports need to cover not just cost issues, but medical, physician, patient, and family issues as well, and also individuals consulted, actions agreed upon, actions taken, and the results.

Case management needs to put its principles and guidelines on record. I feel that too many case managers go along with every whim of their clients, putting themselves at risk. Far too many people are willing to conduct case management according to someone else's agenda. This is not to say that clients should have no input or be unable to restrict the length of time taken on a report, but case managers must do their job responsibly.

Regardless of the client's (payer's) needs, the report a case manager creates should follow a certain format. It should adequately catalog the generic information and capture the specific nature of the case as well. The case manager serves as an objective observer, weaving the role of case management into the picture. Although most case managers tailor their reports to meet the special requirements of clients, each report should include the same basic information: the name of the referral source, the mailing address and phone number for reporting, the line of insurance, the date of occurrence of the accident or injury, the name of the insured, a code for and the name of the claimant or patient. Each report also includes data obtained from the payer source, the patient and family, medical records, the treating physician, and other medical professionals; a review of the policy coverage and limits; any suggested alternative treatment program; and a discussion of relevant community resources. If an emotional or psychological component of the case is powerful enough to affect other care issues, it must be included as well.

Documentation attached to a report might include copies of the patient's past medical records, consulting reports, reports transferred from another treatment facility, questionnaires the case manager might have sent the treating physicians, letters confirming the agreement of the treating physicians with recommendations made by the case manager—anything that substantiates the case manager's activities and the unfolding of the treatment plan. In addition, the case manager should add information (e.g., brochures on diagnostic conditions, equipment, facilities) that might help the claims department or plan administrator better understand the patient's condition and needs, and should append the patient authorization form affirming the patient's permission for the information to be shared.

I usually suggest to newer case managers that each time they write a report, they first ask themselves, "Why am I not writing my successful closure report today? Why is this case still open?" This can help clarify the case's most pressing issues. The short-term situation should be presented along with solutions or responses, and then long-term needs should be cited.

A case management report should present the basics in a brief format using statements that leave room for clarification or follow-up. The first assessment report might be in outline form, but there should be a clause affirming that as the potential for case management involvement becomes more defined or the patient's condition becomes more stable, a more complete report will be filed. Perhaps the client was anxious to receive something on paper for a synopsis to the home office before the case manager was able to speak with the patient or before all medical personnel involved could be contacted. In such cases, the case manager should describe the situation ("This information was gathered in an interview with the family; the patient was unconscious") and add that a broader report will be forthcoming.

The language of reports is different from phone conversation vernacular. No one would write that a patient's house "was a wreck." Rather, it was "in need of repair." Reports also must consolidate communication. It is impossible to portray the living environment of a low-income neighborhood in a heavily urbanized area to a claims examiner in a small, Midwestern city; a few well-chosen words can convey the needed information. Because a range of people might be reading case management reports, they should be understandable to the layperson. Apnea should be described as "the absence of respiratory activity" or "a frequent respiratory distress of infants with an underdeveloped brain center," not as "a low CO_2 level." A report also might be subpoenaed and have to stand up to scrutiny in court, and, therefore, positive and negative observations should be backed by objective statements. The comment "John is not making progress because he's not motivated" would need to be supported by the fact that John has not attended his physical therapy sessions for the past 2 weeks even though he had transportation and was fit enough to do so. Hearsay should be avoided.

Developing prompt reports requires knowledge of community resources, service costs, and appropriate medical responses. The presentation of a report is particularly important when recommending an alternative to the existing treatment plan. Suppose the patient is in a hospital. The case manager calls the billing department: "John's been in the hospital for 15 days. I'm the case manager. We're working here with a company that really doesn't have a lot in terms of benefits. Could you tell me what the interim bill is right now, the billing to date? What's it likely going to be?" Then, the case manager begins to draft a report taking into account quality of care and cost factors as well as patient and family receptivity to the situation. A day in an intensive care unit in this particular hospital may be $3,400. A physician is going to visit every single day (maybe several physicians every day) at $150 a day, 5 or 7 days a week. Add that. The projected stay in the hospital, if no change is made in the treatment plan, is likely to be another 3 weeks. The case manager calculates the per diem cost and then, multiplying that cost by 3 weeks, presents the cost of Plan A.

Then Plan B is described. "I think we could bring John home, but we can't bring him home with anything less than 24-hour care. His wife can take care of him perhaps for the first 4 hours of the morning, but then she has other responsibilities. We'll need to put in an LPN or a home health aide." Knowing that the patient and family will need someone, either an RN or LPN, to provide assistance around the clock, the case manager investigates the cost per hour of such service in the area and multiplies it by 24 hours a day. That may not be the only needed service. John may also need physical therapy. The case manager might need to rent equipment (e.g., a hospital bed and wheelchair). In analyzing the second scenario, the case manager must include as many of the variables as can be predicted.

The case manager should present every alternative that seems plausible. One might be to put the patient in a rehabilitation center or a skilled nursing facility at a fixed, all-inclusive, per diem cost negotiated to $325 per day. How does the case manager get that figure? By calling the facility and saying, "I'm trying to draw up a plan so I can submit it to an approval source. The last time I had someone in your facility it was x dollars per day. Is that still in the ballpark? I won't hold you to those exact dollars. I realize that this patient may be different, requiring other services, but this is an employer group and it's the first time they're seeing figures. I'm just trying to give them round numbers on which to base a decision."

Is this report communicated by letter, fax, or telephone? It may need to be communicated quickly, which means telephonically. The case manager gets the client on the phone and relates her findings: I called up the billing department. It's $3,400 per day, and if we don't do anything, John will be there another week in ICU, with a possible additional week on a regular floor for $1,500 per day. It will cost $34,300, not including physician visits.

We can move him to St. Jude's Rehab Facility in Yonkers. I had a person there 6 months ago; the outcome was really good. I was able to get a rate of $600 per day, including physical therapy, for a total of $8,400. Obviously, I will make certain the plan is approved by the treating physician.

"There is another possibility. John wants to come home. That's his preference, but to do it, we're going to have to add 24 hours of care because his wife can only do 4 hours. After we add physical therapy, the costs of bringing him home will be less than keeping him in the hospital but not as economical as the rehab facility, where he will get more services and better results. I have to let you know that home is where he wants to be. However, he and his family will have to look at what they want to do and how they want to use his benefit dollars."

When a report is drawn up and all this information is documented, the tone becomes more formalized and the case manager includes a projected analysis of predictable costs. Noting that these quotes may vary due to a change in the patient's condition or an unforeseen complication, the case manager would list costs for the current Plan A and alternate Plans B and C. A paragraph or two would follow offering the case manager's opinion as to what is best for the patient and why.

The body of a case management report should not include an emphasis on costs. If such a report should go to court, the case manager might have a problem defending what appears to be "bottom-line" healthcare. It is more appropriate to incorporate financial information by stating that the provider was selected for its quality, ability to meet the patient's needs, and to make the best use of benefit dollars after a review of several providers was conducted. Other financial data, that is, the range of fees offered by the providers, should appear apart from information on the patient's progress in a Cost-Benefit Analysis Report (see Chapter 12).

Ultimately, the choice is the patient's, but the case manager can present to the patient and family what she believes will be the best in terms of quality, outcome, ease of provision of services, and cost of services. The case manager can make it clear that John has x benefits but will use a greater proportion of dollars by coming home. She should also portray the realities of home care: "It sounds really great, but if the RN or LPN doesn't show up for a shift or gets sick, it can be complicated." Patients, especially when they are in a known and comfortable situation, are threatened by the thought of having to leave, and some will be more vocal than others. "Is this going to be okay with my doctor? Why would you want to have me moved? I really don't know; this is kind of far away from my family." The more vocal ones might be a problem for case managers who are unused to patients becoming so involved.

Introducing the alternative of a less-expensive but equally proficient facility can cause concern when the patient or family is attached to a care center because of its name or price tag. People may equate "less expensive" with "inferior quality." A case manager should never talk about cost eyeball to eyeball with a patient and say, "It's too expensive here and I've got to get you out." That sets up an adversarial relationship and increases the case manager's liability exposure. Family members might counter, "Well, okay, but if anything happens . . ." When recommending a site change, I use the Hyundai/Rolls Royce approach: Everything has a price tag, and it does not necessarily follow that expensive is always good and inexpensive is always inferior.

"Listen, this is a really good center here. I know you're very satisfied. You need to be aware, however, that your wife may need 6 months of these kinds of services. At $1,200 per day, this only buys us 2 months of care. Here's another site, where costs will be $500 per day for appropriate services. I'd like your input; I can't mandate that you go there. But I will assist in helping to see that it gets you the results you need, and I will confer with your doctor about it."

Enabling a patient to focus on long-term gains rather than short-term obstacles can help him or her make a decision. "Yes, the new facility is farther away, but even though you'll be away from home for 3 more weeks, remember that in 3 weeks you'll be so much closer to returning to life as usual." Giving the patient an example can be beneficial. "I hear what you're saying because of another patient I worked with. This was his situation, but actually when he got here . . ." A patient needs to hear some of the positives to be able to appreciate the case manager's vision. If the patient, by looking at a brochure or going on a tour, can see the facility is really nice and designed to meet his or her needs, he or she will be more inclined to "buy in."

No one is really comfortable with change. A case manager has to help people see the pros and the cons and allow them to voice their concerns and problems. If their objections can be dealt with, the case manager should follow through. If someone says, "Absolutely no, under no circumstances," the case manager should not try to force a change. The case manager should also never create a situation in which she, the employer group, and the carrier are at odds, because the patient will be more tempted to say, "Well you said I had to do this and now look what happened. I'm going to sue you." In addition, it is important to be wary of a patient or family who wants to turn over all authority to the case manager, because this also places the case manager at additional risk for a lawsuit. Each patient really needs to be involved in planning and be aware of why decisions are made.

The initial report sells the case management plan. A report can and should be used to bring something else to the picture—to provide the client with a vision, to demonstrate the more complex uses of case management, or to create new opportunities for case management work. Even a brief report can include underlined or bold sections that emphasize the philosophy behind case management and its role in solving problems. Report-writing at its best includes creative, analytical thinking that anticipates objections in order to win approval.

To maintain quality services, to better track our cases, and to assist our case managers in creating reports that served as valuable case management tools in and of themselves, I created guidelines for on-site and telephonic initial evaluation reports (Table 9–19), a sample on-site and telephonic Initial Evaluation Report (Table 9–20), guidelines for writing progress reports (Table 9–21), and a sample on-site and telephonic Progress Report (Table 9–22). The guidelines offer direction on what information is needed and, in some cases, why it is important to include certain references or nuances. The sample reports indicate the content and formats that I have found effective when communicating the process and benefits of a beneficial case management plan.

OBTAINING APPROVAL

After the case management plan has been devised and the report has been sent to the client, the case manager must then obtain approval to proceed with the recommendations in the report.

Case Manager: Betty, this is Pat Sanders with Professional Case Management. How is your morning going?

Case Manager: You sound very busy. I'll be brief.

Case Manager: I just wanted to make sure you got my last report, which was dated March 14th. [If report has been received but not yet read.] Well, good, I'm glad to know you received it. Because you haven't had a chance to read it yet, can I call you back tomorrow? I just wanted to get your thoughts on my recommendations to see if I should proceed. I'll give you a quick call on Thursday.

Case Manager: [When report has been received and read.] As you may have read in the report, Mr. Williams is considerably improved from the time of my last report. I think our physician change was a good idea; he seems to be responding real well. Did my two recommendations look good to you? One involved a personal consultation with Dr. Friedman, and the second was getting three bids on the hospital bed. If Mr. Williams is going to need the bed for more than 3 months, we may come out better by a purchase, but I can make some calls on that and let you know.

Table 9–19 Initial Evaluation Report Guidelines

Initial Evaluation Report
(On-site and Telephonic)

Guidelines for use (*see attached Sample*)

Referral Reason: The *major* reasons why case was identified for case management. Examples: long-term care placement, home uterine monitoring, TPN services, etc.

Current Medical Status: A narrative yet *concise* and *specific* paragraph about the claimant's medical status at the time of referral. If hospitalized, include the reason for that admission, course of treatment, complications, dates, care needs, future treatment plan, and expected outcome. You should also include physical descriptions of claimant (if visit occurred) or current height, weight, race, sex, and other physical characteristics.

Past Medical History: A *short* paragraph that should describe conditions, prior surgeries, etc. Include prior admissions, surgeries, and medications *as they impact* on current status and/or future recovery.

Treating Physicians/Other Professionals: A list of *current* treating MDs and perhaps others *if* they will continue to be involved. List name, specialty, address, and phone number.

Medications: A list of medications that the claimant is or will be taking: name, type (i.e., sedative, chemotherapy), dose, and frequency.

Socio/Environmental: A *short* description of claimant's family/work and home situation. Include marital status, family support, any cultural, language, or religious factors that may impede recovery, *or* those factors that will assist in promoting a favorable outcome.

Financial/Insurance: A statement of those issues or limitations that might adversely (or, perhaps, positively) affect outcome.

Case Management Intervention: A *short* paragraph to describe what you have done since the file was opened. It should include how initial assessment was conducted (i.e., phone, visit), who was contacted, authorization documentation, and receptivity to case management. Also state any particular activities/accomplishments.

Problems Identified: An *extremely important* section that serves as the *basis* for your case management intervention and recommendations. If there are no problems, then we don't need a case manager (. . . *and* if that *is* the case, we need to state so and recommend closure). Assuming that we have done a good job in assessing potential for case management, opened the

continues

Table 9–19 continued

---

file, etc., then *list those problems* that need to be resolved and that, when resolved, will bring us closer to a successful closure. No need to list any and all at this initial stage, just those requiring immediate attention and that you can address until the next report date.

Case Management Recommendations: A list of recommendations that is *action* oriented, defines what you plan to do, and is absolutely the logical connection to the problems you have identified. They should also lead to *measurable* outcomes, that is, improving medical outcomes, appropriate and cost-effective use of services/benefit dollars, empowerment/compliance of patient, etc. These recommendations are those you will or plan to accomplish until next report.

Estimated Hours for Case Management: The number of hours that you will expend until the next report (including time spent on your report).

Source: Courtesy of Options Unlimited, Case Management Services Division, © 2003, Huntington, New York.

Table 9–20 Initial Evaluation Report (On-site and Telephonic Reports)

Date of Report:
SS#:

To: Jane Smith, Acct. Manager	Employer group: ABC Auto Corp.
Claimant: Sara Green	Diagnosis: Cerebral vascular accident
Insured: Same	(stroke), diabetes, hypertension.

Referral Reason: Options Unlimited's services requested based upon multiple diagnoses, need for inpatient rehabilitation, ongoing home care and therapy, and limited benefit provisions.

Current Medical Status

Information in this report obtained by telephone/fax. Signed release in file. The claimant is one week post right CVA at New City Hospital. She had sudden onset of left-sided weakness, slurred speech, and suffered a fall in her home. Upon her admission through the ER, the claimant was also found to be diabetic with blood glucose at 280 and her blood pressure elevated to 200/120. She remained in ICU for 3 days and then transferred to the neurological unit, where she is at present. There is significant paresis (weakness) of left upper and lower extremity, speech remains slurred but understandable. Blood glucose levels responding to insulin but dosage

Table 9–20 continued

---

requires more regulation as does her blood pressure medication. Prognosis is guarded at this time with return to pre-illness status questionable.

Past Medical History

Prior to this hospital admission, the claimant had two previous admissions: in 2000 for cholecystectomy and in March 2003 for hypertension. She acknowledged a "touch of diabetes," a "little problem" with her weight (175 pounds, height 5'4") as per the hospital admission note. As per her daughter, claimant took her antihypertension medication,". . . only when she had a headache. . . . didn't want to get too dependent on drugs. . ."

Treating Physicians

Dr. Al Jones	Dr. Bob Brown	Dr. Sam Smith
(neurologist)	(internist)	(endocrinologist)
120 Main Street	100 Main Street	200 Old Street
Nice Town, USA	Nice Town, USA	Fine Town, USA
400-123-4567	400-123-8910	400-321-9876

Medications

NPH Insulin, 40 U, OD
Reg Insulin, 5 U for glucose level between 160–180 mgm, 4× day
Lasix, 20 mgm, BID
K-Dur, 20 mgm, OD
Lopressor, 50 mgm, BID

Socio/Environmental

Mrs. Green is a 58-year-old Caucasian female, widowed for 2 years. She lives alone in an eight-room home in a rural area. Adult daughters (two) while having a close, supportive relationship with their mother, live 2–3 hours away and with family and work responsibilities, are unable to provide care or assistance other than occasionally and via phone calls. She admits to being shy and private with no real friends in the area, a few close coworkers but they are 1 hour away, close to the supermarket where the claimant works as a cashier. In conversation with the oldest daughter (Mary White, 400-000-0000), it appears that the claimant's house has become "very run-down" since her husband's death, resulting in embarrassment and reluctance to having "outsiders" in the home.

Financial/Insurance

Due to the claimant's long-term employment, she will receive full pay for the next 3 months. Although meeting normal expenses is NOT an immediate problem, there is concern that some benefit limitations and

continues

Table 9-20 continued

apparent need for long-term rehabilitation may give rise to financial concerns (60 home care visits up to 4 hours; rehab $50,000 total lifetime).

Case Management Intervention

Since this case was opened, Options Unlimited has conducted an initial assessment of the claimant through telephone contact with her daughter, the discharge planner, and Dr. Brown; and has begun research for rehab facility admission. Signed authorization has been obtained, and claimant and family are receptive to our assistance.

Problems Identified

1) Needs inpatient rehabilitation services; as per MD, 30–45 day period.
2) Limitation of benefits; @ a nonnegotiated cost/day of $1500 × 30 days—$45,000 would be spent with only $5,000 remaining; home care limit, 60 visits.
3) Somewhat medically stable; in addition to CVA, diabetes, hypertension, and weight reduction will require medical direction.
4) Patient by history is poorly educated about her condition and noncompliant due to lack of understanding.
5) Will need home care and/or physical therapy once home; patient is presently unreceptive, unrealistic regarding future and very anxious.
6) Patient lives alone.

Case Management Recommendations

1) Begin to research and negotiate fees for transfer to rehab facility; with MD and rehab facility, explore feasibility of 1- to 2-week admission to conserve benefits. Assist with discharge/transfer plans to rehab facility.
2) With treating MDs, determine who will provide follow-up medical care and/or referrals to appropriate MDs in claimant's area.
3) Enlist family assistance in preparing home for patient's return to allow for necessary home care in a safe environment.

Estimated case management hours: 6–8 hours.

Mary Smith, RN, BS
Medical Case Manager

Source: Courtesy of Options Unlimited, Case Management Services Division, © 2003, Huntington, New York.

Table 9–21 Guidelines for Writing Progress Reports (On-site and Telephonic)

Date of Report:

To: Jane Smith

	SS#:
Claimant: Sara Green	Employer group:
Insured: Same	Diagnosis: Stroke

Medical Status

This should be a *narrative,* yet short and very specific summary of the claimant's medical status since the last report. Include in this section any hospital admissions, surgeries, complications, new conditions and/or diagnostic findings. If there has been notable progress, quality-of-care issues, or other factors impacting on claimant's medical status, it should be included in this section. See Example.

Problems Identified

In order to assure that case management is goal-directed, rather than a reporting of events, *list* in this section those problems that need to be addressed or resolved and that you will be working on during the next month (or report period if on extended diary). Because goals for case management should be directed toward the improvement of medical outcomes (or stability), appropriateness of care and services, and cost containment, we should be looking at the problems or factors that would interfere with this. See Examples.

Case Management Intervention

This should be a short *narrative* section as to what *you* as the case manager actually did on this case since the past report. There should be a demonstration in this section of your *action* and *involvement* in moving this case toward improved medical outcomes, involvement by the patient and family, interaction with the medical team and providers, and an ongoing ability to achieve quality outcome *and* savings or cost-effectiveness. Note: this is *not* to include date-by-date, activity-by-activity reporting of events, phone calls, etc., but rather a more global description of evidence of your impact on the case. This should clearly illustrate why case management is involved, what we've done and/or need to do. Use of "Options Unlimited" or "this case manager" and action verbs should be evident. See Example.

Recommendations

In this section, list those activities that you will do within the next month (or extended diary report period). Remember that these activities should

continues

Table 9–21 continued

---

have a relation or connection to the issues you have noted in the *Problems Identified* section. What do you need to do to solve the problems? See Examples.

Estimated case management hours: Note here the number of hours (including your report) that you will expend until the next report.

Source: Courtesy of Options Unlimited, Case Management Services Division, © 2003, Huntington, New York

---

Table 9–22 Sample Progress Report (On-site and Telephonic)

Date of Report:
To: Jane Smith

SS#:
Claimant: Sara Green   Employer group:
Insured: Same   Diagnosis: Stroke

Medical Status

Mrs. Green continues to recover from her right CVA (stroke) and is now in the second week of her inpatient rehabilitation at Valley Rehabilitation Center. She is actively participating in the program; however, she remains anxious about her return home. Her diabetes is better controlled with insulin and diet but still requires close medical supervision and a change in her medications has brought her hypertension closer to normal range (last reading 130/90, lower than her prior 180/100). There has been an additional weight loss of 10 pounds since her hospital admission 3 weeks ago, with another 15 pounds to go until her target of 140 pounds.

Problems Identified

- Patient lives by herself and will require assistance once home. Adult children (two) live 2–3 hours away.
- Patient is being cared for by three MDs: Dr. Jones (neurologist), Dr. Brown (internist), and Dr. Smith (endocrinologist). All MDs are 1+ hours from the patient's home and she will require frequent medical follow-up.
- Patient has benefit limits for home care and rehabilitation services (60 home care visits of 4 hours each, $50,000 rehab, lifetime).
- Patient is a very private person and resists "outsiders" in her home.

Table 9–22 continued

Case Management Intervention

Since our last report, Options Unlimited was able to expedite Mrs. Green's discharge from New City Hospital to Valley Rehab Center. This case manager researched the facilities in the area, assisted the family in evaluating each and then, upon agreement of all and selection of Valley Rehab, negotiated cost-effective, all-inclusive daily rates. Because of the Plan limit (lifetime) for rehab benefits ($50,000 total), Options Unlimited is working very closely with the staff of Valley to extend these available dollars. We are discussing a shorter inpatient stay in order to use the remaining dollars for a longer period of treatment once the claimant is home. We have also begun to research home care providers and DME dealers in her area.

Recommendations

1) Obtain progress reports from rehab team within next week; determine potential and date for transition to community-based day program and then home physical therapy.
2) Determine level of function and assess home care needs, for example, equipment care, services, etc. Arrange care, negotiate fees, and prepare provider agreements.
3) Contact all MDs. Determine current medical status, share concerns regarding follow-up, and obtain recommendations for appropriate medical care.

Estimated hours for case management: 5 hours

Signature
Medical Management Consultant

Source: Courtesy of Options Unlimited, Case Management Services Division, © 2003, Huntington, New York.

Case Manager: OK, great, I'll go ahead and get started on this tomorrow, and I'll probably have another report to you in about 3 weeks. I'll also check on those medications you questioned and give you a call when I have some answers. Thanks for your time.

There are always going to be times when case managers have to use their own judgment and consider who they are representing. A case manager might receive direct communication from an employer or referral source: "I want John out of that facility; it's too expensive." If the case manager feels that the patient is in the most appropriate center and there is no less-costly setting, she cannot allow the employer or client to override her professional judgment. The case manager cannot serve the client first and the patient last; the interests of the patient must always predominate. Case managers are not in the business of slashing away at the federal or corporate health budget at the sacrifice of patients' well-being and safety.

COORDINATION: PUTTING THE PLAN INTO ACTION

Plans are sometimes put in motion as early as the initial evaluation stage. The case manager may not have completed gathering all the information or submitted a report when she gets the go-ahead to put services in place. When a big, involved case has been referred by a client company the case manager has worked with before, the company might request a verbal report from the site. During that telephone call, the case manager might say, "This person could go home. I could set up some services. Do you want me to continue with case management intervention?" And the response will come, "Yes, go ahead. Do what you have to do."

Whatever the working arrangement is, whether the case manager is representing an insurer, HMO, PPO, TPA, or is part of an independent case management company, she should be aware of the voluntary guidelines that have been issued to promote consistency in managed care, including case management. Jointly developed by representatives of the American Hospital Association, the American Managed Care and Review Organization, the American Medical Association, the Blue Cross and Blue Shield Association, and the Health Insurance Association of America, these guidelines for the most part cover the conduct of concurrent review (see Chapter 10).

Although the concurrent review guidelines may be voluntary, such protocols are becoming part of the case management practice, and case managers could be held responsible in court for applying and utilizing them. In 1986, *Wickline v. State of California* established that any professional involved in making a healthcare recommendation could be held liable for damages or harm to a patient that occurs when services in a managed care environment are not provided in accordance with accepted standards of care. In 1989, Congress created the Office for the Forum on Quality and Effectiveness within the Agency for Health Care Policy and Research (AHCPR), now known as the Agency for Healthcare Research and Quality (AHRQ), and gave it a mandate to publish and disseminate national clinical practice guidelines. Cutting across populations, ages, problem areas, and delivery sites, these national guidelines, now developed for more than 19 clinical subjects, are systematic statements of what is appropriate in specific clinical terms when delivering care to patients. They are accessible on-line through the National Library of Medicine's Medline service. The last areas of care covered included low back pain problems, cardiac rehabilitation, depression, management of cancer-related pain, evaluation and management of early HIV infection, cataracts, and postoperative pain management. What case manager has never worked on cases involving these areas of care? Another task force at AHCPR developed a methodology to translate clinical practice guidelines into medical review criteria—guideposts used to judge the appropriateness of healthcare decisions.

AHCPR looked to the Institute of Medicine (IOM), an arm of the National Academy of Sciences, for advice on how to implement its guidelines program. The IOM, defining the standards for guideline development, devised eight attributes of good clinical practice guidelines: (1) validity (do they lead to the health and cost outcomes projected for them), (2) reliability/reproducibility (a similar group of experts would incorporate the same elements within their guidelines), (3) clinical applicability (the guideline specifies applicable populations), (4) clinical flexibility (details common, expected deviations for the clinical condition), (5) clarity (the language is clear, terms are defined precisely, and the presentation is logical and easy to follow), (6) multidisciplinary process (the guideline reflects input from the various practitioners who treat the condition), (7) scheduled review (guidelines are regularly reviewed for medical advances and new treatments), and (8) documentation (statements clearly addressing the evidence, assumptions, and rationales used to develop the guidelines).

There are, however, any number of practice guidelines and standards of practice that have been developed that do not directly address all of those eight criteria. The AMA's directory of guidelines estimates that over 1,700 different practice guidelines are in circulation.

In 1995, the CMSA published its first Standards of Practice, guidelines for practicing case management. Although they are not clinical in substance, these nationally recognized standards define case management, case manager functions, settings for case management services, relationships with clients, purposes and goals of case management, standards of care, and standards of performance. The standards of care identify activities incorporating assessment/case identification, problem identification, planning, monitoring, evaluating, and outcomes measurement criteria. Within the standards of performance are included measurement criteria for quality of care, education/certification qualifications, collaborative activities, legal compliance, ethical conduct, advocacy, resource utilization, and research utilization. When examined in light of the IOM definitions, these CMSA standards hold up as standards of conduct for case managers, illuminating the role, describing functions, and setting boundaries for appropriate behavior.

Aetna Health Plans and the ICMA (now merged with CMSA) developed Case Management Practice Guidelines, published by Mosby-Year Book in 1996. These guidelines come closer to the IOM's definition of clinical practice guidelines. Like the CMSA standards, they offer general case management guidelines, but also provide condition-specific case management recommendations for 10 clinical or practice areas: AIDS/HIV, brain injury, high-risk neonates, high-risk pregnancy, low back injury, oncology, pediatric care, spinal cord injury, transplants, and workers' compensation.

In addition, there are the Standards of Practice for Case Management (CMSA), a section of which appears as Appendix 9–A, CMSA Statement Regarding Ethical Case Management Practice, Code of Professional Conduct for Case Managers (CCMC), Code of Professional Conduct (Certification of Disability Management Specialists Commissions; CDMS), Code of Ethics (American Nurses Association; ANA), the Standards of Occupational and Environmental Health Nursing (American Association of Occupational Health Nurses; AAOHN), Code of Ethics (AAOHN), Code of Ethics (National Academy of Social Workers; NASW), and standards of care in several practice settings from the NASW.

With legal precedent for potentially holding case managers accountable even though they are not hands-on care providers, it behooves every case manager to become familiar with these practice guidelines. Alice G. Gosfield, a lawyer very familiar with health law issues and a board member of the National Committee for Quality Assurance, said at a Medical Case Management Conference that guidelines such as the AHCPR offerings are readily available to practicing case managers; no one has an excuse for not applying them, when appropriate. However, they are not rigid rules, but rather standardized suggestions for actions given a certain diagnosis or clinical condition. For example, a past Milliman and Robertson (M&R) cataract guideline engendered such resistance and disagreement that major insurers who otherwise used the M&R guidelines refused to apply it as issued. Gosfield suggests that case managers should document both their adherence to and reasons for deviations from guidelines. If a case manager can demonstrate that she has conscientiously followed a national case management guideline or national clinical guideline, she provides herself with an additional shield against potential claims of negligence. The question asked in cases of professional liability is, did you behave as a similar practitioner would under similar circumstances? Attorneys are not attracted to cases in which the fact of negligence can be disproved by documented guideline adherence.[7]

Although we need guidelines and should certainly practice in accordance with the high level of standards in our fields, I caution case managers to call on their professional knowledge and experience in translating guidelines into action. I have seen any number of requests for proposals that call for "state of the art," "best in practice," or "best in class" procedures. A guide is a guide; it is not a mandate. Some guidelines are restrictive; some are dangerous. We all remember the swift outcry when the "drive-through" mastectomy guidelines were published and the legal actions that were taken to require more reasonable time frames for inpatient care following the procedure. The key point regarding use of guidelines is to apply them wisely, fully document your choices and actions, and clearly communicate your reasoning to the appropriate parties.

FOLLOW-UP

Attention must be paid to each detail. Any time a case manager has any responsibility for making recommendations for services or putting services in place, the case manager owes it to herself, the patient, and the client company who referred the case to make sure that what has been put in place is working, remains quality in nature, is cost-effective, and is necessary. Obtaining approval for monitoring from a client company can be difficult; managing a case without monitoring it can lead to liability exposure.

Sometimes a client company wants a case manager to make a one-time visit, put services in place, and be done with the case. No one is watching for changes in the patient's needs or tracking and assisting with increases or decreases in services. No one is gauging the continued effectiveness of the physician's treatment plan. What worked well in the hospital may not work at home. After 5 days, the patient is readmitted to the hospital. What happened? It may be that the patient initially followed the physician's recommendations to the nth degree, then became lax with dressing changes, and now has a dangerous infection. Especially when involved in helping a patient make the transition from one care setting to another, the case manager must make sure that the outcome for the patient will not become compromised.

The monitoring process varies from case to case. It may include semi-monthly home visits by the case manager or periodic phone calls placed by the patient to the case manager. In active cases in which multiple services are in place, the case manager must make monthly on-site visits. It may be that there are no services in place but the patient has been discharged and asked to take specific medications or dress a wound a certain way. The case manager will not go out and watch the patient take pills but will ask for a check-in call to see how the patient is coping. If the patient sounds poor or acknowledges problems, the case manager should call the physician and assess the situation. Perhaps the treatment plan needs to be reevaluated.

When there are multiple services in place, the patient continues to recover, or the family resists any suggested decrease in service hours, the case manager may need to make an on-site visit to ascertain the true situation. It may be that the family members are not good communicators and things have taken a rapid turn for the worse. Without access, the case manager cannot determine whether continuing to adhere to the treatment plan is in the best interest of the patient.

Continuing follow-up and reports are especially important because they help maintain the case manager's link to the patient and support the case manager's role throughout the case. Rather than simply someone who sets up services or assists with hospital discharges, the case manager is perceived as someone who contributes to the entire treatment plan.

EVALUATING THE PLAN

Along with monitoring the medical treatment plan and its effectiveness, the case manager evaluates and reevaluates her own case management plan over the course of the intervention. Is the treatment working? Is the patient cooperating? There will be a flux in case activity and intensity.

Periodically (at least once every 30 days), the case manager should review the treatment plan and the patient's progress. Short-term referrals, which generally run less than 3 months and are characterized by intense activity at the outset that tapers off as the patient improves, are always reassessed prior to the patient's discharge from a facility or program. Long-term programs, such as geriatric care, are evaluated at intervals of 3, 6, or 9 months, or as in a brain trauma or SCI (spinal cord injury) at 1-year intervals. Long-term care evaluations can become challenging because the goal of case management is stability; in some cases, things can hum along for quite a while and there will seemingly be nothing to report.

Further, quality of life is less easily measured than the quantity of money spent on care. Is a continuation of the program warranted? Are the dollars spent on John's care every day worth it? What can the case manager use as a yardstick to measure care progress? Is John experiencing big gains? Perhaps the first month John could not walk alone; this month he walks unaided but his gait needs correction. Or, the first month John remained comatose; the second month he was alert but experienced memory loss. As long as improvements are ongoing, the treatment course can be justified.

The patient might be in a facility for a proposed 6- to 9-month stay at a cost of $1,000 per day. A monthly visit by the case manager can be extremely effective in monitoring the need for continuing placement. (If the patient has been placed in a facility in another state, the case manager may rely on the facility's case manager to keep her updated rather than making a personal on-site visit.) Treatment might be necessary for a 6- to 9-month period, but the patient might not require facility services for the entire time. Although making great strides the first 2 months, the patient may show no further improvement after 3 months. Perhaps the patient has hit a plateau and needs a break from the rigorous therapies. This is something the case manager cannot ascertain from facility reports. The case manager might have to decide whether a $1,400-per-day facility fee is justified when there is a day program available to the patient that costs $500 per day. The next step might be to place the patient in the day program, then perhaps return him or her to the inpatient facility for another round of more intensive therapy if improvement again becomes noticeable.

Over the course of care, the case manager maintains communication with the treating physicians to share concerns and observations regarding developing conditions. The case manager may need to reestablish ties to a specialist to request assistance. As a treatment facilitator, the case manager keeps in touch with everyone who can make a contribution toward the desired outcome for the patient, including physicians, physical therapists, social workers, employers, and community center personnel.

REPEATING THE PROCESS

Each case goes through modification, redevelopment, and reevaluation stages. Changes in patient status will require new measures of care.

I do not think a case manager can ever be certain that a case that appears short-term is not going to become problematic. Some conditions seem very straightforward, and then, for whatever reason (family dynamics, financial difficulties, new symptoms), the initial diagnosis is changed. Case managers should always allow for extenuating circumstances, unforeseen events, and as much as possible, they should try to prevent complications from occurring. Yet, despite the best of care and intentions, short-term problems can become long-term problems.

SPECIFIC CASE MANAGEMENT ACTIVITIES

Throughout the course of care, the case manager will be working in four major areas of activity: medical, financial, behavioral/motivational, and vocational. In "Job Descriptions and Standards of Care" in its *Case Management Practice* publication, the Foundation for Rehabilitation Certification Education and Research included the following descriptions.

Medical Activities

Into this category fall all those activities a case manager performs to ensure that the patient receives the most effective medical and nursing care, including the following:

- Contacting the patient in the hospital, in the rehabilitation unit, or at home.
- Contacting the members of the medical treatment team (the physician, nursing staff, rehabilitation therapists, etc.) to discover the patient's course of progress and needs and utilizing the information in discharge planning and the initial needs assessment.
- Arranging for all services required for discharge or relocation (equipment, home nursing care, therapy, transportation, transfer to another facility, home utilities, etc.), and coordinating efforts with the primary RN, discharge planner, or social service administrator to eliminate duplication of service and conserve benefit dollars.
- Visiting with the family.
- Checking the home for safety factors and architectural barriers and arranging for any needed safety aids and modifications.
- On follow-up, reevaluating equipment, ensuring supplies are replenished, monitoring home nursing services, and arranging for equipment repair; evaluating activities of daily living, home programs, and modifications to treatment.
- Identifying problems, providing health instruction, and referring the patient back to the physician or other health team member when appropriate.

- Identifying plateaus, improvements, regressions, and depressions; counseling accordingly or recommending help.
- Making personal visits or contacting the physician to clarify the diagnosis, prognosis, therapy, activities of daily living, expected permanent disability, limitations, and so on.
- Assisting in obtaining payer authorizations for any modalities of treatment recommended.
- Acting as a liaison between the physician and the insurance company when necessary.
- Sharing pertinent information about the patient with the physician and working together with the physician to achieve the best outcome.

Financial Activities

Some of the specific services a case manager might perform on behalf of a patient are as follows:

- Assessing the benefit plan for coverage and limitations; negotiating out-of-plan coverage to conserve dollars.
- Negotiating for more cost-effective rates for supplies and services.
- Counseling the patient or family on budgeting and notifying creditors.
- Identifying financial distress and referring the patient or family to appropriate community resources.
- Helping the patient or family sort and prioritize unpaid bills.
- Acting as a liaison between the insurance company, referral source, and patient to alleviate financial and other problems or misunderstandings.

Behavioral/Motivational Activities

Behavioral/motivational activities include these:

- Exploring the patient's feelings about him- or herself and his or her injury or illness and helping the patient with the associated trauma and frustration.
- Monitoring the family's feelings regarding the patient's illness and observing the family's ability or inability to manage under new emotional stress.
- Offering reassurance and information about the patient's condition.
- If qualified, counseling in the areas of marital discord, role reversal, dependency, and sexual problems arising from the injury or illness.

Vocational Activities

Possible vocational activities include the following:

- Obtaining a history of past education, employment, hobbies, and job skills and uncovering vocational interests and future goals.
- If appropriate, overseeing psychovocational testing, work evaluations, schooling, transportation, on-the-job situations, and anything else needed to assist the patient in becoming or remaining gainfully employed.
- Assisting the patient in using the recuperative period in a constructive fashion (studying, upgrading skills, preparing for job interviews, etc.).
- Visiting the patient's place of employment and talking with the personnel director or immediate supervisor about the employer's expectations and the patient's needs.
- Completing a job analysis and discussing the possibility of the patient's return to work in the same job, perhaps after job modifications or lightening of duties.
- Sharing the previous information with the physician at an appropriate time.

STAY ON POINT

Case managers always need to remember why they are part of the health-care system. They are there to empower patients, to involve patients in their own treatment and destiny, and to help the very young and the very old live as best they can. During an initial assessment, a case manager might foresee some difficulties in affecting change for the better. The adult children of an elderly patient might be arguing among themselves regarding the best course of care; an HIV-positive patient or a patient with terminal cancer (some companies will not refer a cancer patient until he or she is a hospice candidate) is to be interviewed; a family might be devastated by their child's spinal cord injury. Often, the more catastrophic and irreversible the situation, the more strategic the case manager's planning has to be. Can that family remain intact as a unit? In the face of these odds, sometimes the best thing a case manager can do is ask the patient and family, "What is it you want? What do you hope to get from this care? If you could change the patient's care, how would you do it?" By finding out where their heads and hearts are, the case manager can often make an important difference in their ability to cope with a tough situation.

CASE MANAGEMENT SCENARIOS

Following are several brief case management scenarios, all involving employee–employer relationships that outline the case management process and when and how the various elements of the process take place.

Case #1

A 32-year-old office administrator has been out for 5 days due to exacerbation of pain in her wrists over the last 4 months and a sensation of her wrists falling asleep at night. She is currently 12 weeks pregnant and has a history of being hypothyroid and overweight.

Case Analysis

From the information provided, it would appear that this woman may have carpal tunnel syndrome. This condition's predisposing factors include pregnancy, hypothyroidism, and obesity, all conditions that this employee also has. Our goal would be to obtain an accurate diagnosis, appropriate treatment (which would not interfere with her pregnancy), and facilitate a timely return to work.

Further Information Needed

From the employee. The case manager (following explanation of our role) would determine employee's physical status, what testing or treatment has occurred, how pregnancy is progressing, prior medical history (including obesity and hypothyroidism), and treatment for these conditions. We would also discuss return-to-work issues (i.e., transitional assignments), and then determine response to these questions. We would advise her that we will be conferring with her physicians and working with them to assist her in resolving these problems, keeping her healthy during her pregnancy, and returning her to work.

From the physician(s). We would obtain medical information from her obstetrician, internist, and/or neurologist or orthopedic physician who may be treating the wrist pain. We would request objective information from any diagnostic examinations, laboratory testing, and other significant findings. We would determine the treatment plan, duration of disability, ability to return to work, and physician's willingness to cooperate in a return-to-work process. There would be discussion of her obesity as well because this is problematic for her pregnancy and her probable carpal tunnel syndrome.

From the employer. We would briefly discuss medical issues (respecting patient confidentiality) that are present and explore potential for a transitional assignment that would allow for early return to duty. We would enlist cooperation in this and assure that we would continue to be involved to assist with problems and eventual return to full duty.

If the employee had not yet been referred to a neurologist to evaluate her for carpal tunnel, we would suggest this and assist with this evaluation for appropriate treatment. Other than suggestion for further evaluation for carpal tunnel, no other referrals would be made.

Using *The Medical Disability Advisor* guidelines (by Presley Reed, Reed Group), we would estimate a maximum period of 3 weeks' length of disability/duration with conservative medical treatment; however, with transitional employment, a return much sooner is possible. If diagnosis of carpal tunnel is confirmed and assuming conservative management with splinting, compression, and localized treatment, the case manager would negotiate avoidance of prolonged and repetitive activities, brief rest periods to elevate hands intermittently, or reduced hours.

We would advise employer that employee is being evaluated and, hopefully, treated and suggest that work restrictions may be necessary. If known, we would advise as to possible return-to-work date. This case would not qualify for leave under FMLA and would not require consideration for reasonable accommodation under ADA because the condition is assumed to be temporary.

The next case management follow-up would be made with the patient, physician, and employer, who would be contacted within 5 business days. To facilitate return to work and case closure, we would maintain ongoing communication with the involved parties.

Case #2

Approximately 1 month ago, a 48-year-old boiler repair/field tech was lifting a box weighing approximately 50 pounds at a neighbor's yard sale and developed nonradiating low back pain. He has been working, but now has lost 4 days of work due to progressive back pain. He has had occasional backaches in the past; however, he denies any previous back injuries. He had a previous work-related shoulder injury, which was settled under workers' compensation. His past medical history includes peptic ulcer and obesity. His doctor has advised he be off work for the next 2 weeks to rest, start physical therapy, and use Tylenol for pain relief and a muscle relaxant as needed for back spasm. The physician has told the employee that he may need to be off work for as much as 6 weeks. The employee is concerned about his ability to work with his back pain and reports that his supervisor is not sympathetic. He states that he often drives his repair truck into desolate areas and is required to lift and move heavy boiler parts weighing upwards of 60 pounds.

Case Analysis

From the information provided, it would appear that this man has sustained a back strain in a non-work-related lifting incident. His prior history of occasional backaches, peptic ulcer, and obesity are factors to be addressed, as is his work, which would be classified as "heavy." Because of his prior peptic ulcer, treatment with nonsteroidal medications may be contraindicated, and conservative treatment needs to address back strengthening and weight reduction. Due to the physical demands of his job, a period of disability seems warranted to allow for healing and treatment of the strain. However, an extension of 6 weeks is excessive at this stage.

Further Information Needed

From the employee. The case manager would explain her role and inquire as to current status. Is the pain subsiding? How often is he taking a muscle relaxant and Tylenol? Are they effective? What is he doing now? (watching television, walking, resting). Has he started physical therapy, and what is his perception of it? She would determine his current weight and discuss weight factor influence on his back problems; she also would encourage weight reduction. In addition, she would discuss potential for early return to work and his response to this, and encourage contact with supervisor.

From the physician(s). Determine specialty (if not an orthopedic physician, consideration for referral may be warranted). Obtain objective findings noted during physical exam, reports of any diagnostics (i.e., X-ray, MRI), type of physical therapy program recommended, frequency and duration, and name and dosage for muscle relaxant. Inquire as to feasibility of release to light or sedentary work and when this may occur. Provide MD with job analysis for employee position and alternate or transitional position as well. Discuss/suggest back strengthening programs as part of the physical therapy.

From the employer. Advise as to role of case manager; determine impression of employee (Is he a satisfactory employee? Any other problems? Willing to return him to alternate job?). Encourage contact with employee. At this stage, no further medical evaluation is warranted.

Using *The Medical Disability Advisor* and the information obtained (assuring these are objective findings), the estimated length of disability/duration is 1 week (less if appropriate alternate or light-work position is available). We would advise employer as to current status, plans for return to work, estimated time frame, and suggested alternate position(s). We would recommend a transitional position with no heavy lifting, bending, climbing, etc. No consideration for FMLA; however, reasonable accommodation may be appropriate. If there is no improvement, referrals to orthopedic/ neurologist for further diagnostic evaluation and treatment would be considered.

The next case management follow-up would be made with the patient, treating physician, and employer within 1 week. To facilitate return to work and case closure, we would encourage appropriate treatment of condition, communication between employee and supervisor, and provide support and direction to employee.

Case #3

A 28-year-old secretary slipped on a wet floor and twisted her neck and upper back. She's been out of work for 6 days and reports pain in the posterior cervical area and left upper back. She has vague complaints of discomfort going into her left arm. Her doctor has told the patient she should avoid using her left arm and "take it easy." Her doctor's lines state: "Employee may return to limited duty: no excessive use of left arm, no lifting over 15 pounds, no excessive phone use, sitting or reaching above her head." She wants to get back to work but feels she may not be able to meet her department's performance expectations if allowed back to work with these restrictions.

Case Analysis

It would appear from the information provided that this young woman has sustained a cervical strain, similar to a "whiplash" injury following a slip/fall accident. The case manager would have to ascertain whether treatment with her physician is ongoing and the diagnosis that was made. Because of her young age, we can assume that this is an acute problem and that with appropriate treatment, her ability to return to preinjury state and productivity is excellent. Although the doctor has released her to work, there are limitations, which are vague and in need of more specifics (i.e., what is meant by "excessive").

Further Information Needed

From the employee. Following an explanation of our role, we would inquire as to the current status, treatment to date, and results—is condition improving? Any cervical collar? Medication and results? We would also determine prior problems with neck or back, other medical problems, any other lost-time incidents, how she relates to her supervisor, and whether there's been any contact since the accident. (We would encourage this.) We would also discuss return-to-work issues, possible transitional assignment until she feels better (for example, perhaps as a receptionist—assuming she's right-handed, she would have use of this arm—with use of telephone headset, etc.), and determine her response to this. Advise her that we will be contacting her physician and supervisor and will follow up with her as well.

From the physician(s). Explain role of case manager and our interest in assisting with resolving medical problems and an early return to work. Determine diagnosis, results of any diagnostics, treatment to date, plan for future treatment, etc. Discuss limitations as stated in release to limited duty note, offer to send job analysis for review or share actual physical requirements of employee's job as well as a modified or transitional one. Obtain more definitive information. Determine when employee is scheduled for next visit and advise that we will follow up after that.

From the employer. Determine relationship with employee (i.e., is she a good worker, length of employment). Obtain physical requirements of position (Job Analysis, if available) to be able to share with treating MD. Determine willingness to have employee return to work in a transitional assignment (i.e., reduced hours, varied job duties—employee could use calculator with right hand—perhaps a project involving adding columns of numbers, or filing, taking dictation). Discuss reduced hours/days (which would also allow for treatment), avoidance of typing, use of headset for phone time, etc. Advise that we will be back in touch as soon as we have additional information.

Using the *Medical Disability Advisor* as a guide for estimated length of disability/duration, this woman has approached the estimated 1-week duration. However, if no treatment has occurred, then additional time may be warranted. If no improvement has occurred, discuss with MD the possibility of referral to orthopedist or neurologist for further evaluation. There is no consideration under FMLA and no protection under ADA because injury is of limited duration and does not interfere with major life activity.

The next case management follow-up would be made with the patient as soon as information is obtained from the MD and employer, with the treating physician following the employee's next appointment and with the employer as soon as more is known regarding a return to work (3 to 5 days). We would encourage the supervisor to contact employee and vice versa.

Case #4

A 40-year-old male began an absence 2 days earlier after a driving while intoxicated (DWI) episode. The patient reports he has been ordered by the court to undergo treatment for a cocaine and alcohol problem of some 20 years' duration. In speaking to the patient, the case manager learns that as a result of angry and threatening outbursts against several coworkers and his manager, he was referred 3 months earlier for outpatient assessment and treatment. A psychiatric consultant concluded the patient suffers from a personality disorder in addition to chemical dependency. The employee indicates that after several weeks he discontinued outpatient treatment and resumed his use of alcohol and cocaine. Recently, he has had increasing displays of anger both at home and on the job, and his wife of 18 years is planning to leave him. There are no friends or family who are close to the employee, who reports that he has always preferred solitude. At the present time, the employee is experiencing disappointment and anger against company management in general, indicating they have not been supportive. He adds that he feels his anger would be overwhelming were he to lose his job.

Case Analysis

From the information given, it would appear that this 40-year-old man has a long-standing history of alcohol and cocaine abuse with at least one episode of treatment that was terminated by the employee. With a diagnosis of personality disorder, DWI, arrest and court-ordered treatment, this man is clearly a danger to himself, others, and a threat to the workplace. The goal here would be to determine whether potential exists for treatment, rehabilitation, and return to work. Clearly, more information is needed in order to assess viability of this case. We do not know if this individual is a union employee, nor is it clear how long this individual has been an employee or whether his substance abuse problems have resulted in work-related problems. In this instance, and to determine extent of the problem prior to contact with the employee, the employer would be contacted first.

Further Information Needed

From the employer. We would determine prior lost-time incidents, any involvement with an employee assistance program, union versus management status, any prior alcohol/substance abuse treatment, length of employment, and any prior disciplinary actions. Assuming that there have been no prior disciplinary actions, we would attempt to proceed with resolving the multiple problems.

From the employee. We would contact the employee, explaining our role and the purpose of our intervention. We would express our concern for him, emphasizing the seriousness of the situation and its impact on his well-being and his job. We would determine his interest in accepting help and pursuing discussion of an inpatient program to address his substance abuse and other emotional issues. Because he has been ordered by the court into a program, we would assist him with compliance and entry into an appropriate program. An outpatient program will not be successful, and it will be important for him to recognize this and the responsibility he must now assume to confront and resolve these issues. We would assure him that our involvement will continue and, when appropriate, a return to work would be considered.

From the physician(s). We would contact the treating psychiatrist and obtain prior history, treatment, etc., explaining our role and expressing the concerns of the employer and its interest in attempting to assist in expediting appropriate treatment and possible return to work. We would determine the duration of inpatient and outpatient treatment needed and advise that we would assist as indicated. We would also contact the court officer to determine whether a specific facility/program was mandated and coordinate referrals as needed.

We would suggest 4 weeks to allow for treatment. At this time, the employee is not an appropriate candidate for return to work; he is a danger to himself as well as his coworkers. Assuming his supervisor has been advised of the DWI and related problems, he or she would be told of the planned treatment and probable duration of disability. This individual would not qualify for leave under FMLA; however, if he successfully completed treatment, he may qualify for ADA reasonable accommodation.

The next case management follow-up would be made with the patient in 1 week or sooner, as indicated, and with the treating physician and employer in 1 week. To facilitate return to work and case closure, we would maintain contact, encouraging communication among all parties.

Case #5

A 42-year-old male employee has been absent for 7 days. The employee is being treated by a psychiatrist who indicates he is "not fit for duty" because of stress. Upon initial contact, the employee states he had worked as a manager for 5 years, applied for a manager's position with the same company but at another location within the state, and was hired. However, his local management stated they couldn't transfer him for business reasons. The employee decided to return to his former craft position, which was approved by management. After the employee worked as an operator for approximately 3 months, he announced his intentions of running for a union position. A week after this announcement, local management informed him they had erroneously approved his retreat to his craft position and that he must be reinstated to his former managerial position. The employee feels angry and humiliated. He states "this situation is a conspiracy" and that both "management and the union are after me."

Case Analysis

It would appear that the employee's disability status is interestingly related to a labor relations matter. "Not fit for duty" is an ambiguous term and would not support a continued period of disability. The case manager would work quickly to address and hopefully resolve the issues. However, further information is needed. This would appear to be a nonmedical issue with the potential for being problematic without prompt resolution.

Further Information Needed

After we have spoken with the employee and explained the role of case manager, we would proceed with a call to the employer. We would discuss the information as told by the employee with our contact at the employer and/or its labor relations person (if known), and advise that this is a possible labor/management issue requiring some mediation. We would request employer assistance with this prior to further involvement. Because the employee is already feeling that "management and the union are after me," further contact with his treating psychiatrist may be viewed by this man as "harassment."

If the labor/management issue was irresolvable or would be over a protracted period of time, then, as directed by the employer, we could proceed with disability determination. We would advise, however, that an independent medical exam, etc., could heighten employee anger. There is no consideration for FMLA or ADA.

The next case management follow-up would be made with the employee and the treating psychiatrist as directed by the employer, and with the employer within a few days. We would continue to assist the employer with mediation efforts as directed. If indeed this is a labor issue, we would close the file.

NOTES

1. Foundation for Rehabilitation Certification, Education, and Research, "Interpersonal Skills for Case Managers," in *Case Management Practice*: Foundation for Rehabilitation Certification, Education, and Research, 1993), 120–122.

2. Reinertsen Group, *Doing Well by Doing Good: Improving the Business Case for Quality* (Alta, WY: Reinertsen Group, 2003).

3. Foundation for Rehabilitation Certification, Education, and Research, "Interpersonal Skills," 118.

4. Dearing G, "Improving Patient Compliance in the Best Interests of All," *Managed Healthcare News* 12, no. 12 (1996): 1, 15–16.

5. Hoffmann L, "Practical Tips to Help You Master Telephonic CM," *Case Management Advisor* 8, no. 2 (1997): 29–30. (For more information, please call 800-688-2421.)

6. Foundation for Rehabilitation Certification, Education, and Research, "Interpersonal Skills," 119.

7. Gosfield AG, "The 1995 Legal Clinic," presented at the Medical Case Management Conference VII, New Orleans, LA, October 1995; Gosfield, "Guidelines," 106.

APPENDIX 9–A

CMSA Standards of Practice for Case Management

II. Standards of Care

A. Client Identification and Selection for Case Management Services

The first step in the case management process is to identify those individuals who can most benefit from case management services. Identification of clients for case management services is accomplished through methods and tools that include, but are not limited to, health-risk screening tools, evidence-based criteria, risk stratification through data management, and referrals.

Determining whether a client is appropriate for case management services is achieved by gathering and critically assessing relevant, comprehensive information and data, so that clients are selected according to case management potential to influence positive outcomes. The case manager may or may not participate in client identification or in determining whether the client meets criteria for case management services. Rather, clients may be mandated to receive case management services based upon disease state, age, payer, potential for high cost, etc.

MEASUREMENT GUIDELINES

The case manager will seek to:

1. Evaluate pro-active triggers (such as criteria related to diagnosis, clinical condition, complications, or cost) to identify potential clients suitable for effective case management intervention

2. Consider strategies of predictive modeling, when available, including emerging technologies (i.e., neural networks that predict high-cost populations)

3. Conduct a thorough and systematic evaluation of the client's current status using standardized tools when appropriate, including the following components:

    - Physical/functional
    - Psychosocial
    - Behavioral
    - Environmental/residential
    - Family dynamics and support
    - Spiritual
    - Cultural
    - Financial
    - Vocational and/or educational
    - Recreational/leisure pursuits
    - Caregiver(s) capability and availability
    - Learning capabilities/self care
    - Health status expectation and goals
    - Transitional or discharge plan
    - Legal

4. Assess resource utilization and cost management; the diagnosis, past and present treatment course and services; prognosis, goals (short/long term), treatment, and provider options

5. Engage reliable and valid assessment steps to identify and select clients for case management services

B. Problem Identification

Utilizing objective data gathered through careful assessment and examination of the potential for effective intervention, the case manager identifies problems requiring case management intervention, reflecting practice patterns and trends wherein client outcomes can be positively influenced. Client/family participation is an essential element in problem identification.

MEASUREMENT GUIDELINES

The case manager will seek to identify opportunities for intervention, i.e., when there is:

- Lack of an established treatment plan with specific goals

- Compromised patient safety

- Over-utilization of services or use of multiple providers/agencies

- Under-utilization of services

- Premature or delayed discharge from appropriate level of care

- Use of inappropriate services

- Ineffective treatment plan

- Permanent or temporary alterations in functioning

- High-cost injuries or illnesses

- Non-adherence to treatment or medications

- Medical/psychological/functional complications

- Lack of education of disease course/process

- Lack of resolution in meeting health needs

- Lack of family/social support

- Lack of financial resources to meet health needs

The case manager will also seek to determine patterns of care that may lead a client into a case management program, which may include involvement in analysis of the patterns of care or behavior that may be associated with progression to severe disease.

C. Planning

The case manager, in collaboration with the client/family and members of the healthcare team, identifies immediate, short-term, and ongoing needs as well as develops appropriate and necessary case management strategies to address them. The case manager communicates with the client/family about which case management strategies will be implemented in the plan of care. The case manager assists the client/family in making informed decisions when developing this plan of care. The case management plan identifies measurable goals and time frames for achieved goals that are appropriate to the individual, his/her family, and agreed to by the client/family and treatment team. Distinction should be made between process and end-point goals. The case manager identifies funding and/or community resources that are available to implement the plan.

MEASUREMENT GUIDELINES

The case manager will seek to:

1. Interview, research, and otherwise gather relevant, comprehensive information and data to establish the factual and clinical basis upon which to develop an appropriate plan of care

2. Understand the client's diagnosis, prognosis, care needs, and outcome goals of the plan of care

3. Implement cost-savings strategies when possible, while considering the policy/benefits available to the client

4. Proactively identify situations that are, or may become, barriers to goal attainment

5. Work toward resolution of conflicts and problem solving

6. Involve the client/family and the healthcare team in the ongoing plan of care

7. Identify goals and related indicators for successful planning and implementation, such as clinical stability or client adherence to treatments and medications

D. Monitoring

The case manager employs a process of ongoing assessment and documentation to monitor the quality of care, services and products delivered to the client to determine if the goals of the plan of care are being achieved, whether those goals remain appropriate and realistic, and what actions may be implemented to enhance positive outcomes.

MEASUREMENT GUIDELINES

The case manager will seek to:

1. Maintain professional collaboration and communication with the client and family to the extent possible, so that important information regarding the client's health status and the impact on the goals and outcome of the care plan can be disclosed

2. Maintain professional collaboration and communication with the members of the healthcare team so that the plan of care can be discussed objectively, problems can be identified, and adjustments can be made to the plan as needed

3. Maintain regular communication with pertinent healthcare providers regarding client transition across settings, barriers to care/services, and strategies or plan revisions that are needed. Ascertain that the goals of the care plan are appropriate, understood, documented, and are being met. Also advise the providers of adjustments or revisions to be made in the care plan

4. Compare the client's care plan to evidence-based guidelines, when available, to determine variances and offer solutions or adjustments to the plan of care when variances exist or when otherwise appropriate

5. Review pertinent statistics to perform a comprehensive and independent assessment of the client's status and progress toward reaching the goals set forth in the care plan

6. Implement a data-tracking mechanism, when available, to determine goals that were met versus not met and to review safety indicators

E. Evaluating

The case manager employs a methodology designed to measure healthcare and case management processes focusing on the client's response to the case management plan. The evaluation process occurs over specific time frames and is a continuous process. The evaluation engages the client/family whenever possible, as well as the healthcare team, to appropriately determine the impact of case management and healthcare interventions on outcomes.

MEASUREMENT GUIDELINES

The case manager will seek to:

1. Identify when a client's condition has reached a static or regressive situation and proactively facilitate adjustments in the care plan, providers, and/or services, when possible, to promote enhanced outcomes

2. Focus efforts on maintaining the stability of the client's/family's home environment

3. Utilize knowledge of patterns in the stabilization, recovery process and resource use of individual clients to help revise standards of care for populations of clients

F.   Outcomes

Case management is a goal-directed process. The case manager identifies and implements changes in practice patterns and in the plan of care to produce outcomes that are positive, measurable and goal-oriented.

MEASUREMENT GUIDELINES

The case manager will seek to:

1. Plan with the client/family using a goal-oriented care process that analyzes and gives direction to a plan of care that moves the client toward health, wellness, safety, adaptation, self-care, and/or (re)habilitation

2. Establish measurable case management goals which promote evaluation

of the access, cost, and quality of the care provided

3. Identify the achievement of goals and differentiate those goals that directly resulted from the case manager's interventions

4. Report quantifiable impact, quality of care, and/or quality of life improvements as measured against the case management goals

5. Focus on accountability for quality care and/or cost benefit to clients that are reasonably consistent with payer, provider, and consumer expectations

6. Recommend referral sources based on evaluation of the provider's quality of care and the ability to meet the client's needs

7. Maximize client outcomes through incorporating community-based and non-benefit related services whenever possible

Source: Reprinted with permission, Case Management Society of America, 6301 Ranch Drive, Little Rock, AR 72223; www.cmsa.org.

Chapter 10

Integrated Case Management: Preadmission, Concurrent Review, Utilization Review, Disease Management, and Case Management

There are several methodologies available to identify individuals who could benefit from case management intervention. The line of insurance and the structure and sophistication of a claims department affect which "red flags" are used. Some claims departments contract for review services, whereas others depend on in-house capabilities.

Generally speaking, reviews are either prospective (before the event, called preadmission or precertification), concurrent (during the event), or retrospective (after the event). All these types of reviews are basically forms of utilization review. The purpose of utilization review is to evaluate the necessity, appropriateness, and efficiency of the use of medical services.

Each type of review utilizes certain criteria to determine whether there is a need for further action, decision, or intervention. For instance, an organization that provides retrospective claim review services might review all surgical claims that are over $10,000 and include more than three Current Procedural Terminology (CPT) codes. These factors suggest a potentially unbundled claim, and the action warranted is a review by a utilization review nurse or physician. Another indicator might be an inpatient hospital bill with a disproportionately large pharmacy charge, which suggests a potential overcharge; the action warranted is a hospital bill audit. The review process itself can also be used to identify cases for case management if the organization reviewer is aware of the red flags (e.g., multiple hospital admissions, certain ICD-9 diagnostic codes, claims for apnea alarms, electric hospital beds, infusion care services).

The problem with retrospective reviews is that the services have already occurred and are now being billed. Occasionally, the best that can be gained is a minimal discount, perhaps for a prompt-pay arrangement (invoices earmarked by the case manager to be paid within 2 or 3 weeks). It is always preferable to be positioned from strength, and this is the case if one is aware of services *before* they are implemented rather than after. From a case management perspective, the opportunity to explore alternatives is already absent when the case manager is confronted with a claim for $60,000 resulting from a hospital stay of 28 days. Could the patient have gone to a skilled facility for two of those weeks? Were nursing and other services in the home a possibility? And with these as alternatives, would there have been fee negotiations as well? These are now questions without answers. What to do with the $60,000 bill? Can the carrier get a prompt-pay discount? Was there overbilling? These savings, if possible at all, pale by comparison to what could have been!

Review of services prospectively and concurrently, on the other hand, presents the best opportunity for a successful case management intervention. How this process works varies from company to company, but in my mind there is no reason to have preadmission or concurrent review other than to identify at the earliest opportunity potentially high-cost cases and then intervene.

It is amazing to me that carriers, Third Party Administrators, managed care organizations, and employer groups often set up a precertification or preadmission review* program without linking it to some kind of case management program. They perform reviews in a management vacuum and then assume that there are no savings to be gained. Several companies have discontinued their use because "they didn't save us any money." And, indeed, they will not, other than those possibly realized through the denial of a few days in a hospital or avoidance of an inpatient stay when a day-op procedure is indicated. (However, day-op procedures at ambulatory surgicenters are often much more costly than an inpatient

---

*In my former company, we avoided the use of the term *precertification* because it implies approval or denial of the proposed admission and related services and payment for them. As we believe the Plan makes these decisions, ours is an advisory notification program.

stay would have been. This is because of the lack of reasonable and customary charges for surgicenter facilities.) Without a connection to case management, preadmission review accomplishes nothing more than maintaining a census of inpatient admissions. And preadmission review alone, without concurrent review, is incapable of reducing lengths of stay or allowing alternative care plans to be considered.

Let us assume that there is an understanding of the value of preadmission and concurrent review and a case management program, which is now the case where managed care is well-established. Many companies are looking for care networks in which utilization review is offered as part of a healthcare package, including some type of preadmission review and case management, and many UR providers that began as companies offering retroactive review of medical bills now offer case management, disease management, demand management, and provider profiling. Who should provide the services, how should they be provided, and what, if any, should the guidelines and procedures be? Are there standards of practice, and what should the results be? Fortunately, there are some established standards and guidelines as well as organizations that continue to evaluate and review existing and developing programs. *Milliman Care Guidelines* includes clinical indications, care pathways, benchmarks, nationally recognized guidelines, and current medical research. Other groups providing care guidelines include the National Institutes of Health, the National Committee for Quality Assurance, Value Health Sciences of Santa Monica, California, and Interqual. The Agency for Healthcare Research and Quality web site (www.ahcpr.gov) offers an online database of healthcare quality measures (National Quality Measures Clearinghouse), studies and projects on measuring healthcare quality and quality indicators.

I believe that the maximum opportunity for success exists when one organization provides preadmission and concurrent review along with case management services. Too often, one company does the reviewing and another provides the case management. The delays that inevitably occur between identifying a high-cost case, referring it to a case management vendor, assigning the case, and actually managing the case make the system ineffective, rather than an ongoing process of evaluation, identification, assessment, planning, and implementation that could be the ideal. The key in case management is how the case manager gets involved and how soon. For example, one has missed an opportunity if a case manager starts working with a spinal cord-injured patient 20 or 30 days after the initial hospitalization. Earlier involvement could have resulted in a transfer of this patient to a spinal cord injury treatment center and the prevention of some of the complications that have now occurred, which will be more costly to treat and prolong the period of rehabilitation.

So, let us once again make some assumptions and create the ideal program within one organization. To illustrate how this process could work, let's "take a walk through" the system.

INTRODUCING UTILIZATION REVIEW TO CLIENT GROUPS AND PLAN PARTICIPANTS

Let us suppose that a single organization intends to offer a combination preadmission review, concurrent review, case management, and disease management program. The first step in selling and implementing this program is to explain it to potential clients and the plan participants. If these individuals do not understand its purpose, its full benefits will not be realized. Over the years, I have seen various techniques utilized in an effort to implement such programs. These range from mandating cooperation, to penalizing by reducing the percentage of benefit reimbursement, to denying benefits altogether. Although the policy language needs to have some "teeth" to encourage participation, I think proactively positioning the services has a better chance of achieving success in the long run.

In today's environment, in which virtually everyone appreciates not just the cost of the healthcare system but its complexity as well, communicating the concept of a preadmission, concurrent review, disease management, and case management program is not really difficult. The intent very simply is to very proactively identify at the earliest opportunity patients or situations that could benefit from the intervention of a case manager. The program should be flexible and fast-moving enough to move the patient who needs it into case management as soon as possible. If concern for patients is seen as the focus, then enlisting cooperation becomes easier.

Case managers should be positioned as advocates and facilitators who have the expertise to understand and the ability to effect change. They assist patients by getting information and expediting the delivery of services. To perform their functions effectively, they need a system that allows involvement to occur at the optimum time. Because a seemingly simple admission or "routine" operative procedure can unexpectedly become complex and expensive, each admission needs to be reviewed as it occurs. This does not mean that each will require intervention by a case manager; in fact, most will not. But the strategy of reviewing each leads to the best outcomes for patients and payers.

Not long ago, I was meeting with two client groups. The first was considering having their claims staff handle all of the preadmission notification calls; they would refer to our case management department those cases they thought would be appropriate for our case management services. The second client group was prepared to suggest to its employer groups that they should notify its preadmission and concurrent review providers only of "serious conditions." It became clear to me that we, as the case management providers, were going to be disadvantaged by this incorrect perception of the process. Some further education was obviously necessary.

I took a sampling of the first client group's preadmission forms. It was soon apparent that some of the cases it would have identified were not appropriate for case management, whereas others that would have been overlooked required intervention. As an example, one admission for "abdominal pain" turned out to be a malignancy of the pancreas; the patient eventually went home after a 3-week hospital stay, with nursing and infusion care services arranged by the hospital (the infusion care services were referred to a physician-owned provider). Appropriate case management intervention would have served both the patient and the payer in this case.

The second client group, after a similar discussion, soon realized that each individual has a different perception of what constitutes a "serious condition" and that, in fact, it was not only the "condition" that might signal a problem, but other factors as well (e.g., multiple admissions, several seemingly "minor" medical conditions but only one admission, prior history). Through an education process, both client groups were soon able not only to understand the scope and value of an integrated preadmission and concurrent review and case management approach, but also to develop an appreciation of its complexity, which allowed them to implement a total and integrated system.

Whether by brochure, newsletter, flyer, meetings, or some other format, a program overview needs to be communicated. The sample cases presented in Figure 10–1 and Figure 10–2 were created for our clients to illustrate what would probably occur with and without an integrated system in place. Table 10–1 is a letter designed to be sent to plan participants to acknowledge notification of hospital admission and explain the advocacy role of the case manager and the nature of the case management process. Table 10–2 is a description of our company and its services that we send to communicate to employees, in layman's terms, the process of case management when a union, TPA, or insurer puts case management services in place. This always accompanies a letter such as the one shown in Table 10–1.

Figure 10–1 Case Sample with and without Preadmission Review, Concurrent Review, and Case Management.

Exhibit A

Mr. Jones enters the hospital as recommended by his physician for diagnosis of pneumonia. As prescribed by his medical plan, he contacts ABC Insurance Co. to advise of his scheduled admission. ABC's representative obtains basic information concerning hospital, treating physician, and possibly the proposed length of stay for this admission (5 days).

The notification procedure is completed, there is no follow-up of this patient, and eventually this individual will be discharged.

The hospital claim is eventually received by ABC, and it is then noted that the actual stay was for 21 days at a cost of $45,000.

Exhibit B

Mr. Jones, as prescribed by his medical plan, contacts ABC Insurance Co. to advise of his scheduled admission, and the representative obtains information concerning diagnosis, length of stay, name of treating physician, hospital, etc. This information is then faxed to Options Unlimited, where it is screened for follow-up.

The Options Unlimited nurse contacts the patient and treating physician, and obtains additional information, including prior medical history, other hospital admissions, etc. She is in agreement with the treating physician for length of stay (LOS for this man would be 5 days).

Now on day 5, Options Unlimited nurse contacts hospital utilization review nurse to determine if, in fact, patient will be discharged. Utilization review nurse advises that there was not a good result thus far with current antibiotic and further hospitalization was indicated. Options Unlimited nurse confers with treating physician, who discusses further and hopes that an additional 3 days will result in success.

Options Unlimited nurse contacts treating MD who reports continued lack of response and additional complications. He will try a different antibiotic, will need perhaps another 7–10 days of hospitalization.

Due to extended stay, requests for additional days, and uncertain treatment plan, decision made to refer for on-site case management assessment.

Figure 10–1 continued

Visit by case manager to patient and treating physician uncovers additional problems but result is that MD agrees to discharge patient home on IV antibiotics (rather than continue inpatient stay).

The patient is discharged to his home on day 9 of this hospital admission. Antibiotic therapy and nursing services are provided in his home. The Options Unlimited case manager has arranged the services with the input from the MD, negotiated the fees for these services, and monitored the patient for the desired outcome and eventual discontinuation of these services. Following a 10-day course at home, he is switched to antibiotics by mouth and permitted to return to work.

Results

Action: Pay claim (obtain discount if possible, audit the claim) of $45,000.00
Savings: None
Questions: 1) Were all the costs necessary?
2) Was a 21-day stay necessary?
3) Were there other alternatives?

Results

Pay: Hospital claim of $19,278.00
Pay: Claim for home antibiotic therapy and nursing services of $3,000.00 ($300/day × 10 days).
Pay: Case management fees of $800.00
Total: $23,078.00
Savings: $21,922.00
Questions: Were the costs appropriate? Yes
Were the patient and the plan well served? Yes

Source: Courtesy of Options Unlimited, Case Management Services Division, © 2003, Huntington, New York.

Figure 10–2 Case Sample with and without Preadmission Review, Concurrent Review, and Case Management.

Exhibit A

Mr. Jones sustains an injury to his right knee following a fall from a ladder and reports the injury. He is out of work for 1 week and his supervisor has not heard from him or when he is coming back. The worker's family MD is treating the injury conservatively with rest and minimal activity. It is 3 weeks later and the supervisor now hears from the worker's coworkers that there is now an infection in the knee and the worker is scheduled for a surgical procedure. No date for return to work is known. Another week passes, the worker is out of the hospital but still having problems. The supervisor does not know what the problems are but the worker's prolonged absence is increasing the workload on the department, and the supervisor is behind on his work (trying to keep peace and help out himself). It is now 6 weeks since this "little fall" (as per the supervisor) and it has gone on "too long." The treating MD has told the worker that he can go back to "light duty" and maybe his old job in another month. The supervisor tells the claims examiner there is no "light duty" and the worker continues to remain home. Someone sees the worker mowing his lawn, word reaches the employer, who notifies the claims examiner and requests surveillance. We all know where this is going, don't we?

Exhibit B

Mr. Jones sustains an injury to his right knee following a fall from a ladder. As is required, he reports the injury to his supervisor. The supervisor advises him that a case manager will be contacting him to help him get appropriate care, answer questions he may have, and assist him in returning to work. Options Unlimited's case manager contacts the injured worker and learns that he has sustained a 4-inch laceration to the knee, which required several stitches in the Emergency Room. She also learned during her phone assessment with the employer that he was unclear as to the care of the wound, what dressing was needed, or how often it should be changed. He also did not know the signs of infection to check for and had not yet scheduled a follow-up visit with his family MD. Because the case manager asked about prior medical history, she discovered that the worker had a "little bit of diabetes" (this as per the worker) and was lacking knowledge about this disease and, in fact, was told he had cataracts and that his vision is a little "blurry."

The case manager assessed the following as problems:

• A large laceration, requiring daily dressing changes and inspection of the wound
• Condition of cataracts that resulted in blurred vision and the inability to detect subtle changes in the wound
• Unmanaged diabetes, which prolongs and complicates the wound-healing process

Figure 10–2 continued

The case manager implemented the following:

- Skilled nursing visits daily to inspect wound, change the dressing and assess diabetic care needs
- Referral to physician the following day (after explaining risk factors for infection to office nurse)
- Call to supervisor apprising him of status of employee. During this call, obtained description of employee's job (physical demands, etc.), discussed some possible modifications to be considered, and suggested a call to the worker by the supervisor to "touch base," assure concern, and wish well.

Within a week, healing was progressing well and following calls to employee and treating MD, it was determined that worker could return to work as long as he did not have to use a ladder or work in a crouched position.

The supervisor was able to modify worker's position (climbing the ladder was needed only occasionally and another worker could do this; crouching position was done rarely and this, too, could be done by another). Employee could also be checked daily by the company nurse, who will also monitor his diabetes.

Eleven days after the injury, the employee returned to a modified form of his job. The case manager maintained contact with all parties, insured that the wound was completely healed in 3 weeks, and the worker could return to all of his duties.

continues

Figure 10–2 continued

Exhibit A

Costs:
Medical: Hospital admission for wound
   infection and IV antibiotics; wound
   incisions and drainage.
Hospital @ $1500 × 7 days = $10,500
Surgery: $2,500
Physical therapy, 3 times a week × 4
   weeks (and continuing) = $900.00
IV antibiotics @ home following hospital
   stay @ $550/day plus nursing visit
   @ $140/visit × 7 = $4,830
MD fees = $2,000
Replacement of earnings @ $450/week
   × 6 = $2,700
Medical: $20,730.00 and continuing
Lost earnings $2,700.00 and continuing
Total costs $23,430.00
Indirect costs:
Decreased productivity
Litigation
Employee morale
AND IT'S NOT OVER.....!

Results

Increased costs
An employee with continuing medical
   complications
Adversarial relationship between
   employer/employee
Pending litigation
Decreased productivity
Decreased morale

Exhibit B

Costs:
Medical: Nursing visits for wound
   care/dressing changes @ negotiated
   rate of $75 × 10 days = $750.00
MD fees—2 visits for wound
   care/diabetic management = $200
Replacement of Earnings @ $450/week
   × 2 = $900.00
Total Costs: $1,650.00*

Results

Savings (Net): $20,780*

Actual costs and case management
fees were deducted from costs of case
that would have occurred **as in
Exhibit A.**

A **productive employee** with a better
outcome and the recipient of a true
advocacy program.

A business that can return to its own
business needs and goals.

*Case management is another cost consideration, but in this kind of case, managed early would be less
than $1,000.00.

Source: Courtesy of Options Unlimited, Case Management Services Division, © 2003,
Huntington, New York.

Table 10–1 Letter Acknowledging Prenotification of Hospital Admission and Explaining Case Management to Plan Participants

---

Employee's ID#:
Physician:
Hospital:
Date of Admission:
Employer Group:

To:

We received notification of the above hospital admission on _____. Please be advised that this is an advisory notice only and does not imply payment of the claim/bill that will be received for this hospital confinement. It further does not imply payment for any of the services that may be related to the confinement, for example, surgeon, anesthesia, and so on.

A Nurse Case Manager will be following the patient's progress during the hospital stay. It is also possible that a Nurse Case Manager may be in contact with you either via telephone or in person, should this seem appropriate.

All claims received by the plan administrator for _____ will be reviewed and considered and will be subject to the terms of your medical plan. This includes but is not limited to preexisting conditions, plan limitations and exclusions, cosmetic vs. medical need, uncovered services, etc., co-payments and deductibles.

If there are any changes in the case-related information above, please notify the Nurse Case Manager at 1-800-555-1212. If you have any additional questions or concerns about this or other medical matters, please feel free to call us.

Thank you in advance for your anticipated cooperation.

Very truly yours,

_____

Nurse Case Manager, Options Unlimited
cc: File @ S.L.01437

Source: Courtesy of Options Unlimited, Case Management Services Division, © 2003, Huntington, New York.

Table 10–2 Sample Description of Case Management Services for Employee/
Patient Populations

OPTIONS UNLIMITED

Solving Problems Is What We Do Best

At Options Unlimited, we've been helping people across the country understand their medical choices, evaluate their care options, and find solutions
in tough medical situations for over 20 years. We're a full-service medical
case management and benefits consulting firm. We work with you, your
employer, and your insurer to make sure your medical treatment is appropriate and progresses as it should.

You might talk to one of our nurses on the phone regarding a hospital
admission of an anticipated birth. In complex cases such as cancer, cardiovascular disease, AIDS, a stroke, transplant, head or spinal cord injury, or a
high-risk pregnancy, one of our case managers will arrange to meet with
you personally to help coordinate care for you or someone else covered by
your healthcare plan.

You don't pay for our case management services; they are offered in conjunction with your healthcare plan. And our services are voluntary. We *can
help* you get the best, most appropriate, and most cost-effective care, but
you do not have to use our services. Most important to you, we keep all
personal information regarding you and your health in strictest confidence.

We work as advocates for patients, focusing on each individual case to
explain the diagnosis and what it means for today and tomorrow. We take
the lingo out of insurance plans and forms, arrange for home-care services,
locate alternate treatment facilities or rehabilitation service—sometimes we
even help sort out all the medications, or the bills! The one thing we don't
do is provide hands-on care. We don't take the place of your physicians; we
work as partners with your physicians, making sure that you and your family members get all the care you need when you need it.

We look forward to helping you receive more personalized medical care.

Source: Courtesy of Options Unlimited, Case Management Services Division, © 2003,
Huntington, New York.

THE PREADMISSION AND CONCURRENT REVIEW PROCESS

Each preadmission and concurrent review process differs depending
upon client group specifications and the line of insurance involved. For
example, a nurse reviewer for workers' compensation may inquire as to
the estimated return-to-work date or work restrictions (e.g., no lifting),

whereas a nurse reviewer for a group medical plan does not need such information. (However, some information is requested in both types of review.) It is essential to develop a format to gather the necessary data and organize them so that they will be useful in evaluating and identifying cases with potential for case management intervention. There are software systems that have been developed for this purpose, although an organization might elect to develop its own system.

Each system, manual or computerized, should allow for the input of a professional (nurse or physician). Although standardized questions and data are useful, each patient presents unique problems and symptoms. There needs to be sufficient flexibility to accommodate the differences. If a form or artificial intelligence (computer) system includes only set questions, it is impossible to discover all the situations and variables that might demand special attention. Even some very sophisticated software programs do not, unfortunately, allow for a patient-specific approach, thereby preventing consideration of the kinds of factors that would indicate the need for additional intervention.

All too often, we see utilization reviewers in a care management department talking to the utilization reviewers in the hospital. Most UR reviewers never see the patient. Utilization management looks at fees, access, frequency, and duration of care and services, and identifies which services, providers, and patients are most costly. To do this, standards, guidelines, and criteria are used to authorize and manage the delivery of services. Among the drawbacks of utilization management without preadmission review is that it is reactive and often retrospective. It invites litigation, lacks consistency in administration from company to company and region to region, and views the service and costs (benefit management) rather than patients (care management). No one is talking to the patient, getting a history of the case, learning what the prognosis is, or introducing the role of a case manager.

Notification that a patient is about to enter the hospital, or that a physician has called in for a plan member's hip replacement, is an ideal time to bring in a case manager. A hip implant is not, generally speaking, emergency surgery; however, the case manager might discover that this individual is also a diabetic with hypertension, and at risk for deep vein thrombosis or a pulmonary embolism. She can help prepare the patient for surgery, discuss expectations and post-op recovery time frames, and educate him toward compliance with the treatment plan.

If a healthy baby program is not in place, or the preadmission plan requires only that patients call 2 weeks before their due date, the care management team misses a chance to assist mother and fetus. A quick conversation during the first trimester can uncover any risk factors and identify those pregnant women who should be in case management.

Each case will not call for case management intervention, but being part of the review process early on allows a case manager to determine this in a timely manner.

A key to success is the reviewer's skill in conducting a more comprehensive questioning process. Beyond the general concern (and regrettably, sometimes the only concern) for length of stay, it is important to look for comorbidities. Is there another condition already present that might lead to difficulties or episodes that can be prevented before they happen? What is the medical history attached to this case? Is this a readmission for a chronic condition? We will want to assign the same reviewer to a case that has frequent readmissions; this person knows the patient, family, and history, and can be more effective more quickly than someone taking the information for the first time.

Some plans include a prenotification requirement for certain high-cost equipment and services: all monitors, oxygen contractors, apnea alarms, infusion services, chemotherapy, and more. The emphasis today, and the reason behind the requirement, is eligibility for coverage. Our reasoning should be, is this the beginning of a problem? With a call for such types of equipment, we know something is going on. Get behind the request. Is the equipment needed for a lung cancer patient or is it for short-term use? Perhaps the equipment or service is for therapy, but it might be for someone in the final stage of cancer whose family is actively seeking admission to a hospice program.

After the basic information is obtained (including admitting diagnosis, length of stay, and treatment plan), there needs to be a determination as to follow-up in the review process. If a length of stay is estimated to be five days, there should be a follow-up call on day four, or certainly day five, to determine whether, in fact, the discharge will occur as planned. Although some management groups review every case every single day, I believe this to be extreme and, in many cases, a waste of time almost bordering on harassment of the hospital staff, especially when individuals designated as "case managers" are doing nothing more than tracking LOS for the sole purpose of denying days. Further, an administrative clerk lacks the expertise to recognize possible red flags in the hospital nurse's responses, ask the appropriate follow-up questions, and get more involved in the case. In both cases, every opportunity has been lost for intervention and potential improvements in patient care and expenditures in the long term.

We want to review the appropriate case at the appropriate time for the appropriate reasons. Could anything different be done toward a positive result? A diary system, whether electronic or otherwise, helps schedule and manage hospital reviews. If it becomes obvious during the first call that the patient will require ICU care for the next 3 days, a call can be "diaried" for day 4.

If discharge is scheduled, will there be a need for any further services at home (e.g., nursing visits, physical therapy, or chemotherapy)? How was the hospital stay? Were there any problems or new conditions discovered? Is further testing required? What are post-discharge arrangements? Is a transfer to a different facility now scheduled? Is a follow-up call to the patient or to family members indicated to determine their understanding of the diagnosis or ability to cooperate with the discharge instructions? Were they, in fact, even aware of follow-up care instructions?

This kind of involvement by a nurse reviewer can often prevent a hospital readmission resulting from the patient's lack of knowledge. Two studies reported in *The New York Times* showed that nurse home-visit programs had lasting and positive effects. In one, visiting nurses discussed nutrition, prenatal care, child development, and other issues over a 2.5-year period with women following the birth of their first child. The home visits resulted in fewer and less closely spaced pregnancies, fewer cases of child abuse and neglect, and fewer emergency room visits. In a second program, nurses visited young, poor, unmarried, pregnant women and discussed prenatal health, parenting skills, birth control, education, and job skills. At age 2, the children were less likely to be injured or hospitalized, and mothers were less likely to have pregnancy-induced high blood pressure. Overall, compared with other poor, unmarried mothers, the women in the study had 69% fewer arrests, 46% fewer reports of child abuse or neglect, 44% fewer behavioral problems linked to drug or alcohol abuse, and used 30 months less of Aid to Families with Dependent Children.[1] The benefits consulting firm Hewitt Associates reports 77% of companies offering programs including well-baby or child care, prenatal care, disease management, and flu vaccinations, up from 71% in 1996.[2] (For every $6 flu vaccination, $40 is saved because employees are at work, not home in bed.[3])

A follow-up call to the treating physician by a nurse reviewer to share a discovered problem is always welcome and helps establish a productive collaboration between two professionals who want a good outcome for the patient. Necessary services can be arranged with the client group's PPO network or at a negotiated rate. Continued case management involvement additionally provides the ability to oversee treatment effectiveness and continued need.

As noted earlier, it is not necessary to review every hospitalized patient every day, especially in a routine case such as a C-section or hip replacement.

It is understood that the length of stay will be more than 1 day, and progress will follow a certain sequence. The situation in a catastrophic case is quite different. Here, day-by-day review is appropriate and beneficial, as patient events often lead to changes in treatment.

In situations in which the planned discharge will not occur, the nurse reviewer must uncover the reasons for the continued stay. Perhaps the patient developed a postoperative complication or the diagnostic studies have revealed other conditions that need further evaluation. Perhaps the patient remains medically unstable and requires the services and monitoring that only an acute care hospital could provide. For these and many other reasons, continued hospitalization is certainly warranted. Most review groups today inquire at this point as to the expected length of time that hospitalization will be necessary. Again, there are some software programs that have "built-in" norms for typical admissions, and as long as the responses fall within the norms, the stay continues to be "approved" or "certified." For the most part, hospitals and physicians are no longer guilty of overutilizing inpatient stays. There are those patients who for a variety of very understandable reasons do not fall within the "norms." It is for these patients that discussion between nurse reviewers and/or physician reviewers and the treating physicians becomes extremely important. It usually resolves confusion and leads to a better understanding of a complex treatment plan.

Occasionally, however, a continued hospitalization is requested because of factors that could be addressed using an alternate care plan. The patient, for example, may need IV antibiotics or has no one at home to change dressings or monitor medications. Solutions in such situations include arranging for home infusion services, skilled nursing visits, and home health aide services. The expense is considerably less than a continued stay in the hospital. If the nurse reviewer determines the need and proposes an alternative to the treating physician and patient, more often than not it is approved. Knowledge of the case's status at the right time is crucial, however, to the solution and the realization of savings. Without case management review, notification of circumstances might occur but the ability to alter events will be lacking.

I have seen employer or insurer groups that have preadmission and concurrent review and case management programs but also have language in their benefit plans that works against the goal of better management of patient outcomes. For example, a plan might offer unlimited benefits for inpatient stays, payable at 80% for the first $5,000 and at 100% thereafter, but limits nursing visits to only 20 per year, 4 hours per visit, or allows nursing only if implemented within 3 days following a hospital stay. Although the group might have intended to prevent overuse of nursing services, its self-funded plan language pushes claimants and providers toward overuse of the much more expensive hospital services. An experienced case manager recognizes this as an obstacle and can assist in a modification or revision to the plan that allows more cost-effective solutions. For example, a plan could stipulate that with case management approval, certain benefits may be made available to participants. Other groups have preadmission and concurrent review nurse reviewers continue to track a lengthy hospital stay week after week, but provide no mechanism to refer patients to case managers who could implement changes.

TIMING DISEASE MANAGEMENT AND CASE MANAGEMENT INTERVENTION

At what point in the review process should a referral be made for disease management and/or case management intervention? There are some basic indicators or red flags to look for, and there are other less specific, more individualized considerations for both of these interventions. Some indicators may actually be evident during the very first call from a hospital admissions department, treating physician, or patient's family to a preadmission review department or company. Once a red flag surfaces, it is necessary to apply an amount of risk assessment to move the case into the care management program that best matches the need.

A preterm delivery, a high-risk pregnancy, a cerebral vascular accident suffered by a teenager, a spinal cord injury, or a traumatic brain injury with coma are all conditions for which there is a high probability of a lengthy hospital stay, a need for additional care and services upon discharge, high costs, and benefits to be gained through case management. For the most part, it is appropriate to refer any of these as soon as possible to case management.

Other conditions and circumstances also merit an early referral, not necessarily because of a particular diagnosis but because of surrounding circumstances. For instance, diabetes is not by itself a condition that would prompt a case management referral, but the fourth hospital admission in 2 months of a patient with diabetes might. Why are these admissions occurring so frequently? Is the patient noncompliant or noneducated? Has the patient been treated in a clinic by a different physician each time? Is the treating physician a retiring family practitioner? Perhaps an endocrinologist is needed. Is it reasonable to wait until there are additional complications? A referral to case management at this point does seem appropriate and indeed should be made.

A newly diagnosed diabetic exhibiting no problems and experiencing no episodes is a prime candidate for disease management. This program will provide the kind of assistance, resources, and education that can help avoid escalation into the following situation.

A patient with an admitting diagnosis of cellulitis may not at first glance seem appropriate for referral to case management. However, imagine that as the patient's stay in the hospital continues, more becomes known about this 46-year-old woman: She is also hypertensive, had a coronary bypass 2 years earlier, is diabetic, and weighs 320 pounds, clearly morbidly obese for her height of five feet six inches. The case is obviously complicated. For one thing, the woman eventually might require a below-knee amputation secondary to her multiple conditions. Doesn't the potential of this occurrence at least warrant an assessment by a case management professional? This patient is an ideal candidate not only for case management, but also for disease management, where she could benefit from a combination of ongoing education and behavior modification, in addition to regular, ongoing case management. Patients like this woman would likely be overlooked by a system for case management referral that was driven solely by one ICD-9 code or one set dollar limit. Yet each similar case presents such substantial opportunities for improved outcomes, prevention of complications, and reduction of expenses that not referring becomes a costly risk.

When approval for a case management referral is needed, a presentation of all pertinent information should support the request. A claims examiner or other approval source might be inclined to refuse case management for the cases just described, for example, because they do not fit the notion of an appropriate case. To avoid refusal, the case manager should be prepared to outline the problems, the costs that will be incurred if nothing is done, the solutions that could be applied, the approximate costs of the solutions (including case management fees), the length of time intervention will take, and the results that will be obtained. The object is to make the rationale clear, the savings obvious, and the approval much easier to justify.

When preadmission, concurrent review, disease management, and case management functions are provided by one organization, the transfer of information and concerns is better coordinated and can actually provide ongoing knowledge and improved control of cases. Such coordination can also avoid duplication of involvement, help a claims department manage its workload, assist in the development of prevention and wellness programs, support the evaluation of benefits use, and expose the need to redesign plans. When a nurse reviewer who has been involved throughout a complicated patient admission can share the background information she has acquired, the case manager is able to "hit the ground running."

On the other side of the "effectiveness" spectrum are disease and case management programs working in two separate silos with no coordination or communication between them. The case managers don't ask if the patient is in the disease management program, and vice versa, depriving both groups and the patient of timely intervention. Unable to track the patient fully, the potential optimal benefit from both is lost. If an organization or plan elects to use two different providers for these services, every effort should be made to integrate the knowledge and activities of both.

As a case manager, I once received a referral from a claims department after it was notified by a provider who had conducted the preadmission review 7 weeks prior and noted a diagnosis of cancer of the stomach. The end-of-the-month printout was now in the hands of the examiner, who had also just received a claim for 1 week of TPN and "other" services costing $25,000. The examiner thought a case management referral was appropriate. It was, but it came a little too late. The services continued for a second week as arranged. The provider refused to negotiate retrospectively to lower costs; he knew the services were payable at 100%. (He knew the patient's benefit plan would pay the full price for his services because he called the claims department and learned this from a customer service representative.) The patient expired following a second and final admission to the hospital. Perhaps the TPN services could have been negotiated more cost-effectively; perhaps a hospice program could have been arranged, allowing the patient to die at home with his family around him; perhaps money could have been saved, too. Perhaps, but the lack of an integrated approach prohibited the pursuit of these options. In this instance, there was preadmission and concurrent review and case management and a benefit plan that would have permitted alternatives, yet because each system functioned independently of the others, in a vacuum, realizing the alternatives was not possible.

It is clear that these utilization management functions (preadmission, concurrent review, case management) need to exist side by side, with cognizance of each other's role and an ability to interact when necessary. In addition, the newer model, disease management, needs to be an integral part of such a quality-of-care and cost-containment program.

PREADMISSION AND CONCURRENT REVIEW REPORTS

Preadmission and concurrent review summary reports (see Figure 10–3) and other documentation of case events constitute an ongoing profile of a case. Case-specific reports that include nurse case manager or case manager notes establish a case history and can be used to track the details of

Figure 10–3 Preadmission and Concurrent Review Summary Report.

Group # - 001   Third Party Administrator   1/1/03-1/31/03

Date Reported	Emp ID#	Diagnosis	Type	Admission Date	Discharge Date	Status
1/2/03	000	Fracture	Emerg	1/1/03	1/2/03	Closed
1/3/03	000	Norm Delivery	Emerg	1/25/03		Open
1/5/03	000	Lump in Breast	Sched	1/8/03		Open
1/7/03	000	Myocardial Infar	Emerg	1/11/03	1/18/03	Refer CM
1/12/03	000	Herniated Disc	Sched	1/21/03	1/25/03	Closed
1/14/03	000	Miscarriage	Emerg	1/13/03	1/14/03	Closed
1/16/03	000	Appendicitis	Emerg	1/15/03	1/18/03	Closed
1/18/03	000	Derangement Knee	Sched	1/25/03		Open
1/25/03	000	Depression	Sched	1/28/03		Psych
1/28/03	000	Pregnancy	Sched	3/25/03		Open

Total Admissions for Period = 9   Total Discharged = 5
Total Referred for Case Management = 1
TOTAL CASES FOR PERIOD = 10

Source: Couresy of Options Unlimited, Case Management Services Division, © 2003, Huntington, New York.

a case, which is especially helpful if the case changes from being low risk to being high risk. Produced for all hospital admissions, all scheduled pregnancies, and all emergency cases, case-specific reports incorporate ongoing notes made by nurse reviewers. They are valuable for internal use in a preadmission and concurrent review department, provide the rationale for case management referral, contain the background for the case manager assigned to the case, and are also forwarded to the claims examiner. (Options Unlimited developed the software for the computer-generated report presented in Figure 10–3. Not all case management departments and companies have similar computer capabilities, but the form itself is a useful tool whether it is created by a computer or not.)

The review summary report (Figure 10–3) shows that only one patient out of ten was referred for case management. One review summary report showed that there was a surprisingly high incidence of admissions for complications of pregnancy for this employer group, consisting mostly of women, and it led to the development of a maternity screening and management program and the prevention of two premature babies. The savings to the group far outweighed the costs of the managed care program.

ESTABLISHING AN EFFECTIVE PREADMISSION REVIEW, CONCURRENT REVIEW, CASE MANAGEMENT, AND DISEASE MANAGEMENT SYSTEM

To be effective, a preadmission and concurrent review and case management system or department requires flexibility and cooperation on the part of payers and providers, benefit plan language that supports case management, and a claims administrator who understands the difference between managing benefits and managing cases. As stated previously, the only way case reviewing and case management can become truly potent is when each element is applied as part of a unified system. How should the system be set up? The first step is to look at what is in place in order to determine what is needed. Whether one is working with a Third Party Administrator, an insurance company, or a self-administered plan, the signs of a benefit and claims system in trouble are the same.

Most health insurance plans today (and with growing frequency, workers' compensation plans as well) have some form of review system in place, especially for hospital admissions. Unfortunately, too often the "notification of an admission" is the only step rather than the first step in an integrated system of review and case management. What value is it to those companies who pay for such services to require individuals to call an "800" number prior to entering a hospital or within 48 hours of an emergency admission? What purpose does it serve and what should be the result of such a notification system? It is interesting how many claims departments, Third Party Administrators, and employer groups require such a system, put one in place, and then have great difficulty describing the results. Over the last several years, it has almost become a "we have to have it" kind of service, but run with little accountability, and showing still less in terms of results.

So how can one determine whether a company or department needs a better preadmission and concurrent review and case management system? By asking the direct questions listed in the following sections.

Preadmission Review Services

Are patients required to call someone before entering the hospital? If the answer is no, then you know that there is no system in place. The result is that individuals can enter the hospital as often as they or their physicians want, stay until someone questions the hospitalization, and spend as much as may be available for hospital services.

If a notification call is required, to whom is it made? If it is to a claims department, does a claims examiner or a medical professional take the call? If it is a claims person, is the information intended to be used to decrease lengths of stay or costs, improve outcomes, or identify high-cost, complex cases? If the call goes to a medical professional in the claims department, what is done with the information? Are potential long-term cases flagged for any kind of action? Does the person taking the call have the ability to authorize case management, or is there a mechanism established to suggest a referral for case management? Dehydration or vomiting will not be a certain "red flag" to a nonclinical administration person, but an RN or case manager hearing that would pursue it with the caller to get more information, just in case there is a deeper problem.

If this kind of preadmission call is directed to a review organization, what are the results? Is the organization simply advised of the admission? Does anyone review the admissions as to their appropriateness? Are patients allowed to remain in hospitals for a fixed number of days, are they allowed to remain as long as their physicians want them there, or is each stay checked every single day, every other day, or after 7 or 10 days? In my mind, a call to the hospital every single day is a waste of time. If there is a day one, you can be assured there will be a day two.

Prenotification for all high-cost services, even if hospital admission does not occur (e.g., pregnancy monitoring, apnea alarms, IV therapy), is valuable because such services frequently signal other problems that can be successfully resolved by case management.

Proactive management of cases in the preadmission/concurrent review stage helps identify potential cases before they spiral out of control. All high-cost/problem cases eventually enter the hospital. This is an opportunity to speak to the patient, family, and physician from the start, introducing and explaining the role of case management, and if appropriate, disease management.

Concurrent Review Services

Does anyone review a hospital stay during the confinement? If so, how often are such calls made?

Does anyone from the review group ever speak with the claims department staff? Are reports available to indicate the number of admissions and readmissions and the average stay? Does a review of these reports indicate any problems (e.g., unusually long stays, unusually frequent readmissions)?

Does anyone authorize continued stays and, if so, what criteria are utilized? Again, some review services have a software program that uses a series of questions; depending on the answers, the system allows or denies extra days. Other review services utilize predetermined medical criteria and a professional reviewer. Use of software systems alone may result in arbitrary decisions and prevent consideration of individual patient needs. The ideal review program assessment combines industry standards and norms and professional interaction with the patient, physician, and family.

What happens beyond hospitalization, when the patient returns home? Is concurrent review extended? Does anyone track the patient's progress to prevent readmission?

Case Management Services

Assuming that the preadmission and concurrent review services are appropriate, what happens when a "red flag" indicating a possible need for case management is identified? What are the red flags? To whom is the information communicated and when? Is the claims department notified by phone or by report? What then is done with the information?

If there is some kind of notification, is the case referred to case management services? Are the case management services affiliated with the review group or provided by another company?

How long does this process take? Too long an interval reduces the opportunities for timely intervention and cost containment.

How many cases are actually case managed? Does this match the industry standard (3% to 5% of a group have potential for case management), or is the number higher or lower than would be expected?

What kinds of cases are managed? What are the results and the costs? Are any arranged services discounted or are fees negotiated? Are savings reports submitted? What are the costs for case management compared with the savings attained? If several nurses in several departments are each performing an activity of case management for one or a series of patients, case management is not being practiced. Case management is practiced when all activities of case management are integrated into one care plan, directed by one case manager across the continuum of care for an individual. (Working as a consultant, I met a hospital case management team "working with" an insurer case management team. The hospital team used Interqual's standards for length of stay and reasonable and customary fees; the insurer team referred to Milliman's standards. Relationships were strained, as you can imagine.)

Critical care paths, "best in practice" plans, care maps, and guidelines all help us to know about appropriate and successful procedures. However, systems can't manage all people appropriately and successfully all the time. Case management addresses those issues that care paths and care maps can often overlook: multiple conditions, financial funding problems, social/cultural issues, etc.

Exploring the answers to these questions one at a time will be effective in determining the structure, function, and, more importantly, the results of any cost-containment program. Obviously, when the answers indicate a poorly designed or managed program, they also indicate minimal savings. The lack of savings places the review group in the unenviable position of trying to justify the costs to their clients without being able to point to significant performance results. Again, this does not mean that these services do not yield savings, but they do not produce the savings that a well-designed, well-managed, and fully integrated program does.

Let us assume that the claims department, Third Party Administrator, or employer group has determined that there is a need to design and implement a fully integrated preadmission and concurrent review and case management program. One question that then needs answering is whether to do the work in-house or hire an outside company or freelance professionals to develop a program to meet specific client group needs.

In-house programs usually offer greater control, but the expense and increased management burden of adding review and case management professionals to existing staff may not be justified. Some considerations for in-house programs include these:

- Who will hire the staff?
- Who will train and supervise the staff?
- Who will define the responsibilities?
- Who will integrate claims and medical activities and responsibilities?

Employer-funded and employer-administered plans, whether workers' compensation or medical, tend to be better suited for the in-house staff approach. The companies that have such plans have already made the commitment to actively participate in their benefit plans. Larger employer groups are moving steadily toward integrating all of their employee lines of insurance, including short- and long-term disability and workers' compensation insurance, for reasons other than direct control. They are finding that a well-coordinated benefits philosophy and integrated 24-hour coverage are necessary elements of a truly cost-effective care management program. Third Party Administrators and insurance carriers are exploring the feasibility of coordinated, in-house programs as well.

For groups that choose not to use in-house staff, collaboration with a full-service managed care organization provides cost-containment capability and the flexibility to design company-specific programs. As employer groups have become knowledgeable about cost containment, they have become more vocal about what they want and do not want for their employees. The ability of a review organization or case management service to be responsive to these requirements or preferences is one factor to consider in designing a program.

Disease Management Services

Case managers are the creative minds of healthcare, monitoring those who otherwise fall through the cracks, making the best use of dollars spent across the provider continuum, and maintaining an unwavering commitment to quality care. The benefits of case management increase exponentially when CMs integrate their programs across utilization management, disease management, discharge planning, rehabilitation, outpatient, transition to home, hospice, and other services.

Although the majority of case management programs have focused on the management of the sickest and costliest individuals in a group, most would agree that earlier, more creative, and nonepisodic management presents far greater opportunities to prevent these healthcare disasters. Healthcare organizations and the payers have been striving to improve the quality of care, to control costs, and to actively involve plan members in this process. Whereas case management focuses efforts on an individual patient, disease management (also called population health management or condition management because of the discomfort that the term *disease* may present to participants of these programs) targets groups of individuals with diagnostic conditions that have historical and financial evidence of being costly and that will be significantly improved with more integrated and systematic management. It can assist in identifying cases earlier, an important asset to care, and pulls people who might otherwise go undetected back into the healthcare system for needed attention, using standards and guidelines to educate and help individuals better manage their disease state.

Several diseases have already been identified as having the greatest potential for change: asthma, diabetes, high-risk pregnancy, cardiovascular, and chronic neuromuscular. Companies are now looking at a broader spectrum of degenerative conditions, including diseases such as multiple sclerosis, amyotrophic lateral sclerosis (ALS), hemophilia, and cystic fibrosis, as well as chronic back pain and arthritis. In fact, because of the presence of comorbidities in so many high-risk patients, the approach of enrolling individuals in single-state programs becomes operationally challenging, if not impossible to execute. Programs have been moving toward a whole person model, where all the conditions a patient has are managed by the program. This should be welcome news to case managers who have long held beliefs that holistic management is one of the keys to successful management and improved outcomes for their patients. Pharmacy benefits are also a growing field under the disease management umbrella. Disease management programs can also benefit those with behavioral disabilities and substance abuse or addiction problems.

In 2002, URAC approved national accreditation standards for disease management programs, a sign that it is becoming a fundamental part of managed care offerings. In its 2005 Industry Report, URAC acknowledges that national trends are revealing a medical management industry in a dynamic period of transition. URAC supports the Disease Management Association of America (DMAA; www.dmaa.org) definition of disease management, which is "a system of coordinated healthcare interventions for populations with conditions in which patient self-care efforts are significant." The URAC standards in the accreditation of disease management programs note that six components are essential: population identification processes; evidence-based practice guidelines; collaborative practice models to include physician and support service providers; patient self-management education (may include primary prevention, behavior modification programs, and compliance/surveillance); process and outcomes measurement, evaluation, and management; routine reporting/feedback loop (may include communication with patient, physician, health plan, and ancillary providers and practice profiling).[4]

Disease management programs seek to target these individuals at the earliest stages of known high-cost conditions. By providing ongoing information and intervention, these programs can prevent, or at least minimize, the problems that eventually result in chronic and costly complications. Among the drawbacks in disease management as it is now practiced are the following: It more often addresses a group profile rather than an individual's needs; it often does not track patient's progress or lack of progress; it lacks consistency in administration from provider to provider and region to region; it does not show all comorbid conditions; and in many cases it does not provide for the neediest cases, those who are noncompliant, unable to respond to phone calls, or illiterate.

The three cases described in Figures 10–4, 10–5, and 10–6 are examples of the benefits to both the patient and payer when precertification, case

Figure 10–4 Level I Integrated Precert/Disease Management Program.

Mr. B, 30-year-old African-American male
DX: DM2

PRECERT	CASE MANAGEMENT	DISEASE MANAGEMENT
01/08/03 - Precert nurse contacted by patient to advise of elective admission for inguinal hernia repair. Questioned patient as to etiology. Patient states is "loader" at factory and recently felt "pull in groin" while loading truck at work. Precert nurse advised patient to report to worker's comp through employer as most benefit plans do not accept responsibility of coverage for work-related injuries. Further assessment of medical status revealed 30-year-old African-American male was diagnosed with type 2 diabetes 8 months prior. Has strong family history of same (both parents and two sisters with diabetes). Is currently under excellent control with oral medication, diet, and exercise program. Patient has no comorbidities. Precert nurse contacts plan to notify of information received from patient regarding work-related injury. Precert nurse initiates referral to disease management due to diagnosis of diabetes.		01/08/03 - Disease manager contacts patient to provide thorough assessment and learns was referred by primary care physician to endocrinologist who practices out of diabetes center affiliated with local hospital. Received appropriate education from CDE and RD. Attends weekly diabetes support group at center where receives ongoing education. Exercises 5/7 days per week by walking 5K. However, assessment revealed patient experiencing hypoglycemic episodes frequently during walk. Has tried adding snack to prevent episodes to no avail. Very good knowledge base regarding self-management. Supportive wife and family. Compliant with plan of care. Disease manager initiates referral to endocrinologist requesting visit with RD and/or CDE regarding hypoglycemic episodes. Disease manager contacts patient after visit to verify understanding of treatment plan.

continues

Figure 10–4 continued

Mr. B, 30-year-old African-American male
DX: DM2

PRECERT	CASE MANAGEMENT	DISEASE MANAGEMENT
		Disease manager will monitor patient on a level I tier through telephonic contact every 6 months, receive seasonal condition-specific participant education materials, and be given access to condition-specific 24/7 nurse line.
		RESULTS
		Effective disease management prevented an acute episode from occurring by promptly intervening and coordinating appropriate measures to address the patient's hypoglycemic episodes early on. This serves both the patient and the plan well.

Figure 10–5 Level II Integrated Precert/Disease Management Program.

Mrs. M, 55-year-old white female - DX: DM2

PRECERT	CASE MANAGEMENT	DISEASE MANAGEMENT
03/31/03 - Precert nurse notified by hospital of admission for uncontrolled blood sugars. Precert nurse contacts UR and requests clinical review. Precert nurse contacts physician and requests C/B. Precert nurse contacts patient at bedside and learns this 55-year-old white female was diagnosed with type 2 diabetes 1 year earlier. Further conversation revealed good glycemic control initially. However, recently developed problems. Had appropriate referral to endocrinologist year prior and she continues to see every 3 months. Has received past education from CDE and Registered Dietitian. Checks blood sugars 4×/day and keeps log. Verbalizes understanding of diabetic self-management and meal plan. Subscribes to diabetes magazine and reads religiously. However, has had recent lifestyle changes which are adversely affecting glycemic control. Was not working when originally diagnosed,		03/31/03 - Disease manager contacts patient to conduct thorough assessment. Through this intervention it is learned the patient was recently widowed, necessitating her need for employment. She states she is under the care of an endocrinologist whom she sees regularly. Mrs. M has had adequate diabetes education in the past and has a good knowledge base of diabetes self-management. Feels she would benefit from a "refresher" class and behavioral modification training. Both are available through her endocrinology office. In addition, she is interested in a support group and agrees to level II tier participation. Disease manager sends assessment report to primary care physician and endocrinologist identifying need for additional education and support group. Disease manager contacts physician to verify receipt of assessment report and obtain agreement to facilitate appropriate referrals.

continues

Figure 10–5 continued

Mrs. M, 55-year-old white female - DX: DM2

PRECERT	CASE MANAGEMENT	DISEASE MANAGEMENT
but recently accepted job as cook at local grade school. Often is too tired to take her usual walk after work. Also, states job as cook has presented a problem with dietary compliance as she often "tastes" too much. Has gained 20 lbs. and blood sugars have been recently elevated to 160–200 range. However, today elevated to 405 and experienced acute visual changes and headache which caused her visit to the ER. Precert initiates referral to disease management.		Disease manager contacts patient within 1week to confirm arrangements for recommendations are in place. Reinforces availability of 24/7 nurse line. Educational materials sent. Disease manager will monitor patient's plan of care to prioritize and manage identified problems and risks as needed. Patient will receive appropriate nurse follow-up based on clinical activity and personal care goal status. Disease manager will send patient seasonal condition specific education and risk specific materials as needed, customized to her unique needs. Evaluation for case management will be assessed on a quarterly basis. **RESULTS** By addressing identified problems early on, disease management was able to greatly decrease the risk of current and future diabetic complications. This action enhances the efficiency and effectiveness of delivering health care. Again, the patient and the plan were well served.

Source: Courtesy of Options Unlimited, Case Management Services Division, © 2003, Huntington, New York.

Figure 10–6 Level III Integrated Precert/Disease Management Program.

Mrs. S, 58-year-old white female
DX: CVA, DM2, Obesity, Tobacco abuse, Hypothyroidism

PRECERT	CASE MANAGEMENT	DISEASE MANAGEMENT
11/27 - T/C from hospital; gave admit info. Admitting diagnosis right hemiplegia. 11/28 - T/C to hospital UR and clinical review requested. T/C from hospital UR: patient admitted 11/25 with c/o numbness face, jaw & right arm. Dizziness, right hemiplegia. MRI = left thalamic CVA. B/P 149/99 Rehab eval done. Diabetes mellitus type 2 diagnosed 3 years ago. Has not seen a physician in 1 year. BS on admission 525. Diabetic teaching started. Cholesterol 221, triglycerides 450. Heparin drip, Plavix started. Social: Single, lives with daughter, son-in-law, grandchildren. Prior to event employed as factory worker on evening shift. Precert nurse verified rehab benefits. Supplied network participating rehab facility with needed information. 11/29 - Precert nurse received and reviewed PT, OT, ST evals. Medical necessity for acute rehab verified. Secondary Medicaid verified.		

continues

Figure 10–6 continued

Mrs. S, 58-year-old white female
DX: CVA, DM2, Obesity, Tobacco abuse, Hypothyroidism

PRECERT	CASE MANAGEMENT	DISEASE MANAGEMENT
11/29 - Precert nurse contacts patient at bedside. Only medical care from local D.O. Lives in rural area of Tennessee. Had been on oral antidiabetic (Glucophage) but stopped taking it 1 year ago because thought was causing diarrhea. Never notified MD of problems. Also stopped all other meds at same time, including thyroid medication. There has been no medical management of her diabetes. States she would occasionally check her blood sugar. Received no formal diabetic teaching at time of diagnosis. Current weight 179, height 5'. Smoked 1 ppd prior to admission. Precert nurse noted claimant has no understanding of the impact uncontrolled diabetes has on body or disease process. She is agreeable to case management. T/C from Rehab. Patient transferred from acute care to network participating rehab. 11/30 - Assigned to case manager.		

Figure 10–6 continued

Mrs. S, 58-year-old white female
DX: CVA, DM2, Obesity, Tobacco abuse, Hypothyroidism

PRECERT	CASE MANAGEMENT	DISEASE MANAGEMENT
	12/1 - Learns from rehab case manager family is bringing food to patient. Rehab MD was notified and he discussed this with patient.	
	Case manager contacts patient to discuss status, care plan, and compliance. Reinforces education and asks questions to verify understanding of same. Patient unable to verbalize understanding of meal plan. States "they gave me a piece of paper with my diet on it. I will read it when I get home."	
	Case manager contacts rehab case manager and requests RD see patient/family to continue meal plan education.	Case manager verifies patient and family educated regarding meal plan and importance of same. Stressed need for compliance to decrease risk of future complications.
	Case manager contacts attending physician. Learns admitting HbA1c was 14.3% (N=≤ 7%). Learns diabetic teaching is continuing daily by CDE and RD. Discussed plan of care for diabetes management. Case manager asks if endocrinology consult might be helpful.	Case manager notes that MD agrees insulin will likely be needed to achieve glycemic control and reduce risk of future complications. Discussed triad of diseases DM, HTN, Hyperlipidemia and difficulty to control any if all are not in control. Will order endocrinology consult.

continues

Figure 10–6 continued

Mrs. S, 58-year-old white female
DX: CVA, DM2, Obesity, Tobacco abuse, Hypothyroidism

PRECERT	CASE MANAGEMENT	DISEASE MANAGEMENT
		Case manager learns Endocrinology consult done and aggressive medication management started, including insulin regimen.
	12/4 - Case manager contacts rehab case manager. Learns patient does not have own glucometer with her. Requests family bring and that at least one family member is taught to check blood sugars, as well as patient.	
	Case manager learns family/patient cannot locate glucometer. Requests RX for new one be given to family.	Case manager verifies new glucometer/supplies purchased by family and brought to facility. Education done. Successful demonstrations returned by patient and family member.
	12/7 - Case manager contacts attending physician regarding medical status and care plan.	
	Case manager contacts endocrinologist and discusses current control and plan of care. Agrees with plan to increase insulin.	
	Case manager contacts rehab case manager and recommends family member learn insulin administration as well as patient.	Case manager verifies patient and daughter have learned to administer insulin.
		Case manager has frequent discussions with claimant regarding level of diabetic management needed at discharge and importance of same to decrease risks.

Figure 10–6 continued

Mrs. S, 58-year-old white female
DX: CVA, DM2, Obesity, Tobacco abuse, Hypothyroidism

PRECERT	CASE MANAGEMENT	DISEASE MANAGEMENT
	Case manager learns compliance improving and BS readings improved. 12/7 - Case manager locates outpatient diabetic center/classes and verifies benefit for same. Verifies clinic is ADA recognized. 12/10 - Case manager learns patient's blood sugars under excellent control. Has been compliant with management and able to verbalize understanding of same. Case manager contacts endocrinologist and obtains orders for outpatient diabetes class. Diabetes center contacted and patient enrolled. Case manager receiving ongoing status reports regarding PT, OT, ST progress. Arrangements finalized for continued outpatient therapy in anticipation of upcoming discharge. Case manager contacts network participating home health agency and arranges for f/u visit after discharge to monitor status.	Case manager contacts patient to discuss need for continued outpatient rehab and diabetes education after discharge. Patient verbalizes understanding of importance of same and agrees to comply. Has stopped smoking since admit. Verbalizes understanding of relationship to stroke and plans to remain smoke free. Declines offer of nicotine patch.

continues

Figure 10–6 continued

Mrs. S, 58-year-old white female
DX: CVA, DM2, Obesity, Tobacco abuse, Hypothyroidism

PRECERT	CASE MANAGEMENT	DISEASE MANAGEMENT
	12/13 - Patient discharged home. Rehab LOS = 14 days	
	12/14 - Case manager contacts patient at home. Learns blood sugars remain under control. Patient able to verbalize principals of diabetic self- management and importance of maintaining compliance with outpatient plan of care.	Case manager learns patient compliant with appropriate and medically necessary MD appointments with specialists, including endocrinologist and gastroenterologist who will evaluate problems with chronic diarrhea. Patient attending outpatient PT, OT, ST.
		12/19–20 - Case manager notes patient attends two-day diabetes class at center with family member. Remains smoke free.
	12/15–2/20 - Case manager maintains regular contact with patient, physicians, and therapists to monitor medical status, coordinate care, and intervene as indicated.	
	02/20 - Patient has met outpatient rehab goals and is discharged by PT, OT, ST. OT from rehab will meet with patient and Occupational Health Nurse at plant to evaluate work station for safety in anticipation of returning to work.	

Figure 10–6 continued

Mrs. S, 58-year-old white female
DX: CVA, DM2, Obesity, Tobacco abuse, Hypothyroidism

PRECERT	CASE MANAGEMENT	DISEASE MANAGEMENT
	03/06 - Patient returns to work half days.	Case manager learns patient continues to be compliant with outpatient care. Blood glucose remains under control. Remains smoke free.
		04/08 - Case manager learns patients current HbA1c reported at 7.8%.
	04/08 - Case management closed. Case manager initiates referral to disease management.	
		Disease management continues to contact patient periodically to monitor status, identify potential problems early, and identify case management needs.
		RESULTS
		Had Options Unlimited not been involved with this case the patient would have continued to poorly manage her diabetes and not receive appropriate care. This would have placed her at a high risk of developing further life-threatening complications. In addition to the significant cost savings recorded by aggressive utilization management in this case, it is likely multiple future hospitalizations were avoided.

Source: Courtesy of Options Unlimited, Case Management Services Division, © 2003, Huntington, New York.

management, and disease management services are integrated. Figure 10–4 illustrates how a Precert nurse, asking questions that dig deeper to elicit more than a simple "yes" or "no" response, can uncover and address a problem when working with a patient who seems to have a good understanding of his disease and was practicing effective self-management. In Figure 10–5, the importance of knowing about a patient's current lifestyle and any recent changes in it become clear. The combination of precertification and disease management programs assists this individual in taking better care of herself.

The role that integrated precertification, case management, and disease management programs can play is shown in Figure 10–6. The case management intervention continues for 5 months, and when combined with disease management, effectively removes the patient from a high-risk status for developing further, life-threatening complications.

We have assisted several clients by adding a disease management program to the services we were already providing to them, such as preadmission, utilization review, and concurrent review. To introduce the disease management program to employees, a letter describing the service is sent to each individual (Table 10–3), accompanied by a questionnaire we developed to gather preliminary information regarding those with diseases or conditions that require self-management. The letter states very clearly that the program is voluntary, and that all health information they share will be kept strictly confidential. Our questions were carefully worded to help us design a disease management program that would meet the needs of the employees, given their disease, its progression, and need for additional education and possible case management intervention.

The major thrust of effective disease management programs is in the prevention of acute episodes. According to Margaret Flaum, RN, Director of Population Care Client Management at McKesson Health Solutions in Broomfield, Colorado, the care providers in McKesson's Disease Management program have seen a 33% increase in glucose monitoring among diabetic participants, a 33% decrease in hospitalizations, and 28% fewer missed workdays. For enrolled individuals with congestive heart failure, the disease management program has lowered readmissions for cardiac-related symptoms by 30.4% and inpatient readmission rates have plummeted 73%.[5]

In 1997, the Diabetes Treatment Centers of America in Nashville, Tennessee, successfully reduced hospital admission rates for patients enrolled in its program to 67.3% below the national average for diabetics nationwide.[6] Another successful program at the Denver-based National Jewish Center for Immunology and Respiratory Medicine reported in 1995 that asthma hospitalizations decreased 83%, emergency department

Table 10–3 Letter Introducing Disease Management Program to Client Employees

Dear _____,

Options Unlimited, on behalf of Tele Electro, Inc., is very pleased to offer *Healthy Options*, a wellness program that provides a personalized approach to those patients with conditions that require self-management. *Options Unlimited* is the organization that provides Tele Electro with hospital prenotification, case management, and other services. We are the 800 # on the back of your medical card. The goal of the *Healthy Options* program is to assist you and your family in enjoying optimal health by providing information, resources and, in some instances, coordinating healthcare services. In these busy days, we don't always take the best care of ourselves, as we should.

Healthy Options is designed to help you better understand and manage some conditions and illnesses you might have. This program is entirely voluntary and strictly confidential. Enclosed is our Health Assessment Questionnaire. We hope that you will take this opportunity to fill out the questionnaire and return it in the stamped envelope provided. This assessment will come directly back to *Options Unlimited* and be reviewed and evaluated by our professional staff to determine if one of our programs is right for you. You will then be given the option of participating in this program. If you choose to participate in one of the targeted programs, you will receive communications on a continuous basis so that you can become more proactive in your care.

Some of the conditions covered in our programs are diabetes, heart disease, asthma, obesity, and cancer. It also covers pregnancy with its *First Breath* program. *First Breath* is designed for women who are pregnant or thinking of becoming pregnant. It offers personal care plans, a 24/7 nurse hotline, access to specialized care materials, articles, and more.

We hope that you will take advantage of this added benefit and complete the enclosed questionnaire. Please remember this is strictly confidential and personal information will not be shared. The sole purpose of this program is to assist you and your family with resources and tools to make sure you enjoy the best health you possibly can.

So, please fill out the questionnaire, return it in the envelope provided, and get started in taking charge of your health! If you have any questions about this program or filling out the questionnaire, please give us a call at 1-800-555-1212.

Sincerely,

Catherine Mullahy, RN, BS, CRRN, CCM

President

Source: Courtesy of Options Unlimited, Case Management Services Division, © 2003, Huntington, New York.

visits decreased 45%, and hospital days decreased 82% for this high-cost patient group.[7]

Given such good statistics in its early days, it is surprising to learn that less than one in ten employers now use disease management programs, although there is great interest and growing demand.[8] On the other hand, that fact will sound sweet to any case manager or case management company looking to build its book of business by offering disease management services.

Admittedly, the design and implementation of disease management programs will necessitate substantial commitment of resources and a true partnership among providers, payers, and plan participants. Change will be necessary at every level; for those case managers (working with the sickest individuals) who may be frustrated by the referral of patients too late for either prevention or effective management, these programs are certainly welcome news.

Risk assessments and the stratification of services play a significant role in a successful disease management program. Thoughtful assessment of risks to the patient and to the plan allow departments to apply the program at the level that best meets identified needs. Here are simple guidelines:

Level 1: Low-risk individuals can get by with frequent mailings and occasional phone contact. Basic information about disease and community resources should be made available.

Level 2: Medium-risk individuals often require frequent phone contact, alone. Determine level of understanding of disease (beginning, midway, end knowledge), impact of the disease and consequences, and the ability of the patient to be compliant. This level might last 3 to 6 months.

Level 3: This patient is suffering a more severe or chronic disease, or the consequences of noncompliance in managing the disease. High-risk individuals receive more frequent telephone contact, as well as occasional home visits and medical monitoring, reeducation, and coordination.

PREADMISSION REVIEW, CONCURRENT REVIEW, DISEASE MANAGEMENT, AND CASE MANAGEMENT CHECKLIST

The ideal program has the following elements and characteristics:

- Full integration of preadmission, concurrent review, case management, and disease management services, with coordinated communications and integrated databases between departments

- Knowledge of the plan and its provisions and restrictions
- Consensus on how and when cases are opened
- An outside company or an in-house department with nurses, physicians, and clerical and administrative staff who understand each other's role and function, have ongoing interaction, and operate as a unit in pursuit of quality outcomes and cost-containment results
- An established communications link with the claims examiner or claims staff administering the plan
- The ear of the CEO or a decision maker regarding specific allowances to be made on a case-by-case basis
- Preventive interventions (interventions at regular intervals) to catch problems before they happen; most DM programs have little or no interface with the enrolled population
- A regular reporting system charting active case management cases by type, duration, expenses, outcomes, and savings
- A process of continual program evaluation and the capacity to revise the program year to year. If, for example, the program initially included only cases over $100,000/year, criteria might be refocused to target another specific disease, red flag, goal, or group.
- A case management closure protocol. It is highly unethical to keep patients in disease management for the revenue stream, but it is commonly done. Only the truly catastrophic cases will have a case manager on board long-term. Once a case is stabilized, the patient no longer deemed at risk, and savings are no longer realized, the case manager should consider closure. The patient and family become, in essence, their own case managers. That being said, a periodic reevaluation of closed cases would seem appropriate as a continuing risk assessment tool to protect both patient and payer.
- A schedule to evaluate the computer systems that are used to capture potential cases or target needy patients, allowing program managers to improve the case selection basis
- A mechanism to direct cases into disease management programs. Not all diabetics need DM; some are well-educated, compliant, and self-manage very well.
- A mechanism to learn from past experience. Has the company or department ever had a preadmission and concurrent review and case management system in place before? If not, there should be a mechanism to track one year's performance against the next and determine how well the program has functioned.
- A mechanism that stratifies and allows for change in the level of disease education and behavior modification. Most individuals enrolled in disease management programs do not remain at the level

at which they entered the program. In many cases, we expect to see a person move from a higher rate of management to a low-maintenance level of intervention as he becomes his own case manager and healthcare advocate.

- A schedule of preenrollment or postenrollment goals so that a person's progress is tracked

FEES: CAPITATED, HOURLY, OR PER CASE

Once the hurdle of setting up the preadmission and concurrent review and case management system is gotten over, there is another potential stumbling block—the fees. Companies accustomed to buying preadmission and concurrent review services customarily purchase these services at capitated rates (a predetermined per-employee, per-month cost) ranging from $.85 per employee per month to $2.00 and on up. These become set fees, varying only by the number of employees or covered lives, and have nothing to do with office visits or hospital admissions. Therefore, fees for a group remain relatively constant if there are 20 or 60 or 200 admissions to a hospital. It is important, therefore, to determine an expected hospital experience for a group prior to establishing fees so that the fees charged will at least meet the expenses incurred in providing services (e.g., payroll, phone, computers, software).

Capitation as a system for reimbursement is gaining popularity among payer groups. Getting its start with HMO plans, capitation certainly places all kinds of risk on those who accept it as payment, rather than its predecessor, the "fee-for-service" arrangement. In a fee-for-service system, providers charge for a service as it is rendered, whether offering hospital, surgical, home health, pharmaceutical, or other medical care. With the inception of HMOs, there was a change in how service fees were paid. Given a certain number of employees and/or covered lives, HMOs consulted actuaries to review the group's prior health history, healthcare activity, and group demographics and to estimate the percentage of the group that would need certain services. The actuaries help set a capitated fee—a charge per employee or covered life for care or services to be provided over a period of time (usually 1 year).

Capitated fees are now applied by the range of managed care providers, including case management services. Many smaller case management companies break out preadmission/concurrent review services on a capitated basis, but because they do not feel as skilled in setting capitated case management fees—predicting how active a case is going to be or how much of a nurse reviewer's time it will need—case management remains a fee-for-service arrangement. Within larger managed care organizations such as HMOs and PPOs, where it is standard to have capitated arrangements with insured groups for purchased services (whether it be a mail-order prescription plan, a vision plan, or case management), capitated fees are more the norm.

Moving from fee-for-service to a capitated rate structure in case management is not easy. There may be considerable risk to the case management provider unless there is knowledge of the insured or self-funded group. In case management, especially with a new patient population or client, and considering marketplace volatility, we are seeing employer groups that are not staying with a particular insurer for any length of time. Therefore, the caseload is inherited with little knowledge about previous experience; the case managers don't have the ability to look back and review prior experience from 2 to 3 years for big cases. The patients may be coming to an HMO, PPO, or POS plan from another company, and the first company's claims department is not going to be sharing its claims information. The case manager then has to project, using standardized information, that perhaps 3% to 5% of the group may require case management; she also must know what her expenses might be to manage a case for the life of that case. Is the average case open 3 months or 6 months? How much activity does a case manager expend on a case? How is it charged out?

In capitated structures, if the industry norm shows that 3% to 5% of the group will be responsible for spending the larger share of the health benefits dollars, those are the individuals to manage. One must decide if it is best to manage all of them or manage 1% of the group very intensively with on-site case management and another 3% telephonically. Rates are then set based on how much it would cost to pay a case manager by the hour to manage those cases. That total fee is then broken into months and divided by group members to determine a capitated fee structure.

Industry norms for preadmission/precertification programs average $1.50 per person per month. Concurrent review services range from $1.50 to $4.00 per person per month, depending on the depth of the follow-up (telephonic or personal visit, for example). The per-person per-month fees for disease management programs (level 1 and level 2 intervention) vary with the disease state. Although diabetes disease management might be charged at $90 per person per month, the cost for chronic obstructive pulmonary disease (COPD) disease management might approach $130 per person per month.

Fees range widely, to put it mildly. Some companies use physicians as case managers, and their fees obviously are going to be higher when figured into a capitated rate, possibly throwing the per-member per-month rate considerably higher. Those companies that do all their case management telephonically may quote fees to manage the life of a case at a lower rate because a case manager can manage many more cases, there is no time on the road or in the hospital, caseloads tend to be higher, and the amount of time spent per case tends to be less. The capitated fees will reflect those givens.

Capitation does seem to be the wave of the future, but it is not without its problems. If those running the department and negotiating the contracts do not have an actuarial or underwriting background, it is very problematic to project group experience. An individual might know case management but not be able to predict group experience and set fees. However, reasonable projections can be made. If prior group experience is unknown, it is advisable to place some risk projections into the contract or to consider the purchase of stop-loss or reinsurance coverage. (HMOs, payers, providers, and case managers may take responsibility for a certain dollar threshold when providing or paying for health services, and purchase stop-loss insurance or reinsure themselves to protect against financial risk and loss. A group might set a specific stop-loss threshold, with a payer covering perhaps $50,000 per case, or an aggregate stop-loss threshold, with the same payer saying it will pay up to $2 million in healthcare fees for the entire covered group. The payer then purchases stop-loss insurance for a predicted caseload above that threshold, as determined by an underwriter or actuary.)

Another fee system is modified fee-for-service. In this system, providers are paid on a traditional fee-for-services basis, with specified maximum fees for each procedure.

The following examples are offered as illustrations. The cases used are for illustrative purposes only, because the range and complexity of case management services may vary from company to company.

It is reasonable, and I strongly recommend, that at a *minimum*, 1% of covered lives in a group be case managed. For one union plan that my company managed, we quoted a capitated rate structure based on numbers from the union's records compared to our other groups with similar experiences. Let us assume the group contained 2,500 members. Using 2.3 as a factor to determine covered lives, and multiplying by the 2,500 members, we determined a given of 6,250 covered lives. One percent of this group (the minimum to receive case management services) is 62 cases. Given assumed lifetime case management fees of $2,500 per case per year, multiplied by 62 cases, we have a total of $155,000 for the year. To structure this contract on a capitated basis, we took the total of $155,000, divided it by 2,500 employees, and divided it again by the 12 months in a year. This determined a capitated rate of $5.16 per employee per month—the fees we would receive to case manage the covered lives associated with this employee group. (This fee could be quoted with one "carve-out," which would occur when capitated fees would be dropped for a fee-for-service structure, perhaps for an extraordinary experience such as more than the projected number of cases or cases requiring more intensive or lengthier intervention, such as transplants, traumatic brain injury, or preemie babies.)

My company had a year's experience with this particular group, so we were relatively comfortable moving into a capitated arrangement with them. Compare this with a smaller group with which we have a contract. Less than 4 months after we assumed responsibility for its case management services, the group had an extraordinary experience. The group of 350 employees provides services to nursing homes in the New York metropolitan area as nurse's aides, housekeepers, and porters. Using the same 2.3 as before to factor our covered lives, we set 805 lives as our covered group. One percent of this group (the minimum to receive case management services) is 8 cases. Given our formula, we would expect to manage 8 cases a year, give or take a few. We have already identified 10 cases and placed them into case management. There are 8 more months in our contracted year, however, and this group appears to be sick!

Had we made our usual assumptions and set capitated rates (1% of covered lives with case management fees of $2,500 for the care lifetime of the case), we could be experiencing a substantial loss. We would have set our fees to manage 1% of the covered group or eight cases for the year, with average fees of $2,500 per case, for a total of $20,000. A capitated rate would be $4.76 per employee per month ($20,000 divided by 350 employees, divided by 12 months, equals $4.76). If the experience of this small group continues as it has, there could be another 20 cases by year's end, with a total count reaching 30. For 30 cases at $2,500 each, we might be providing $75,000 worth of case management services for a capitated rate based on a projected experience costing $20,000, at a loss to us of $55,000. One can easily appreciate how financially problematic capitated rates can be, as well as the importance of establishing a fee structure based on a group's previous experience.

We were contracted to provide services for another group that had a substantial language barrier. Although communication materials were distributed to the members informing them of the need to notify our preadmissions department prior to all hospital admissions, calls were few. Perhaps the language barrier, or culture barrier, was greater than anticipated, or preadmission was not recognized as important. The union's experience, although it should have been the same or greater than other of our groups, was one quarter of the caseload we expected. I informed union management that our capitated rate was set too high. I took back the capitated rate structure and proceeded on a per-case basis until we discovered the true caseload experience for that group. We must be fair. Every company wants to make a profit. If case managers make an unearned profit, and the client company discovers the inflated charges, as companies will, the service provider loses all credibility and trust in the relationship.

Another trend instituted by HMO plans is to put a portion of their fees *at risk*. In most arrangements, the managed care company sets capitated fees assuming the experience of the group. Customarily, if the group has a worse experience than anticipated, the onus is on the managed care company to oversee the costs or perhaps create a carve-out arrangement and renegotiate the fee. An option is to risk a portion of the MCO's fee payment. This means that if quality assurance goals are not met, if patient satisfaction surveys are not completed, if outcomes do not improve, or if costs do not decrease as established in contract negotiations, the client does not pay the MCO fee in full. For example, a company with an HMO that has a disease state management program for asthma patients may go in saying we are going to reduce the cost of your asthma cases by 15%. If we do not, we will risk 2% of our fees. They will have examined their abilities and outcomes and the client's history and will have drawn a line in the sand, saying we can do this and if we do not, you do not have to pay us.

Case management companies are being asked to put a portion of their fees at risk. Setting fees at risk or setting capitated rates can both be risky maneuvers. It is unwise, to say the least, for a case management department or program to blindly set a capitated rate structure with no idea of what the group's experience has been or can be. We once managed two groups of the same size—2,500 members. One group had 40% more hospital admissions than the other group due to age and industry demographics. The first group's members tended to be more sickly, less educated, did not take care of themselves, did not have continuous medical care, did not follow diets, and were not compliant with medication. This again illustrates how a smaller group can have a worse experience history than a larger group. A case manager or department can choose to manage a certain percent of the high-cost cases or go back to the client and renegotiate based on their experience. We have done both. I recommend that case managers leave some room to negotiate either up or down when setting fees, capitated or otherwise.

Common problems of our immature capitation market include the use of multiple carve outs, which becomes an administrative nightmare. Some providers, seeking to keep their services in line with the capitated fees they are receiving, might opt to eliminate services for the problematic, catastrophic patients. And what happens when all the services provided within a facility are not included in the capitated contract? Does the case manager have to pick from the list of available options?[9] For example, a case manager may be instructed by a payer to use ABC Rehabilitation because a contract exists with that group. When the case manager is preparing to place a traumatic brain-injured patient in the facility, she discovers that this diagnosis is not covered under the capitated rate structure. She must address the issue straight on and negotiate coverage and fees or negotiate for approval of another rehabilitation facility. As patient advocates, we must remember that we manage care. Included within that job is our responsibility to consider benefit restrictions, allocations, and their impact on patient care and outcomes.

Some companies, believing that their employee groups (including dependents) are basically healthy, may elect to purchase services on a "per-case" basis. Fees may be calculated on an hourly basis for the time each reviewed case would take or on a flat-fee basis (i.e., a set fee is established for each review).

This covers the fees for the "small stuff." When such fees are quoted, they seem almost painless to the client groups. And, in fact, many client groups consider preadmission and concurrent review services to be case management. They truly believe that "review" and "manage" are one and the same, so discussions about case management fees often generate resistance. If a client group already thinks it is getting review and case management services for a capitated rate of $2.00 per employee per month, then it is necessary to redefine the terms, explain the differences, and determine the services actually being provided. Case management services are usually billed on an hourly basis or deemed "out of contract" or "extracontractual" services. When the services and fees are discussed, the group may decide to forgo them or to use them sparingly, only for catastrophes. ("We've only had one or two of these, thank God, our people are healthy!") Quite apparently, the group needs a little more information about case management, the kinds of cases typically managed, and how case management differs from preadmission and concurrent review.

Case management fees, if billed hourly, do get noticed. A case manager needs to discuss the fee structure and reach an agreement on it with the potential client group or payer prior to invoicing for these services. Hourly fees vary depending on the geographic location, whether services are provided telephonically or on-site, as well as the size of the case management company or department, and its client base. Case management provided within a specific market niche, such as oncology or premature babies, may warrant higher hourly fees due to the expertise and experience of the practitioner. In general, case management hourly fees can fall between $75.00 and $150.00.

Full acceptance of these fees is not automatic, nor is explaining them an easy process. They need to be presented as individualized and time intensive. A description of the kind of work that is involved is helpful and provides an understanding not only of the process, but also of the time required for visits, arranging for services, negotiating fees, monitoring, and so on. It should be pointed out that if a case is unmanaged, the costs will go unchecked and might indeed prove to be catastrophically expensive. A side-by-side comparison of patients that are case managed and those that are not is extremely valuable in demonstrating potential savings. Because some cases can generate thousands of dollars in invoices, there needs to be a thorough discussion and acceptance of the case management concept before work begins.

Trusting that a payer will automatically perceive the value and accept the costs of case management services is not a risk worth taking. It often results in having to justify expenses after the fact, which places one in the position of "putting out fires." There may be resistance or lack of understanding, but it is better to confront problems before services are initiated than to be well into a program and faced with a client who feels misled.

Because case management is largely intangible, educating prospective or current client groups takes time, energy, and verbal skills. One successful method of education involves the sharing of cost-benefit analysis reports. When these reports are reviewed case by case, it becomes evident that the investment in case management is worthwhile. Presenting case management as "the" solution to high-cost cases allows even the dubious to consider it, if only on a one-case-at-a-time basis.

Once aboard, "converts" become "zealots" as success after success is documented. Of course, there will be cases that do not yield as large a savings as others, but overall effective case management programs will always result in considerable savings. The bottom line should be that the dollars spent on case management are far less than the savings realized.

NOTES

1. "Studies Show Nurses' Visits in Pregnancies Helped Later," *New York Times,* 27 (1997): A18.
2. Reuters News, "Most Employers Still Offer Health Programs," *Bio/Analogics* 1, no. 5 (2001), http://www.imakenews.com.
3. Bliss K and Mischler E, "Planting the Seeds for Improved Health and Productivity: Disease Management Programs," *Continuing Care* 21, no. 6 (2002): 22–25.
4. URAC, "What Is Care Management?" http://www.urac.org/resources/careManagement. aspx (accessed January 2, 2009).
5. Flaum M, "Comorbidity and DM," *Health Management Technology* 22, no. 10 (2001): 28.
6. "Proactive CM Improves Outcomes for Diabetics," *Case Management Advisor* 8, no. 3 (January 1997): 1, 22. (For more information, please call 1-800-688-2421.)
7. "Asthma Program Slashes Hospitalization Costs," *Disease State Management* 1, no. 3 (October 1995): 31.
8. Ceniceros R, "Employer Interest in Disease Management Growing," *Business Insurance* 36, no. 6 (2002): T4, T7.
9. Bliss K and Mischler E, "Planting the Seeds,".

Chapter 11

Working Effectively with Claims Departments: Case Managers in Consulting Roles

There have been many changes in the ways healthcare claims are paid, yet in some fields there are still few incentives to watch out for costs. As long as there is coverage available and a doctor's prescription or a letter of medical need accompanies a claim, it will be paid because most claims examiners and departments do not have the sophisticated medical knowledge to know whether a procedure is really necessary. Once coverage starts, who in the claims department can say when it should stop? Is the claims staff supposed to decide the beginning and end points in medical care? One would not assume so, but in terms of payments for healthcare delivery, much has been left in the hands of the providers and claims personnel. Certainly neither individuals nor corporations really want to turn over their checkbook, especially in areas in which there are no reasonable and customary charges established for medical services, yet they do, daily. When a bill comes in, it gets paid at 100% or 80% of the submitted amount despite the fact that charges are all over the map; some people are paying what they should be and others are billed far above what is even deemed profitable. So, do we leave everything to the free market—let the buyer beware and hope that care costs eventually stabilize? I don't think so.

Let the buyer beware? Patients are often too weak, too compromised, or too distraught to look out for themselves. Savvy corporate managers, as well as smart homemakers, get thrown into the middle of the convoluted delivery-payment system and must gear up to act as self-advocates. The more complex their needs, the less likely it is they will be well-served by the system. The more providers involved, the less likely it is that there is one person looking out for the patient. Fortunately, all kinds of state, federal, and independent organizations, as well as consumer advocates, are providing healthcare financial information to patients via books, newsletters, and the Internet. Employers across the country are ramping up their initiative to encourage their employees to be educated consumers. Still, we work within a system in which, despite dollars being spent, no one person has the responsibility of trying to ensure that the outcome will be desirable and the services will be quality.

This is the case manager's opportunity to create collaborative roles with employers, payers, and providers as they work in their patients' best interests. With a better understanding of the claims world, joined with their knowledge of how the healthcare delivery system works, case managers can get the most and best use from plan dollars and often extend the length of time care can be provided through the judicious use of available funds.

A nurse in a hospital would never decide to get involved in a patient's care just by reviewing the case while sitting at a desk. The nurse would walk down the hall and visit that patient, talk to the physician, and talk to the family. A case manager would do no less. There are too many liabilities and too much at stake. Similarly, shuffling claims (or even speeding claims) through the system for payment is not enough. Patient information is not enough. A physician's operative report is not enough. It is the combination of information and what the case manager does with that information that makes case management a valued service.

Understanding the roles and responsibilities of claims personnel and working in concert with claims staff can help a case manager improve patient outcomes and enhance a payer's bottom line. It can help her build a more successful case management program and achieve a better position in the marketplace. The line of insurance, the entity retaining the case manager's services, and the case manager's position dictate how close a case manager's contact is with a claims department. Some case managers never talk to a claims person, ever. They might converse with the case management department in XYZ insurance company, and that department then perhaps communicates with a claims department. Unfortunately, for far too many companies, the case managers work in a vacuum with no claims interface at all.

The amount of interaction with a claims department also depends on the structure of the case management department or company. The individual case manager may have more or less freedom to communicate directly with a claims department, benefit examiner, or claims adjustor.

The bigger the company and the more case managers there are, the less likely it is a particular case manager will have ongoing contact with a claims adjustor. Sometimes, the supervisor of a case management company is afraid that a case manager will get too close to accounts and decide to start her own company, taking the accounts along. Case management and claims services are rarely integrated, and both the patients and the program suffer.

In short, the ideal does not exist. Not every case manager has ongoing communication, nor does every case manager who makes a recommendation see it put into place. A report may go to claims supervisor Jane Jones, but never past her to the claims examiner. Or, the report may go directly to a home office, because in this particular company only the home office assigns cases for case management; the local claims department may never see the report or know about it. There is no universal ideal for the interface between case managers and claims departments. However, this does not mean that case managers should ignore the benefits of this liaison or hesitate to establish it. The "norm" does not free a case manager from the responsibility to know claims issues and claims personnel, because whatever work a case manager does is eventually forwarded to a claims department.

CLAIMS DEPARTMENT STRUCTURE AND OPERATIONS

To make the most of their relationships with claims departments and to benefit patients and payers, case managers should distinguish the main players in the claims arena. What are the reporting relationships within the office? How does this person fit into the loop? A person's title may convey how much or how little control he or she has over processing a claim. It is also vital to determine the concerns of the claims staff: What is the real reason a claim was referred for case management? What is the claims manager looking for from the case manager? How can the case manager get timely, accurate answers to her questions in an effort to address claims concerns? Finally, case managers will want to discover their own process of working with claims staff to get the best for their patients and clients while creating more advocates for case management.

The Players

Job functions vary from claims office to claims office. Titles such as *processor*, *examiner*, and *adjustor* may be interchangeable, or each may denote different jobs with different responsibilities. In general, there are some titles and activities that are fairly consistent across organizations:

- A customer service representative is the first person an insured speaks to regarding eligibility, coverage issues, and plan allowances.
- A claims processor may not be a decision maker, but does put claims into the system. Edits to claim entries may occur after processing. This title is usually used in a high-volume claims environment.
- A claims examiner is a claims processor who has the necessary skills to examine claims and make decisions whether to approve, investigate, or deny them.
- A claims supervisor is usually in charge of work flow, examiner production, and the first level of management decision making.
- A claims manager usually makes the final decision regarding claims. Directors and vice presidents may be involved in decisions.
- A plan administrator has responsibility for overall administration of the plan, handling appeals and plan design and changes. Within a self-funded plan, there is a designated management-level person with responsibility for stop-loss advisories. This person notifies the stop-loss carrier when a call point is reached, usually when 50% of the dollars allotted to the primary insurance plan have been spent, and is the person responsible for allowing an override of the cover to pay a high-cost claim. The case manager is often involved in some of the conversation between the stop-loss carrier and the claims department liaison.
- An account manager with insurance and marketing skills is the direct interface between the client group and the claims department. This individual handles service issues, complaints, funding issues, and may report regularly on the claims experience.

These are the people charged with making claims payments and enforcing whatever insurance benefit contract might be in effect. Their responsibilities include the accurate and timely payment of claims in a manner that follows contract language and documents their activities. In most claims offices, there is also a productivity quota that must be met. When working for a self-insured employer group (in-house or self-administered claims), the staff reports to the employer's CFO or CEO. In the case of a Third Party Administrator, the claims staff answers to the Third Party Administrator's CEO or vice president. Claims personnel employed by an insurance carrier report to the insurance company's CEO or president.

The expertise and background of claims personnel vary widely. Some claims examiners have minimal experience in claims; some processors are experienced in data entry and are trained as they work their way up the claims staff ladder. In larger companies, an individual may begin as a file clerk, take on data entry, become a processor, and then become, over the course of several months, an examiner adjudicating and paying claims. Most claims personnel have a high school degree at least. Again, the bigger and more established companies tend to have many more in-house people experienced in claims issues. Newer firms and groups often begin their claims operations on a smaller scale, bringing in more expensive, more experienced senior people once their client base is more stable.

Broadly speaking, claims examiners have no background in medical terminology, and any experience they do get will come from day-to-day jobsite training or from courses they attend in medical benefits administration. There are videos and seminars available covering workers' compensation, liability, and group medical coverage as well as the more complex topics (e.g., co-payments, coinsurance benefits, and statutes and regulations) they will encounter as they move up to become senior-level examiners.

Case managers and examiners view each case from totally different perspectives. Whereas case managers view a case globally and consider the patient's entire medical history and experience, claims examiners are presented with cases on an item-by-item basis, checking one ICD-9 or CPT code or R & C charge at a time. Further, examiners are productivity driven. The money that is going to be made by their employer is made by getting the claims in, getting them quickly and fairly administered, and getting them out. There is not a lot of time to be spent on the phone or deliberating over single claims.

Unaware of this, case managers sometimes get exasperated at the gaps in claims examiners' knowledge of cases. Claims examiners rarely get the opportunity to handle all the claims for one patient, never mind the claims for one entire family.

There is no staffing pattern common to all claims departments, and there may be little true account dedication. A claim comes in and anyone in a room of examiners may process it. Some companies do set up account-specific groups; an insurance company handling 500 different employer groups may have one set of individuals processing claims for ABC, Inc., but they handle the auto, group medical, and workers' compensation claims for all of ABC's 1,200 employees. Another department may section its staff by procedure; surgical claims staff, dental claims staff, and anesthesia claims staff, for example, administer surgical, dental, and anesthesia claims for the entire covered population.

The case manager trying to find out "why was this claim paid this way?" might have a long wait, depending on the claims department's line of business. Because it has direct contact with the employer, a Third Party Administrator usually has many more customer service and account representatives right in the claims department. The Third Party Administrator's representative may be in daily contact with the employer's human resources manager. In a large insurance firm, however, contact may be far removed. The employer group might call its insurance agent or broker, who in turn calls a customer service representative, who brings it to the attention of an account representative, who hopefully talks to a claims manager.

The diversity of claims operations makes a case manager's job more difficult; any assumptions she makes about a claims department usually turn out to be erroneous. Whereas a nurse in a coronary care unit in New York is likely to have had the same experience as a coronary care unit nurse in Nebraska, a claims examiner paying medical claims in a building in Chicago may not have had the same experience as the claims examiner at the next desk. Adding to the challenge for case managers are the reams of claims forms and the computer technology endemic to claims departments.

The Paper Trail

A claims department is a paper-intensive environment. One claims history can have hundreds of pieces of paper and electronically submitted documents, along with actual claims submitted by various providers. And, depending on the structure of the department, one claimant may have his or her claims paid by no fewer than 5, 10, or 20 individuals, none of whom may have any understanding of what is going on in the case. Because these pieces of paper and e-mails relate to only a small segment of the patient's overall condition, and because claims departments can be huge, it is a paper trail that is virtually impossible to track. Who has which claims, how were they processed, and what does this claimant's record look like when it is all assembled? The payment system is convoluted and fraught with regulations; every claim has to be submitted with this attachment and that notice, and because a consensus is lacking on how to handle claims, it takes one person minutes just to decide how to process a claim, which slows down the whole payment sequence. This is what the industry is complaining about, it is what providers are complaining about, and it is what the federal government and the states are complaining about.

And if the payment system is a challenge for the claims industry, it is a source of confusion and anxiety for the patient. For the most part, there is no one person to speak to if a patient has a problem. John Jones says, "Last month, I got my claims paid fine, and 2 weeks later I sent in a claim from the same provider, but now it's been paid differently. Why did that happen?" There do not seem to be any hard-and-fast rules, and claimants seemingly have no redress. And because of cutbacks in most companies, John can only "speak" to a telephonic mail system. The non-computer-savvy person or the person with a language barrier or a disabling condition is left hanging with no way to resolve major problems.

COMPUTERIZATION

The growing use of computers has alleviated a portion of this mess for some individuals. A patient's entire claims history can be keyed into a computer system and be pulled up on a computer screen. Many claimants, especially those insured by large plans, can see their plan on-screen and check coverage. People can enroll on-line and make changes in their enrollment as the plan allows. Technology is allowing enhanced access to check the status of a claim, whether it has been submitted, and where it is in the claims system.

Computers ease some of the confusion, but there are issues remaining that must be reviewed with a live person. This is why more patients are bringing case managers into discussions about claims. Sometimes, the case manager is the only person the patient feels he can talk to because she knows all his medical needs. I would advise all case managers to increase their understanding of insurance operations, plans, and the claims process. It is another area in which case managers can make themselves indispensable.

The majority of today's computer systems are set up in such a way that the problem has worsened. Claims examiners are no longer looking at actual pieces of paper. A claimant, who has been told to save a copy of everything, might have a copy of the claim but is talking to someone who is looking at a computer screen containing numbers, ICD-9 codes, and that is all. Even if the claimant had attached an explanatory note to the claim, there will be no corresponding explanation on the screen. So the claimant might have gone through laborious steps to clarify his or her situation but no one has recorded it. This is extremely frustrating for everyone involved.

Yet most lines of insurance today, including long-term disability, workers' compensation, and group medical insurance, are administered by software programs. Some insurance company departments and Third Party Administrators still administer claims by hand, but most large, competitive companies have computers assisting in the processing of claims. Various indicators can be programmed into the software to alert a claims examiner or consultant to a claim that may be problematic. Insurance companies or administrators handling claims for several employer groups need to be able to report back to those employer groups when an individual appears to be filing high-cost claims consistently. This allows the insurance company to control their present claims experience better and also plan for their future benefit needs. Actuarial professionals have been using these same techniques for years, garnering information from software programs to rate groups more appropriately and accurately. These reports also highlight information of interest to risk managers.

Employers in a particular industry purchase insurance at rates based on the industry's experience. In some industries, there may be an abnormal number of back injuries or a high incidence of lost-time accidents anticipated due to the type of work employees perform. Risk managers advise employer groups and insurance underwriters on how to decrease employee risk, prevent accidents from occurring, and contain the associated costs once they occur. Can a different therapy be used to shorten the rehabilitation period? What preventive or safety mechanisms can be installed to decrease the incidence of injury at that work site?

Most often, risk managers are consulted by companies that offer property, casualty, and liability insurance, yet are rarely approached by group medical carriers. To my mind, it makes good sense to apply risk management principles to all lines of insurance. I am certain that the trend toward moving patients from high-cost care settings to outpatient settings resulted from the examination by consultants of data runs showing the average length of hospital stays. A consultant would look at a benefit plan, see that there was little coverage available for outpatient care, and approach the company about ways to change the plan language to integrate outpatient care and make the whole experience a better one for the employer and insureds alike. In this way, software programs and risk management principles can be utilized for every line of insurance.

In some respects, there is an overreliance on software by managers and employer groups, who are understandably impressed by software capabilities. But software programs can tell just so much about what is really going on. No matter how sophisticated, software cannot keep up with all the elements involved in claims payment. Sometimes, employers rely on software to tell them what the problems are and how to solve them. They create great reports that give the percentage of people who generated a certain percentage of benefit dollars, but the software provides no clues on how to help those people or lower costs.

There is a common misconception that the speed and efficacy of a software system will now solve the problems that insurers thought they had (e.g., the relatively long time it might take to pay a claim). Now, perhaps claims are paid too quickly. They do get paid faster, but more important pieces fall through the cracks because of the speed. For example, fraudulent claims are less apt to be picked up. Examiners are no longer looking at a claim and saying, "This looks doctored to me." We have lost some of the familiarity and hands-on knowledge regarding problem claims or people who might benefit from a one-on-one relationship with the claims examiner, but we have gained the ability to process the volumes of simple and complex claims that are submitted. Nothing would ever get paid in some cases without the use of software, yet perhaps it is relied on too much in the identification of problem cases. Software alone cannot really tell us what the problems are.

CLAIMS ISSUES

Case managers need to be aware of the concerns of claims personnel. These individuals have their own set of criteria that they must meet on the job, and case managers can create much better relationships by taking the time to understand claims issues. Some of these issues are preexisting conditions, the funding vehicle (self-insured, fully insured, administrative services only, reinsurance, cost plus), insurance contract language, and coordination of benefits (if there are two medical plans in a family). Is COBRA coverage involved? Is the claimant in the midst of an eligibility change: active to retired, active to disabled, active to Medicare eligibility, or active to COBRA? If the insurer is an employee group, return-to-work issues are important to the claims staff, as are ERISA concerns.

INDICATORS FOR CASE MANAGEMENT

Sometimes, the best teachers for a case manager are the cases that came to her too late, in which she envisions all kinds of possibilities, if only she could have had this case earlier, when the home care first started. Now, it's 6 months later and she's wondering how to get the family unhooked from their services. Some services are difficult to "undo." By looking back at some of those cases, a case manager can develop her own red flags. The "I could haves" turn into red flag indicators.

Cases that benefit most from case management commonly involve the most expensive services. Use of these services is, thus, a red flag. Other indicators include a high frequency of admissions in a short period and an unusually long hospital stay. It is usual, perhaps, for certain surgical procedures to require 5 to 7 days hospitalization. (A stay of 10 days or longer for a surgical hospitalization indicates multiple problems or complications now and points to problems down the road as well.)

This is where a case manager's clinical knowledge comes into play, her feel for what constitutes a big case. Having developed a set of indicators, the case manager then needs to communicate them to claims personnel. The object is to get them to understand which cases to bring to the case manager's attention so she can at least follow up with a phone call and find out what is being recommended. If the treatment plan includes 12 hours per day of home nursing services or infusion care services for someone with a chronic infection, the result could be 30 days of services at $700 or $800 per day. With negotiation and appropriate service arrangements at the beginning, the case manager can get the patient what is needed and really demonstrate cost savings as the service is being put in place. It is very difficult to renegotiate a bill for $24,000 after the fact.

One new client handed me bills for $24,000 and $50,000 and asked, "Can't you do anything about this?" I informed the client that it is hard to do anything about such bills once the services have been provided. I said that similar cases, however, if referred early on, would benefit from case management and the costs could be reduced. The claims department, for example, was confronted with a claim for payment of monitoring services provided in the home of a woman with a high-risk pregnancy. They were looking at a red flag but did not know it. Instead of asking if the woman was covered, the claims personnel should have been asking if it is normal for a pregnant woman to be monitored at home. I needed to educate the claims department. Fetal monitoring is not usual for most pregnancies, and by informing the claims personnel of this fact, and showing them that abnormal means big costs, I was able to get them to tell me about such cases upfront, when case management could have a more positive impact.

It is important to let the claims personnel know that they really can make a difference. I have tracked a case without case management, run it through the case management process of negotiation and active intervention, and then shared the results with the claims staff. I tell the managers of the Third Party Administrators I work with, "Listen, if you get your people involved, if you give them some kind of incentive, let them become the ones who refer cases, who are given the credit for savings, you will see a marked difference in the reports to your clients." Empowering everyone and giving each person insight into his or her role in the team effort makes for a better claims team and more effective claims administration.

With regard to another service our company provides, claims review, we faced a problem with the wrong kind of incentive. There was an administration quota, and for every claim that claims personnel paid over and above a certain number, they were given a monetary bonus. Obviously, this encouraged them to pay claims quickly. I said, "Do you understand what you're doing here? You're pushing things through the system. It takes your examiners time to pull aside a claim and give it to me for possible case management intervention or review. Yes, you want prompt payment of claims but you don't want to pay everything without consideration. If you can put a monetary incentive in place for those claims examiners who refer claims that actually result in savings, you'll have the proper emphasis. As a Third Party Administrator, you're charged with the responsibility to save money, and your people should be rewarded. Not only is it part of their job, but ultimately it will be part of whether or not you get a contract renewed to pay a client's claims again."

The education process continues, little by little, case by case. Figure 11–1 is a "tip sheet" I developed for the claims department of one client Third Party Administrator. It includes red flags for case management intervention as well as indicators for claims review.

Figure 11–1 CareSolutions™ Red Flags and AccuClaim™ Red Flags.

CareSolutions™ Red Flags

• **Diagnosis:**	Cancer	Alcohol and	Chronic Respiratory
	AIDS	Substance Abuse	Conditions
	Stroke	Cardiovascular	Psychiatric
	Transplant	Head Injury	Multiple Trauma
	Neuromuscular	Hepatitis C	High-Risk Infant
	Diseases	Severe Burns	Lyme Disease
	Spinal Cord	High-Risk	
	Injuries	Pregnancy	

• **Potential Treatment:**	Ventilator-dependent	Extended ICU
	IV Antibiotics	Home Care
	TPN/Enteral	Chemotherapy

• **Frequent Hospitalizations:** Three Admits Same Year/Same or Related Problem

• **Cost of Claim:** Same Illness over $25,000 Year-to-Date

• **Location of Claim:** Complex Care Delivered in Rural Setting, Small Hospital, or Facility with Poor Outcome History/Diagnosis

• **Patterns of Care:** Failed or Repeated Surgeries, Hospital-Acquired Infections, Malpractice Concerns

• **Diagnostic Codes:** ICD9CM - Case Management Referral Indicators

continues

Figure 11–1 continued

042–044	HIV infection	330–337	Hereditary and degenerative diseases of CNS (Alzheimer's, Huntington's chorea)	644	Early or threatened labor
140–239	Neoplasms (cancer)			655–656	Fetal abnormality
250	Diabetes with complications			710	All collagen (SLE+)
277	Cystic fibrosis, polyarthropor-phyria, metabolic disorders (mult. hosps.)	340–349	CNS disorders, MS, CP, quadri-plegie, paraplegic, anoxic brain damage	714	Rheumatoid arthritis w/ inflammatory polyarthropathies

042–044 HIV infection
140–239 Neoplasms (cancer)
250 Diabetes with complications
277 Cystic fibrosis, polyarthropor-phyria, metabolic disorders (mult. hosps.)
279 Immunity deficiency disorders (repeat hosps.)
286–287 Coagulation defects (repeat hosps.)
290–299 Psychoses
300–316 Neurotic personality and other nonpsychotic mental disorders
850–854 Intracranial injury excluding those with skull fracture
860–869 Internal injury of chest, abdomen, and pelvis
870–879 Open wound of head, neck, and trunk

330–337 Hereditary and degenerative diseases of CNS (Alzheimer's, Huntington's chorea)
340–349 CNS disorders, MS, CP, quadriplegie, paraplegic, anoxic brain damage
358 Myasthenia gravis (repeat hosps.)
359 Muscular dystrophy (repeat hosps.)
430–438 Cerebral vascular disease, car. hemorrhage
496 COPD
501–503 Asbestosis and silicosis
584–586 Renal failure
925–929 Crashing injury (may involve extensive trauma)
948 Burns over 25% of body
952 SCI without spinal bone injury

644 Early or threatened labor
655–656 Fetal abnormality
710 All collagen (SLE+)
714 Rheumatoid arthritis w/ inflammatory polyarthropathies
740–759 Congenital anomalies, spina bifida, cardiac septal defect
760–763 Maternal causes of perinatal morbidity and mortality
765.1 Premature birth
800 Fracture vault of skull
806 Fracture of vertebral column w/SCI
994 Effects of external causes—lightning, drowning, strangulation
996–999 Complications of surgical and medical care

AccuClaim™ Red Flags

- **Surgical and Anesthesia Claims:** All provider claims over $10,000 and all cases with more than two line items should be referred for a medical review. Alert for GYN, Orthopedic, Plastic Surgery. If the surgical claim is referred, corresponding anesthesia claims should be referred also to verify complexity of claimed procedure. Information to obtain: 1) Operative report; 2) Anesthesia time; 3) R&C charges for each CPT code.
- **Podiatrists:** All claims that exceed $1,000 should be referred. Information to obtain: 1) Operative report if a surgical procedure is being billed; 2) R&C charges for each CPT code.
- **Physical Therapy and Occupational Therapy:** Claims that exceed 6 weeks of treatment should be referred. Information to obtain: 1) PT evaluation; 2) Therapy progress

Figure 11–1 continued

notes that include long- and short-term goals and the range of motion results; 3) Letter of medical need from treating MD with diagnosis, frequency of treatment, and estimated duration.

- **Chiropractic Care:** Claims that exceed $500 should be referred. Information to obtain: Complete copy of the medical records; NO summaries. Include diagnosis, treatment plan, frequency of treatment, estimated duration.
- **Durable Medical Equipment:** This is an area of extreme abuse and overutilization of services and fees. The following claims should be referred: oxygen concentrators and related equipment, hospital beds, wheelchairs, any monitors, respirators/ventilators, bone stimulators, insulin and lymphedema pumps, requests for home modifications (ramps, etc.).
- **Home Health Services:** All claims for nursing, aides, or related services should be referred. Information to obtain: 1) Itemized bills; 2) Nursing notes.
- **Infusion Care Services:** All claims for the following infusion services should be referred: IV antibiotics and other medications, TPN (total parenteral nutrition), chemotherapy, and analgesia (pain medications). Information to obtain: 1) MD's prescription; 2) Itemized billing for medications, nursing, and related services and supplies.
- **Any of the following should be referred:** 1) Appeals; 2) Difficult providers; 3) Ambulatory surgical centers; 4) Large hospital bills: over 7 days LOS; to review for LOS, medical needs vs. custodial.
- **Procedure Codes:** CPT AccuClaim Referral Indicators

Integumentary System
11000–11044 For cosmetic vs. medical
15780–15791 For cosmetic vs. medical
15810–15840 For cosmetic vs. medical
17304–17310 For cosmetic vs. medical
19318–19500 For cosmetic vs. medical
Musculoskeletal
27590–27598 Amputation
Pulmonary System
30400–30630 For cosmetic
31300–31660 Laryngectomy-
tracheotomy, etc.
32310–32545 Lung surgery
Cardiovascular
33200–33220 Pacemaker surgery
35450–35458 Vascular vs. cosmetic
37799 Unlisted procedure
38999 Unlisted procedure
39599 Unlisted procedure
Digestive
41100–41155 Mouth, tongue (for cancer)

43600–43630 Stomach (biopsy, etc.)
44100–44340 Intestinal
47100–47135 Liver
Urinary System
50200–50380 Kidney, including transplant
51550–51597 Bladder (especially for cancer)
Maternity
59000–59100 High-risk procedures
59120–59140 High-risk procedures
Nervous System
61340–61576 Craniectomy
62180–62258 Spine
64999 Unlisted procedure
Eye and Ear
65771 Radial keratotomy
69300 Cosmetic
69399 Unlisted procedure
68899 Unlisted procedure

Source: Courtesy of Options Unlimited, Case Management Services Division, © 2003, Huntington, New York.

Different red flags should be used for different lines of insurance. Looking for case management indicators, a case manager will not apply the same dollar limit per claim in a workers' compensation case as in a group medical case. In workers' compensation, for each lost-time injury there is an established guideline, and if the injured person is still out of work a month beyond the date calculated using the guidelines, then that fact becomes a red flag. (Physicians use the reference *The Medical Disability Advisor: Workplace Guidelines for Disability Duration*, written by Presley Reed and published by Reed Group Ltd., to find out about injuries common to different job descriptions, including typical recuperative periods and return-to-work time frames.) On most workers' compensation claims forms, physicians are usually asked to note the date the claimant can return to work. If a physician has left the space blank or puts down "undetermined" month after month, that is a definite red flag. To my mind, a physician avoiding a return-to-work date indicates a problem. On the other hand, the physician might write in that a workers' compensation claimant should be able to return to work in 4 to 6 weeks. Four to 6 weeks go by, then another 4 to 6 weeks, then the patient needs another month of physical therapy three times per week. This kind of extension of treatment also indicates a problem. (Further, if the physical therapy is provided in a physician-owned facility, it may be a red flag.) Other indicators are: if the case continually passes by established goals; if the claimant is going to one doctor, and a month later he's going to another doctor who provides a similar service; or if the patient is receiving physical therapy and chiropractic manipulation at the same time. Or, the case manager might discover the patient is taking large numbers of pain medications and antidepressant medications, indicating the existence of new emotional components such as depression or lack of concentration, or that a seemingly simple injury has assumed grandiose proportions, with the patient seeing a variety of practitioners.

Other cases that need to be watched include those in which a new employee suffers a serious injury. One major concern is that the employer might not feel a commitment to get the employee back on the job, especially if modifications are required. New injuries to persons with prior claims for back or other workers' compensation injuries should be treated as red flags. (There is usually a state data bank that claims departments can use to research a claimant's prior workers' compensation injuries with other carriers or with other employer groups.) Indicators also include injuries to claimants nearing retirement age, injuries to part-time employees who might also work full time someplace else, or injuries to employees who could do work off the books. The insurer may be paying for an injury that occurred but not on the site the insurer is responsible for, or the claimant might still be able to work his or her main job but not the secondary job. For example, the claimant might work full-time as a file clerk in a corporation and part-time as a supermarket bagger. While recuperating, the claimant may be able to do filing but not stand for 4 hours and bag groceries, yet the workers' compensation carrier is still responsible.

Personnel issues can become reasons for people to go on short-term or long-term disability, and case managers need to devote attention to cases involving employees who are nearing retirement age or have both short-term and long-term disability policies (allowing a short-term leave to turn into a long-term leave, which is especially common in departments or companies facing layoffs). Employees who are at risk for being laid off or who have been passed over for promotion sometimes stay on short-term or long-term disability for security, using the insurance payments as a salary replacement. Obviously, the higher the salary replacement within a long-term plan, or the longer the HISOCC clause (see Chapter 4) in a long-term disability plan, the more quickly a case manager should review the claims. On the whole, the higher the policy benefits offered, the more bells and whistles should be going off.

In group medical coverage, the concerns are different. Group plans cover employees and their dependents, and a case manager might target catastrophic illnesses, premature deliveries, cancer cases, plus other chronic and devastating long-term diseases, such as AIDS or multiple sclerosis. Other things to watch for include multiple hospitalizations, multiple physicians, expenses beyond a certain threshold (e.g., $10,000), and particular kinds of services such as chemotherapy, radiation therapy, and infusion care.

Because medical professionals do not staff most claims departments, I encourage case managers to include visual aids or informative material to help illustrate the conditions of claimants when they are first introducing red flags and when they are working on a weekly basis with claims personnel. A case manager can discuss ICD-9 codes and CPT codes until next week and never make the impact that one good picture will create. For example, imagine a case involving body burns. The case manager may say, "There are substantial body burns, but they are confined to the trunk and upper extremities," and then shade those areas in on front- and back-view line drawings of the type supplied by most medical companies. The case manager, without spending much time, has enabled the claims staff to feel they know what the case is about.

I see articles all the time in consumer publications such as *People, TIME, Newsweek,* and *The Ladies' Home Journal* that can serve as terrific teaching aids. I might tear out a piece on breast cancer or cystic fibrosis and send it along to a claims examiner with a note. I have also purchased medical dictionaries and reference books designed for laypersons and handed them to my claims associates. Specific examples include *The Pill Book, Tenth Edition* (Bantam Books), *The Merck Manual of Medical Information, Second Edition* (Simon & Schuster), and the *Mayo Clinic Family Health Book, Third Edition* (Harper Resource).

The more complex and complicated the medical picture, the more user-friendly the explanation has to be. The goal is to get claims personnel to understand the reasons behind the need for case management and the decisions of the case manager. I have gone to the extent of taking a claims representative to a rehabilitation facility. I have also used videos from a rehabilitation facility showing pieces of equipment as well as videos taken by parents showing their child in a walker. I use videos and photos to give a clear impression of a given situation. I do not do this for every case or claim, only for those requiring special attention while we try to resolve their problems. Sometimes, word pictures suffice: The patient is down a country road six miles from his nearest neighbor, his family is dispersed across the nation, and he lives alone. Word pictures can humanize a case.

I have found all these methods of education extremely beneficial. They not only improve my relationships with referral sources but also enable me to do a better job for my patients, because I now have the understanding of the people who sent me out in the first place.

THE CASE MANAGER AS CONSULTANT

Case managers are an asset to a claims department. Bringing to the table their knowledge of clinical needs, medical procedures, and costs, they are a significant support toward maintaining cost-effective healthcare programs.

Claims Software

Working directly with a claims department on specific limit reports, group claims runs, and individual claims runs is a facet of the case manager in a consultant role. She becomes a hands-on team member, sitting alongside the employer group, the Third Party Administrator, or the insurer to capture those claimants in need of case management intervention. Using these tools, computer-generated claims runs, and creating the reports that follow from them, the case manager expands upon her case management activities and involvement with clients. These activities constitute the next step beyond noting red flags, but it is not a step every case manager may want to or be able to take (due to restrictions in her job description, the level of her interaction with the claims department, or the lack of computer technology sophisticated enough to generate claims runs). I include it here because I believe such consulting work is a vital part of case management capabilities, profile, and marketing strength.

Specific limit is the term I use to signify a computer-generated report that consolidates a particular type of information or claims run from all the claims experiences of a group of covered individuals. Such reports help pinpoint problem areas in which case management can effect a great change in case outcomes and dollar expenditures. If a company's employee base is predominantly female, I might want to see a specific limit report tracking pregnancy-related claims and benefit dollars spent. From this report, I could tell if there was a high incidence of problem pregnancies or premature births among these women. Perhaps the company needs to offer prenatal counseling or well-mother and well-baby seminars. At the least, it needs to make sure its female employees know they should be seeing a physician or nurse-midwife throughout their pregnancies, and it should give them clear information on what their benefit package covers regarding childbirth and infant care.

A case manager or claims manager can set a specific limit "marker" for any time, dollar, or medical treatment indicator. A specific limit report can cover any dollar amount one wants to establish, or it can be a hospital report with three admissions or more. Ideally, because everyone is concerned about dollars, the marker is a dollar amount, but it could also be time or an ICD-9 code. It might be appropriate to spin off a report on everyone in a group who has a diagnosis of cancer. Perhaps the case manager notices cancer cases are typically expensive and, in her role as consultant, wants to see who else in the group is likely to draw substantial benefits.

I might see that I seem to have an unusually high number of diabetes risks. In this situation, I will want to hone my data and look at everyone with diabetes who has spent $5,000, for example. I will want to know if they are in good systems of care. Is there something that should be done? Should the company establish a diabetic management program? Why is there such a high number of cases? This puts the risk management principle into case management, exactly where it belongs.

The object of tracking claims is not to dump a report in an employer's lap that announces that the firm has experienced *x* number of lost-time accidents in the past year, each requiring a recuperation period averaging 6 months and running up benefit expenses averaging $15,000. The purpose of claims tracking is to assess the information and utilize it proactively to design solutions. Case managers can help employers and Third Party Administrators create cost-containment claims administration programs to meet their particular needs. Does a company or a community have a particularly high rate of oncology claims, due perhaps to environmental conditions or job-site chemicals? Is a company experiencing an unusual rate of complex pregnancies or premature births? Once the presenting problem is pinpointed, a software program can be created to help find potential cases before complications are manifested.

A case manager consultant looking to interface more directly with claims personnel as a way of increasing cost-management capabilities first needs to understand the client company's claims system and computer and software systems. Five workers' compensation carriers may each have a software program capable of manipulating data in distinct ways and creating various report printouts. Can the system generate a report that breaks out cases with claims totaling over $10,000 or $20,000? Can it separate out all claims paid for lost-time injuries? Can it provide a run (list) of all claims filed by one claimant in the last 18 months?

The person to contact for this type of information is the claims manager. The claims manager may not be the programmer or the in-house computer wiz, but he or she is first in the line of communication. If the company has purchased software from an outside consultant, there may be reports already produced for the client that the case manager can use as a resource. There also may be an in-house capability to design almost any report the case manager might request. The extent of this capability varies from company to company and from line of insurance to line of insurance.

I sometimes ask to look at a run of workers' compensation cases in which the employee is still on salary replacement after 3 months, for example, regardless of the injury. Then I often note the amount of dollars that have been spent. If there is an explanation for big dollars spent, everything is fine. It is understandable that someone with a serious injury will be out of work a long time and will have high medical bills. On the other hand, if someone has only claimed a few hundred dollars in workers' compensation medical benefits yet is still off after 3 months, I want to know what is really going on. So, sometimes low dollars can be an indicator. Is the person really being treated? Is the person just sitting out there waiting for someone to say, "Hey, go back to work"?

In group medical coverage, a case manager can ask for a run of all claimants with three or more hospitalizations in a calendar year, all claimants with multiple medical procedures, or all claimants with home health services in place. The marker or specific limit might be a claims total of $50,000 or more (or $25,000 or $15,000). It doesn't take several years for some claimants to reach the $75,000 level; costs of this nature can add up within 1 or 2 months, and these cases would be among the ones called up for review.

TRACKING CLAIMS BY GROUP

The real key to consulting in case management is demonstrating to a client that only a small percentage of any employee group is responsible for generating the majority of claims and the bulk of benefit payouts. A case manager cannot attend a client conference, announce this fact, and expect the client to jump on the case management bandwagon. The case manager must be prepared to present concrete and objective information and offer a way to identify the relevant cases and improve the overall claims experience for the entire group. Nothing speaks louder to a client than a report taken from its own group experience. With a claims run, the case manager can show that out of a group of 500, with total claims paid of $200,000, fewer than 20 individuals (4%) filed claims totaling 80% ($160,000) of that sum. And nothing positions a case manager better than to work with a client as part of a team dedicated to helping better the claims experience.

With documentation, the case manager works with the claims department or Third Party Administrator to sell case management to the employer group. Because corporations often assume case managers work on all cases, it is important to emphasize that they focus on just a few; not everyone can benefit from case management. It is also appropriate to remind CEOs that case management is not a punitive investigative process, but a service whose purpose is to recognize and resolve healthcare delivery problems.

A computer run can be conducted to include all individuals covered by a policy. Perhaps a case manager is working with a company on its workers' compensation coverage. The first step is to define a benchmark, a worst-case marker, to find the cases in need of case management intervention. The class picked out might include those who have been out of work for 2 months or longer or those who had a lost-time accident resulting in a year or more of disability leave. (Employers with workers' compensation coverage pay medical as well as lost-wage expenses, so long absences are a big issue for them.) If there are no year-long cases, the case manager searches for absences lasting 9 or 6 months. To create a report, the case manager needs to work with the total number of covered lives, the number of individuals with major claims, and the kinds of injuries typical of the group. Are the injuries often catastrophic, such as traumatic brain injuries, or are they mostly unresolved back injuries? Using the data from a computer run, the case manager can determine that indeed 5% of the workers' compensation cases accounted for 83% of the claims dollars and that the majority of the individuals filed claims for complex, unresolved back injuries.

Figure 11–2 is a group claims run, a "hospital claims register," that includes all claims for hospital admissions. This run was requested as a

Figure 11–2 Hospital Claims Register.

Cert #	Rel	Claim #	Type	Days	Incur	Paid	Charges
11355	4	1025022919	I/P	4	02/01/12	02/04/05	5,137.66
42093	4	1026501411	I/P	6	02/02/09	02/04/05	4,484.93
62164	4	1023703222	I/P	4	02/01/16	02/04/05	4,101.34
36014	4	1024502223	I/P	12	02/01/14	02/04/05	2,827.41
36014	4	1026602508	I/P	4	02/02/10	02/04/05	5,021.73
47794	4	1023021212	I/P	4	01/12/31	02/04/05	2,840.07
91247	4	1026502210	O/P	1	01/12/18	02/04/05	829.58
92247	4	1026502211	O/P	1	01/12/12	02/04/05	101.02
42376	4	1026602617	I/P	3	01/12/29	02/04/05	3,372.96
60170	4	1022021123	I/P	3	02/01/07	02/04/05	3,492.97
02136	4	1025701314	I/P	2	01/12/19	02/04/05	1,530.28
02136	4	1026502028	I/P	21	02/01/17	02/04/05	3,845.77
81182	6	1027202404	O/P	1	02/01/14	02/04/05	236.60
39464	1	1024501916	I/P	6	02/01/21	02/04/05	3,033.81
52052	5	1024402713	I/P	2	02/01/18	02/04/05	2,580.59
67116	4	1022020309	I/P	6	01/12/28	02/04/05	3,840.88
01212	5	1024502323	I/P	3	02/01/22	02/04/05	1,914.24
11093	4	1024402712	I/P	4	02/01/28	02/04/05	2,206.92
62129	4	1025021223	O/P	1	02/01/21	02/04/05	367.02
74120	5	1025802404	I/P	7	02/02/05	02/04/05	2,922.12

Figure 11–2 continued

Cert #	Rel	Claim #	Type	Days	Incur	Paid	Charges
23269	5	1024402202	I/P	2	02/01/26	02/04/05	1,705.08
88196	5	1025802408	I/P	5	02/02/06	02/04/05	2,063.55
67198	1	1026601017	O/P	1	02/02/10	02/04/05	185.02
43282	1	1027302218	I/P	2	02/01/10	02/04/05	5,085.52
08551	5	1026601523	O/P	1	02/01/05	02/04/05	261.53
06055	6	1026701502	I/P	3	02/02/18	02/04/05	1,645.75
06055	4	1026701504	I/P	3	02/02/18	02/04/05	3,110.40
11038	6	1027302508	I/P	3	01/12/20	02/04/05	1,352.50
46230	4	1026701402	I/P	3	02/02/08	02/04/05	2,181.82
41144	5	1027202102	I/P	3	02/02/15	02/04/05	4,366.21
02812	4	1027101011	I/P	4	02/02/09	02/04/05	4,355.95
06326	4	1028102021	I/P	2	02/02/26	02/04/05	1,763.56
21139	1	1024502309	I/P	11	02/01/11	02/04/05	19,462.06
64552	4	1026602517	I/P	5	02/01/08	02/04/05	12,848.09
30252	4	1026602519	I/P	5	02/01/19	02/04/05	6,102.62
52232	1	1025021124	O/P	1	02/01/12	02/04/05	1,011.10
10102	5	1026602812	I/P	3	01/12/10	02/04/05	2,103.41
10301	6	1023703010	I/P	2	02/01/16	02/04/05	1,852.32
64984	1	1024402705	I/P	5	02/01/15	02/04/05	3,270.81
88292	1	1027302406	O/P	1	02/02/15	02/04/05	78.02
10283	4	1025021714	I/P	5	02/01/10	02/04/05	3,075.54
Month Total							132,568.76

Source: Courtesy of Options Unlimited, Case Management Services Division, © 2003, Huntington, New York.

means of focusing on those patients in need of case management intervention; a broad net (all hospital admissions) was used for the first cast. Such a run could also be conducted using length-of-stay data. The computer run could then be narrowed and patients be better targeted by adding a specific limit (e.g., hospital admission stays of 10 days or more only).

Figure 11–3 is a report generated from a group run. This type of quarter evaluation report breaks out the high-cost cases over a calendar or fiscal

Figure 11–3 Quarter Evaluation.

Medical Claims—ABC Corporation - April   843 Employees—2,213 covered lives

Claim Number	Amt. of Claim	Diagnosis
0421160	$3,800	OBS-GYN
0743221	2,100	Deceased—in C.M., ovarian cancer
(W) 1501617	4,028	Psych—ALC
(H) 2214689	3,615	Anthroscopy
1821041	6,437	OK
1847756	4,100	OBS
1523314	4,580	Vasc. dis., diab. in C.M.
1015252	1,800	OK
5830764	3,958	Fx nose
0962140	9,200	HIP, CVA in C.M.
	$43,618	

Total claims: $129,575

1% of group generated 34% of claims

Medical Claims—ABC Corporation - May   858 Employees—2,262 covered lives

Claim Number	Amt. of Claim	Diagnosis
(M) 1356602	$ 2,732	
(W&D) 1516758	5,008	
(M) 2083312	25,571	
(M&S) 4373029	1,881	
(M&W) 0917462	4,923	
(M) 1503327	3,100	
(M) 2543178	1,644	
2594622	1,522	
1296654	7,521	Referred to case management but pt. declined
3601744	2,320	
3237161	1,500	
5237708	1,646	
*1523318	3,918	
(D) 3541006	25,073	We have in C.M.
(M) 0929763	7,770	
*(M) 0962143	1,800	
	$97,929	

Total claims: $146,800

16 employees (2%) generated $97,929, or 67% of total

*Also in April report.

Figure 11–3 continued

Medical Claims—ABC Corporation - June   864 Employees—2,291 covered lives

Claim Number	Amt. of Claim
(S) 0543112	$6,417
(W) 0677896	2,324
** (M) 1371818	3,907
(M) 5221021	1,459
(M) 1147786	17,103
** (W-Heidi) 2594638	2,914
(M) 1821053	3,451
** (M) 1296685	2,675
Miller, M. (M) 1703217	1,690
** (W&S) 1814437	3,085
(W&D) 1516992	4,682
** (W) 5237718	7,525
*** (M) 1523319	1,452
** (D) 3541008	14,632
(M) 3202772	2,050
(M) 2567131	4,328
*** (M) 0962144	50,737
(W) 5818753	2,280
(M) 2501763	5,692
	$138,403

Total claims—$188,704
*In April report
**In May report
***In April, May & June
Note: W = wife; H = husband; M = member; D = dependent; S = spouse
19 employees (2% of group) expend $138,403, or 73% of total
3 employees, .3% expend 44% of total

ABC Corporation - 2nd quarter

		Employees	Covered Lives
April	$129,575	843	2,213
May	$146,800	858	2,262
June	$188,704	864	2,291
TOTAL	$465,079		

34 Employees (4% of group) expend $280,121, or 60% of total.

Source: Courtesy of Options Unlimited, Case Management Services Division, © 2003, Huntington, New York.

quarter and can be used to demonstrate that only a handful of claimants need case management intervention. If these few cases are properly managed, the whole group benefits from lower claims costs. In April, 1% of the group generated 34% of the claims; and in May, 2% generated 67% of the total. In June, 2% of the group was responsible for 73% of the benefit dollars paid, and .3 percent (three employees) actually accounted for 44% of the total. This run also tracked cases that continued to require costly care from one month to the next. It clearly shows the need for case management.

Regardless of the reimbursement system or type of policy, once the case manager has identified a group of patients that could benefit from case management intervention, the focus turns toward setting up a preventive cost-containment program to reform the group as a whole. After intervening at an early stage in the treatment of a complex, unresolved back injury, for example, the case manager, by pointing to the improved outcome, shortened time, and reduced cost, can gain the confidence of the claims department.

TRACKING CLAIMS BY INDIVIDUAL CLAIMS HISTORIES

A case manager can also track individual claims histories. In particular, she may want to look at the claims histories of the few individuals responsible for the bulk of the claims for a given period.

In looking at a particular claims history, the case manager may first identify the dollar amount and then fine-tune the review to see if this is a case in which case management could make a difference. Suppose the individual has reached the specific limit of $75,000. The case manager might note that the claims were for one hospitalization and one major surgical procedure, a colostomy. The procedure is completed, there were only minor post-op problems, so there is no real opportunity for case management to have an impact. Another individual who has reached the $75,000 specific limit may have a series of claims for treatment of an unresolved ulcer of the foot, diabetes, hypertension, and vascular disease. Taken together, these claims indicate a healthcare time bomb. What is the real problem here? Why isn't the ulcer resolving? Is this person getting appropriate care?

Figure 11–4 presents an excerpt from an individual claims report. This report, which breaks out the claims history by ICD-9 and CPT codes, was requested because a set dollar limit had been reached. The question was, what were the charges for? By checking each diagnosis, it was discovered that the medical problems ranged from a stroke to respiratory

Figure 11–4 Subscriber History File Accessing Report.

Worksheet Inquiry

Group   930656 Hampshire Cty (Actv/Ret/COBRA)
Enrollee   e123-45-6789
Member   e123-45-6789
Enter latest incurred to date   _____

Claim no.	Statuses	Incurred dates	Benefit	Diagnosis
e 94009618-01	f f	01/11–01/11	M1	CVA/EQU/ACERMAN MED SUPPLY
e 93051425-11	f f	08/11–12/31	M0	93¢RX/X-8 FARMING, FPO PHARM.
e 93099250-02	f f	12/01–12/31	M0	RB/MS/ATLANTIC REHAB/CVA
e 93086701-13	f f	12/22–12/29	M0	CVA/PTHD/ROCHE LAB
e 93086701-12	f f	11/29–12/21	M0	CVA/PTHD/ROCHE LAB
e 94004825-01	f f	12/20–12/20	M1	GI TRACT DIS/ERH/ KIMBALL MC
e 94004825-02	f f	12/20–12/20	M1	GI TRACT DIS/ INEL 12/KIMB PHY
e 93086701-14	f f	12/01–12/15	M0	CVA/PTHD/ROCHE LAB
e 94001820-01	h	12/05–12/05	M0	TRACHEST/ERH/ KIMBALL MED CT
e 94001820-02	h	12/05–12/05	M0	TRACHEST/ERD/ KIMBALL EMERDR
e 94001820-03	f f	11/16–12/05	M0	TRACHEST/VARIOUS PV'S
e 94001820-04	f f	12/05–12/05	M0	TRACH/INEL#12/MOOSA JAFFARI,M
e 93086701-15	f f	12/01–12/01	M0	CVA/XRAY/JERSEY SHR MC
e 93086701-09	f f	11/30–11/30	M0	HEMIPLEGIA/INEL#69/ JERSEY SHORE
e 93099250-01	h	11/26–11/30	M0	RB/MS/ATLANTIC REHAB/CVA
e 93086701-08	f f	11/22–11/26	M0	HEMIPLEGIA/PVIM/AHN
e 93086701-10	f f	11/04–11/26	M0	RB/MS/RUSK INST/ HEMIPLEGIA
e 94004825-04	f f	11/02–11/26	MI	GI TRACT/XRYD/JERSEY SHORE R
e 93086701-16	h	11/25–11/25	M0	CVA/CON/LOUIE MD

continues

Figure 11–4 continued

Claim no.	Statuses	Incurred dates	Benefit	Diagnosis
e 93067106-72	f f	10/07–11/24	M0	VASCULAR/RDO/ NYU RADIOLOGY
e 93086701-11	f f	11/23–11/23	M0	ABDOM PAIN/ SRI/PTI/ASHA MD
e 93094583-02	f f	10/11–11/22	M0	DEPRESS/MPVO/ OLLINS, MD
e 93086701-07	f f	11/08–11/19	M0	HEMIPLEGIA/PVI/ AHN, MD
e 93091059-02	f f	11/16–11/18	M0	CHOLELITH/PVI/ PFEFFER, MD
e 94004825-03	f f	11/12–11/12	MI	GI TRACT DIS/PVO/ PARRY, MD
e 93094583-01	f f	11/02–11/11	M0	DEPRESS/MPVI/ FRANK, MD

Enter worksheet to inquire into (r)estart or (c)ontinue Alt-Z=Help COM1 9600 8N1
VT102

Source: Courtesy of Options Unlimited, Case Management Services Division, © 2003, Huntington, New York.

and vascular difficulties to depression. By reading this history, the case manager is in a much better position to provide assistance.

Another step in the case management consultation process is to review the actual claims in particular files. (Access to files might be possible if the case manager and claims manager have a good relationship.) A computer provides just so much information: coding information, dollars, and where the money was spent. By looking at an actual file, the case manager might discover that the patient is on several medications, each prescribed by a different physician. Are the physicians aware of one another and of the other medications the patient is taking? Admissions and complications can be caused by interactions between medications. Perhaps the patient is having difficulty describing his or her symptoms or understanding the prescribed treatments and is consequently going from physician to physician. This is the type of case in which the case manager might be able to make a major contribution.

Although helpful information is usually plentiful, a case manager has to know exactly what data are available and how they can be used to help patients, providers, and payers. The claims department should ideally perceive case managers as a tool to better their service, whereas case managers use the tools of the claims department to help them resolve some case management problems.

MOVING INTO THE CONSULTANT ROLE

I have had terrific opportunities to put these theories into practice in my associations with Third Party Administrators. As a consultant, I help Third Party Administrators track claims and increase the efficiency of their administration services. We have become a value-added service in ourselves, and are now part of the Third Party Administrator's marketing strategy in reaching new clients.

My development and use of claims tracking reports and computer runs was motivated by my frustration at not being able to reach claimants who needed case management in time to make a difference. After convincing the TPA president to allow my company's staff to show how case management can resolve problems and reduce payouts, we were given access to the Third Party Administrator's claims staff and began training them in case management concepts and delineating the kinds of cases we wanted to see. I created red flags and the claims review tip sheet shown in Figure 11–1 as well as a "Request for Service" form (Figure 11–5). The claims personnel were to fill out this request form and leave it in my in-box whenever they came across a claim fitting the red flag profile or had a question concerning a case's suitability for case management or claims review. (I made it a practice to be in the Third Party Administrator's office once a week to review these requests and to be available to the claims staff as an associate and assistant.) Figure 11–6 is a form we designed for TPAs to use when they have a question or a claim to review on a case now in case management, or when they question a possible reentry into case management for a case that has been in the program.

When a case is referred to us for case management or claims review, a letter similar to the one appearing as Table 11–1 is sent to thank the claims examiner and to give him or her the name of the case manager assigned to the case. This promotes a more open and communicative association.

How did we convince the Third Party Administrator's president of the benefits of case management? We selected our trial group by requesting a quarterly report with a specific limit run of $100,000. (This was the stop-loss insurance benchmark for one of the Third Party Administrator's client companies.) When preparing a "mock" report like this to explain the value of case management, I've found it makes a deeper impression if we use the client's own cases and actual dollars spent to show the potential savings when case management is applied.

Figure 11–5 Request for Service Form.

ΟΡΤΙΟΝS
UNLIMITED
HEALTH CARE & DISABILITY MANAGEMENT SERVICES
76 East Main Street, Huntington, New York 11743
(631) 673-1150 FAX (631) 673-8369

	DATE

------------ REQUESTED BY: --

NAME	PHONE	YOUR FILE # (SS #)
COMPANY NAME	LOCATION	INSURED
CLAIMANT		INSURANCE COVERAGE & STATE
DATE OF DIS.	DIAGNOSIS	EMPLOYER GROUP

REQUEST FOR

PLEASE CHECK ONE
❑ CareWatch - UTILIZATION REVIEW: PREDETERMINATION, PRE-ADMISSION, CONCURRENT
          REVIEW, IDENTIFICATION FOR CASE MANAGEMENT, SPECIFIC LIMIT REVIEW
❑ CareSolutions - MEDICAL CASE MANAGEMENT
❑ CompSolutions - WORKER'S COMPENSATION
❑ AccuClaim - CLAIMS REVIEW
❑ Other Questions _____

IF NECESSARY, HAVE YOU INCLUDED:
❑ PRE-AND POST-OP PHOTOS   ❑ MD/PT OR CHIRO OFFICE NOTES (ATTACHED)
❑ OPERATIVE REPORT (ATTACHED)   ❑ R&C CHARGES (LIST HERE):
❑ ANESTHESIA REPORT (ATTACHED)   CPT CODE   R&C CHARGE
❑ ITEMIZED BILLING   _____
❑ NURSING NOTES (ATTACHED)   _____
                                          _____

CONSULTANT RESPONSE

SAVINGS:
SIGNATURE: DATE:

Send Original and one copy to   REFERRAL SOURCE COPY - YELLOW
                                 OPTIONS UNLIMITED COPY - WHITE

Source: Courtesy of Options Unlimited, Case Management Services Division, © 2003, Huntington, New York.

Figure 11–6 TPA Claims Review Sheet.

OPTIONS UNLIMITED CLAIMS REVIEW SHEET
FOR

Date: _____   Claims Examiner: _____
                        (Last, first name, ext:)
                        _____

Employer Group: _____   Network: _____

Insured: _____   Please check one:
                           ☐ CareWatch - To Identify Case Mgmt.
Patient: _____   ☐ CareSolutions-Case Mgmt.
                           ☐ AccuClaim-Claims Review
S.S.#: _____

Address: _____   City: _____   St. _____   Zip: _____

Provider In or Out-of-Network: _____   Is this an appeal?   Yes   No
How much was paid on claim? _____

Please Circle:
Reason claim is being reviewed: Chiro PT - Surgery - Pre-Determination - Dental - Cosmetic
HHC/Nursing - Worker's Compensation - Coverage/issue - Podiatry - Diagnostic - Other

If Any: Please include: Pre- and Post-op Photos - Operative Report - MD/PT or Chiro Notes/Itemized
                         Billing/Other

CPT CODE	AMOUNT CHARGED	R&C	REPRICED AMOUNT

Is there a co-pay? Y N   How much? _____   Deductible Remaining: _____
What would the claim normally be paid at: 70% 80% 90% 100% Other: _____
Has the deductible been satisfied? Y N

Questions/Comments for Reviewer:

Source: Courtesy of Options Unlimited, Case Management Services Division, © 2003, Huntington, New York.

Table 11–1 Claims Contact Letter

Date

Ms. Sue Ying, Claims Examiner
Third Party Administrator
One Chamber Plaza, Suite 1413
Cheyenne, WY 82001

Claimant: John Doe
Insured: Susan Doe
Group: Seventy-Seven Slides
S.S.#: 999-99-9999

Dear Claims Examiner:

Please accept my appreciation for referring the above captioned file for case management services.

_____ [Case Manager] will be handling this case. She will conduct an initial evaluation and will contact you with a verbal report to be followed by a complete written report with our impressions and recommendations.

Should you have any questions about this file, please don't hesitate to call me at (516) 555-5555.

Very truly yours,

President

KB:cs

Source: Courtesy of Options Unlimited, Case Management Services Division, © 2003, Huntington, New York.

We as case managers were looking for all claims over $25,000, which is our company's own marker. We looked at every month to see whether the total number of cases over $10,000 increased and if the same individuals were consistently filing the larger claims. Once we identified several cases, we asked to see the actual claims files. In one instance, we found that the claimant had run up a claims total of $30,000, most of it in pharmaceuticals. There were pages and pages of claims on file for drugs prescribed by different physicians. Reviewing the prescriptions, we searched for drugs recommended for the same or related conditions, side effects, drug interactions, and drug combinations, and we also tried to determine whether the drug combinations were contributing to the patient's medical problems. In this case, we found there was reason to be concerned for the patient's safety. Because the Third Party Administrator fully supported our endeavor, we contacted the individual and his physicians to share our concern, finding that the physicians were unaware of each other and the prescription "overdose." We were then able to establish one primary physician who acted as the sole dispenser of medication. The example proved a perfect one for showing the benefits of case management to both patients and the bottom line.

In another instance, we saw a total of $50,000, but what really caught our eye were the three inpatient hospitalizations. Dollars are a case management indicator, but the truly important factor is always going to be how those dollars are spent. What is driving expenses up? Did these three admissions occur over a long period of time, or were they a series of closely spaced, short-stay admissions? When I see three or four admissions within a short time period, I wonder whether there is something wrong with the discharge plan or whether the individual cannot sustain the level of stability at the time of discharge once he or she reaches home.

Case managers working with claims departments become detectives. Using curiosity, instinct, and a paper trail, they look for items to uncover potentially serious cases. Obviously, the more experienced the entire team, the better they are at following the paper trail. But any case manager and any group of claims personnel can make a difference, a major difference, for their clients and the covered patients.

Part III

Case Management Administration and Outcomes Management

Chapter 12

Financial and Quality Assurance Reporting

Everyone flinches at the very sound of the words "the cost of healthcare." Not far behind the direct costs are the administrative or management expenses that are impacting all of us as we attempt to brake this "running train." While we individually and collectively grapple with these fees, those of us providing or managing case management services need to realize that our interventions are an addition to an already costly system. Cost of care is an issue that has to be faced head on. Case managers need to deal with the financial ramifications of care and alternatives. To make recommendations for care that the benefits dollars will not cover is ridiculous, and to not know how costly one facility is in comparison with another is not doing one's job.

If a case manager is going to put together a set of recommendations or alternatives, she needs to cite costs. Further, the case manager needs to involve the patient, family, physician, and other members of the healthcare team in financial matters. I think we have all been insulated from financial concerns for far too long. At some point early on, it is essential to sit down with paper and pencil and a family and say, "If your dad has three more hospitalizations at $1,500 per day, this is how quickly his benefits are going to be eaten up. If we can keep him out of the hospital longer and put services in the home, if you'll be willing to help with some of the care as well, we can get him care and services over the projected length of this illness, which is certainly what our goal needs to be here. We don't want to run out of benefits before he runs out of problems."

Although it would be nice if all consumers and healthcare professionals perceived the medical and monetary value of case management, unfortunately not everyone does. To avoid being seen as merely part of the "medical-insurance bureaucracy," case managers need to play an active role in communicating the benefits, in health management and dollar terms, of their services. Because most case managers come from nursing or social work backgrounds, they tend to resist talking about the financial aspects of healthcare.

DOLLARS AND HEALTHCARE

The majority of healthcare professionals today probably entered the field with a desire to help others. We were the actual hands-on providers of the services deemed necessary. No one questioned our motivation, methods, or outcomes. We were acknowledged as professionals and were generally assumed to adhere to the strictest of practice standards and to want only the best for our patients. But then money got in the way, and healthcare professionals were called upon to balance treatment and cost. Why healthcare costs became so unmanageable will, I suspect, be left to historians. In any case, there are now so many interest groups that sorting out truth from fiction will perhaps be an insurmountable task. Clearly, the healthcare system is undergoing profound changes. The system many of us trained in is a thing of the past. Cost is an issue for all of us, consumers (employers and employees) and healthcare professionals alike. And because cost is an issue, the transition for healthcare professionals continues to be a struggle. Why is it such a problem?

To develop a better understanding of the current situation, it may help to examine the healthcare system of yesterday. Those who entered medical and related fields had much in common. They shared, among other things, a desire to help, a need to contribute, and a willingness to comfort and counsel others in distress. They did not share, by and large, an interest in or talent for financial management. In fact, most healthcare businesses or practice settings have someone other than the physician, nurse, or therapist keeping the books. It was generally accepted that if medical professionals did have responsibility for financial matters, it might influence their decisions and cloud their perceptions of what was best for their patients. For many, many years, it was considered perfectly all right to protect professionals from having to deal with money issues.

Add to this society's idealized view of medicine and healthcare and its tendency not to question healthcare costs. Interestingly, we demand to know the price of almost everything, from houses to cars to airfare to hotel rooms and college tuition. Some of these items, when advertised, have their price tags clearly visible. Other items, such as designer clothing or jewelry, have their price tags more discreetly placed, but the prices are still discoverable through a little effort. This is not the case with healthcare services, undeniably among the most expensive commodities.

When was the last time you saw a price tag on an MRI (magnetic resonance imaging), saw, or were quoted, the fee for a specific surgical procedure, or chose Hospital A or Hospital B because the service was equal but one was more reasonably priced? Although most of us are facing higher deductibles and co-payments, we are still not asking the dreaded question, "How much will this cost?"

For example, imagine someone who needs surgery. The medical plan providing benefits reimburses at 80% of the reasonable and customary charge for the procedure. The surgeon selected has quoted a price of $9,200; the plan has established that the reasonable and customary fee is $7,500; the reimbursement, at 80% of $7,500, is $6,000; and the remaining balance is $3,200. Quite clearly, the time to resolve the discrepancy between the price and the payout is before the surgery takes place, not after. What can be done? The person can choose another qualified surgeon who charges less; discuss the matter with the current surgeon, who might be willing to negotiate or reduce the fees; or decide to proceed with the current surgeon despite the additional costs. But at least the decision will be an informed one, with all results and consequences evident.

When I hear providers criticizing case managers for "talking about money" and "asking prices," I realize they may resent having to compete and having to defend their prices. The old days of automatic acceptance of charges are gone forever. And this really is better for all of us. Medical professionals are intelligent consumers, and they do know how to make decisions that benefit their patients while preserving valuable medical resources.

The merger/acquisition activity among providers has created somewhat of a monopoly in healthcare, with the advantage to make more money weighted to the providers. Hospitals and specialists are following the direction of pharmaceutical coverage, offering boutique and "concierge" service in several tiers of healthcare packages. These out-of-network examinations and follow-up are for those patients who can and will pay a higher price. Case managers can look into such high-end marketplaces. The "sandwich generation," caring for their children and parents at the same time, needs elder case management, too.

Case management does become involved not only with the outcomes of care, but also with the many alternative levels of care and with the financial aspects of care. In fact, to address quality and outcomes and the alternatives without paying attention to the costs is doing a disservice to patients, payers, and, yes, even providers, who will also be losers if costs go unchecked.

Because of its role in cost containment, case management focuses on catastrophically ill patients (acute and chronic) and high-cost cases, as well as those predicted to be, for example, disease management cases. As defined and practiced, it addresses costs, but never at the expense of patient safety or quality of care. If case managers do not communicate both its cost-containment benefits and its quality-improvement benefits, case management could well become eliminated as a tool in the treatment of patients.

There are many experienced case managers who initially worked hard to demonstrate their effectiveness to their client companies. After their clients became believers, the case managers no longer felt the need to push the potential benefits. Case management departments were created, staffed, and supplied with computers and other equipment by major insurance carriers and Third Party Administrators, and hundreds and thousands of dollars were spent, month after month, until another someone at the senior level closely examined the figures. Then, questions were asked: "What does this department do?" "Is it making us any money?" "Does it save us or our clients any money, and if so, how much?" There were no answers because the case managers had stopped documenting their efficacy.

Discussion of fees and costs should be part of any case management program. Financial issues need to be examined and debated before a company implements such a program or contracts with a case management provider, or before a professional decides to be a provider of case management services. There must be an acceptance of financial accountability for the costs being added to the system. Individuals or departments who are not able to demonstrate cost-effectiveness will not survive, and their demise will be their own doing.

So, how do case managers prepare information or reports that will support continued case management involvement? How can they consider or suggest alternative care plans if they do not know the costs involved in the current system of care? How should the subject of costs be approached? What questions need to be asked and to whom should they be directed? Are prices negotiable? Should discounts be requested? How do case managers know what is reasonably priced and, at the other end, what is an exorbitant fee? Does cost have anything to do with quality or outcome? Just as with other products and services, it is best to be prepared with information beforehand. How is this information acquired? By acknowledging that the whole subject of healthcare costs is uncomfortable, especially for practitioners, and by asking questions over and over to compile provider cost-of-service lists.

There are several ways to obtain pricing information while learning about a company and its services. One of the easiest is to attend local, regional, and national conferences. Most conferences include provider exhibits as well as sessions conducted by provider companies. Such sessions offer marketing and educational opportunities for those who might either have influence on or direct purchasing capabilities. For example, a firm might present a session titled "Respiratory Management of the HIV Patient at Home." Although the information may be generic, the presenters are typically available afterward to provide specifics regarding the credentialing of staff, the accreditation of the firm, the location of its offices, the scope of its services, plus all of the other "need to know" information, such as "How much will this cost? Are there additional considerations for all-inclusive, for prompt-pay, for volume, for exclusive, or for PPO arrangements?" (And are these questions not the same kinds of questions we all ask before making other kinds of purchases? Is anything here "unprofessional"?) Most providers have ranges of fees and negotiating options and are better prepared today than 10 years ago to discuss fees. So go ahead, ask.

The larger the conference or the more diversified the subject matter, the more opportunity there is to meet with multiple providers of a wide range of products and services. A conference titled "The Rehabilitation of the Alcoholic Adolescent" will include presentations on topics of interest, such as "Peer Pressure," "Tough Love," or "Family Dynamics." Further, the exhibit hall is likely to feature providers such as inpatient programs, day treatment centers, and residential long-term centers, all utilized in the care of the alcoholic adolescent. If teenage rehabilitation is going to be a strong component of one's practice or department focus, this is an important conference to attend. On the other hand, a conference titled "Managed Care: Healthcare Reform and Self-Insured Groups" will provide the opportunity to acquire an incredible amount of information in one setting. Featured will likely be HMOs, PPOs, home care agencies, rehabilitation facilities, head injury programs, pharmaceutical companies, equipment manufacturers and dealers, hospitals, computer software and hardware companies, consulting firms, infusion care services, and so on. This type of conference offers a nonstressful environment in which to learn about the whole range of services and providers available to case managers and, equally important, to begin discussions about costs. (One way of mitigating some of the anxiety caused by having to discuss fees and other costs is to examine the decision-making process for other purchases and then apply some of the same skills and methods to purchase agreements for healthcare services. This is a very concrete way to demystify some of the fear that has crept into this arena. I believe that this transition is possible if one approaches it in increments of time and information. In the process, our decisions will not only be safe and quality-assuring ones, but will also be cost-conscious and cost-effective.)

When the necessary cost information is acquired, what should be done with it? For the small company or independent practitioner, perhaps keeping a separate "provider book" will be sufficient. Dividing the book into sections by provider type or service or location allows easy access to the data. For instance, under "Infusion Care Services" should be listed companies that are quality providers; their strengths, weaknesses, and areas of expertise; special offerings that are of particular interest; and the costs of the services. Other categories might be high-risk pregnancy management, home care, subacute hospitals, durable medical equipment dealers, and so on. The information should be updated continually, eliminating providers that are no longer viable, adding new services, and changing contact names or the location of offices. Provider information needs to be current so that the time spent selecting providers and services is kept to a minimum.

In a larger organization or case management department, serious consideration should be given to putting such information in a computer database. Each case manager would then have access to it and would be able to update and change it according to departmental guidelines, obviously adhering to provider selection criteria applicable to that particular area. The accumulated information would not only be useful in actual case management activities, but could also serve as the database for cost-benefit analysis reports (discussed later in this chapter).

In addition to conferences, there are several other resources that can be utilized in developing provider information: government organizations and publications, travel and professional associations, and periodicals that publish data on costs and trends. Publications such as *Business & Health* (now online at businessandhealth.com), *Business Insurance*, *The Wall Street Journal*, *Medical Economics*, and *The Case Manager* frequently list costs of hospitals per day, average lengths of stay, fees for procedures, and high-cost organizations. They also sometimes publish lists of rehabilitation facilities, skilled nursing facilities, and other types of organizations and evaluate rates, services, and so on. *Newsweek* and *Time* run special issues on healthcare as a whole and often examine a disease state in-depth.

NEGOTIATING SKILLS

Once armed with information about services and fees, a case manager is better able to arrange for services and negotiate fees. Negotiating is an acquired skill and does require thought, and there are books written on the subject and guidelines developed especially for case managers (see Table 12–1 for a list of gender-related communication problems). William Ury, cofounder of the Program on Negotiations at Harvard Law School, has written two of the definitive books on negotiation: *Getting to Yes: Negotiating Agreement Without Giving In* (Houghton Mifflin Company and Penguin Books editions) and *Getting Past No: Negotiating with Difficult People* (Bantam Books). *Getting to Yes* is also available in a video workshop format. National conferences almost always have a session or more devoted to negotiating skills. The newsletter *Case Management Advisor* as well as journals *Harvard Business Review* and *Continuing Care* frequently incorporate tips for case managers.

The first thing to keep in mind in negotiating is that there are ranges in price for everything in healthcare. This does not mean that we aim for the least expensive category or that selecting a "Rolls Royce" price tag guarantees excellence—high price tags only guarantee a big bill. The goal is to try to fulfill the patient's equipment and service needs in a cost-justified manner.

The first roadblock case managers and product or service suppliers commonly confront is the difference in background, orientation, and industry jargon each party brings to the negotiations. For example, a home medical equipment supplier may be well-versed in the features and functions of the equipment, but may not understand why certain models are problematic or inappropriate for a patient. The case manager knows the patient's diagnosis and needs, but is not necessarily familiar with the technical capabilities of equipment. To overcome this and other snags, it is best to take an honest and open approach to communications.

I have found it helpful to work exclusively with one representative at a durable medical equipment, home medical equipment, or home health-care agency. First, this allows me to review equipment, services, contracts, and billing in a single call, and, second, it helps me get answers when I need them. Just as I want to know all the options included with a piece of equipment that might assist a patient, I am also interested in terms— lease, rent, rent with option to buy, and outright purchase and service costs. The various options often affect my decision.

Case managers and product and service providers alike are looking for long-term working relationships. An otherwise good relationship will be undermined if the case manager accepts a price break on a 1-year rental agreement knowing the patient probably has only 3 months to live or if the agreed-upon equipment arrives with expensive optional features that were sold to the patient without the case manager's knowledge. In their pursuit of high-quality healthcare at an affordable cost, both providers

Table 12–1 Common Female-to-Male Communication Obstacles and Solutions

---

Problem: Women tend to take too long to get to the point, using too many details.

Solution: State your main point up front, using few details. Be brief and precise.

Problem: Women tend to use soft, tentative, unassertive voices, especially in talking to men.

Solution: Practice speaking in a firm, moderately loud, confident voice.

Problem: Women often allow themselves to be interrupted by men in conversation.

Solution: Try one or several of these: (1) Keep talking in a firm, louder voice.
(2) Stop in mid-sentence and wait in silence till the interrupter has stopped, (3) Say politely, "I'll be happy to continue when you're finished."

Problem: Women often end statements in a questioning tone of voice, with a rising inflection.

Solution: Speak in firm, declarative sentences that sound like clear statements, not tentative questions.

Problem: Women tend to seek consensus and agreement by ending sentences with "question tags," such as "don't you agree?" or "am I right?"

Solution: Drop most of those question tags from your speech, especially when talking to men.

Problem: Women tend to hedge in conversation instead of stating firm opinions.

Solution: Mentally define your message clearly, then state it assertively.

Problem: Women have learned to communicate in a way that builds friendship and agreement, while men are more action-oriented and directive.

Solution: Be aware of the differences in male-female communications styles and learn to match your communications style to men's when talking to them.

Problem: Women too often preface remarks by actually asking their listener not to take them seriously. ("This probably isn't a very good idea, but . . ." or "I don't know a lot about this; however . . .")

Solution: Never apologize or discount what you have to say. Believe in yourself and your statements and speak accordingly.

Source: Reprinted from *Medical Case Management Conference V,* p. 187, with permission of ICMA and Nancy N. Bell, © 1993.

---

and case managers can benefit by serving as resources for each other. Dealers can take the confusion out of techno-speak; case managers can alert suppliers that certain bed features are not recommended for people with a particular back problem. By working as partners with service and equipment providers, case managers can build beneficial business associations and stronger resource bases.

Negotiating is a specific form of educational communication. As Louis Feuer has noted, negotiation allows for an open discussion of issues at hand, enables all parties to freely discuss their objectives, and helps all parties understand the implications of the plan. The more we know, the better decisions we can make. Here is a synopsis of some of Feuer's suggestions for successful negotiations outcomes:[1]

1. Define the limits, including time limits on a contract and time relative to the patient's illness, financial resource limits, and medical resource limits.
2. Know your power—in personality, expertise, situation, and sharing of information. (I would add the flip side, know your limits.)
3. Be aware of hidden agendas—was a decision made before negotiations began?
4. Know when you will walk away—what is your bottomline?
5. Never take the first offer—go through the process.
6. Know that negotiations have stages: establish the criteria, exchange information, and then reach compromise.
7. If you reach an impasse, set aside that issue and concentrate on smaller issues to create a momentum of agreement that will carry you through the critical issue.
8. Be aware of changes in demeanor, in both you and your "opponent"—physical reactions, need to negotiate, more or less willing to negotiate.
9. Never assume that something will not work.

To assist case managers in establishing a negotiating process and evaluating service providers and facilities, two documents were developed: "Service, Equipment, and Supplies Placement Guidelines" (Table 12–2) and "Program Questionnaire and Facility Review for Case Managers" (see Appendix 12–A at the end of this chapter). These were designed to serve as standard tools for selecting providers and vendors and evaluating facilities, and they include criteria to facilitate the making of informed decisions based on the needs of the patient. The forms should be customized by the addition of the case manager's own criteria. Is there one person to contact for financial questions, or one contact for patient updates? This can save a lot of time otherwise spent playing telephone tag or holding on the

Table 12–2 Service, Equipment, and Supplies Placement Guidelines

1. Evaluate client to accurately determine his needs:
   - Personally assess client/family/home.
   - Review evaluations and recommendations of others—PT, OT, physician, etc.
   - Secure physician's order, if required.
   - Recommend or confirm the correct equipment supply or service.
2. Determine whether rent or purchase is more cost-effective. Consider:
   - Length of service
   - Availability and cost of service/maintenance contracts
   - Comparative costs of rent/purchase
3. Secure payer authorization (approval of claims professional).
4. Bid equipment, supplies, or service.
   - Requests for bids from providers must be uniform.
     —May be requested by phone (occasionally written)
     —Outline:
   - Specific item or service requested
   - Date to begin/deliver
   - Duration of service
   - Means and percent of payment from insurer
   - Date and time bid will be closed
   - Seek to determine the provider's
     —Ability to deliver service
     —Follow-up plan
     —Type of supervision
     —Teaching support
     —Reputation for dependability and quality of service
   - Request that providers convey bid figure by phone—with a written confirmation.
   - Vendors should be contacted once only with an accurate and identical description of the item/service needed. Failure to respond by bid closing time will constitute a "no bid."
   - Provided all key issues (service, delivery, and quality) are equal, the business is awarded to the lowest bidder. If not equal, the decision will be at the case manager's discretion/judgment and will be final.
   - Bid information may be available to participants only after the bid is awarded—and only at the case manager's discretion.
   - Providers should be requested not to actively market their equipment or services with case management clients, but rather to forward observations, suggestions, and recommendations to the case manager for consideration and coordination with the medical team and funding agency.

Table 12–2 continued

---

5. Follow-up to ensure:
   - Item (or service) is appropriate
   - Timely response or delivery is provided
   - Instructions are adequate
   - Service to equipment is available
   - Item (or service) is retained only as long as needed
6. Summarize bids (and logic behind choice if not lowest bidder), with attention to cost saved in report.

Source: Courtesy of Case Management Society of America, Little Rock, Arkansas.

---

line while someone who can answer a query is found. Does the vendor return phone calls? What is their level of service? All these elements play into the making of a good service match.

The following negotiating guidelines originally appeared in *HomeCare* under the title "Simple Negotiations." Although designed for home care providers, they are applicable to the types of negotiations in which case managers engage:[2]

1. For patients on long-term therapies, implement a reverification process.
2. Negotiate the payment terms. A good general rule is the deeper the discount offered, the sooner the provider should be paid.
3. Ask if a fax of the claim or other documentation can be sent to speed claims processing.
4. Always confirm verbal agreements in writing. Include in the confirmation letter the effective date of the agreement, the full name of the person who conducted the verbal negotiation, a complete description of the products and services agreed upon, the agreed-upon discount, the agreed-upon payment terms, the net payment after the discount, the agreed-upon type of claims submission form, and notification that the agreement will be considered mutual unless the supplier states otherwise in writing within a certain number of days.

I would add:

1. Remember to negotiate on a case-by-case basis. No two cases are alike, and no two negotiation processes will be alike. There are

always things you can bring to the table from your past experience. However, each payer and provider has his or her own feelings and concerns, and even these may vary from case to case.

2. Negotiating is a subtle art, and it is all about listening. First, you learn the real concern behind the words when you listen carefully and watch for body language, and second, the people you are working for want to know you are paying close attention to them.

3. Negotiations can get testy. Keep your mind on the overarching goal, and gently position conversations (that is, remind participants) so that all involved are pursuing the best solution for everyone concerned.

4. There is something to be said for using a "most favored nation" negotiating strategy if this is a provider you will be working with on a regular basis.

5. The opposite of that is to negotiate from a one-case basis: "This is a singular need. We are not going to be seeing 20 or 30 more patients in this situation. How can we make it work?"

NUANCES BETWEEN NEGOTIATING WITH PROVIDERS AND PAYERS

Case managers are in a different position and, therefore, employ varying strategies in discussions with payers as opposed to providers. When negotiating with a provider, such as a home care agency, the case manager most often is one healthcare professional talking to another, using similar terms supported by shared understanding. Further, it is assumed that the case manager has the authority to approve or decline the price quote given; if she is not the decision maker, she is certainly a strong influencer in the process. It is also assumed she has a wide variety of providers to access because of the number of quality providers available, although the range of price quotes she receives may or may not be as varied. She may have the time to choose among the various proposals. The gathering of information from providers helps make her a more effective negotiator.

Negotiating with a payer for approval requires a different tack, and tact. The case manager is no longer the decision maker. Whether it is an insurance carrier, self-funded employer, or a Third Party Administrator, the healthcare dollars and ultimately the decision are the payer's. The payer may not have the medical knowledge or expertise to know what it is the case manager seeks, and why. The payer negotiator might be a chief financial officer (CFO) or a human resource manager who is uncomfortable with the responsibility of making the healthcare decision. Case managers have to help them arrive at an understanding of the situation to enable them to feel good about making the decision, which requires skill. They are concerned with a number of issues. How long will this alternative care last? If I do it for this case, will I have to do it for all the others?

Perhaps the case manager wants to place a patient in a subacute facility; this particular payer has no language in its plan to cover such facilities and it is the first time the case manager is approaching the payer to consider the issue. The payer's first reaction might be, "We don't allow for subacute care." To help the payer better understand the case so she can negotiate more effectively, the case manager needs to educate the payer by listing the alternatives and the consequences of not approving the suggested facility in terms that are meaningful to the payer. This means illustrating that financially, approval of another level of care or a more appropriate center for care is in the payer's best interests.

I had a case in which I negotiated with a payer on behalf of a youth hospitalized with a traumatic brain injury. The boy was beginning to come out of his coma but had developed bed sores, pneumonia, and an infection. The payer's plan provided unlimited days of coverage for hospital care and the boy met its criteria to remain there; however, I knew if he did, he would deteriorate further. We hoped to take him to an out-of-state, long-term care facility that had the ability to wean him off the respirator and address his rehabilitation needs. There was no plan language for that type of facility. I had to show the plan that the acute care facility was well equipped to manage his initial trauma but lacked the range of resources to manage his optimum recovery. I introduced the human aspects of the decision. Yes, they had hospital coverage, but this young man's condition would definitely worsen there. He had already experienced far too many complications; I felt we would lose him if he remained hospitalized, and we wouldn't have anyone left to rehabilitate.

I negotiated by being very patient with that payer who had every right to say, "No, there's no language in the plan, and we're not doing it." I had to help them understand that this young man was being harmed by every extra day he was there, that we would have a much better chance of getting him out of any kind of center for care if we brought him to a facility that could more appropriately meet his needs. I explained that hospitals are not set up to do long-term rehabilitation care. I showed them in real dollars how much continued hospitalization was going to cost. If he stayed in the hospital and had a decubiti, and needed skin grafting, he would face more infection and IV antibiotic treatment, and this is what it will cost in dollars and cents. By the time we get him cleared from the skin graft and infections, he will have lost whatever gains he had made. He already had a number of physical problems to overcome. I suggested that the faster we could get him to a place with expertise in managing his complications and rehabilitation needs, the faster he would improve and heal.

If case managers encounter resistance, I encourage them again to "get behind the no." Identify the payer's concern and continue to address it. Help them understand that a case manager is looking out for their interests in terms of medical and financial risk. Payers often buttonhole nurses and social workers as employee advocates and may become concerned that we give equal thought to the employer's needs as well. The case manager must be able to take herself out of the patient advocate role and be a strong advocate for the payer group as well. She can make the decision-making process a little less overwhelming for them, showing the payer group she understands that this is new territory for them and that she respects their questions. Make the payer part of the process; report every 2 weeks on money actually saved and the patient's status, which is what our office did in the previously mentioned case.

Not every case is successful. We explained to one payer that we were aware of its limitation of 60 home care visits in a calendar year, which the individual had exhausted. If we didn't go outside those limits, the patient would be back in the hospital again. The payer held to its plan language. In another instance, we were negotiating with a union for hospice benefits. A few members of its Board of Trustees had personal feelings that in essence set up a roadblock, so a reasonable discussion could not take place. They were almost sending up emotional flares. We knew allowance for a hospice benefit would best meet the patient's desires and needs, while saving expenses for the union. There was no way to win the group over to this decision.

Sometimes, case managers just have to wait for the disaster to happen. Then, they can return to the payer, not to gloat, but to ascertain if the decision remains unchanged.

NEGOTIATING IN A MANAGED CARE ENVIRONMENT

It is becoming more likely for case managers to negotiate an out-of-contract benefit in the managed care environment. HMOs and PPOs are realizing that although they may have contract limits and established contract language, in some very high-cost cases, they may have to do more creative and unusual things. More MCOs have determined that they do not need to change their contract language for all covered lives; however, especially when their dollars are funding a risk-based contract, and when they realize it is their money, they will respond to the best interests of their own bottom-line or profit margin.

A case manager may not receive approval for an alternative to a plan on the first phone call. I have found that a "no" does not mean I cannot get approval; it might mean that I am not speaking to the right person. If I can contact someone who is financially responsible for what goes on in the plan, I meet with greater willingness to negotiate. The key lies in how information is presented. I present the cost-effective care alternatives in financial terms first, and then discuss the fact that it is good for the patient and the right thing to do.

Negotiating in a Capitated Contract

This willingness to listen to options extends to payers and providers in capitated arrangements. Managed care is putting more of the responsibility on the providers to achieve the results. I've talked to nurses in HMO plans who years ago could not negotiate care alternatives. Now, because the HMO is contracting with a physician practice group that receives *x* dollars per month per employee to provide a range of services, these providers are doing whatever they can to keep patients healthier and to minimize hospitalizations.

Hospitals, home care agencies, and rehabilitation facilities all negotiate for services that help their entire organization run more efficiently. Those in home care might notice certain cases requiring a greater portion of its services, more of its nurses' time. The nurses are experiencing difficulty moving these patients toward independence or self-care, and the cases require numerous home visits. It may be that the agency is stretching to provide a service that it does not normally offer. Perhaps the agency does not go into the in-depth educational visits that these patients need to progress into self-care or to reduce the number of hours the nurse is working the case; this service will have to be added.

We will see fewer practice variances among providers, and greater acceptance of critical care paths, because we will have established the best treatment paths for pneumonia, for example (which is now treated differently by every provider in town). In part, this is because of the maturity of the marketplace, the business side of managed care. There is also growing acceptance and recognition among medical professionals, who have had a difficult time with loss of autonomy during the transition to managed care, to accept a medically appropriate, cost-effective option.

Negotiating for Carve-Out Services

Negotiating for carve-out services varies with the practice setting. Large payer groups, such as HMOs, PPOs, or employer groups, have contracts with rehabilitation facilities or hospitals. The hospital provides specified general services at a set rate per day. Services such as an organ transplant or bone marrow transplant are carved out and negotiated directly. We have a network of hospitals we are working with now. If we have an admission in a plan provider hospital, we do not negotiate hospital costs, unless the patient requires care that is not subject to the plan rate (such as head trauma care, certain surgeries, and organ transplants). We then negotiate a plan rate.

The same applies for a nurse's visit by a home care agency. For a patient who presents with complicated problems, requiring more than the standard nurse's visit (or physical therapist's visit), the price would be negotiated separately, or carved out.

In the same way, high-cost procedures, such as a transplant, are sometimes negotiated as carve-outs. Particularly with self-funded groups, the stop-loss carrier might have negotiated separately with Centers of Excellence if there appears to be a potential for one or two employees to have a such a need. These "laser-out" agreements serve as an umbrella policy on insurance, setting coverage at $250,000 and superceding the basic stop-loss agreement of $150,000. A case manager will want to ask about any laser-out agreements that the self-insurer might have struck with its own network providers.

Perhaps the all-inclusive case rate provides 21 days of coverage for a bone marrow transplant. The patient you are advocating for demonstrates a strong recovery rate and is discharged at 14 days, or it goes the other way, and the length of stay increases to 28 days. Worse, the transplant fails and a retransplant is mandatory. If the stop-loss insurer, as the risk-bearer, has negotiated with Centers of Excellence, the carrier might take over negotiations at this point. The case manager will continue providing care management services on the case, as before.

DOCUMENTING NEGOTIATED ARRANGEMENTS

Assuming that a case manager has selected the most appropriate service for the patient and negotiated a different fee structure than the one quoted originally, what is the next step? I believe it is important to document and communicate the terms of agreement that case managers arrange with providers.

It should be reemphasized, however, that prior to negotiating or arranging for any service, the case manager must have received approval to do so from the payer source. To begin with, the case manager needs to check that there is language in the plan contract that allows case management. Reviewing the details of the plan contract is especially important when arranging for services, selecting providers, seeking discounts, and so on. Will what the case manager arranges for actually "hold up" when the claim for services finally arrives in the claims department? Will it be paid on a "prompt-pay" basis (that is, within 2 to 4 weeks of arrival at the department)? Will it be paid even though language in the plan may not mention or may even exclude such services? Will it be paid at 100% of the submitted charge, rather than 80% of what is reasonable and customary? Will it be paid even if the plan maximum for the services has already been reached? Who knew about the services, who approved them, who will pay for them, and if no one else will, is the case manager now responsible?

Failure to get answers to these questions before starting work on a case or for a client company puts everyone at risk—the patient, the provider, the carrier or payer, and the case manager. Acting on mere assumptions in this extremely important area can result in legal consequences for all involved.

When entering into a relationship for the provision of case management services, the case manager needs to describe the scope of the services in sufficient detail to permit a complete discussion of how case management will interface with the department or individuals who will have the ultimate payment responsibility for what could best be described as "alternate care plans." It is essential to lead a potential client group through a typical case, one that illustrates just how case management works. The presented scenario should include referral, assessment, the care setting, the exposure the group has for this particular area of service within the patient's insurance plan contract, alternative care plans, and the details of the insurance plan contract that apply to these alternatives. For example, the alternatives presented might include sending the patient home and providing round-the-clock nursing care at $45 an hour ($1,080 a day) or placing her in a skilled nursing facility at a cost of $285 a day. The plan contract allows a maximum of 40 skilled nursing visits of up to 4 hours each, does not mention coverage for skilled nursing facilities, but does state nursing home custodial care is not covered. The case management proposal is for 30 days of care in a skilled nursing facility at a negotiated rate of $285 a day (not the usual $425) if the claim can be paid within 2 weeks of receipt. The other option is a continuation of the patient's stay in the acute care hospital at a rate of $1,500 a day, minimum, which the treating physician favors and for which there is coverage available. However, once apprised of the skilled nursing facility alternative, the treating physician switches his allegiance, and the patient and family also prefer this option.

The portrayal of a fairly typical case allows a client group to begin to understand the nature of case management and to realize how expensive the restrictions in a given plan contract can be when they prevent certain options from being approved. In the preceding scenario, the difference between 30 days of hospital care and 30 days of skilled nursing facility care is $36,450. Hopefully, such examples give client groups the determination, creativity, and sound business/financial rationale to allow the "insertions" of such solutions not just in one case but for as many times and situations in which not doing so would be deemed as fiscal irresponsibility.

Case managers need to be able to present this kind of information to client groups in order to create the right environment for case management and the system or pathways that will allow it to be used successfully. Healthcare cost "problems" are not without solutions. The important thing is to uncover, discuss, and resolve pertinent issues prior to the institution of an in-house case management program or the establishment of a working relationship between an independent practitioner or small company and a client group. There is no point in developing plans that might work "if only." This is why it is imperative that case managers understand and appreciate the various payer systems, plan contracts, and the claims payment process for the various lines of insurance. Inadequate understanding leaves the case manager functioning in a vacuum outside of the system instead of as an integral player within it.

After the case manager has made the client group understand what is required for the implementation and approval of suggested plans, payment issues need to be addressed again. I developed a heightened appreciation for the importance of developing a good relationship with a client's claims department when some claims for services I had arranged and received approval for (from the claims manager) did not get paid and then were "lost." At the same time, other claims were being paid but not at the rate I had negotiated, nor in the desired time frame. This resulted in embarrassment for me, with the provider and with the client group, who questioned the savings I had reported. On a closer look, a claim for a higher fee came in and was paid, because it was billed from the provider's regional office rather than from the local office with which I had "successfully negotiated." For these and many other reasons, I determined that there needed to be a more formal, accountable, and credible way of securing payment arrangements.

To better track and manage case negotiations and claims processing in my office, I designed provider agreement forms to be utilized for each provider and each service. Psychiatric, durable medical equipment, infusion, nursing care, therapy, rehabilitation hospital, and skilled nursing facility services all have separate provider agreement sheets (see Appendix 12–B at the end of the chapter), which are sent with a cover letter explaining their use (Table 12–3). For our staff, I developed guidelines to assist them in filling out the forms and in applying them to different situations (Table 12–4). All these forms are designed to be revised whenever necessary to meet our own needs or the needs of a client company.

These forms can be used for any number of distinct negotiations. They are not used for every X-ray or every piece of durable medical equipment; rather, they are used for high-priced items, for benefit plan exceptions, and so on. Perhaps the payer has a preferred provider arrangement that allows patients to receive a discount, or we have agreed on a prompt-pay discount of 3% if I can ensure that the invoice will be paid in 2 to 3 weeks (which qualifies as early in claims circles). Especially helpful when an alternative care plan is created, a provider service agreement documents case manager, provider, and payer approval for a specific care procedure so that the claims examiner is not put in the awkward position of having to "authorize" a treatment.

Following negotiations with the provider, the case manager completes most portions of the form, which is sent by fax to the provider for an approval signature. Then, a hard copy of the agreement is sent to the provider with a cover letter, which notes that any invoices must accompany the form. A copy of the agreement is also sent to the claims examiner; that particular claim will then be flagged manually or by computer for special handling so that the negotiated price, time frame, or exception is not lost. Given that five or more different examiners or different claims departments might cover one claimant, such tracking is vital.

My company manages the tracking and payment in two different ways. Sometimes, the case manager becomes the "clearinghouse" for every invoice received on behalf of a particular claimant and will hand the negotiated claim to an examiner for processing. In other instances, the provider company sends in its customary bill, knowing it will be reduced as per our agreement (for example, from $410 to $280).

Whatever type of provider agreement format a case manager uses, it should incorporate specifics of the arrangement: the time frame (beginning and end dates), the fees, and any conditions (for example, "payment at 100%" or "payment within 30 days," or "per diem rate is all-inclusive; no other charges to be billed"). The information needs to be documented and

Table 12–3 Provider Service Agreement—Cover Letter

Service Agreement

Date: _____

Patient: _____

Insured: _____

Emp. Group: _____

S.S. #: _____

Dear _____:

OPTIONS UNLIMITED is a case management consulting firm retained by _____.

Attached hereto is a description of the services and/or supplies that you agreed to furnish to _____ on _____.

In order for you to receive payment from the Plan for the services and/or supplies furnished to the Patient, you must submit each claim/bill to Options Unlimited with a copy of this letter and the enclosed Service Agreement, using one of the enclosed envelopes. This will ensure special handling and payment by the Plan subject, of course, to co-payments, deductibles, and other limitations of the Plan.

Any claim/bill received without a copy of this letter, with Service Agreement, will be returned with a message: "Please resubmit with Service Agreement."

Claims/bills received in amounts greater than allowed by this Service Agreement will be reduced to the agreed amount with the following "explanation of benefits" message: "Claim reduced to amount agreed to in the Service Agreement."

Claims/bills for services and/or supplies not covered by this Service Agreement should be sent to the Patient, who must then submit a claim to the Plan in the customary manner.

If you have any questions regarding this Service Agreement, please contact immediately the case manager identified below.

This Service Agreement is entered into by Options Unlimited on behalf of the Plan. This Service Agreement is a contract between you and the Plan, *not* between you and Options Unlimited, or any other person or entity.

We thank you in advance for your anticipated cooperation.

Very truly yours,

Options Unlimited

By: _____

Table 12–3 continued

Case Manager

(631) 555-1212

I have reviewed and am in agreement with the above arrangement.

Provider: _____

Name/Title: _____

Signature: _____

Date: _____

Source: Courtesy of Options Unlimited, Case Management Services Division, © 2003, Huntington, New York.

Table 12–4 Provider Service Agreement Guidelines

Subject: Provider Agreements

Purpose: To document service agreements with providers with the specifics of the arrangement clearly outlined.

Procedural Guidelines

1. Certain cases may require the utilization of specialized services, equipment, and therapies. Through ongoing assessment and in conjunction with the treating physicians, the case manager will identify the needs, select the appropriate services and providers (using the attached guidelines to assist you), negotiate fees and arrangements, and continually monitor patient status, appropriate use of goods and services, continued delivery of services and equipment, any complications or changes in patient, and timing of possible discontinuation of services and equipment use.

2. Source of Agreements

   —Nursing (RN, LPN, Home Health Aide)

   —Durable Medical Equipment (including apnea alarms, wheelchairs, hospital beds, oxygen, etc.)

   —Infusion therapy

   —Other therapies (PT, OT, Speech)

   —Rehabilitation facility, SNF, Psych, and Substance Abuse programs

continues

Table 12–4 continued

---

3. Responsibilities
   —The case manager will fax form and letter of agreement to provider, requesting their signature to acknowledge acceptance of the terms. When signed, the case manager will send out the hard copy with a supply of envelopes with the case manager's return address.
   —The case manager will receive claims, accompanied by the agreement form, will review for adherence to the agreement, and will forward to the claims department for payment.
   —Note: Once the services are in place, it is the *case manager's* responsibility to monitor for quality/outcome and determine on an ongoing basis the need for less (or more) services.

In addition to requesting the claim for review, any notes related to these services must accompany the claim, for example, nurses' notes, PT evaluation and notes, and so on.

It is also the case manager's responsibility to monitor the reevaluation and/or expiration dates of these agreements and follow through with whatever is indicated. You will be in jeopardy of services being discontinued even if still needed, due to failure to renew an agreement.

Source: Courtesy of Options Unlimited, Case Management Services Division, © 2003, Huntington, New York.

---

communicated to the provider and the payer source (claims department). In addition to all pertinent data, such as the patient's name, insured's name, group policy number, social security number, and physician, the form should include a space for the contact person, the case manager, and phone numbers where they can be reached. Each case management department or company needs to develop a method or system consistent with its administrative capabilities and client base. For case management departments in insurance carrier groups, notes entered into a computerized claims system might suffice. Companies working with several carriers might find that mail or fax communication works best. When established, the system should enable accurate payments to be completed in a timely manner and also allow tracking of some of the savings realized by case management.

COST-BENEFIT ANALYSIS REPORTS

Documenting savings from case management intervention is a necessary component of case management work. One method of documentation is to use cost-benefit analysis reports. These are reports that serve to illustrate in financial terms that the costs spent on case management services (and the services that are implemented as part of an alternate care plan) translate into dollar savings, or dollars spent versus dollars saved. Each case management program should have from its very inception a mechanism in place to demonstrate savings to all who will pay for the services. The report format may vary from company to company, and it can certainly be customized or modified to meet client company needs. Report variables may change as a case management program develops.

A cost-benefit analysis report is so specific that I believe it is best prepared by the case manager who works the case. This individual possesses knowledge about the patient, the problems, and the care plan in place at the time the referral was made. She also identified solutions; prevented additional problems; and selected, arranged for, and negotiated the services that were utilized. As a consequence, she is in the best position to evaluate the intervention's success.

Cost-benefit analysis reports are not extended narratives, nor do they include ongoing documentation. They are concerned with the financial aspects of case management and, in my view, should not be included among the monthly progress reports. Because it is possible for certain cases to be in litigation (in particular, workers' compensation, auto, and disability cases), the financial aspects of case management should generally not be included in the patient-centered reports. Although it is expected that costs will never be the focus of case management decisions, there is concern that any mention of dollars (even alongside all the other reasons for a particular treatment decision, such as higher quality care, patient preference, etc.) might be misconstrued or misrepresented by those who view case management intervention solely as a means to control costs.

Some client groups, claims departments, and other purchasers of case management services would prefer to receive reports that deal exclusively with numbers, but it is my contention that this does a disservice to case management. By only portraying savings, one virtually eliminates all of the other contributions of case management. It would seem highly desirable, therefore, to develop a report format that can not only demonstrate savings, but also communicate the impact of case management and illustrate the process.

The data in these reports can be realigned to provide clients with insight into the workings of their benefits plan, successful or otherwise. They can serve a claims function by signaling a potentially greater risk and spurring a response before it occurs. Monthly, yearly, or reports over 1 or more years can be used to analyze benefit usage, group experience, and possible stop-loss needs. Documents can also be formatted by provider (is one much more costly than the other?), diagnosis (is a disease-state management program indicated?), or hospital claims (is billing accurate for services rendered?).

Whatever format is chosen, it is important that each case within a grouping is presented similarly. Following is a list of items that should be included in each case presentation:

1. Identifiers (file, case, or social security number; carrier; employer group; date case opened; date case closed; total weeks or months in case management; diagnosis)
2. Overview of case management intervention
3. Summary of intervention
4. Case management fees
5. Savings
   - Avoided charges
   - Potential charges
   - Discounts and/or negotiated reductions
   - Reductions in services, products, and equipment
6. Actual charges
7. Gross savings (potential charges minus actual charges)
8. Net savings (gross savings minus case management fees)
9. Status of case (open or closed)

Table 12–5 is a worksheet that can be used for each case, and Table 12–6 is a set of guidelines that explains how the worksheet sections should be completed.

A word about actual versus potential savings: Fortunately, there are many opportunities for case managers not only to improve the quality, outcome, and lifestyles for our patients, but also to become better at attaching value to what we do—as we perfect our skills and realize our worth. To cite an example, new case managers may be comfortable suggesting and then arranging for home care as a way of saving money, but experienced case managers know that they can realize additional savings by asking for prompt-pay discounts, reducing levels of care or hours of care through continual assessment of the patient's progress, and so on. Reductions, discounts, negotiated rates, all-inclusive per diem rates, and "freebies" are examples of actual savings.

Potential savings are more difficult to quantify but also need to be reported. For instance, a case manager is referred to a patient who, in prior months, had an admission every 1 or 2 months for diabetic complications and an emergency hospital stay of 5 to 7 days. At the time of the

Table 12–5 Cost-Benefit Analysis Worksheet

Quarter _____

Re:

File #:

Carrier/Client Group:

Date of Referral:

Date of Closure:

Total Weeks/Months of Case Management:

Diagnosis:

Case Management Fees:

Summary of Intervention:

Avoidance of Potential Charges:

Total of Potential Charges:

Alternate Care and Related Charges:

Total Charges for Alternate Care and Case Management Fees:

Net Savings:

  Source: Courtesy of Options Unlimited, Case Management Services Division, © 2003, Huntington, New York.

Table 12–6 Cost-Benefit Analysis Guidelines

Re: Assigned system number.

File # (SS #): Insured's social security number.

Carrier/Employer Group:

Date Opened: Date opened for case management.

Date of Closure: If applicable.

Total Weeks/Months in Case Management: How long case has been active.

Diagnosis: Major categories only, for example, Cancer of Liver, Right Side CVA (Stroke).

*Remember that these will be utilized by "lay" people mostly, so keep this understandable.

continues

Table 12–6 continued

Case Management Fees: Related case management expenses for report time frame.

Summary of Intervention:

Note: This is not to be a discussion of the patient's entire medical history, symptoms, or surgeries. This will have occurred in initial and progress reports and should not be repeated here.

This is a summary of *your* intervention on this case. How did you make a difference in the quality, eventual outcome, patient compliance, patient and family support, prevention of complications, better/more appropriate use of resources, service, and dollars?

*See example reports for further illustration of this section.

This is the "proof" statement for case management, the justification for it on this case! It is *your* turn to cite *your* accomplishments, and give evidence of the need for our services, and the fees for our services.

Avoidance of Potential Charges: This section lists by specific service *and* possible charges (if there is a range put the range, for example, $750 per day–$1,000 per day) that *could* have occurred if this *case* did *not* have your intervention. Remember that you would not have been there to suggest home IV antibiotics versus continued stay in the hospital, or to negotiate rates for services (for example, fees for home IV and nursing services that could have been charged and paid for because there is no R & C for these, anything goes!), or to reduce RN visits from 3 × per week to 1 × per week to discontinuance. List *each* of these services or hospital admissions for the complications that you prevented or equipment, therapies, etc., that would have occurred and (probably) continued if you did not intervene during this quarter. Your list should look something like this:

1. Continued longer stay in hospital

5 days × $1,500 per day = $7,500

Additional MD visits while patient in hospital @ $150 per visit × 5 days = $750

2. Home care services—discharge planner & MD request hospital-based home care services following patient's discharge.

RN visits 1 per day × 14 days @ $160 per visit = $2,240

HHA 6 hours per day @ $20 per hour × 14 days = $1,680

PT 3 × per week × 2 months @ $115 per visit = $2,760

Total of Potential Charges: This should be a combined dollar figure for the preceding charges, e.g., $14,930.

Table 12–6 continued

Alternate Care and Related Charges: This is a list of *specific* services and charges for each that *you* put in place, negotiated rates, effected purchase versus rental, usually instead of the potential charges. For example:

Home care services by community-based, Joint Commission-accredited agency at following rates and with MD approval:

RN visits 1 × per day × 7 days @ $100 per visit = $700

then RN visits 3 × per week @ $100 per visit = $300

HHA 6 hours per day @ $18 per hour × 7 days = $756

then HHA 4 hours per day @ $18 × 5 days (family helped on weekends) = $360

PT 3 × per week × 1 month @ $85 per visit = $1,020

then PT 2 × per week × 1 month @ $85 per visit = $680

Total Charges for Alternate Care and Case Management Fees:

The sum total of charges compiled from preceding listing, e.g., $4,666.

Net Savings: This is a *dollar* figure to be calculated from the potential charges *minus* the charges incurred from the "Alternate Care and Related Charges," e.g., $10,264.

Note: Occasionally, it will not be possible to claim savings; you may not yet have had an opportunity to reduce the level of care or services, because the patient's condition worsened or the patient had to be readmitted to hospital, or you have just put the services in place, but no claims are in yet and savings are "to be determined." You may, however, state an approximate dollar figure that you expect will occur.

Actual Savings

Fortunately, there are many opportunities not only to improve quality, outcome, and lifestyles for our patients, but also (as we perfect our skills and realize our worth) to become better at attaching value to what it is that we do. To cite an example—experienced case managers may be comfortable suggesting and then arranging for home care versus continued hospital stays, but newer case managers may not know that there is still an ability to realize additional savings by asking for prompt-pay discounts, reducing levels of care or hours of care by assessing patient progress and needs frequently, etc. Such reductions, discounts, negotiated rates, all-inclusive per-diem rates, "freebies," etc. are *actual* savings.

continues

Table 12–6 continued

Potential Savings

This is more difficult to quantify and qualify but *needs* to be stated. For instance, you have been referred a patient who in prior months of referral had an admission of 1–2 months for diabetic complications and the emergency hospital stay was 5–7 days. At the time of your initial evaluation, you determined that this patient lacked the understanding of his diagnosis, had minimal compliance, and, in fact, frequently ignored dietary restrictions, urine and blood testing requirements, etc. During the 3 months of case management intervention, you have communicated the problems to his MD, referred the patient for formal education and a diet counseling program, and involved the patient in a daily monitoring of his own progress. You have successfully resolved what *would* have been a continuing pattern of admissions and complications; in fact, in the 6 months of case management involvement, there have been *no* hospital admissions. The potential charges that *would* have occurred without case management intervention and savings could be stated in the following manner.

Summary of Case Management Intervention:

Case manager during this quarter identified and then implemented solutions for this man who had been referred due to recurrent hospital admissions. Patient was poorly informed and because of this was noncompliant following a diagnosis of diabetes. Further complicating this was prior history of increased blood pressure and angina. Case manager advised treating physician and with his cooperation arranged for diabetic education and counseling program; patient was directed to monitor his own progress and report problems to case manager and MD. Programs were available through community hospital outpatient program with considerable savings and good results. There have been no further admissions during this 3-month period and the patient feels more in control. This man was at absolute risk for increased problems and costs.

Avoidance of Potential Charges:

2 hospital admissions @ 5 days for each × 1,500 per day = $15,000

MD visits while patient in hospital @ $150 per visit × 10 days = $1,500

Diabetic Management Program @ $1,000 per private outpatient program

Total of Potential Charges = $17,500

Alternate Care Charges:

Diabetic Management Program @ $750 per program = $750

MD visits—1 per month @ $75 per visit = $225

Total Alternate Care Charges = $975

Total Savings $17,500 – $975 = $16,525 plus additional savings over several more months.

Table 12–6 continued

The preceding is an example of what a group might determine to be "potential savings"; *however,* positioned with expertise and stated strongly and authoritatively, it becomes highly credible.

Note: If there are *no* savings to be claimed, either actual or potential, then state *none* or *to be determined,* with a brief (few word) statement; for example, patient still in hospital, savings will be realized next quarter.

Source: Courtesy of Options Unlimited, Case Management Services Division, © 2003, Huntington, New York.

---

initial evaluation, the case manager determined that this patient did not understand his diagnosis, was minimally compliant, and, in fact, frequently ignored dietary restrictions and urine and blood testing requirements. During the 3 months of case management intervention, the case manager communicated these problems to the physician, referred the patient for formal education and a diet counseling program, and involved the patient in the daily monitoring of his own progress. She successfully resolved what would have been a continuing pattern of admissions and complications. In fact, in the 6 months of case management involvement, there were no further hospital admissions. This is the kind of potential savings that should be noted in cost-benefit analysis reports.

THE COST-BENEFIT ANALYSIS SUMMARIES

After each client case has been outlined, there needs to be a summary of the case management program for the particular client group—a total financial analysis of dollars saved versus dollars spent for case management services for the quarter, 6 months, or year. Examples of such summaries are provided in Appendix 12–C and Appendix 12–D at the end of the chapter; these are expanded versions prepared for two different clients, one a union group and the other a self-funded employer utilizing a TPA. The former shows an annual summary as well as semiannual summaries and reports. The latter shows a quarterly summary and cost-benefit analysis reports, including a difficult pregnancy case, which is discussed in the sections that follow: "Quality Assurance Programs," "Explaining Difficult Situations," and "Feedback from Patients." The reporting format that should be used for each client depends on the needs of the client group and the structure of the case management program, among other factors. These serve as a representative sampling of cases worked; not all cases that were worked are reported for this time frame.

These reports are tools that help make case management services more vital to a client. Pulling a diagnosis summary report allows a case manager to show a CFO the costs of a specific disease state, perhaps caused by an upswing in diabetes among the worker population, indicating the need for disease management or a wellness program. What is driving hospital admissions? A diagnosis summary report correlated to a hospital admissions report (using numbers, not names, to indicate cases) might reveal that there are a select few with that disease who are at the top of the group's benefits outlay. These few need to be in a case management program; the others might improve their health with the help of an educational program. A case manager delivering this type of report is pointing out the areas in which the employer is vulnerable to risk, a constructive and looked-for service.

It is recommended that some kind of financial analysis of case management programs be performed on a regular basis, whether quarterly, semiannually, or annually. Because dollars can add up quickly, especially in very active cases, preparing cost-benefit analysis reports on a quarterly basis is appropriate. Frequent reporting not only makes the compiling of information a more manageable task, but also allows on-line case managers and the supervisor or program director to evaluate the effectiveness of services before too much time has passed and too many dollars have been spent. Not all cases yield savings, and some are more successful than others. What is important is that a timely evaluation of services (which in essence is what this is all about) allows for earlier recognition of problems and the prevention of bigger ones. If case management fees are high and savings on several cases drop each quarter, the problem may be a case manager who is not using time appropriately or does not know how to capture savings. She may require additional training. It might also be a signal that some cases need to be closed.

Preparation of cost-benefit analysis reports is one of the more difficult tasks for many case managers. For several years, I assumed the responsibility for my staff. However, as business increased, this reporting became a larger part of my job, and I learned that I no longer had the kind of day-to-day knowledge of the cases that allowed for a more accurate capturing of savings. Eventually, it was decided that the best person to prepare each individual cost-benefit analysis report was the case manager who was working the case. Instruction in cost-benefit analysis writing became necessary and has now become a part of our training program. (Depending on the size of the case management company or department, preparation of the client group summary is probably a management task, which is relatively straightforward if all the case managers' summaries are in hand.)

QUALITY ASSURANCE PROGRAMS

Financial accountability is perhaps the greatest contribution that cost-benefit analysis offers. Although the reports are appreciated by clients and are useful as marketing tools, they are also useful as quality assurance tools. Further, the process utilized in the preparation of cost-benefit information becomes an empowering experience. Individuals come to appreciate the real value of case management and recognize their own contribution to each success. In instances of limited success, they are able to understand the reasons and develop different strategies to meet them. This kind of self-evaluation promotes excellence and allows the ongoing monitoring of case management services.

EXPLAINING DIFFICULT SITUATIONS

Almost every case manager will at some time be called upon to explain case management fees. Why are the case management fees so high this year compared to last year? Why does your time cost so much? Cost-benefit analysis reports can be a very effective tool for addressing such queries.

In one such instance, my company was providing case management services for a self-funded employer (Sam's, the firm in Appendix 12–D) through a TPA. One day, my contact at the TPA called, very disturbed. The human resources manager at Sam's had called her, ready to terminate his contract with the TPA due to our "increasing" case management fees. He was indignant that our fees had risen substantially in one year, and he and the TPA were looking for an explanation.

A review of several months from the previous year against our current experience with the Sam's employer group provided immediate, clear reasons for the increase in our fees. My letter to the TPA, along with a comparative analysis of the two blocks of time, appears in Table 12–7. The problem was more sick people and greater medical costs. The company's employees and their dependents had experienced a 51% increase in hospital admissions, a 120% increase in pregnancies, and a 400% increase in cardio/respiratory conditions. Using the cost-benefit analysis reports we had prepared, I was able to support the fact that the financial exposure to the employer's plan without case management intervention would have been disastrous.

I outlined one case in particular (included in Table 12–7 and listed as Case 0003 in Appendix 12–D) in which a diabetic woman, already diagnosed with kidney and eye damage due to years of noncompliance, became pregnant against the advice of her physician. This high-risk case

Table 12–7 Sample Letter Addressing Client Cost Concerns with Comparative Analysis

---

MEMO

DATE:

TO: Tami Monk

FROM:

RE: Case Management Fees and Group Experience for Sam's

Following a telephone conversation, and your expressed concerns regarding our case management fees, I researched the situation thoroughly and have prepared an analysis of my findings.

It was said that these increased costs were of concern to Sam's, and there was discussion of terminating their contract with the TPA.

Following is a more detailed breakdown; however, the major problem *does* appear to be one of more sick people and more costs. I reviewed the hospital admissions for the same period of time for last year and this year (January 1–May 16). **Sam's had a 51% increase in the number of admissions, a 120% increase in the number of pregnancies, and a 400% increase in cardio/respiratory conditions.**

The individuals who are in case management have extremely complex cases, and, unfortunately, have required a good bit of professional time. The financial exposure to the Plan *without* this intervention would be disastrous.

Consider the following . . . of the cases we now have open, there are:

1. A 17-year-old, now on dialysis awaiting a kidney transplant. Because of language and cultural differences and the multiple providers involved, we have had to maintain extremely close connection in order to ensure appropriate treatment and cost-effective use of services (we are negotiating/reviewing dialysis claims).
2. Two premature infants—one that we successfully closed with savings and one that was born prior to group coming to TPA that is now closed and has a conservative savings estimate of $101,491.
3. A 35-year-old gentleman for whom we expedited hospital discharge and successfully transferred safely and with no interruption in services or care from Georgia to N.Y. (for extended recovery at his mother's home). We coordinated airlines, physicians, continuous oxygen therapy, and transition to specialists using network providers. **This man weighed 454 lbs. at time of our initial involvement and was in hospital with heart failure, pneumonia, morbid obesity, and pulmonary emboli (life-threatening blood clots in the lung). This claimant to date and with our ongoing intervention is more medically stable and has lost 115 lbs.**

Table 12–7 continued

4. A 22-year-old woman, native of Guam with longstanding history of diabetes, pregnant with her second child who was admitted to hospital in her second month with markedly high blood sugar. She is known (prior to pregnancy) to be noncompliant and was advised not to become pregnant. We have needed to follow her extremely closely due to risk factors (claimant already had kidney and eye damage due to years of noncompliance) and religious and cultural differences. She requires Insulin 4× daily (she often fails to administer this), and medical monitoring (several medical emergencies have occurred, and with our intervention these have been resolved). She lives in remote, rural area of Washington (1-hour drive plus ferry ride to closest university hospital). Case manager has maintained contact with multiple specialists and has arranged for nursing and monitoring services. Delivery date is 6/20 and we are cautiously optimistic of safe delivery. We are also considering placement of this young woman in hospital for duration of pregnancy if noncompliance continues . . . because of risks to infant and mother.

5. A 23-year-old woman with a brain tumor, for whom we have already obtained more appropriate treatment and expertise with renowned neurosurgeon, who will perform surgery with expectations for favorable prognosis. Claimant was being treated in community hospital and we were concerned about the appropriateness of her care. Through our intervention, we have avoided several hospital admissions and an extended inpatient rehab program, as well as obtained significant savings in fee negotiation with providers. Although this has been time-intensive, the exposure to the Plan was significant and, certainly, consequences for this young woman with inappropriate treatment could be devastating.

Tami, I hope you can appreciate that each one of these cases is far from "routine" and *none* can be resolved with just a few phone calls. We have already achieved significant savings and do what we can to provide *our* intervention in the most cost-effective manner.

I trust that the aforementioned will allay your concerns. Should you need further information, please feel free to call me.

Sam's
Analysis of Medical Experience

continues

Table 12-7 continued

Last Year: January 1–May 16

39 Admissions
14 Employees
16 Spouses
9 Dependents

Diagnostic Breakdown

10 Pregnancy & Related Conditions (26% of the admissions)
3 Cancer Admissions (on same patient) (8% of the admissions)
5 Psych/Alcohol (13% of the admissions)
2 Cardio/Respiratory (5% of the admissions)
2 Kidney-related (on same patient) (5% of the admissions)
17 Miscellaneous Surgeries/Medical (44% of the admissions)

This Year: January 1–May 16

59 Admissions
22 Employees
22 Spouses
15 Dependents

Diagnostic Breakdown

22 Pregnancy & Related Conditions (37% of the admissions)
2 Cancers (2% of the admissions)
4 Psych/Alcohol (7% of the admissions)
10 Cardio/Respiratory (17% of the admissions)
3 Kidney/Urinary (5% of the admissions)
18 Miscellaneous Surgery/Medical (31% of the admissions)

Conclusions

- Sam's had a 51% increase in the number of admissions.
- Sam's had a 120% increase in the number of pregnancies.
- Sam's had a 400% increase in cardio/respiratory conditions.

Source: Courtesy of Options Unlimited, Case Management Services Division, © 2003, Huntington, New York.

included emotional/marital, cultural, and religious issues that had to be addressed. In addition, she lived in a remote, rural area of Washington State, 1 hour plus a ferry ride to the closest university hospital. Our total net savings for this case alone were $168,625, to say nothing of the improved life expectancies of this woman and her newborn.

FEEDBACK FROM PATIENTS

Owing to their lack of understanding of case management services and to their perception that employees might view such services as intrusive or interfering, carriers and employer groups have been concerned about and occasionally have resisted implementing case management programs. When my office began working more directly with corporate decision makers on group health cases, I could better appreciate the employers' position. Although interested in cost containment, they did not want to upset the favorable employer–employee relationships they had established. There was also unease expressed about the potential for liability. Would case managers or treating physicians be directing care? What if something negative happened to an employee as a result of a case manager's recommendations?

Case management requires direct interaction with patients and in some respects does interrupt their access to care and services. Frequently, the arrangement for case management services occurs too late for maximum benefits. For instance, one referral to our office was made because for more than 1 year postinjury the claimant was still in active medical treatment and had not returned to work. The claimant viewed this "reactive" referral by the claims department somewhat disdainfully. Where were we before when he needed us? For the most part, however, patients and their families have welcomed case managers. It is important for others to know this.

I first began conducting surveys of patients when I worked primarily in the areas of workers' compensation and auto insurance, prior to my expansion into the group health market. I wanted to be able to improve the delivery of our services not just for our client groups, who were satisfied as long as we were able to save money, but also for the recipients of our services—claimants and their families. We developed a questionnaire that was sent at the close of each case; for those cases that remained open for a long time, one was sent out every 6 months. The questionnaire, which has been revised in light of our increased experience, has helped assure our client groups that case management does make a difference, is well-received, and, as a valued employee service, can be used to improve public relations.

The questionnaire is sent with an explanatory letter (Tables 12–8 and 12–9). It combines a "check the box" format with blanks where individuals can enter their own responses, suggestions, or criticisms. It does not have to be signed but most are, and we further encourage a response by including a self-addressed stamped envelope. Over the years, we have reworked this letter and questionnaire, designing questions that encourage patients and their families to respond with examples of how and

Table 12–8 Quality Assurance Questionnaire Cover Letter

Date

xxxxxxxxxxxxxx
xxxxxxxxxxxxxx
xxxxxxxxxxxxxx

Dear _____:

In an effort to improve the quality of our services, OPTIONS UNLIMITED is conducting periodic surveys.

_____, RN was assigned to your case to provide case management services as requested by _____, the company administering benefits for _____. At the onset of Case Management Services, our goal is for you to have a better understanding of your health needs and management and to assist you and your family to have better communication with your healthcare providers. The goal is also for you to be able to access appropriate healthcare as required.

In order to assess the quality of our services and our patient's satisfaction, we are asking that you complete the enclosed questionnaire and return it in the self-addressed, stamped envelope. Your candor and cooperation is appreciated.

If you have any questions, please call me at (xxx) xxx-xxxx.

Very truly yours,

_____

Catherine M. Mullahy
President

CMM:mm
Enclosure

Source: Courtesy of Options Unlimited, Case Management Services Division, © 2003, Huntington, New York.

---

when the case manager made a difference, and whether the case manager affected an improved understanding of their disease/condition and treatment plan, health, outlook on life, and quality of living. These are views that we can gather as percentage points and present to clients, showing

Table 12–9 Client Satisfaction Survey

OPTIONS UNLIMITED CLIENT SATISFACTION SURVEY

Was your first contact with OPTIONS UNLIMITED:
_____ Friendly
_____ Supportive
_____ Helpful
_____ Informative
_____ Other   Please check all that apply.

At what point of your healthcare status were you contacted by OPTIONS UNLIMITED:
_____ Newly diagnosed
_____ Hospitalized
_____ At home
_____ Presurgical
_____ Other   Please check all that apply.

	Strongly Agree	Agree	Disagree	Strongly Disagree	Not Applicable
1) The case management services were helpful for me.	5	4	3	2	1
My family	5	4	3	2	1
2) Case management helped me with the needs I feel are important.	5	4	3	2	1
3) The role of case management services was explained to me, my family, and my physician.	5	4	3	2	1
4) My case manager was helpful in thoroughly explaining my diagnosis and treatment options.	5	4	3	2	1
5) My case manager was helpful in obtaining the services I required.	5	4	3	2	1

continues

Table 12–9 continued

6) My case manager and providers worked well together caring for me.	5	4	3	2	1
7) Using what I learned from my case manager, I believe I am more able to access medical services on my own.	5	4	3	2	1

My case manager paid attention to my needs:
_____ Physical
_____ Safety
_____ Communication
_____ Nutrition
_____ Emotional
_____ Spiritual
_____ Understanding of medications   Please check all that apply.

What did you like about case management services?

What areas do you feel would have made a difference in your care?

Thank you for taking your time to complete this survey. We appreciate your input and we value your comments.

_____
Printed Name (optional)

_____
Signature of Claimant or
Significant Other (optional)

Source: Courtesy of Options Unlimited, Case Management Services Division, © 2003, Huntington, New York.

that a certain percentage of our patients who answer do so with positive comments. For employers, the employees' feedback often indicates that case management is viewed as a value-added benefit. Combined with cost-benefit analysis reports, such patient/family responses give us records on the benefits case management brings to healthcare, family support, and financial outcomes.

Table 12–10 is a quality assurance cover letter we use in cases in which the patient has passed away. We always make certain an appropriate amount of time has gone by before sending this on to the family.

We are also working on a "Preinvolvement of Case Management" questionnaire to give us a "before case management" history that can be compared with the "after case management" perceptions. We anticipate that this will reveal a more in-depth and accurate look at the differences case management makes.

I am hearing more questions and demands from consumers, yet I do not believe our industry has recognized that they have a right to their questions and to carefully considered responses. The attitude has been, "Well, we're providing this highly sophisticated care, we're sharing what we've created, why seek their counsel?" We have been very late in the game to ask ourselves, "Is this really what a patient wants?" For instance, consider shortened maternity stays in a facility: This decision was not in the patients' best interests, and it was dangerous. This is a very clear-cut and simplistic example of how policy is established in hospitals, HMOs, insurance carriers, and employer groups across the country with little regard for the patient. It was quite obvious that no one had consulted new mothers, women who had experienced the birthing process, regarding the 24-hour return to home.

If we really are operating with an awareness of those characteristics that constitute healthcare ethics—respect for the patient, patient autonomy, dignity, veracity, beneficence, nonmalfeasance—we need to actively solicit patients' input in the health delivery process. And we must seek their comments before and during the process, not only after they have left us, after we've had all the control and authority over their lives at a point when they were very emotionally and physically vulnerable.

Particularly within critical care settings, case managers often minister to a substantial number of patients who are, in addition to their physical challenges, emotionally and cognitively impaired due to a head injury, stroke, multiple sclerosis (MS), and other neurological conditions. As difficult as it may be to meet the healthcare needs of our more able hospital or clinic patients, how much is our obligation heightened when the individual is struggling against communication deficits, including aphasia or locked-in

Table 12–10 Quality Assurance Cover Letter Used When Patient Has Passed Away

---

Date

XXXXXXXXXXXXX
XXXXXXXXXXXXX
XXXXXXXXXXXXX

Dear _____ :

We are aware that _____ has passed away and if we have not yet conveyed this to you, please accept our sincere sympathy. OPTIONS UNLIMITED had been providing medical case management services to _____ in order to assist with the coordination of care and services, to provide information and support, and hopefully, to ease some of the other burdens that often accompany illness. At the onset of Case Management Services, our goal was for _____ to have a better understanding of his/her health needs and its management and to assist _____ and your family to have better communication with your healthcare providers. The goal is also for you to be able to access appropriate healthcare as required.

These services were provided at no cost to the patient (or insured) and were at the request of _____, the Plan Administrator for the employer group medical plan. It is our hope to continually assess the quality of our services and, as needed, to improve or change certain aspects of them.

_____, RN was the case manager who was assigned to _____ and we are interested in any comments you may wish to offer regarding her role, as well.

Once again, thank you for your assistance and should you wish to contact us directly, please feel free to do so.

Very truly yours,

Catherine M. Mullahy
President

CMM:xx
Enclosure

Source: Courtesy of Options Unlimited, Case Management Services Division, © 2003, Huntington, New York.

---

syndrome? We must recognize that these persons have little or no ability to express their degree of satisfaction or dissatisfaction, and should expand our efforts to communicate as we design patient satisfaction question- naires and incorporate patient/family responses into our programs.

To better plan a course of treatment, we need to ask, before patients are admitted or as soon as possible upon admission: What are your goals? What do you hope? Your doctor thinks that you should be here for 4 weeks. What do you think you will be able to accomplish in 4 weeks? What kind of care do you expect? What kind of professionals do you think are going to be working with you? Do you want an explanation of your therapy or the test? Would that make you feel better?

The answers to these kinds of questions help us understand what a patient knows about his condition and also what his prior education has taught him, what his prior experience in a healthcare delivery system has prepared him for, and how much you need to address some of his mis- understandings or misperceptions before you can create what both patient and provider hope will be a successful outcome. Our treatment is not ethically sound if we once again operate in a vacuum, as we in health care tend to do, outlining our best practice program, our state-of-the-art care maps and plans for day one and day two, without taking into con- sideration the needs of the patient. Addressing patient concerns when planning our programs elevates quality of care while elevating the ethics of care because we have asked, is this care palpable to patients?

A physiatrist (a specialist in physical medicine and rehabilitation) may have what he or she deems to be the ideal program to address a stroke, MS, or traumatic brain injury patient, but is that what the patient and his family are expecting? Is it in their best interests? The physiatrist may feel that 3 weeks or 4 weeks is enough to stabilize that patient, but does the patient see that? Maybe the patient's perception is based on an experience with a parent years before who was in a facility 2 or 3 months. Shouldn't that be addressed? Because of new technology or improved therapeutic moralities, or because he had a better surgical result than his parent, you are going to be able to move this patient along much faster. Here is the opportunity to calm any alarm, the chance to say, this is now the normal treatment program.

The patient questionnaire becomes a quality assurance tool, a marketing tool, an outcomes report tool, and a business tool. These are strong play- ing cards in this very complex system. From an operating perspective, it is an invaluable indicator to help fine-tune a program, to better train profes- sionals, to more adequately meet the needs of patients, and to address the expectations of payers as well. With these uses in mind, it is appropriate to conduct segments of a patient questionnaire before admission, upon admission, midway through treatment, at discharge, and at postdischarge to discern how well the patient's needs were met.

The design of a questionnaire must be made as objective as possible. Anyone can create a market survey instrument without ever placing the facility or service in an unfavorable light by asking questions that elicit only favorable responses, never enabling a patient to give "undirected" input that might include negative comments. Perhaps the patient satisfaction questionnaire design group should include persons outside the facility itself, other providers such as physicians who refer to the facility, selected staff members, patients and family members who have been in your facility, and certain payers who meet the expenses of your facility. Anticipate what some of the negatives might be, and allow for that kind of response from a patient. We have a responsibility to make the survey instrument as patient-focused as possible. This is achieved by incorporating statements such as, "We would appreciate any comments you may have to improve our service. What would you like us to have done differently? What things that you experienced were not positive for you?"

SHARING QUESTIONNAIRE RESULTS

Care is a collaborative process, so survey results should be shared with internal staff. If responses are funneled only to the public relations or marketing department, for instance, how do people ever know whether they are improving? How do you evaluate the success? How do you propose change unless you have a benchmark? After the information has been applied during internal evaluation and planning, then it is appropriate to communicate selected comments and how the facility or service responded to prospective consumers; they need to understand that a group is invested in its patients, that services are patient-driven.

A sensitive area regarding implementation of the patient questionnaire involving both patients and staff is confidentiality. It is now a legal responsibility, as well. Patients should feel free to say negative things without a fear of untoward recriminations or legal action. Elements of the satisfaction survey might be completed anonymously, or the instrument might include a statement verifying that all information is confidential and will only be used to improve programs. Patients, especially those who will return, should be welcome to share whatever concerns they have. You also want to receive honest answers. Some groups code patient surveys so that they are completed anonymously but allow the patient or staff member to be identified should something problematic occur.

In the same way, staff confidentiality can become an issue. Positive feedback from a patient in a questionnaire can be shared; we want people to know when they have done a good job. However, when it is negative feedback, it should be handled between supervisor and staff member, never naming the patient. The information becomes an instructional vehicle; the patient might have a real issue with a staff member, a legitimate complaint that needs to be addressed. Patient questionnaires become the vehicle giving further assurance to both current and future patients that quality-of-service standards will remain high.

Effective means for linking patient satisfaction surveys back to the planning and provision of services include written documentation and regularly scheduled planning meetings among appropriate individuals. Results can be made part of a monthly or quarterly review of all programs. Beyond that is the peer review concept. A patient advisory board might be a huge asset. How often have hospital space planners designed a whole new wing without ever asking a head nurse about patient- and workflow on the floor? An ad for an HMO organization announced evening and Saturday hours and invited community members to stop by for a visit. This HMO is reaching out to meet local families where they are by making the medical staff available when the potential customers have free time. Instead of once again getting all the medical professionals together in a room to redesign a program, why not invite patients in? Tell them that the response to the orientation program was 50% favorable, and ask their opinion on how to raise that to a 98% positive response rate.

Ongoing methods of communicating the results of patient questionnaires to your staff professionals are a newsletter or bulletin board posting complimentary or grateful letters from patients so everybody can see them. Letters might be forwarded to a unit or program via administration or department directors. Negative comments should be handled in a different way. The need to communicate patient concerns may be fulfilled in a departmental meeting or performance review. Perhaps some comments can be used as a teaching or supervisory tool so staff becomes more aware of how their actions are being perceived by others.

Those preparing a patient questionnaire must think very carefully about the range of questions asked, and be prepared for the responses. Patient input on operations and the resulting internal review can prompt staff morale problems, liability, and issues of risk management, purchasing, profitability, and public relations.

After a problem is disclosed, a company or case manager has an ethical responsibility to address it. Criteria should be established for possible liability situations. No one wants to find out years later that a serious charge was reported and just left on file. Although patient confidentiality must be respected, a case manager is also charged with the additional responsibility of correcting injustices or infractions. Should a similar incident occur and be reported publicly while a former patient's comment on his previous similar experience was reported and went unheeded, the department or group might be held liable. To prevent such problems, the decision might be made to send reports through a risk manager, to corporate counsel, department heads, or a peer review. The choice of procedure is less vital to the health of the case management department or company than the fact that there is such a plan in place.

Questionnaire surveys are useful not only from a marketing perspective, but also in the evaluation of staff members and in the identification of problems with service. Many suggestions offered by our patients have become incorporated into our current services. When our case managers are given praise for their assistance, they receive a copy of the document for their records and it becomes part of their personnel file. Criticisms are also taken seriously, obviously allowing for personal preference, personality clash, or a situation that places the case manager in a position of reducing home care services or confronting noncompliant behavior. Criticisms also sometimes point to areas in which additional training or supervision might be helpful.

Whenever a questionnaire is returned, everyone is eager to see the results. Staff and administration want to know the positives and the negatives. If 80% of respondents thought a program was good, it means that 20% found it lacking, and some individuals will be very concerned about that 20%. What if a company delivers quality services and is the most cost-effective act in town, but patients have legitimate concerns about their care at the facility? Corporate counsel might well be up in arms. What if someone says something? Then we are required to take action. You mean we actually have to record negative comments? How many negatives are we getting? What is our insurance cost going to be like if x number of patients report an accident in our facility? How happy will our underwriter be about writing liability insurance now?

We provide summaries of the responses to the client groups and usually include actual samples. This has been most helpful, especially with those groups that were initially concerned about the receptivity of their employees. After seeing employee reactions, they soon start calling to suggest cases they now think should be case managed.

COMMUNICATING SUCCESS

Cost-benefit analysis reports and quality assurance surveys need to be communicated appropriately. They should be provided on a regular basis and ideally are presented in personal meetings. Cost-benefit analysis reports in particular need to be explained, because the information, when taken out of context or reviewed by individuals unfamiliar with the process or results, can easily be misinterpreted. Certain terms (for example, *avoidance of potential charges* and *prevention of complications*) and the method of calculating savings (*gross* and *net*) should be discussed. Reviewing a few or all of the individual cases within a group is also helpful. It enables a client to understand the case management process and raise questions regarding the accuracy of the figures and the credibility of the savings—all important steps. If case managers are not willing to explain and inform, then the whole purpose of reporting is subverted.

Usually, the individual representing a client group in its relationship with a case manager is the CFO, an insurance professional, or a human resource professional. In most instances, this individual does not have a medical background and is unwilling to accept everything the case manager feels justified in claiming as savings. To illustrate, several years ago one of my first major clients was a large health insurance carrier that contracted with my company to develop a case management program for it and its client groups. As part of the program, we obtained early discharges from hospitals, negotiated fees with facilities and providers, arranged home care, and prevented the kinds of complications that would have occurred had case managers not been involved.

Feeling very positive about our services and the results, I looked forward to sharing our first quarterly report with this group. The results were impressive, a 1:23 ratio (that is, for every dollar that this group spent on our case management services, we were able to save $23). Quite respectable, I thought, especially as we were somewhat conservative in our calculation.

At the meeting, the carrier's representatives included an underwriter, an actuary, the corporate counsel, and the claims director. Not one case manager! I started with the summary page, concise data, and the kind of "number crunching" that this group could really get into. Questions began: Where were the actual claims that we got these savings from? If we were saying that they never had claims (avoidance of potential charges), then how could we calculate a savings? How could we prevent a hospital admission or complications? This was going to be harder than I thought. How could I help them understand?

Case by case (fortunately, there were only eight that quarter), I led them through the case management process. I described each case at the time we received it, gave the claims history prior to our involvement (three hospital admissions for 3 to 5 days each on a noncompliant diabetic), reported what we learned at the time of our assessment (this patient had been treated in a city hospital, had a different physician each time, no family physician, was trying to stretch his insulin to last because finances were tight, never did get around to getting his glucometer), and described what the case manager did (referred him to a local endocrinologist, arranged for insulin and supplies to be billed directly to the carrier instead of the patient having to pay first and then wait to be reimbursed, obtained a glucometer at a discounted rate, arranged for diabetic training and diet plan by a nurse clinician in a physician's office, and referred him to a local diabetic support group, which he could participate in at no cost).

Finally, I summarized the results. There were no admissions during the quarter. With this scenario as described, was there any doubt that without case management intervention, the revolving-door admissions to the hospital would have continued and additional complications occurred due to noncompliance? This overview and walk-through demonstrated the problem, the solutions, and the savings.

We discussed all eight cases, and although there was some disagreement over whether something would or would not have occurred, at the end of this meeting all the representatives were enthusiastic about the accomplishments, including the containment of costs. For several quarters thereafter, interest in case management increased and more people attended the meetings, often contributing their own ideas as to what else could have been done and reporting that more of the client groups wanted this case management "stuff." This carrier group became so convinced of the merits of case management that it eventually developed its own department and retained us to work cases it could not handle.

Case managers are experts in assessing and resolving problem cases. Others cannot be expected to understand the case management process as well as we do. It is not enough to manage the case; we need to manage our relationships with clients as well. Educating clients allows them to "buy into" case management and helps avoid micromanagement discussions (for example, questioning whether the 5 minutes spent on a phone call was really necessary). To make case management more successful and established as an industry, each case manager not only needs to work effectively but also needs to articulate her achievements—walk the walk and talk the talk.

NOTES

1. Feuer L, "Manipulative Negotiations: Winning and Loving It!," presented at the Medical Case Management Conference VIII, Orlando, FL, September 1996.
2. Thomas-Payne L, "Simple Negotiations," *HomeCare* 14, no. 11 (1992): 104.

APPENDIX 12–A

Program Questionnaire and Facility Review for Case Managers

PROGRAM QUESTIONNAIRE

Name: _____

Address: _____

Phone: _____

E-mail: _____

Contact Person: _____

Medical Director/Specialty: _____

Number of Beds: _____ Age Range of Patients: _____

Specialty Areas: _____

Per Diem Cost	$ _____	Cost varies per program and per individual need. Case managers call the facility for an estimate of cost for care.
All Inclusive	$ _____	Following an evaluation of specific need, the facility can issue a letter confirming cost for care.
Room & Board Only	$ _____	

Approximate Therapy Cost per 30 Minutes

Physical	$ _____	Vocational	$ _____
Occupational	$ _____	Cognitive	$ _____
Speech	$ _____	Psychological	
Recreational	$ _____	Counseling	$ _____
Prosthetics	$ _____	Drivers Ed	$ _____
Respiratory	$ _____	Audiologists	
		(Screening)	$ _____
		Therapeutic Recreation	
		Outings	$ _____

Comments:

Accredited by: _____ Joint Commission _____ CARF

Written Reports Rendered:

Insurance Company Representative included at staffings
_____ Yes _____ No
Case Manager or Insurance Representative permitted to:
_____ Attend staffings _____ Participate in staffings

Will the facility provide statistical data on length of stay, average costs, distribution of discharge placements?	( ) Yes	( ) No
Will the facility negotiate costs?	( ) Yes	( ) No
Does the facility have fax capability?	( ) Yes	( ) No
If so, fax #: _____		
Will the facility provide written reports no less often than 30 days?	( ) Yes	( ) No

Staffing

Board-certified medical director?	( ) Yes	( ) No
Physician/psychiatrist team leader?	( ) Yes	( ) No
Is the physician (the team leader) on premises?	( ) Yes	( ) No
Is the physician out-of-facility consultant?	( ) Yes	( ) No
24-hour skilled care available directed by RN?	( ) Yes	( ) No
Team is multidisciplinary, including representatives from all therapies?	( ) Yes	( ) No
Do patients have the same therapists and team members throughout their stay?	( ) Yes	( ) No
Are the majority of employees on staff and not contracted from an outside agency?	( ) Yes	( ) No
Are therapists registered or certified?	( ) Yes	( ) No
Does the facility have access to consulting physicians?	( ) Yes	( ) No
Is list of consultants available?	( ) Yes	( ) No

Additional questions for subacute facility:

Board-certified medical director with acute care experience?	( ) Yes	( ) No
Is there 24-hour physician coverage?	( ) Yes	( ) No
24-hour acute care nursing specialists directed by nurse/clinician?	( ) Yes	( ) No
(Nursing staff may include RNs specializing in medical/surgical care, critical care, home care, pulmonary rehabilitation, and oncology.)		
Is there 24-hour access to medical specialists certified in internal medicine?	( ) Yes	( ) No
pulmonary medicine?	( ) Yes	( ) No
critical care?	( ) Yes	( ) No
family practice?	( ) Yes	( ) No

Does the on-site support staff include

registered dietitians?   ( ) Yes   ( ) No
respiratory therapists?   ( ) Yes   ( ) No
physical/occupational therapists?   ( ) Yes   ( ) No
speech pathologists?   ( ) Yes   ( ) No
social workers?   ( ) Yes   ( ) No
grief/bereavement counselors?   ( ) Yes   ( ) No

Clinical Care Available

Is a rehabilitation plan tailored for the patient's
specific needs?   ( ) Yes   ( ) No

Are team conferences held: ____ weekly ____ every two
weeks

Do all members of the team, including patient, family,
and insurance representative, attend?   ( ) Yes   ( ) No

How many hours of therapy/rehab services does patient
receive per day? _____

Are personal hygiene assistance and meals considered
therapy?   ( ) Yes   ( ) No

Are the patient's therapy prescriptions appropriate?   ( ) Yes   ( ) No

Are therapies offered daily, and if patient conditions warrant,
are therapies offered twice a day?   ( ) Yes   ( ) No
Weekends?   ( ) Yes   ( ) No

Check therapies available:

Physical _____   Speech & Language _____
Cognitive _____   Orthotic Services _____
Occupational _____   Psychological Counseling _____
Recreational _____

Additional questions for subacute facility:

Check treatment categories available:

Pulmonary care _____   Infectious disease _____
Wound management _____   Pediatrics _____
Rehabilitation _____   Oncology _____
Orthopedics _____   Cardiovascular _____
Neurology _____   Nutritional support _____

Check 24-hour capabilities for:

Laboratory services _____   Radiology _____
Pharmacy _____

Check service capabilities for:

Pain management _____   Hydrotherapy _____
Superficial wound debridement _____   Bowel/bladder training _____

Electrical stimulation _____

Check equipment capabilities for:

Telemetry _____   Piped-in suctioning _____

Ventilator support _____   Hemodialysis _____

Piped-in oxygen _____

Discharge Planning and Coordination of Follow-up

Is discharge planning instituted early in the hospitalization? ( ) Yes   ( ) No

Is there a tentative discharge date set early in the
hospitalization?   ( ) Yes   ( ) No

Is patient/family education ongoing throughout the
hospitalization?   ( ) Yes   ( ) No

Does the family education include assisting the family to
realistically consider the client's long-term physical and
cognitive prognosis?   ( ) Yes   ( ) No

Is there a prescribed continuum of family ed?   ( ) Yes   ( ) No

Is there continuity of care and follow-up after discharge?   ( ) Yes   ( ) No

Will staff perform on-site evaluation for home
modification needs?   ( ) Yes   ( ) No

Will equipment and home modification needs be discussed
with insurance representative before purchase or direction
to the family?   ( ) Yes   ( ) No

Will several bids for DME be acquired if requested?   ( ) Yes   ( ) No

Will physician team leader refer patient to a local physician
for follow-up and act as a resource as needed?   ( ) Yes   ( ) No

Are outpatient services available?   ( ) Yes   ( ) No

Please detail living arrangements for outpatient program
below.

Are patients encouraged to complete trial home visits
prior to discharge?   ( ) Yes   ( ) No

Will the facility provide a written discharge plan, including
level of care required, number of hours per day assistance is
required, abilities in ADLs, equipment needs, medications,
return-to-work/vocational potential, specific follow-up
care required?   ( ) Yes   ( ) No

Additional Comments:

Reviewed by: _____

Office: _____

City, State: _____

FACILITY REVIEW

Does the facility have pre-admission criteria?	( ) Yes	( ) No
Is the facility clean and cheerful?	( ) Yes	( ) No
Does the facility admit only those patients with rehabilitation potential?	( ) Yes	( ) No
Does the facility offer an evaluation program to determine rehab potential?	( ) Yes	( ) No
Does the facility have a designee in the business office to deal with the insurer/case manager?	( ) Yes	( ) No
Do patients look well cared for?	( ) Yes	( ) No
Is there a family education program?	( ) Yes	( ) No
Is there a patient/family information guidebook?	( ) Yes	( ) No
Are there other patients with the same diagnosis? How many? _____	( ) Yes	( ) No
Are there dedicated treatment teams per diagnosis?	( ) Yes	( ) No
Are the facilities and equipment appropriate for the patient's needs?	( ) Yes	( ) No
Do patients have access to dining area, nursing units, grounds, elevators, etc.?	( ) Yes	( ) No
Are there well-defined policies and procedures in place for medical emergencies?	( ) Yes	( ) No
Can the facility adequately treat minor/moderate medical complications on-site?	( ) Yes	( ) No
Will the facility notify insurance representative of upcoming conferences/staffings?	( ) Yes	( ) No
Are goals reset as patient status changes?	( ) Yes	( ) No
If patient no longer shows significant gains, is discharge proposed?	( ) Yes	( ) No
Is there a staff coordinator or internal case manager assigned to each patient who acts as a liaison for family and insurance representative?	( ) Yes	( ) No
Are there well-defined quality assurance programs in place?	( ) Yes	( ) No
Are there outcome criteria? Is the effectiveness of services measured?	( ) Yes	( ) No

Additional questions for subacute facility:

Is this a dedicated environment?	( ) Yes	( ) No
Is there significant use of agency nurses?	( ) Yes	( ) No

Average Length of Stay:
By diagnosis—the figures for preceding year (if available)
CVA _____
SCI (NEW) _____
SCI (OLD) _____
Referral Procedure:

Source: Courtesy of Case Management Society of America, Little Rock, Arkansas.

APPENDIX 12–B

Provider Service Agreements

Initial _____
Renewal _____

CLAIMS NOTIFICATION—PSYCHIATRIC/SUBSTANCE ABUSE
SERVICES

To: _____ Date: _____
Re: Patient: _____
   Insured: _____ Group: _____
   S.S. #: _____
   Physician: _____ Phone: _____
   E-mail: _____
   Type of Services:
   Inpatient Services _____
   Outpatient Services _____
   Day-Hospital Services _____
   Long-Term Residential _____
   Other _____
   Date to Start: _____ Date to End or Reevaluation Date:
_____

   Provider: Name: _____ Telephone: _____
      Address: _____ Ext: _____
      City, State, Zip Code: _____
      E-mail: _____
      Contact Person: Service: _____ Telephone: _____
            Billing: _____ Ext: _____
      Billing Address, if Different: _____
      E-mail: _____
      Fees: Per diem: _____ All-Inclusive? Yes _____No _____
          Per week: _____ If no, state other charges.
          Per month: _____
Special Arrangements: _____

Claims Person: Name: _____ Phone: _____
Advised: Yes _____ No _____
Arranged by: Case Manager: _____ Phone: _____
      Company: *Options Unlimited on behalf of the Plan identified in
      the attached Service Agreement.*
Accepted by: _____ Title: _____

Initial _____
Renewal _____

CLAIMS NOTIFICATION—DURABLE MEDICAL EQUIPMENT FORM

To: _____ Date: _____

Re: Patient: _____

Insured: _____ Group: _____

S.S. #: _____

Physician: _____

Equipment:	Purchase Price	Rental Price
Wheelchair: Manual:	_____	_____
Electric:	_____	_____
Hospital Bed:	_____	_____
Walker:	_____	_____
Commode:	_____	_____
Alarm:	_____	_____
Oxygen & Related Equipment:	_____	_____
Other:	_____	_____

Arrangement Made: _____

Length of Time: _____ Date Started: _____

Date to end or reevaluation date: _____

Discussed with claims department: Yes _____ No _____

Name: _____ Phone #: _____

Provider Agency: _____

Contact Person: _____

Address: _____

Telephone #:_____ Fax #: _____

E-mail: _____ _____

Arranged by: Case Manager: _____

Company: *Options Unlimited on*   Telephone #:_____
behalf of the Plan identified on the   E-mail: _____ _____
attached Service Agreement.

Accepted by: _____

Title: _____ Date: _____

Initial _____
Renewal _____

CLAIMS NOTIFICATION—INFUSION SERVICES

To: _____ Date: _____
Re: Patient: _____
    Insured: _____ Group: _____
    S.S. #: _____
    Physician: _____ Phone: _____
    E-mail: _____
Type of Services: _____ Fees: _____
TPN: _____
Chemotherapy: _____
Pentamidine: _____
Antibiotics: _____
Antivirals: _____
Enteral Feedings: _____
Pain Management: _____
Nursing Services Required: (For patient education, site care, etc.)
Describe: _____
Equipment Required: (Pumps, supplies, etc.)
Describe: _____
Frequency of Services:
Continuous: _____ Daily: _____ Hours per Day: ____
Date to Start: _____ Date to End/Reevaluation Date: _____
Provider Agency: _____ Phone #: _____
Address: _____ Fax #: _____
Contact: Service: _____ Billing: _____
E-mail: _____ E-mail: _____
Address: _____
Advised: ____ Yes ____ No
Arranged by: Case Manager: _____
    Company: *Options Unlimited on*   Telephone #: _____
    behalf of the Plan identified on the   E-mail: _____
    attached Service Agreement.
Accepted by: _____ Title: _____

Initial _____

Renewal _____

CLAIMS NOTIFICATION—NURSING CARE SERVICES FORM

To: _____ Date: _____

Re: Patient: _____ Group: _____

Insured: _____

S.S. #: _____

Physician: _____

Type of Service:

Nursing:

R.N. _____ L.P.N. _____ Aide _____ Other _____

Hours per Day: _____ Hours per Week: ____ Fees per Hour: _____

Provider: Name: _____ Telephone: _____

Address: _____

City, State, Zip Code: _____

Billing Address, if different: _____

Contact Person: Service: _____ Phone: _____

Fax: _____ E-mail: _____

Billing: _____ Phone: _____

E-mail: _____

Note: If more than one agency will be used, enter identifying information.

Name: _____ Phone: _____

Address: _____ E-mail: _____

Contact Person: Service _____ Billing: _____

Date to Start: _____ Date to End or Reevaluation Date: _____

Claims Person: Name: _____ Phone: _____

Advised: Yes _____ No _____ E-mail: _____

Arranged by: Case Manager: _____

Company: *Options Unlimited on behalf of the Plan identified on the attached Service Agreement.*

Phone #: _____

Accepted by: _____ Title: _____

Initial _____

Renewal _____

CLAIMS NOTIFICATION—THERAPY SERVICES FORM

To: _____ Date: _____

Re: Patient: _____

    Insured: _____

    S.S. #: _____

    Physician: _____

Type of Therapy:

P.T. _____ O.T. _____ Speech _____ Respiratory_____ Other _____

Frequency of Therapy:

Daily _____ Weekly _____

Fees per Hour: _____ Estimated Duration of Therapy: _____

Date to Start: _____

Date to End or Reevaluation Date: _____

Name of Therapist(s): _____

Address: _____

City, State, Zip Code: _____

Phone #: _____ Tax I.D. #: _____

E-mail: _____

Claims Person: Name: _____

            Phone #: _____ Fax #: _____

            E-mail: _____

Advised?: Yes _____ No _____

Arranged by: Case Manager: _____

Company: *Options Unlimited on behalf of the*   Phone #: _____
Plan identified in the attached Service Agreement.

Accepted by: _____ Title: _____

Initial _____

Renewal _____

CLAIMS NOTIFICATION—REHAB HOSPITAL/ SKILLED NURSING FACILITY

To: _____ Date: _____

Re: Patient: _____

    Insured: _____ Group: _____

    S.S. #: _____

    Physician: _____ Phone: _____

                               E-mail: _____

Type of Services:

Inpatient Services: _____

Outpatient Services: _____

Therapies: OT: _____ PT: _____ Speech: _____

Other: _____

Date to Start: _____ Date to End or Reevaluation Date: _____

Provider: Name: _____ Telephone: _____

        Address: _____ E-mail: _____

        City, State, Zip Code: _____

Contact Person: Service: _____ Telephone: _____

           Billing: _____ Fax: _____

                             E-mail: _____

Billing Address, if Different: _____

        Fees: Per diem: _____ All-Inclusive? Yes ____ No ____

           Per week: _____ If no, state other charges: _____

           Per month: _____

Special Arrangements: _____

Claims Person: Name: _____ Phone: _____

                             E-mail: _____

Advised?: Yes _____ No _____

Arranged by: Case Manager _____ Phone: _____

                             E-mail: _____

        Company: *Options Unlimited on behalf of the Plan identified in the attached Service Agreement.*

Accepted by: _____ Title: _____

APPENDIX 12–C

Expanded Cost-Benefit Analysis Summary

Summary of Savings for Case Management Services—Calendar Year
Local 123 Welfare Fund
January 1, xxxx–December 31, xxxx Year End Summary

Cases open at beginning of year	7	
Cases referred this year	49	
Cases closed this year	46	
Total cases worked this year	56	
Total fees for the year		$102,335
Average fees per month		$ 8,528
Average fees per case/year		$ 1,827
Average fees per case/month		$ 152
Total savings for the year		
Gross		$816,131
Net		$713,796
Average Savings per Case for the Year		$ 12,746
Ratio of Dollars to Savings	1:8	

Local 123 Welfare Fund
First Half-Year Summary of Cost-Benefit Analysis for Case
Management Services
January 1, xxxx–June 30, xxxx

Cases open at beginning of period	7	
Cases referred this period	29	
Cases closed during the period	22	
Total cases worked during period	36	
Total number of open cases	14	
Total fees for the period		$ 61,571
Average fees per month		$ 10,262
Average fees per case/period		$ 1,710
Average fees per case/month		$ 285
Total savings for period		
Gross		$402,990
Net		$341,419
Average savings per case/period		$ 9,484
Ratio of dollars to savings	1:7	

Note: To evaluate the benefits of a program for a client, we use total fees billed for all cases worked and the saving resulting from our intervention, whether savings were realized in every case, one case, or several cases.

SAMPLES OF CASES FROM JANUARY 1, XXXX – JUNE 1, XXXX

CASE MANAGEMENT COST-BENEFIT ANALYSIS REPORT

Re: 0002

Carrier/Client Group: Local 123

Date of Referral: 1/11/xx

Date of Closure: 1/31/xx

Total Weeks/Months of Case Management: 3 weeks

Diagnosis: Cancer of the Colon

Case Management Fees: $1,313

Summary of Intervention:
Options Unlimited conducted a thorough assessment and expedited discharge from acute care to subacute care. Once at subacute level, progress was monitored closely. In this way, discharge to home was expedited 1 week earlier than anticipated. Home care visits were negotiated and provided to determine if additional services (HHA, PT, OT) would be necessary. A full report from home care RN was obtained by the case manager and evaluated. Through involving claimant and family, additional services were avoided.

Potential Charges:
Expedited discharge from 1 week acute care at $1,500/day × 7 days = $10,500
Surgeon fees at $100/day = $700
Primary MD fees at $100/day = $700
Subacute care nonnegotiated × 8 days at $900/day = $7,200
Expedited discharge of 1 additional week subacute care at $400/day = $2,800
BLS transportation 1 way at $260 + $8 mile = $324
2 home care visits at $150/visit = $300

Total of Potential Charges:
$22,524

Actual Cost and Related Charges:
Subacute care at $400/day negotiated × 8 days = $3,200
BLS transport at $120 + $5 mile = $160
2 skilled RN visits at $100/visit = $200

Total of Actual Charges and Case Management Fees:
$3,560 + $1,313 = $4,873

Net Savings: $17,651

CASE MANAGEMENT COST-BENEFIT ANALYSIS REPORT

Re: 0003

Carrier/Client Group: Local 123

Date of Referral: 2/9/xx

Date of Closure: 5/12/xx

Total Weeks/Months of Case Management: 2 months

Diagnosis: Total Hip Replacement

Case Management Fees: $1,514

Summary of Intervention:
Options Unlimited implemented home health aide, nursing, and DME services. The claimant was discharged unsafely from the hospital without Options Unlimited's knowledge. The claimant had a knowledge deficit regarding her medication and ambulation regime. Through nursing intervention, it was determined that the claimant was taking two medications that cross-reacted. Through prompt intervention, an emergency visit was avoided. The claimant's teenager was taught to be independent with her mother's injections thus avoiding nursing visits. Physical therapy was implemented in a timely manner as client was at high risk for falls. DME was monitored for appropriate discontinuance of services. The physician was not cooperative with returning case management and home care agency calls. No on-call physician was available.

Claimant's physician answering machine instructed all patients "to go to ER if problem arises."

Potential Charges:
ER visit due to cross-reaction between medication = $750
Unnecessary nursing visits for injections at $150/visit × 2 weeks = $1,500
Home Health Aide services at $18/hour × 2/hrs day × 18 days = $648
PT home visit at $150 × 5 visits = $750
PT visit outpatient via Care Provider

Total of Potential Charges:
$5,148

Actual Cost and Related Charges:
Negotiated:
PT visits × 6 at $85 = $510

Home Health Aide at $15/hr \times 2$ hrs/day $\times 18$ days = $540
Nursing visits at $100/visit $\times 12$ = $1,200

Total of Actual Charges and Case Management Fees:
$2,250 + $1,513 = $3,763

Net Savings: $1,385

CASE MANAGEMENT COST-BENEFIT ANALYSIS REPORT

Re: 0005

Carrier/Client Group: Local 123

Date of Referral: 12/8/xx

Date of Closure: 3/7/xx+1

Total Weeks/Months of Case Management: 3 Months

Diagnosis: Hepatic Encephalopathy

Case Management Fees: $1,064.15

Summary of Intervention:
This quarter, with physician input, case manager formulated a comprehensive plan of care to provide infusion therapy, with skilled nursing, to monitor the claimant's status on a continuous basis during an acute exacerbation of hepatic encephalopathy, thereby providing for a medically safe home environment in lieu of hospitalization. Extensive research was required to select qualitative providers of specific services at cost-effective rates; however, the claimant's husband, a resident physician, strongly objected to home care and maintains that the hospital setting is the only appropriate setting in the event of acute exacerbation. Nutritional counseling was provided in the last quarter. Through the claimant's increased level of understanding of nutritional restrictions and dietary allowances, she has a greater level of compliance to dietary regimen and greater awareness of symptoms of hepatic encephalopathy. As a result, claimant intervenes more readily with oral hydration and complications have been averted. Case closed due to relative stability of status and present refusal to consider option of home infusion therapy.

Potential Charges:
February 1–March 7, xxxx
2 hospital admissions for IV hydration at $1,500/day, 3 days each
  admission = $9,000
  Daily MD visits at $150/day = $900

Total of Potential Charges:
$9,900

Actual Cost and Related Charges:
Nutritional counseling (last quarter) resulted in greater dietary compliance and no acute exacerbations of symptomatology. No hospital admissions since November.

Total of Actual Charges and Case Management Fees:
$1,064 Case Management Fees

Net Savings: $8,836
Lifetime Savings $13,275

CASE MANAGEMENT COST-BENEFIT ANALYSIS REPORT

Re: 0006

Carrier/Client Group: Local 123

Date of Referral: 12/30/xx

Date of Closure: Remains open

Total Weeks/Months of Case Management: 2 months

Diagnosis: Preterm labor, preterm membrane rupture

Case Management Fees: $1,286

Summary of Intervention:
Options Unlimited expedited the claimant's hospital discharge following two hospitalizations through placement of home care services in lieu of prolonged hospital stays. Expedited hospitalization discharge through the placement of home care services for IV hydration, fetal stress testing, and home uterine monitoring at negotiated rates for considerable savings to the benefit provider.

Expedited hospitalization II through the placement of home care services for skilled nursing for wound care and home health aide services due to claimant's C-Section incision opening when wound staples were removed 4 days after surgery. Services were provided at rates negotiated with two providers, Healthcare and Metro Home Care.

Potential Charges:
33 days in hospital at $1,500/day = $49,500
Associated MD visits at $150/day × 33 = $4,950
Nursing visits 2 × day at $150/visit × 14 days = $4,200
Home Health Aide at $160/day × 5 days = $800
Note: Also avoided birth of premature infant

Total of Potential Charges:
$59,450

Actual Cost and Related Charges:
33 days home uterine monitoring at $125/day = $4,125
14 days hydration at $100/day = $1,400
7 days infant nonstress testing at $125/day = $875

14 days wound care at $100/visit × twice day = $2,400
5 days home health aide at 4 hrs/day × $15/hr = $300

Total of Actual Charges and Case Management Fees:
$9,070 + $1,286 = $10,356

Net Savings: $49,094

CASE MANAGEMENT COST-BENEFIT ANALYSIS REPORT

Re: 0009

Carrier/Client Group: Local 123

Date of Referral: 11/27/xx

Date of Closure: 2/6/xx+1

Total Weeks/Months of Case Management: 5 weeks

Diagnosis: Recurrent asthma

Case Management Fees: $652.55

Summary of Intervention:
This claimant has had recurrent hospitalization for asthma. Through case management intervention, the claimant was referred to a pulmonologist and a more aggressive treatment plan was developed. Options Unlimited intervened to coordinate delivery of prescription plan medication. Family and physician were contacted as claimant did not receive medication delivery in a timely manner resulting in noncompliance with medication regime and increasing symptomatology of an asthma attack. Family was directed to contact MD immediately for an interim prescription to obtain medication avoiding an ER visit and hospitalization. Since case management intervention, no further hospitalizations have occurred.

Potential Charges:
Avoidance of ER visit at $750
Avoidance of hospital × 3 days for asthma at $1,500/day = $4,500
Associated MD fees at $100/day × 3 = $300

Total of Potential Charges:
$5,550

Actual Cost and Related Charges:
None

Total of Actual Charges and Case Management Fees:
$652.55 Case Management Fees

Net Savings: $4,897.45

CASE MANAGEMENT COST-BENEFIT ANALYSIS REPORT

Re: 0022

Carrier/Client Group: Local 123

Date of Referral: 12/6/xx

Date of Closure: 2/10/xx+1

Total Weeks/Months of Case Management: 12 weeks

Diagnosis: Coronary Artery Disease/Diabetes

Case Management Fees: $2,430

Summary of Intervention:
During a recent visit to this claimant, this consultant noted that claimant's blood sugars were extremely high. This consultant noted that claimant had stopped taking one of her diabetic medications just prior to a recent procedure, was due to resume taking this following this procedure and never did. Claimant resumed taking this medication after this consultant pointed out this error. This consultant continued to monitor claimant's progress after she resumed her prescribed diabetic medication. Claimant's blood sugars remained moderately high. This consultant recommended that claimant visit her endocrinologist, which she did. Claimant's endocrinologist increased the dosage of claimant's diabetic medication. Claimant had also complained of intermittent midsternal chest pain and did not have a prescription for Nitroglycerine (helps to reduce the workload of the heart, reducing the incidence of heart attack). This consultant directed claimant to contact her cardiologist and notify him of these symptoms, which she did. Cardiologist ordered Nitroglycerine, which relieved the chest pain. This consultant educated, supported, and guided this claimant toward improving her health status. Initially, this claimant had little knowledge of her cardiac or diabetic condition. This consultant was instrumental in the claimant returning to her endocrinologist whom she had not seen in more than 6 months (claimant's blood glucose levels were extremely elevated at this time). This consultant encouraged the claimant to contact her physician when she was experiencing chest pain, which was relieved. Through contact with Dr. M and the Cath Lab, this consultant was able to reschedule this claimant's cardiac cath procedure following a cancellation due to a misunderstanding. This consultant also alerted Dr. M of this claimant's uncontrolled diabetic state. This resulted in better preparation for the catheterization procedure, possibly averting another cancellation.

Potential Charges:
Cardiac Complications:
Two Emergency Room visits at $750 each visit = $1,500
Two admissions to rule out M.I. × 10 days each admission:
C.C.U. × 3 days each admission at $2,000 per day = $12,000
7 days on medical floor each visit to ensure stability on medication at
  $1,500 per day = $21,000
Diabetic Complications:
Two Emergency Room visits at $750 each visit = $1,500
Two MD Emergency Room charges at $125.00 = $250
Two admissions to stabilize diabetic crisis × 10 days each at $1,500
  per day = $30,000

Total of Potential Charges:
$66,250

Actual Cost and Related Charges:
None

Total of Actual Charges and Case Management Fees:
$2,430 Case Management Fees

Net Savings: $63,820

Local 123 Welfare Fund
Second Half-Year Cost-Benefit Analysis for Case Management Services
July 1, xxxx–December 31, xxxx

Cases open at beginning of period	14
Cases referred this period	20
Cases closed during the period	24
Total cases worked during period	34
Total number of open cases	10
Total fees for the period	$ 40,764
Average fees per month	$ 6,794
Average fees per case/period	$ 1,199
Average fees per case/month	$ 200
Total savings for period	
Gross	$413,141
Net	$372,377
Average savings per case/period	$ 10,952
Ratio of dollars to savings	1:10

Note: To evaluate the benefits of a program for a client, we use total fees billed for all cases worked and the savings resulting from our intervention, whether savings were realized in every case, one case, or several cases.

CASE MANAGEMENT COST-BENEFIT ANALYSIS REPORT

Re: 0001

Carrier/Client Group: Local 123

Date of Referral: 3/19/xx

Date of Closure: 7/20/xx

Total Weeks/Months of Case Management: 4 1/2 months

Diagnosis: Liver transplant

Case Management Fees: $1,900 ($4,267 Lifetime Fees)

Summary of Intervention:
Options Unlimited spent a great deal of time on negotiations for hospital-ization and transplant services. Initially, the reimbursement manager was noncompliant with this consultant's multiple phone calls. Contact was made with transplant coordinator to resolve this issue. The facility was also initially not open to negotiations. Through persistent intervention by Options Unlimited, a 30% discount was finally obtained for hospital-ization and transplant services.

Potential Charges:
Hospitalization at $97,324
Transplant services at $122,391

Total of Potential Charges:
$219,715

Actual Cost and Related Charges:
Negotiated rate of $153,800

Total of Actual Charges and Case Management Fees:
$153,800.50 + $1,900 = $155,800

Net Savings: $64,015
Note: Prior net savings of $2,357 = lifetime savings of $66,372

CASE MANAGEMENT COST-BENEFIT ANALYSIS REPORT

Re: 0002

Carrier/Client Group: Local 123

Date of Referral: 7/3/xx

Date of Closure: 9/30/xx

Total Weeks/Months of Case Management: 12 weeks and 4 days

Diagnosis: Coronary Artery Disease

Case Management Fees: $1,349

Summary of Intervention:
Options Unlimited conducted a thorough assessment and expedited this claimant's discharge from acute care to home in a prompt fashion utilizing safe and medically appropriate plan of home care services. These services included a visiting nurse who specializes in diabetic care and teaching as well as postoperative management of home care patients. Home physical therapy was added to this claimant's home program because he was found to have decreased strength and mobility upon initial visiting nurse assessment. The mentioned services were arranged at a cost-effective rate. All services were monitored closely and discontinued once the claimant was medically stable with MD's approval. Options Unlimited coordinated and negotiated cardiac rehabilitation services at a cost-effective, all-inclusive rate. These services included continued monitoring of diabetes and continued education focusing on preventive measures. This consultant researched and encouraged claimant to have a consultation with an endocrinologist for guidance regarding effective diabetic management. Claimant took our advice and is currently under the care of an in-network endocrinologist for diabetes management. Options Unlimited has reviewed claims on an ongoing basis. Claimant is very grateful toward our intervention.

Potential Charges:
Emergency room visit because of ineffective diabetic management = $750
Nonnegotiated visiting nurse services at $150/visit = $1,200
Nonnegotiated home physical therapy services at $150 per visit for
4 visits = $600
Nonnegotiated cardiac rehab services at $200 per visit × 3 days per week for
12 weeks = $7,200

Total of Potential Charges:
$9,759

Actual Cost and Related Charges:
Negotiated visiting nurse service $100 per visit × 8 visits = $800
Negotiated home physical therapy services at $100 for initial eval and $85 per visit thereafter × 4 visits = $440
Negotiated cardiac rehab services at $100 per visit all inclusive × 3 days per week for 12 weeks = $3,600

Total of Actual Charges and Case Management Fees:
$4,840 + $1,349 = $6,189

Net Savings: $3,561 Lifetime Savings

CASE MANAGEMENT COST-BENEFIT ANALYSIS REPORT

Re: 0003

Carrier/Client Group: Local 123

Date of Referral: 6/18/xx

Date of Closure: 10/4/xx

Total Weeks/Months of Case Management: 15 weeks

Diagnosis: Cerebral Aneurysms

Case Management Fees: $2,989

Summary of Intervention:
This consultant monitored this claimant's progress through contact with Dr. S and Lisa C. The claimant's care was monitored for appropriateness and effectiveness. Suggestions were made for changes when appropriate and necessary.

This consultant was able to expedite this claimant's transfer from Brook Memorial Hospital to St. John Rehabilitation Center as soon as Dr. S wrote orders for the same. This avoided additional hospital days that would have been spent by the social worker in an attempt to have completed all of these arrangements (on short notice) independently.

This consultant arranged cost-effective inpatient rehabilitation services through St. John Rehabilitation Center. This claimant's progress was monitored closely and the services provided were assessed for effectiveness.

This consultant was able to arrange for cost-effective skilled nursing services through St. John. This was for a 2-week period following permission from the group to flex benefits for the same.

This consultant was able to arrange cost-effective ambulance and ambulette transportation services when the claimant was transferred from the hospital to the rehabilitation center and back, and again when the claimant needed transportation for a CT scan. This consultant avoided the need for a more expensive ambulance transport by arranging for the claimant's daughter to accompany her in an ambulette.

Potential Charges:
Three additional hospital days spent while the hospital social worker/ discharge planner made arrangements for transfer at $2,000 per day = $6,000
Inpatient rehabilitation services at $1,500 per day × 30 days = $45,000

Ambulance Transportation × 2 at $450 each = $900, plus $9.25 per mile × 36 miles = $333

Total $52,233

Two additional weeks of inpatient rehabilitation services at $550.00 per day = $7,700

Total of Potential Charges:
$59,933

Actual Cost and Related Charges:
Inpatient rehabilitation services at $550 per day × 30 days = $16,500
Ambulance transportation × 1 at $185 plus $3.75 per mile = $252.50
Ambulette transportation × 1 at $25.00 each way plus $1.00 per mile = $68
Two additional weeks of inpatient rehabilitation services at a reduced rate of $300.00 per day = $4,200

Total of Actual Charges and Case Management Fees:
$21,020.50 + $2,989 = $24,009

Net Savings: $35,924 Total Lifetime Savings

CASE MANAGEMENT COST-BENEFIT ANALYSIS REPORT

Re: 0004

Carrier/Client Group: Local 123

Date of Referral: 4/6/xx

Date of Closure: 9/16/xx

Total Weeks/Months of Case Management: 5 $\frac{1}{2}$ months

Diagnosis: Lung Cancer

Case Management Fees: $332 ($1,051 prior fees = $1,383 Lifetime Fees)

Summary of Intervention:
Options Unlimited worked closely with the claimant's oncologist and encouraged the claimant's chemotherapy be administered in the physician's office, 3 days a month for 3 months, when it was demonstrated that the claimant suffered no severe reaction from same during the first 3 months of treatment when it was administered in a more costly hospital setting. Options Unlimited monitored the claimant closely for chemotherapy side effects and complications.

Potential Charges:
9 days hospitalization at $1,500/day = $13,500
9 MD visits at $100/visit = $900

Total of Potential Charges:
$14,400

Actual Cost and Related Charges:
9 days of chemotherapy at $269.47 = $2,425.23

Total of Actual Charges and Case Management Fees:
$2,425.23 + $332 = $2,757

Net Savings: $11,643.00
Note: Prior savings of $8,100 = $19,743 Total Lifetime Savings

CASE MANAGEMENT COST-BENEFIT ANALYSIS REPORT

Re: 0008

Carrier/Client Group: Local 123

Date of Referral: 11/20/xx

Date of Closure: 8/28/xx+1

Total Weeks/Months of Case Management: 10 months

Diagnosis: Cancer of Nasopharynx

Case Management Fees: $3,075.33 ($4,104 Lifetime Fees)

Summary of Intervention:
As claimant's condition deteriorated, we sought and obtained approval to set up hospice services at home. A per service arrangement was negotiated rather than a per diem as the claimant needs were limited and this was much more cost-effective. Timely and appropriate intervention and support by Options Unlimited case manager avoided hospitalization or the need for inpatient hospice. The claimant expired on 8/26/xx+1.

Potential Charges:
2 hospital stays at 5 days each or 10 days at $2,000/day = $20,000
Associated MD visits at $100/visit × 10 = $1,000
Inpatient hospice at 14 days × $450/day = $6,300
Per diem rate for home hospice = $125/day × 20 days = $2,500

Total of Potential Charges:
$29,800

Actual Cost and Related Charges:
Home hospice at per service rate for a total of services of approximately =
  $1,500

Total of Actual Charges and Case Management Fees:
$1,500 + $3,075 = $4,575

Net Savings: $25,225
Note: Lifetime Net Savings $21,121

CASE MANAGEMENT COST-BENEFIT ANALYSIS REPORT

Re: 0026

Carrier/Client Group: Local 123

Date of Referral: 6/12/xx

Date of Closure: 7/13/xx

Total Weeks/Months of Case Management: 1 month

Diagnosis: Status Asthmaticus

Case Management Fees: $608

Summary of Intervention:
Options Unlimited expedited the claimant's discharge from the hospital through the placement of skilled nursing visits provided by a Spanish-speaking nurse from a home care agency in order to provide the claimant and her mother with the necessary knowledge base of her disease process and compliance with her plan of treatment in order to prevent unnecessary ER visits and/or hospitalization due to disease exacerbation. The claimant has been compliant and returned to school full-time. Previous to Options Unlimited intervention, the claimant had missed 102 days of school this school year.

Potential Charges:
1 ER visit at $750
3 days hospitalization at $2,000/day = $6,000
3 MD visits at $100/each = $300
4 SNV nonnegotiated rate of $150/visit = $600

Total of Potential Charges:
$9,650

Actual Cost and Related Charges:
4 SNV at negotiated rate of $100/visit = $400

Total of Actual Charges and Case Management Fees:
$400 + $608 = $1,008

Net Savings: $8,642 Lifetime Savings

Source: Courtesy of Options Unlimited, Case Management Services Division, © 2003, Huntington, New York.

APPENDIX 12–D

Expanded Cost-Benefit Analysis Summary for Self-Funded Plan

July 1, xxxx–September, 30, xxxx
Third Quarter Cost-Benefit Analysis for Case Management
Services for Sam's

Cases open at beginning of period	4	
Cases referred this period	0	
Cases closed during the period	5	
Total cases worked during period	7	
Total number of open cases	2	
Total fees for the period		$ 5,325.00
Average fees per month		$ 1,775.00
Average fees per case/period		$ 761.00
Average fees per case/month		$ 254.00
Total savings for period		
Gross		$59,946.00
Net		$54,621.00
Average savings per case/period		$ 7,803.00
Ratio of dollars to savings	1:11	

Note: To evaluate the benefits of a program for a client, we use total fees billed for all cases worked and the savings resulting from our intervention, whether savings were realized in every case, one case, or several cases.

CASE MANAGEMENT COST-BENEFIT ANALYSIS REPORT

Re: 0001

Carrier/Client Group: Sam's

Date of Referral: 1/10/xx

Date of Closure: Open

Total Weeks/Months of Case Management: 9 months

Diagnosis: Congestive Heart Failure; Pulmonary Emboli; Morbid Obesity; Psoriasis

Case Management Fees: $1,475

Summary of Intervention:
Through case management intervention, the claimant continues to be provided with durable medical equipment at negotiated monthly rental. During this quarter, Options coordinated the claimant's relocation to another area in Georgia, without interruption to care or services and by researching quality and cost-effective providers in his area. With our ongoing and continuous support, the claimant has been compliant with all physician visits and his plan of treatment, which has resulted in an additional *27-pound weight loss,* with a total weight loss of 180 pounds in a 9-month period. The claimant continues to work full-time without need for hospitalization since our involvement. Our intervention will continue, although to a lesser extent, in order to ensure that the claimant reaches his target weight.

Potential Charges:
3 months nonnegotiated rate for CPAP respirator at $475/mo. = $1,425
3 months nonnegotiated rate for Oxygen Concentrator at $450/mo. = $1,350
1 ER visit at Georgia rate = $500
3 days hospitalization (for respiratory/cardiac complication) at $1,300/day = $3,900
3 MD visits at $100 = $300

Total of Potential Charges:
$7,475

Actual Cost and Related Charges:
3 months CPAP Machine rental at $225/month = $8,675
3 months Oxygen Concentrator at $175/month = $525

Total of Actual Charges and Case Management Fees:
$1,200 + $1,475 = $2,675

Net Savings: $4,800

CASE MANAGEMENT COST-BENEFIT ANALYSIS REPORT

Re: 0002

Carrier/Client Group: Sam's

Date of Referral: 5/22/xx

Date of Closure: 8/22/xx

Total Weeks/Months of Case Management: 3 months

Diagnosis: Status Asthmaticus; Asthma

Case Management Fees: $398

Summary of Intervention:
This 1-year-old girl was identified for case management during her admission to the hospital for a severe asthma episode. NOTE: This little girl had three hospital admissions last year for the same diagnosis and was identified at that time; however, the mother did not respond to our letter or phone calls. This time, she was more receptive and we have been able to direct her to appropriate medical care as well as advise her of the necessity to rid the home of the causative factors, for example, a cat, smoking adults, etc. Our case manager also reviewed with the parent the importance of seeking treatment at the first signs of respiratory distress. The child appears to be medically stable and the mother more compliant, and our file has been closed. There have been no further episodes.

Potential Charges:
Avoidance of hospital admission for asthma at $2,000/day at 5 days = $10,000
MD visits at $100/visit × 5 = $500

Total of Potential Charges:
$10,500

Actual Cost and Related Charges:
None

Total of Actual Charges and Case Management Fees:
$1,200

Net Savings: $9,300

CASE MANAGEMENT SECOND QUARTER
COST-BENEFIT ANALYSIS REPORT

Note: This second quarter report for case 0003 is included to illustrate previous intervention and savings, which are then added to savings in the third quarter to reflect lifetime savings on this case.

Re: 0003

Carrier/Client Group: Sam's

Date of Referral: 11/17/xx

Date of Closure: Open

Total Weeks/Months of Case Management: 7 $\frac{1}{2}$ months

Diagnosis: High Risk Pregnancy; Uncontrolled Diabetes

Case Management Fees: $4,320

Summary of Intervention:
Our case manager was intensely involved with this woman for this 3-month period of time. The patient, because of emotional/marital problems, cultural differences, and lack of education, was extremely noncompliant with prescribed medical appointments. In order to avoid premature delivery of her baby (which was highly likely) and to prevent long-term confinement of this mother in the hospital for the protection of her and the unborn infant, Options arranged for home care visits (with favorable negotiated rates) and visits by a Public Health Nurse (at no cost to the plan) in order to collaborate strategies to manage this case. It was also necessary to research a pediatrician who would work with the treating obstetrician in minimizing the risks for this infant *and* who would be covered by the network and Medicaid. Despite all of this intervention, the patient, after an upset with her husband, did not take her insulin or check her blood sugars and required hospitalization. Options, in discussion with MD and nursing staff, recommended extended stay to allow for medical and emotional stability. Following a nine-day stay, she safely delivered her healthy baby on 5-29-97. Our involvement will continue for a while longer to ensure that the mother's diabetes returns to a safer status and to monitor the infant for diabetes as well.

Potential Charges:
Avoidance of premature delivery of infant 3 months prior to expected date of confinement:
3 months in Neonatal ICU at $3,000/day = $270,000

MD visits (2 specialists at $100 ea. × 90 days) = $18,000

OR

Continuous confinement of mother in hospital at $2,000/day × 90 = $180,000

MD visits at $100 × 90 = $9,000

Total of Potential Charges:
Range from $189,000 to $288,000

Actual Cost and Related Charges:
Hospital confinement at $2,000/day × 9 days = $18,000
MD visits at $100 × 9 = $900
Nursing visits at negotiated $100/visit × 6 = $600

Total of Actual Charges and Case Management Fees:
$19,500 + $4,320 = $23,820

Net Savings: Range from $165,180 to $264,178

CASE MANAGEMENT THIRD QUARTER
COST-BENEFIT ANALYSIS REPORT

Re: 0003

Carrier/Client Group: Sam's

Date of Referral: 11/17/xx

Date of Closure: 8/30/xx+1

Total Weeks/Months of Case Management: 9 $\frac{1}{2}$ months

Diagnosis: High-Risk Pregnancy; Diabetes

Case Management Fees: $755 (prior fees of $6,458 results in total fees of
   $7,213 for life of case)

Summary of Intervention:
During the last 2 months of case management, Options monitored the status of the claimant and her infant daughter to ensure stability and compliance. Because of our case manager's close follow-up, the newborn received appropriate care, and the claimant became much more aware of the need to seek medical treatment for herself. Because of this awareness, the claimant avoided a lengthy hospitalization when she sought treatment after developing a hematoma (collection of blood under the skin surface). The incision and drainage only required an overnight stay instead of a much longer one that would have occurred had she delayed treatment (which had been her usual behavior). Home care services were discontinued in a timely manner. The claimant and infant are receiving the public assistance they are eligible for and the claimant's marital/domestic status appears to be stable. Options was able to contribute significantly to the successful outcome of this extremely medically volatile case, a safe delivery and healthy baby, and *tremendous* savings to the Plan (presented in prior 1st- and 2nd-quarter reports). NOTE: Claimant has expressed a high degree of satisfaction with Options case management services . . . Patient Satisfaction Survey response included.

Potential Charges:
Additional 3 days in hospital due to complications following hematoma
   @ $2,000/day = $6,000
MD visits at $100/visit = $300

Total of Potential Charges:
$6,300

Actual Cost and Related Charges:
Overnight hospital admission at $2,000
MD visit = $100

Total of Actual Charges and Case Management Fees:
$2,100 + $755 = $2,855

Net Savings: $3,445
Note: Prior net savings of $165,180 results in total *net* savings of $168,625 for life of this case.

CASE MANAGEMENT COST-BENEFIT ANALYSIS REPORT

Re: 0004

Carrier/Client Group: Sam's

Date of Referral: 6/6/xx

Date of Closure: 7/30/xx

Total Weeks/Months of Case Management: 7 weeks

Diagnosis: Depression

Case Management Fees: $700

Summary of Intervention:
This file was identified for case management following claimant's admission to a facility for treatment of depression. Options immediately began negotiations in order to maximize the use of available benefits. We were able to expedite the claimant's discharge by 10 days and continued to monitor the effectiveness of the treatment plan as well as his compliance with recommendations. He became medically stable and continued with the necessary outpatient services in a county mental health program.

Potential Charges:
30 days hospitalization at a nonnegotiated daily rate of $1,500 = $45,000
    (paid at 80% as per plan would have exhausted his lifetime benefit of $36,000)

Total of Potential Charges:
$45,000

Actual Cost and Related Charges:
21 days at negotiated rate of $750/day = $15,750

Total of Actual Charges and Case Management Fees:
$15,750 + $700 = $16,450

Net Savings: $28,550

CASE MANAGEMENT COST-BENEFIT ANALYSIS REPORT

Re: 0005

Carrier/Client Group: Sam's

Date of Referral: 5/28/xx

Date of Closure: 8/14/xx

Total Weeks/Months of Case Management: 10 weeks

Diagnosis: Anxiety Disorder

Case Management Fees: $682

Summary of Intervention:
This case was referred directly by Total Plan Administrators, Inc., the TPA, after they received a request to flex inpatient benefits for outpatient benefits. Had benefits not been flexed, the claimant would have been admitted to Willowtree Hospital. After discussion, it was determined that the claimant would benefit from a full-day program in lieu of inpatient hospitalization. This consultant negotiated a cost-effective rate for the day program. Options monitored the claimant's status for effectiveness of her treatment plan and gradually decreased services, working in conjunction with the recommendations of MD. Clinical updates were reviewed on a weekly basis. As the claimant's condition stabilized, this consultant discussed the feasibility of the claimant attending half days in lieu of full days in the program. A cost-effective rate was agreed upon and the claimant transitioned to the three-hour morning program on June 24th. The claimant was discharged from the program on July 5th. Since the claimant's condition has stabilized, this case was closed to case management intervention.

Potential Charges:
Inpatient hospitalization at $1,500/day × 30 days = $45,000 (exhausting plan limit of $25,000)

Total of Potential Charges:
$25,000

Actual Cost and Related Charges:
Day hospital program at 300/day × 15 days = $4,500
Partial hospital program at $150/day × 10 days = $1,500

Total of Actual Charges and Case Management Fees:
$6,000 + $725 = $6,725

Net Savings: $18,275

CASE MANAGEMENT COST-BENEFIT ANALYSIS REPORT

Re: 0006

Carrier/Client Group: Sam's

Date of Referral: 6/12/xx

Date of Closure: 7/2/xx

Total Weeks/Months of Case Management: 3 weeks

Diagnosis: Traumatic eye injury

Case Management Fees: $600

Summary of Intervention:
The claimant, being an adolescent and having lost his left eye secondary to trauma, exhibited emotional problems that impacted his follow-up care. The claimant refused a psychological evaluation. This consultant contacted the claimant's mother and encouraged her to contact the psychologist for strategies in dealing with her son. The claimant refused to see the surgeon postoperatively. This consultant instructed her to inform her son of the potential damage to the "good" eye if an infection develops. She followed the advice resulting in appropriate follow-up care, thus avoiding inpatient hospitalization and treatment secondary to complications.

Potential Charges:
Emergency Room visit due to infection at $700
MD fees at $125
Inpatient treatment to stabilize and treat infection:
   $1,500/day × 5 days = $7,500
   MD fees = $625

Total of Potential Charges:
$8,950

Actual Cost and Related Charges:
None

Total of Actual Charges and Case Management Fees:
$600 Case Management Fees

Net Savings: $8,350

CASE MANAGEMENT COST-BENEFIT ANALYSIS REPORT

Re: 0007

Carrier/Client Group: Sam's

Date of Referral: 1/24/xx

Date of Closure: Remains Open

Total Weeks/Months of Case Management: 8.1 months

Diagnosis: Brain Tumor

Case Management Fees: $896

Summary of Intervention:
This quarter, case manager monitored the claimant's course of recovery since undergoing brain surgery in June; prior to this time, her mother-in-law attended to all the medical issues, as well as assisted the claimant with her ADLs; however, her husband underwent CABG surgery and she returned to her home upstate. Postoperatively, the claimant was seizure and headache free. She underwent surgery for an ovarian cyst with uneventful recovery. Case manager intended to close file, but claimant began experiencing seizure activity again. Claimant has apparently developed a suspicious lesion that will be investigated further. She will also be evaluated by a seizure specialist. Case manager will obtain all pertinent medical data to determine if further surgical intervention is indicated and formulate appropriate level of care if needed. Case manager also intervened when home care agency submitted billing in excess of terms of provider agreement for claims that had already been paid.

Potential Charges:
Home occupational therapy/excess charges = $750

Total of Potential Charges:
$750

Actual Cost and Related Charges:
Occupational therapy paid as per provider agreement.

Total of Actual Charges and Case Management Fees:
$896 Case Management fees

Net Savings: None

Source: Courtesy of Options Unlimited, Case Management Services Division, © 2003, Huntington, New York.

Managing a Case Management Department: Your Role as Department Head or Independent Case Manager

REDEFINING CASE MANAGEMENT

In insurance companies, hospital systems, claims departments, and managed care service organizations I have visited across the country, case management is adrift. Many programs lack clear goals, departments manage the distribution of provider services rather than identifying and managing patient problems, and cursory preadmission review masquerades as case management. Effective case management is the foundation for successful managed care. To make it work, we must take stock of our case management programs and get back to the basics.

How Did We Get Off Track?

We stopped—or never began—managing the care of a patient across the continuum of care, in multiple settings, addressing the ongoing needs of the individual. Instead, I see the management of benefits and/or services a patient uses within the system (physicians, infusion, pharmaceutical benefits, rehab, home care); episodic management, in which only a single setting (rehab, home care, hospital) is even recorded, much less managed; nonintegrated programs, where one patient's case is "managed" both by Jane in Home Care, by Alice in Rehab, and by four different precert nurses who log in multiple hospital admissions (so no one is able to say, "Wait, he was only home three days, let's see what the problem is"); or redundant review, in which *all* home care services are tracked, with no distinction made for those patients who only need an occasional skilled visit. Too often in my role as a consultant, I find that the measure of success in some departments is shortening the length of stay.

Not every AIDS case or high-risk pregnancy needs a case manager, but every case should be screened by a professional to determine whether it poses a significant health and financial risk. Does this person require an intermediary to make sure she receives appropriate care to prevent potential problems from occurring? By the same token, if cardiac cases are managed in the hospital, but no one reaches beyond discharge to coordinate care outside the hospital or to verify patient compliance, that's not true case management.

The principle behind effective case management remains: Only a *small percentage* of people using expensive services are driving up costs. To provide high-quality, appropriate care, and rein in costs by curtailing clinical risks and dollar exposure, we must address the individual with the problem. Until the patient is contacted, how can one determine what the problems really are?

Nurses have good instincts. They know a problem when they see it, but sometimes corporate structure with its approval requirements makes it impossible for personal insight to have an impact. Overreliance on system-generated "guru guidelines" that make sense to no one also drive up costs. Remember the widely decried mastectomy as a day-op procedure? Or, think of today's day-op prostatectomy. Several red flags indicating a need for further case review and follow-up might well be present, but go unremarked because they don't fit into the boxes to be checked on a survey. What is the incidence of readmission? Infection? Are there signs of bleeding into a catheter or blockage of the catheter?

Back to Basics

Effective case management requires a well-designed case identification methodology, flexibility in management options, the ability to move a person quickly through a system, and prompt decisions and exceptions to benefit plan language as needed. A case manager can begin to realign a case management program by evaluating the group's healthcare issues and then gradually tailoring a program that targets them. One solution implemented over a wide expanse of cases is not the answer. No one would deluge a patient with multiple drugs and then try to sort out the side effects.

Whether a case manager is heading up a hospital's case management program, an insurance carrier case manager, or a home care agency's case management supervisor, she should consider the organization's mission statement. What are its goals, what is senior management looking for? Are the goals reasonable for her staff? Would they benefit from additional training? As a nurse, she would not intervene with a patient unless she understood his problems and needs. That same principle should be applied in this business/medical environment.

I firmly believe that we need to do more to demonstrate our success for ourselves, our staff, and those supervising our departments. We must define our role and contribution. When management understands the contribution of nurses and case managers, there is no question of their value. Create a report format that shows how case management intervention impacted the healthcare outcome and the cost of care. Continue to "get smart." The entire healthcare field has moved into the world of business. We must educate ourselves and our nurses on the clinical, managerial, and financial aspects of healthcare at the graduate and undergraduate level. We have already waited too long.

Evaluating a CM Department

1. Where are your high-cost cases? Identify the type of cases (diabetes, cancer, high-risk pregnancy) that require management within your employee group, hospital, admissions group, or covered lives.
2. Why are you managing those cases? What is the clinical risk to the patient and financial risk to your group (that is, how much more will it cost if you do not manage this case)? Are you discriminating between long-term, chronic illnesses, and the person who only needs IV antibiotics for 5 to 7 days?
3. Is there a sound system in place to identify cases for case management? Do nurses talk to patients and evaluate their needs? If an administrative assistant scans paperwork, a computer system flags certain diagnoses, services are based on LOS alone, or patients are automatically moved into case management only after they have exhausted their standard contract benefits or require an exception to plan language, you need to revise your mechanism.
4. How flexible are your case management red flags? Is it easy to identify and bring someone into case management? If it takes weeks or months, you do not have an effective case management program. Are multiple layers of people consulted to resolve problems, or do you and your staff have authority and autonomy to act?

5. What have you done to improve patients' overall outcomes? You should be able to record the clinical steps taken and why, and the patients' experiences. You should also see clear contrast in patient care improvement and in benefits spent among cases that are not managed and those that are.

6. Have you set goals? You must know what success looks like in order to implement the steps to achieve it, and then evaluate it. Highly important and often overlooked are the outcomes that are actually communicated to the payer. There is a need for case managers to be willing to be completely accountable; to take credit for our successes, we must continually evaluate our work. The days of an employer thinking, "If I'm paying for it, it must be working" are gone.

BECOMING AN INDEPENDENT CASE MANAGER

As in other entrepreneurial endeavors, there are advantages and disadvantages in "going it alone," and one should evaluate these carefully before hanging out one's shingle. Thanks to some very important changes, both in healthcare and our economy, small businesses are on the rise. Although many succeed, some do not fare so well. Being given the opportunity for success does not automatically guarantee it, nor does being a truly excellent case manager guarantee profits.

Why then should one consider taking this step? The benefits are numerous. As the statistics bear out, case management has been and will continue to be one of the most effective tools in the growing array of cost-containment and quality assurance tools in the marketplace today. Following mergers and changes in our economy, the large corporate giants are downsizing, and this trend has resulted in the creation and growth of numerous, smaller competitive companies. These companies are facing the same need to contain the costs related to illness and disability and are likely to use the services of smaller case management companies and even independent practitioners. Likewise for the growing number of midsized corporations that are increasingly dissatisfied with lack of attention to their needs and a gap in provision of services. These smaller and midsized companies are facing accelerating concerns; employee ill health and disabilities often have a greater impact and increased risk for these firms, regardless of their funding arrangements. Independents are certainly able to capture a share of this market, as these companies are not necessarily looking for the giants in the case management community.

To case managers who have worked in corporations, hospitals, and healthcare facilities, some of the problems that characterize large bureaucracies are evident: too many layers of management, too many meetings, too many delays. ("I'll take that suggestion under advisement," "Let's table that for our next meeting.") Are these reasons for becoming an independent practitioner? Perhaps not, but bureaucratic aggravations frequently lead individuals to at least consider starting their own companies.

Autonomy is one advantage, but there are others. Creating and expanding a company provides an opportunity to develop and use talents and skills, including marketing, public relations, financial management, negotiating, risk management, sales, accounting, personnel development, and human resources.

Then there are the financial considerations. No longer is it necessary to wait to be given a raise or a promotion; just write a check! Sound too good to be true? It is, but the opportunity for financial gain is most definitely there.

Given all of these wonderful advantages—autonomy, growth, creativity, and opportunity for success and wealth—what reason could there be for not going it alone? Unfortunately, the disadvantages are almost as numerous as the advantages.

Large organizations may have their problems, but they would not exist if they lacked value entirely. Their very size means that many outstanding professionals work side by side and are able to share their knowledge. When case managers leave this type of environment, they usually miss the camaraderie.

Those individuals were not only colleagues, but many became friends. Friends to have lunch with, discuss goals and dreams with, commiserate with, and have fun with. In addition to those who shared a profession (be it nurse, social worker, rehabilitation counselor), the case managers had other departments and their personnel and resources to draw from while learning and developing an area of expertise. The kind of isolation that comes with independence can truly be overwhelming when cases are not progressing as hoped, when client companies are upset about the time billed on a case, and potential clients, after extensive wooing, select another case management company. These things do happen and sometimes all in one day. Who can one share this with? Not with clients, who would feel anxious if they learned about such problems, nor with colleagues, who may also be competitors. A certain amount of isolation is unavoidable and needs to be addressed. It is easy to keep going when all is well but tougher when it is not.

Although starting a case management company provides an opportunity to create a business from the ground up, it does require learning about things that were of little use before but are now very important. Remember that big company? Aside from the medical staff, it also had departments and services that were probably taken for granted: purchasing, personnel, communications, public relations, and a business office. An independent case manager assumes other roles and performs other functions necessary to keep the business afloat. Remember also the security of knowing that a payroll check will come every 2 weeks? This, too, is no longer a "given." Neither is a 2- or 4-week vacation, paid holidays, or a medical and dental benefits package. In short, the financial security of being an employee has been traded for the opportunity for substantial gains—an opportunity that may never be realized.

FOR YOUR BUSINESS OR DEPARTMENT

So much for the pros and cons of becoming an independent practitioner. After consideration of these factors and others, if there is still a determination to take the next step, what should that be? Whether working to revitalize a case management department or start an independent business, the creation of a business plan should be the first move. Just as in case management, the strategy is to gather all of the necessary information, evaluate the situation, and identify the steps that will ensure a successful outcome. Looking at incorporating long- and short-term goals, strategy is then implemented, progress is monitored, and problems are identified and solved one by one. Why is a business plan necessary, and does it need to be a lengthy, formal document? Not really, especially if in the beginning the company will essentially be a one-person operation or if the plan is being developed for monitoring of progress within the case management department only. But a case manager trying to coordinate care and services on behalf of 20 to 25 cases in different lines of insurance for several different client groups needs to have the structure. Every case management business and all case management department operations require some kind of planning—a framework to provide ongoing direction.

DEVELOPING A BUSINESS PLAN

What should a business plan incorporate? Are there key components that every plan should have? Following is a list of important issues to address.

- **Type of company:** Should it be a full-service company? Should it be restricted to medical case management only? One disease state or one type of insurance only (for example, workers' compensation, liability, group medical)?

- **Location:** Will the company provide services in one town or city? In one or several counties? In the entire state?

- **Size:** Some case managers want to work cases themselves. They have no interest in taking on partners or hiring and supervising other case managers. Others are willing to make that next and very critical move: becoming an employer. Establishing limitations regarding size and number of cases right at the beginning is extremely important. A case manager with 25 cases might be offered 3, 5, or 10 more. Does she say "No, I don't want any more work," take them and be unable to work them, or be spread so thin that the quality of her work suffers? Or, does she start thinking about getting a partner?

- **Financial resources:** Most small businesses require some kind of budget. In addition to salary, there are other expenses: telephone, fax, e-mail, rent, utilities, business and professional liability insurance, postage, office supplies, equipment, and furnishings. Depending on personal finances, a small business loan might need to be considered. A loan assists in defraying some of the start-up costs and keeps the business going until payments from accounts start coming in. If a large portion of business will be with insurance companies, TPAs, and other large groups, payment for services may not be received until 60 to 90 days after invoicing. This kind of delay can certainly result in financial strain, but it can be planned for instead of coming as a worrisome "surprise." As new accounts are acquired, assessing their financial status becomes as crucial as knowing one's own. To illustrate, one of my accounts is a TPA with a consistently expanding client base. Although I was very excited to learn that all their clients would be using our case management services, that excitement soon turned to anxiety. Two of these accounts went into chapter 11 (filed for bankruptcy). Another small group had their financial office review each payment before authorizing the TPA to release the checks, and still another only funded its account every 60 days. The combination of lost payments and delays in reimbursement had a definite impact on my business, because I had already paid my staff for the work they had done. This example also demonstrates the need to have not only a financial plan, but also some contingency plans.

- **Short- and long-term goals:** In good case management, it is essential to define goals in order to ensure movement of a case toward a successful outcome. The same applies to business planning.

Establish some attainable and maybe some not-so-attainable goals for the next year, for the next 5 years, and for the next 10 years. Obviously, changes in the healthcare industry and the national or local economy may prevent reaching all goals in the planned time frame, but the goals should be set anyway. They will act as "benchmarks" for evaluating and reevaluating the company's direction. Revising a business plan several times in a year or every few years is not a problem. Not having a plan most assuredly will be.

Following is a checklist of assessments to make and needs to consider:

Assess Your Personal Skill Sets
- Skills from nursing and other business experience
- Skills from family finances management
- Skills from life: soccer moms develop excellent organizational and team-building skills

Know Your Strengths and Weaknesses
- What are you good at? You will be doing the work.
- What do you enjoy? You need to enjoy your role to take you through the hard times.
- What are your business and organizational skills?

What Type of Business Do You Envision?
- Do you want a partner—someone to complement or match your skills, for example, one person who is clinically proficient and one with business acumen?
- Will you do consulting work?
- Will you oversee a CM office or department?
- Will you do the case work yourself, maintaining a workable caseload?

Define Your Nature and Personality
- Can you say no?
- Can you sustain your spirit through the early months of potentially uneven returns?
- Do not start a business just because you are a great case manager and/or RN.

What Role Do You Want to Play?
- Where can you make a difference, so your job will be fulfilling?
- What is the need in your community—growing migrant, immigrant, or elder population?
- What is your niche or specialty—oncology, pediatrics, public sector case management?

- Select a clinical niche.
- Select a practice setting.
- Take your CM skills to your company.

Financial and Business Issues
- How will you finance your start-up?
- Do you have 3 to 6 months of assets to tide you over?
- How will you cost-out your services?
- Can you establish a banking relationship?
- Can you hire an accountant?
- How will you create access to legal counsel?
- How will you create contracts for staff and clients?
- Do you know licensing and business regulations for your state?

PRICING THE MARKET

One of the most difficult tasks a new case manager starting a business will have is determining how much to charge for the services provided. Unfortunately, there are no hard-and-fast rules for setting prices. Some may believe that undercutting the competition guarantees business, but this strategy can backfire. It may net a few cases from those who always look for the "cheapest of everything," but more will wonder why the prices are so low. The tendency will be to think services are probably not as good as those provided by other, more established companies. Pricing services closer to the competition is actually a more astute business strategy, especially if the goal is to grow.

To illustrate further, let us say the going rate for case management services in your locale is $75 per hour. You are just starting out, working out of your home. You have no secretary (preparing your reports on your computer) and are managing all the cases yourself. You were making $27 per hour plus benefits in a case management company when you left to start your own business. You really want business, so you decide to charge $35 an hour and are looking forward to considerable profit. You also believe that if you charge $35 and others are charging $75, then you will definitely get business. And you do.

You continue and soon are up to 25 cases, cannot work any more yourself, and decide to hire your first staff case manager. She is perfect, except for one thing: She is not computer literate. So you also hire a secretary. These two additions to your staff cannot work out of your home, so you move into a new office. You have thus, in a short period of time, increased your expenses more than your income. Now what? You need to raise your rates! How do you explain to your new accounts that you will now have to double your rates to $70 an hour or increase even more? An uncomfortable position to be sure—and one indicative of inexperience in business.

Discussions with your accountant or banker will be helpful in deciding a fair market value for your services. Whatever the rate decided upon, it should reflect your costs and allow you to generate a profit. A profit margin is desirable in order for you to continue to be able to upgrade and expand your business, unless, of course, you want to join the not-for-profit organizations or engage strictly in "pro bono" work.

There are various directories and other publications that list companies and provide information about their services and, in many instances, their current rates. The information is fairly reliable, but keep in mind that many of the listed companies may be large, provide several kinds of cost-containment services, or have a national capability, and the costs of any extra services are built into their hourly rates. So although published rates may be helpful, a company's own rates should reflect its cost of doing business rather than being a mirror image of the competition.

LOOKING AT THE COMPETITION

Every case management company and independent practitioner must consider others in the community who are in the same field. This can be intimidating, but it also provides an awareness that case management is a growing industry. Competition is good. It keeps case managers on their toes and helps them stretch toward excellence. Also, "breaking into" the marketplace may be easier if there are others who have gone before. Being the only provider of a service does *not* guarantee a company the entire market and may, in fact, create more problems. Why? Because there is reluctance on the part of purchasers to buy an unknown, no matter how good it may sound. They are inclined to think, "Let the others buy it first, and then we can see how they like it."

Fortunately, case management is already a tried-and-true service. Others have gone before and have demonstrated its worth. The object, then, is to establish a niche among competitors. Rather than being afraid of what they are doing, learn to seek knowledge about what is already out there. This is not difficult to come by. Attending conferences and visiting the exhibitors' area provides firsthand information. The Internet offers fast access to vast amounts of educational, clinical, statistical, operational, and administrative data and resources, and serves as a guide to other books, associations, foundations, and groups. As case managers are now a target market for pharmaceutical and other companies, it is wise to take the time to sort the reliable information from the marketing language.

When you place an online request for rheumatoid arthritis information, the pharmaceutical companies with products used to treat the condition are likely to top your search engine list of sites.

Large companies usually print brochures and other handouts that describe their services and list their office locations, areas of specialization, and occasionally even their fees. Smaller regional or local companies also have marketing handouts, and these should be reviewed carefully to discover exactly what these companies are selling to potential clients. Similarities and differences in services can be utilized to help define one's own corporate identity.

Being knowledgeable about the competition and their various activities is part of being in business. Although "hot off the press" information is not always available, information about changes in competitors' client base, rate changes, and innovative services and approaches can be gleaned from various sources. Of most importance is how the competition responds to change. Changes in workers' compensation programs, employer involvement in benefit plans, wellness promotion, management approaches to high-cost and chronic conditions (for example, high-risk pregnancies, cancer, COPD, asthma), and outcomes research influence the direction of case management. How each company responds to these changes will obviously be different, and much can be learned from the successes and the failures of colleagues.

The successful approaches will eventually be described in articles in industry publications (for example, *The Case Manager, Case Management Advisor, Inside Case Management, Business & Health Institute* at www .businessandhealth.com [previously *Business & Health* magazine], *Business Insurance,* and *Risk Management*) or in presentations at various conferences. Keeping abreast, therefore, is as easy as attending conferences and reading industry periodicals. Attending conferences, in addition to updating one's clinical and business knowledge, also affords a wonderful opportunity to interact with competitors in a social environment. Sharing experiences and frustrations frequently results in an enhanced ability to view problems and challenges more objectively and to move toward resolution.

For instance, in a breakout session of a case management conference, there were several case managers representing the national and regional companies as well as independent practitioners. This session was focused on the "business" aspects of case management. There was discussion of billing, including the various approaches used to bill for services and client responses to bills. Interestingly, despite the differences in invoice formats and hourly rates, we learned that we did actually have something in common. Each of us at one time had a client who called to question some aspect of a bill. "Did it really take four tenths of an hour to make that phone call?" "Couldn't you have done it in one tenth or two tenths of an hour?" "Company X never charged me for that and you do."

From the conversation, during which we shared the all-too-familiar "war stories" of client objections, it became apparent that case management is being looked at closely. Our results and our costs are being examined. It also was clear that the main cause of client discontent over billing was not skepticism about the efficacy of the services or the reasonableness of the bills but rather lack of documentation. By discussing how to prepare cost-benefit analysis reports, we reviewed how to draft documents that demonstrated the benefits of case management intervention as well as its ability to contain costs. This sharing of information among various case management providers uncovered the solution to a very real problem.

Was this "helping" the competition? Isn't that a business no-no? Aren't we supposed to hope competitors fail and then grab their clients? There was a time when I engaged in that kind of thinking. Although not actively hoping that anyone would fail, I had ambivalent feelings about sharing any of my knowledge with the competition. Experience gained over many years has helped me to view the issue of sharing somewhat differently. If the providers of case management services become better at what they do, then the viability of case management is assured. Because sharing information improves the performance of practitioners, it enhances the status of the entire case management industry and makes it more likely any given practitioner will survive.

A recent example of that kind of thinking put into action was the "Visioneering Case Management's Future" invitational meeting, cohosted by The Academy of Certified Case Managers (ACCM) and CMSA in December 2002. Major players and stakeholders in the case management industry came together to discuss the challenges in healthcare management and case management in particular, and strategies to ensure the viability of our industry. The success of the meeting and its outcomes was and continues to be dependent on the willingness of the sometimes competing groups to candidly share concerns, perceived shortcomings, and the solutions each has found for specific problems. Attending were representatives from a range of practice settings, provider and payer groups, and associations, including the Academy of Certified Case Managers, American Association of Occupational Health Nurses, American Society on Aging, Association of Rehabilitation Nursing, Blue Cross/Blue Shield, CCMC, Health Insurance Association of America, Lippincott's *CM*

Journal, Michigan State University, National Association of Social Workers, St. Vincent's Hospital, Trustmark, University of Arizona, and more.

What about those in our industry who, in our judgment, may be doing it a disservice? This includes those who may have different business practices or who may attempt to garner clients by waging a price war or who just may not be good providers. How should one react when potential clients cite these case managers as the norm? Perhaps a client has had a very bad experience with such a provider and now assumes that all case managers are the same. This certainly is a problem and merely dismissing it does not make it go away. We are all part of the good and not so good in this business. Acknowledging that there are good, mediocre, and even bad providers of case management is no different a consideration than in any other product line or area of service. As in other businesses, it is never a good idea to knock the competition. This tactic does not automatically elevate one's own status. When a case manager is confronted with negative comments, her best strategy is to acknowledge the concern without either confirming or denying the information. This enables her to maintain control of the conversation and discuss what must be communicated, which is her ability to provide competent and appropriate case management services.

In reality, competition should be viewed as just another factor in the world of business. Undue importance given to competitors limits an individual's or company's creativity and ability to survive and excel. There are, of course, plenty of large, well-financed, diversified case management companies, but not every client needs that kind of company. For every big client, there are smaller clients just waiting to hear how a small case management company can help them.

NETWORKING AND THE PROFESSIONAL COMMUNITY

Developing and maintaining contacts in the case management and business community are essential for survival. Having the ability to communicate and share information with members of the professional and business sectors enhances one's capabilities. It is often easy within one's own profession (nurse, counselor, social worker) because one shares a common "language" and similar experiences. These become comfortable associations. Reaching outside the case management profession to individuals and organizations not concerned with healthcare, rehabilitation, or insurance may be somewhat intimidating.

The importance of professional alliances in the workplace is recognized by everyone. In a hospital and other traditional healthcare settings, a healthcare provider in one department may need to consult with someone in another department in order to deal with a particular problem. For example, although nurses may possess an understanding of nutritional needs, few would have the extensive dietary education to care for a diabetic without assistance. A call to the dietary department is all that is needed to arrange for a bedside visit, educational materials, and even classes for the patient from a nutritionist or registered dietitian upon discharge. Again, although nurses can assess respiratory function and detect sounds indicative of impending complications, the actual respiratory treatments most often are administered by a respiratory therapist. A social worker on a rehabilitation unit will have a physician and occupational therapist as members of the team who will provide the input needed for appropriate therapeutic service and equipment for a post-CVA patient. Such associations and contacts are inherent to the multidisciplinary approach in rehabilitation facilities and hospitals.

For case managers, especially those outside traditional settings, professional associations are no less important but perhaps more difficult to establish and maintain. It requires time and research to develop a network and creativity to nurture relationships. Furthermore, the networking process needs to be ongoing. Today, one may have two head-injury patients in a caseload, but 6 months from now these cases may be closed. Who should be contacted to assess the needs of the next head-injury patient? Will the neuropsychologist used for the last assessment still be in private practice or will she have joined the staff of a head-injury facility two states away?

Given all of the mergers, acquisitions, and closings of healthcare organizations, keeping key contacts is a never-ending challenge. Interestingly, however, over the years many of the relationships that I established still exist today. Some of these individuals have moved into new companies or now hold different positions yet continue to be colleagues and invaluable assets.

When I started my own firm in 1983, I was feeling somewhat insecure about its standing as a brand new company. I wondered if any reputable insurance carrier, such as Aetna, would be "allowed" to assign cases to me. The claims manager with whom I had met must have sensed my concern as I nervously inquired, "Don't you have to get this approved?" and "Will your home office have a problem with an unknown?" In reply, he said something that, over the years, has provided me with the confidence to approach potential clients: "We don't do business with Intracorp. We do business with Catherine Mullahy or Jane Doe. A business name may get you in the door but they won't sustain a working relationship."

Strong relationships lead to other relationships, and gradually a business network is created and expands. For example, early in my career I was assigned a man who was rendered quadriplegic at the fourth and fifth cervical vertebrae following an automobile accident. When referred to the company that employed me as a rehabilitation specialist, he was on a ventilator in a small community hospital. He had been in its ICU for 2 months, and the referring carrier requested an evaluation. At the time, rehabilitation facilities were few and far between, and those that would even consider accepting a ventilator-dependent patient were very rare.

This 42-year-old man and his family desperately wanted him home, and the carrier obviously did not relish having him endlessly confined in an ICU. An aggressive pursuit of a pulmonary rehabilitation program began. After many telephone calls, evaluation of records by various facilities in surrounding states, and one refusal after another to accept the patient, discouragement and frustration surfaced. I could not, however, forget the visit of this man's wife and their four children to the hospital. I prepared them for the fact that we might not be able to find a suitable facility. They would not accept defeat and said they just "knew" I would help. I was willing to keep trying, but how long would the carrier allow my pursuit of an appropriate placement? On my own time, I continued the search. I made numerous calls to other nurses, to physicians with whom I had worked years before, and to spinal cord programs on the West Coast to see if they knew MDs on the East Coast who specialized in this narrow field.

One night on the evening news, there was a feature highlighting a young spinal cord victim who was treated in a facility headed by a physiatrist who was also a pulmonary specialist. Here might be the answer to my problem. The next morning, I called the news station and found out the name of the physician and the facility and crossed my fingers as I made a call. After giving an overview of the pertinent factors and the family situation, I asked if the physician would at least see my patient to determine if our rehabilitation goals were even feasible. Thankfully, he agreed to see my patient personally and accepted him into the facility.

It was a highly successful intervention and my patient eventually returned home, using the ventilator only during hours of sleep. The discharge planning nurse worked closely with me in transitioning this man back to his community and into the care of his wife and intermittent nursing services. The physician was compassionate, dedicated, and of great assistance to me. Over the years, he changed hospitals several times but continued to do independent medical exams for me and has been a fellow presenter at conferences and a resource to me in countless situations. And the discharge planning nurse? She, too, has moved several times during these past years. We kept in touch, and several years ago she became a regional rehabilitation nurse with a national insurance carrier. A few years later, she was promoted to home office rehabilitation coordinator and became one of my corporate clients. She referred cases to us for case management services. It is indeed a small and interesting world; I never dreamed that these associations started so long ago would continue to be so professionally fruitful.

Many professional associations turn into friendships, and, just as in one's personal life, such relationships deserve extra consideration. This does not mean lavish gifts, expensive lunches, or other such gestures, which may be deemed as potential causes of conflict of interest. Sending a note to an associate expressing appreciation and an acknowledgment to his or her supervisor or company are always acceptable and should become a standard networking plan. In addition, referrals of other patients or colleagues to an associate, as long as there is no monetary payment in return, is a professional way to express recognition of his or her expertise, quality of service, and willingness to work with you in a case management endeavor. Not all case managers have frequent opportunities to refer, but fortunately there are other ways to nurture professional contacts. These include sharing articles of interest, advising associates of seminars, and extending invitations to associates to speak to professional groups or client companies who would welcome their insight. Professional contacts are an important aspect of the case management practice, but when viewed as another link in the process leading to success, they can be both rewarding and enjoyable.

THE BUSINESS COMMUNITY

Most case managers today have some interaction with individuals in the business community and are with increasing frequency being recognized for their contributions toward the attainment of the goals of increasing quality and containing costs. Because the business sector pays the largest share of healthcare costs, a closer alliance between case managers and this concerned group is essential. The object should be not only to improve individual working relationships, but also to increase the public's awareness of case management in general.

Although most healthcare professionals know about case management, fewer business people do, despite its proven success. Interestingly, however, when business people are told what case managers do and the results they obtain, their response is usually extremely positive. They then ask, "Why isn't my company using this kind of service?" "How come there aren't more case managers?" and "Why has this been kept a secret?" Why, indeed?

Part of the answer is that case managers have failed to communicate the benefits of their services to those in the business community. The actual providers of case management services are usually linked to business organizations by individuals who are not case managers. For instance, an employer group needs a package of benefits for its employees. Depending on several factors, including economic feasibility, medical benefits will be provided through a plan that is either fully insured, partially funded, or completely self-funded (by the group). The group appoints from within or contracts someone to purchase the kind of plan it feels it can offer and afford. An insurance career, a TPA, or the employer group itself administers the plan and pays the claims. None of the individuals involved thus far in this process is likely to be a case manager.

As the plan design evolves, there may be discussion of cost-containment techniques, including those of managed care. However, the terms *case management* and *case manager* may never be heard. PPOs, HMOs, pre-cert, utilization review, and second opinion programs will probably come up in conversation, because they have become relatively well-known and well-understood. But case management presents a challenge.

Those who purchase, use, are recipients of, or interact with case management services may be confused. Many assume case management is a given part of TPA services, and automatically credit the TPA with the benefits case management has produced. When there is a change in TPA, neither the employer, consultant, nor broker knows the case management provider as a separate entity. In a more educated healthcare provider system, carriers and employer groups would know case management is a freestanding service and a working relationship can easily continue beyond the association with a TPA.

Is it any wonder that case management is not a household word? The qualifier that distinguishes case management from other managed care services has not been communicated. Add to this the fact that even though case management finally has been defined, those who market case management services are usually from outside the field. They work in insurance, claims administration, marketing, or finance and tend to tell potential client groups merely that the big cases will be "managed." Unfortunately for the case management professional or company, this kind of characterization falls far short of the representation a case manager would want and is fraught with problems.

Because most managed care tools exist as a system, services are paid for on a capitated basis (per employee per month). Case management services, on the other hand, tend to be billed per hour or per case. In fully insured plans, services such as case management, disease management, and utilization review are often wrapped in a package, with one premium paid on a capitated rate, at x dollars per member per month. When case management services are consolidated into a package, they are no longer as visible as they might be, shining a spotlight on savings. (Of course, the same spotlight illuminates shortfalls, but a well-run case management department will produce more successes and savings than unfavorable results.) Self-funded plans often pay separate rates for services selected from a menu—claims services, reinsurance, an employee assistance program, vision program, and so on.

If employees and their dependents are unaware of a case management program and the case manager role as a health advocate, then when contact with an employee is initiated through a telephone call or a letter, the response might be, "No, thank you" or "I don't think I need you." The employee may call his or her supervisor or the human resource department, who may not know of the program either. The human resource department may then call the broker or insurance company account representative, who will attempt to sort out the confusion. Wouldn't it have been better for everyone to have known about the case management program right from the start? Most assuredly yes, but even knowledge of the program is not enough. What is really needed is communication from case managers.

Case managers should be part of the decision to purchase, marketing directly to the in-between contacts, the consultants and brokers. We must tell our story to the right people, the payers, the human resource managers, the personnel staff overseeing benefits for an employee population. It is the case manager who can best help middle management better position the benefits of our services. We all know that healthcare is a huge issue that can only be solved via coordination among all concerned parties.

To keep their voices in the forefront regarding healthcare issues, case managers need to submit articles to business publications, join community and business group coalitions to address healthcare concerns, and meet with business and healthcare leaders to tell them about the advantages of case management programs. Case managers need to be more involved in positioning themselves as part of the solution to the country's healthcare crisis. As healthcare reform evolves, many segments of society will be examining the details and looking to see how the changes will impact them directly. The business community, too, will be part of this process. Even in small towns, businesses have formed associations and committees. Such groups frequently look for guest speakers or for experts to join a panel discussion on a healthcare topic. Open exchanges lend themselves readily to the exploration of problems and solutions.

By calling or visiting the local chamber of commerce, one can acquire lists of member organizations and information about any special health or insurance committees. Because case management today is utilized by most lines of insurance, employer groups need to know that case managers understand their concerns and can help prevent continuing escalation of costs.

Local and regional business periodicals are available by subscription or may be reviewed at the local library. They provide insight into particular areas or issues of concern and afford opportunities to respond, such as by sending letters to the editor, to the authors of articles, and to individuals mentioned in articles. Initiating correspondence on a topic or issue can lead to an ongoing dialogue and perhaps will create a new client for case management services.

Besides gaining new clients through involvement with the business community, case managers can enhance their ability to manage a business and ultimately achieve success. Because many case managers do not have a business background, relationships with business people are often invaluable. By observing how others resolve business problems, case managers become more comfortable grappling with them. They can also learn about hiring techniques, computers, financial management, recruitment, training, marketing, and legal issues by attending business seminars and meeting with individuals who provide the services necessary for the business operations.

Case management is much like other businesses and has many of the same requirements. It is necessary to be aware of personal and business limitations and contract or arrange for assistance in dealing with critical day-to-day management issues. Obviously, restrictions (usually financial) may prevent the hiring of appropriate experts. For example, a public relations or marketing consultant could assist in the creation and expansion of a business, but, especially in the early days, hiring such a person may not be feasible. Growth might be slower, but not hiring a consultant is unlikely to create a crisis. On the other hand, a lack of understanding of or comfort with the financial aspects of business can indeed pose a serious threat to the viability of an operation. If expenses exceed income or if taxes or bills are not paid in a timely manner, the consequences can be devastating. In short, whereas some aspects of business can be learned and developed over time, others require immediate attention.

The best place to start finding answers to questions and solutions to problems is right within one's own community. The local chamber of commerce helps businesses to network and is always supportive of new owners. So, too, is SCORE, "Counselors to America's Small Business," a group that provides assistance to start-up businesses. The local branch is listed in the government section of the Yellow Pages, with information also available at state SCORE web sites and at www.scorechapter14.org. There are a myriad of government services and resources available to business owners at the federal, state, and local levels. Contact can be made via the Internet, by e-mail, letter, phone, or a personal appointment. Private-sector services are also available, often for free or for a nominal fee. Most newspapers have business calendars that list dates, times, locations, and fees for a wide variety of seminars, meetings, and discussion groups. Attending such forums provides an opportunity to explore (without serious financial commitment) services that may be of interest and to meet the providers.

Case managers try to empower patients (consumers of healthcare services) by furnishing the necessary background and describing the alternatives so they can make informed choices. Because owners of case management companies are consumers of business services and products, it makes sense that they should empower themselves through the acquisition of information so that business decisions are sound ones. Information empowers one to be a more astute business manager. All the assistance required to do this is available; you only need to access it, and today it is often only a mouse click away.

GENERATING NEW BUSINESS

Because even successful businesses experience peaks and valleys, having a plan to generate new clients is always important. Relationships with good clients can extend over many years, of course, and this is indeed fortunate, because known entities are usually easier for both the provider of case management services and the recipient company(ies) to work with. Owing to the complexity of case management, the number of players involved, and the need to individualize each case management program, it is highly desirable to maintain longstanding associations. This ideal, however, is not always possible. Occasionally, even the most successful business association ends. For example, a referral source, who is a branch manager of the claims department and a key contact and focal point of referrals to a case management company, receives a promotion to district manager and moves to a different geographic location. Her replacement is a woman who has had a long and successful association with a different case management group, and it is this company that she will continue to utilize. In this era of mergers and acquisitions, it is also possible that a local referral source (an employer group, TPA, or carrier) may be acquired by another entity that may already have a case management program in place with no need to alter that arrangement.

So, what can be done to prepare for the loss of clients? Realize that it can happen tomorrow. Create a plan to generate new business and integrate the plan with the overall business plan. Like the entire business plan, the plan for generating new business needs to be developed thoughtfully, with a budget in mind, with expected goals and time frames in place, and with a way to evaluate the success of the efforts. The process includes many steps, but the following five are probably the most basic.

Establishing Referral Sources

Who exactly are the referral sources for a case management business? Insurance carriers, employer groups, attorneys, TPAs, counties, municipalities, states, the federal government, and individual consumers are current users of case management services. Following the inevitable reform of healthcare, there are likely to be others.

Various industry and business periodicals provide the names of specific companies that have case management programs. Perhaps there are branch offices or subsidiaries that would be referral sources. Articles citing problems in administering workers' compensation or employee medical plans can be used to identify companies that are probably not aware of the case management solution. It makes sense to get in touch with them and share the good news.

Such an opportunity presented itself to me. I had sent a packet of information to a start-up TPA in my community. With it was a letter congratulating the new company, wishing them success, and providing an overview of case management. I pointed to the win-win scenario that could be created by adding case management to the company's set of tools and even outlined a high-cost case with and without case management. Allowing the claims administrator some time to review my proposal, I followed up with a telephone call about a week later. He thought it was all "very nice" but felt he was dealing with small employer groups with "healthy employees" and probably would not need case management services. He further stated that he had hospital networks and PPOs with "great discounts" and thought he was in great shape. Our discussion continued, but I was unable to change his mind.

However, several months later, the claims administrator saw an article that I had submitted to a publication for self-insurers and TPAs called

"The Self-Insurer." He read it over a weekend, thought it made great sense, and intended to try to contact the author when he got into his office on Monday. He looked at the name, thought it looked familiar, and, sure enough, found the author was the very same person who had sent him information months ago. He did, in fact, call me, related the story, and admitted that he was now having "some problems," as I had suspected he would. We arranged a few meetings, and we now enjoy a mutually beneficial association. So, the direct marketing approach did not initially work, but it did pave the way for an eventual business relationship.

Openings like this really are out there, and one needs to be prepared to seize the moment. Although telephone conversations, articles, and letters are all helpful, marketing materials will be important in creating and sustaining an image, which leads to the second step.

Preparing Marketing Materials

Most case managers will want to contract for assistance in designing and implementing a marketing plan and creating a company image. As with most other aspects in the business plan, marketing will likely be done in stages and within certain financial parameters. A new business will probably not be able to afford multipage and multicolor brochures, yet well-designed business cards and stationery are an absolute must for even the smallest of companies. Selecting a company name and corporate logo is a matter of individual preference, but the advice of a public relations or marketing consultant could be extremely helpful. This does not necessarily mean using the largest and most high-profile public relations or advertising firm in one's community. There are many small consulting companies that specialize in the healthcare market, and they offer many options, even packages of services for discounted fees (for example, a business card, a corporate logo, stationery, and a simple brochure outlining the proposed services). Purchasing a package of services increases the chance that everything will be well-coordinated and focused.

When I first started my company, I only had enough money for the design of my corporate logo, business cards, and stationery. It was almost 2 years later that a corporate brochure was created. At that time, my business was restricted mainly to workers' compensation and auto insurance cases; group medical cases were just starting to be referred. It was my feeling the claimants had minimal understanding of case management and frequently did not hear about us until months after an injury, sometimes only after litigation was also involved. For the group medical insurance referrals, case management was a brand new approach. Because the response to case management by claimants would help make or break us, our first brochure (Figure 13–1) was designed specifically for claimants and their families, not the actual payers. However, I also used it successfully to interest potential clients. It was reader-friendly, had an easy-to-understand question and answer format, and showed us to be proactive (something extremely important to me) and cost-conscious (something extremely important to our clients). It has been modified over the years but remains an integral component of our marketing package. In general, our marketing efforts and direction have evolved and will continue to evolve in response to the ongoing changes in our industry.

Targeting New Business Goals

Although it is important to maintain current business, it is always necessary to identify potential sources of new business. This is a challenging process, one of discovery and innovation. Determining specific new business targets is accomplished through matching one's strengths and areas of expertise with segments of the business community that could utilize such expertise. To be able to capitalize on the many opportunities, one needs to keep current in one's own practice setting (whether this is oncology, AIDS, high-risk pregnancy, etc.) and current within the business community. What are the problems yet to be resolved? How could case management respond? What are the emerging needs that come with our changing population—hospice care, language translation, elder care? What types of partnerships could be created that would facilitate the provision of services? There are immediate targets for case management services today, and on the horizon are potential users waiting to be identified. This is the excitement of our industry!

At my company, we branched out into another area of business, providing Care-at-Home service. Looking to grow this market niche, we created a second marketing piece describing this program and answering the most frequently asked questions for the physicians, social workers, and families with whom we would be interacting.

Since then, we have applied this concept of reaching out to engage the stakeholders in medical care and cost management, whether they are patients, families, physicians, employer groups, TPAs, insurers, brokers, unions, reinsurance carriers, or others. This relationship building serves as a platform to transition into new markets. With information gleaned from questionnaires, we can report that "our patients say . . ." or "brokers say . . ." We have found that a more broad-based appeal leads to greater receptivity.

Figure 13–1 Options Unlimited Patient Brochure.

WHAT DO I DO NOW?

Call us. Every case is unique and will be considered in a FREE preliminary screening.

If you decide to contract for our consulting services, you can be assured that OPTIONS offers a personalized service and medically knowledgeable people who will deal with you as an individual. With OPTIONS, you will have a friend and confidant, as well as a medical expert.

HEALTH CARE AND DISABILITY MANAGEMENT SERVICES

HEALTH CARE AND DISABILITY MANAGEMENT SERVICES
(XXX) XXX-XXXX

Catherine M. Mullahy
President

Catherine Mullahy has thirty-nine years of experience in healthcare management in both hospitals and corporate settings.

Her diversified nursing experience includes work in multiple trauma, medical/surgical, cardiac, orthopedic, and neurologic conditions.

She is the founder and President of OPTIONS UNLIMITED, a healthcare and disability management company. Her consulting firm possesses national capability, and works with corporations, private carriers, government agencies, and individuals. She has written for national publications, serves as a consultant to insurance companies and providers, and lectures frequently on a variety of topics in the disability management field.

Catherine Mullahy and OPTIONS UNLIMITED offer you a timely and cost-efficient program whose specialty is caring.

COST-EFFECTIVE
INDIVIDUAL
CASE MANAGEMENT SERVICES
medical, emotional,
and vocational

CATHERINE M. MULLAHY, PRESIDENT
76 EAST MAIN STREET
HUNTINGTON, NEW YORK 11743
(XXX) XXX-XXXX
FAX (XXX) XXX-XXXX

Figure 13–1 continued

WHAT IS OPTIONS UNLIMITED?

We are a medically knowledgeable consulting firm that serves the special needs of patients and their families, nationally.

HEALTH CARE AND DISABILITY MANAGEMENT SERVICES

WHAT DOES OPTIONS DO?

We act as the patient advocate to ensure an injured or ill person's return to wellness in the shortest possible time at the lowest possible cost.

HOW DO WE ACCOMPLISH OUR GOALS?

We serve as liaison between the patient, physician, therapist, insurance company, and employer, coordinating all facets in order that each patient may return to a productive life.

WHY DO YOU NEED OPTIONS?

When injury or illness strikes, common reactions of the patient and family are shock, panic, and especially confusion.

They don't know who to talk to, what questions to ask, or where to go for help. They are also insecure with the unfamiliarity of medical language at a time when they become completely dependent on the medical community.

A physician simply cannot spend enough time with the family to help them understand the complex problems involved in catastrophic injury/illness cases.

OPTIONS helps the patient and the family to cope with the medical, insurance, social, emotional, vocational and financial problems related to the injury or illness.

SPECIFICALLY, WHAT DOES OPTIONS DO TO ASSIST YOU?

- Secure proper medical care and equipment
- Prevent inappropriate or excessive treatment
- Expedite facility/home placement and care
- Inform insurance company of your condition and treatment
- Help your family to understand and to adjust
- Find community resources to work on your behalf
- Coordinate and provide necessary follow-up treatment
- Remain available to you and your family for reassurance and counseling

WHO WILL PAY FOR THIS SERVICE?

If your insurance company has referred you to us, they will be billed for our services.

If you contact us directly or if you are referred by your doctor or others involved in your care, we will contact your insurance carrier; if there is no coverage, you will be billed. In all cases, we will outline a clear plan for coordinating your care with an easy-to-understand rate schedule.

WON'T USING OPTIONS JUST CREATE GREATER EXPENSE?

Even if your insurance company does not cover case management services, OPTIONS can usually save you money in medical and related costs. We help you get back to the business of living.

DOES OPTIONS SERVE ONLY SEVERE ILLNESS/INJURY CASES?

Although OPTIONS specializes in catastrophic, chronic, and complex medical problems, we have experience in a wide variety of disabilities—pediatric through geriatric.

Source: Courtesy of Options Unlimited, Case Management Services Division, © 2003, Huntington, New York.

Creating and Maintaining Relationships with Referral Sources

Most case management companies initially grow one case at a time and then expand in larger increments as new case management programs are created based on the successful cases. When starting a business, therefore, it is very important to identify and accept the kinds of cases that present the most potential for success, both in terms of medical outcome and savings.

Although we all welcome a challenge and want to be able to demonstrate that we can do what others cannot, we do not want to attempt the "impossible." Some cases are beyond anyone's capabilities—for example, the patient who is 2 years postinjury; who has had two surgical interventions, four hospitalizations, ongoing physical therapy, and psychological counseling; whose employer has no light-duty program; and whose union is in a contract dispute with management. And the claims examiner is already demanding that this case be resolved. This clearly is a challenge to avoid.

This does not mean taking only "easy" cases, because the easy ones do not usually require case management and asking for them sets one up for comments such as "Well, this guy probably would have gone back to work without you." There are, however, many cases in between the two extremes. Case managers also have the potential to create opportunities for success by knowing and then communicating the red flags that indicate the need for case management (see Chapters 9 and 11).

If one referral has been successfully case managed, it should be relatively straightforward to obtain others. Likewise, if one good relationship with a referral source in a company has been established, it should be easier to establish others with individuals in the same company. For instance, following positive outcomes and after proving the value of case management to one claims examiner in a workers' compensation department, a case manager could ask if there were other examiners who might consider using case management services. Does this carrier also write auto or group medical insurance? It would also be a good tactic to ask the initial referral source to write a letter of recommendation or allow him- or herself to be used as a reference. Most individuals who are pleased with the results of case management are only too happy to provide an endorsement, giving credibility to a service that in many cases is still an unknown. Because no one wants to be the first customer, a firm endorsement by one person or company encourages others to try the services being offered.

Expressing appreciation for past and current business is important in maintaining ongoing associations and generating new referrals. If such appreciation is not communicated regularly, client groups soon feel less than valued. Sharing information about conferences or articles that might be of interest is one way to expand relationships. So, too, is seeking expert help from associates, perhaps to clarify a claims matter. I have learned most about the complexities of all the lines of insurance our company is now involved with from individuals who started as clients and over the years have become colleagues.

Initially, I had a need to know, and thankfully there were those who had a desire to share their very specialized knowledge. This collaboration truly was synergistic in that both parties had something to offer and gain from the association; together there was a stronger unit than either possessed as a single entity. With one of these colleagues, I have presented at conferences. She, at my suggestion, was a presenter at a case management conference, and we anticipate coauthoring a book. All these techniques have helped me to expand my own business, and they are quite viable for the new and even established businesses that want to create new markets or expand existing ones.

Reaching Decision Makers

Even the best marketing plan, impressive marketing materials, and savvy marketing strategies do not necessarily generate business unless the individual who can authorize and pay for case management services can be convinced of their value. Case management services, unfortunately, are usually placed in the "loss" column by most companies. Most potential clients are reluctant to pay out additional money for services that, at least until they prove their worth, merely offer the promise of containing costs. Furthermore, the services do not necessarily ease the bureaucratic workload, but may, in fact, require more direct involvement on the part of company staff. Companies also are more inclined to buy products or services that will generate more business and money for them, and case management is not perceived as one of these, at least not in the early stages.

After case management services are established and successful, it is certainly easier to gain work, but what about those first cases? The claims examiner may be a case manager's main contact but is likely not the individual who can create or allow for the expansion of case management programs. How does one identify and get to the decision maker? By keeping alert, asking questions, and paying attention to the market.

Reaching the individual who has overall fiscal responsibility is not always an easy process but is well worth the effort. Start at the very top—by approaching the CEO or president of the group. If the CEO does not have day-to-day responsibility for healthcare matters but someone else does (for example, the chief financial officer or director of insurance), then this other person is usually directed to respond to the approach. If one starts at the middle-management level, then the person contacted often has to go upward to obtain an okay. Not only that, but requesting assistance (and money) is often perceived as a reflection of poor management. It puts the individual in the position of having to acknowledge a problem and an inability to solve it alone. Few will voluntarily place themselves in this situation, so the decision to use case management will likely be deferred.

HIRING ADDITIONAL STAFF

Success brings with it new questions and new issues. Growth for many reasons can be troublesome, so it requires a good deal of planning. The first issue may be whether to hire another case manager and staff or remain a one-person company. The decision to employ others is possibly one of the most difficult for the entrepreneur case manager. It means relinquishing some of the control over case management activities, delegating some of the responsibilities, and, perhaps the most challenging of all, introducing customers to someone who they may perceive as not quite as good as the expert they have become accustomed to working with.

Another possible issue is whether to accept cases in a broader geographical area than previously covered. Let us assume that a caseload of 18 to 25 is manageable: The case manager can effectively direct and support elements required for each of those cases. She can stay on top of each case, make enough money to pay the bills, and take regular days off and maybe even some vacation time. Perhaps a few more cases can be handled by putting in a few extra hours or a few extra-long days. But then several "quiet" cases all of a sudden become very active. At this point, a prospective client calls and says he has 8 to 10 cases put aside. (Where was he when the caseload was down to 10?) The time is *now*; a decision must be made. Should the case manager accept these cases and plan to work 15 to 18 hours a day? Not if she plans to be around for a few years and certainly not if she plans to continue to be able to provide quality, timely interventions and manage cases rather than be managed by them.

Nothing says the case manager must hire staff and build the company. Some case managers are comfortable setting limits, advising customers that 20 or 25 is the maximum number of cases they want, and then suggesting the name of colleagues who might be able to assist. However, there are good reasons to expand—the challenge, the opportunity to provide services to more people in need, the potential to expand the use of case management, and, of course, the possible financial rewards that might be realized.

Hiring individuals who have the necessary expertise and who share the same philosophy, work ethic, and business goals is highly desirable. Finding such individuals, however, is not always easy. One essential step in the process is to clarify just what it takes to be a case manager. Unfortunately, because case management is evolving, it is difficult to succinctly set out all the job's elements. A standard definition of case management has been created by CCMC, the regulatory body responsible for the CCM designation, as described in Chapter 1. CMSA has also revised its Standards of Practice to more fully describe the role, function, and activities of individual case managers as they practice in today's settings. In addition, URAC has established guidelines for case management organizations and departments. These are all good references.

I have developed three position descriptions, one for a nurse reviewer, one for a medical case manager, and one for a director of case management services position. These appear at the end of the chapter as Appendix 13–A, Appendix 13–B, and Appendix 13–C, and incorporate summaries of each role, principal duties and responsibilities, required knowledge, and qualifications. I use evaluation tools during the course of the year that are matched to these job descriptions when reviewing employees' job performance.

Limiting the search to case managers with the CCM credential, as important as this credential is, would exclude many fine candidates from employment. Experienced case managers who understand all the lines of insurance, have had a diversified clinical background prior to case management, and have worked in a variety of traditional and nontraditional settings would be the best candidates, right? Not necessarily. I have hired case management professionals from competitors and carriers, and I have hired nurses who I thought possessed excellent potential but lacked on-line case management experience. For me, it has been easier, though not always trouble-free, to hire and train individuals who have no case management experience. When bringing in individuals with prior experience, I found it was often difficult to convince them to put aside the business practices (billing, need to attain a set number of hours each week) and philosophies of previous employers. Or, they had only handled workers' compensation or liability cases and could not keep the return-to-work goal out of our group medical insurance cases. It has generally been easier to train rather than retrain.

Further, professional experience, credentials, published papers, and a multitude of degrees do not guarantee success. I used to be intimidated when applicants would submit incredibly impressive résumés, would know what our salary limitations were (as a small company they were restrictive), yet would want to interview for a position. A few PhDs in particular stand out in my mind. It did not take me long to realize they would fail to make it. These candidates had assimilated all of the theory, could quote studies and statistics, but in my judgment would not have been able to understand, nor work within the confines of, the workers' compensation law of our state. Does this mean that no one with a PhD can be a case manager? Not at all, but it does mean that one has to look beyond credentials, impressive résumés, and accomplishments. At the same time, when I interview individuals who are not experienced case managers, this does not mean they are perceived as people with no experience. In my judgment, case management work is complex, demanding, and challenging. Not every individual can do it, even with training. There are professional attainments and personal characteristics that increase the likelihood of success in this field and personal characteristics that almost preclude success.

Professional Background

The type of professional background staff should have depends partly on the type of case management services offered. A company that provides a broad range of medical case management services needs staff members with diversified clinical experience. If it works mainly within the group medical insurance area, it should probably hire mostly nurses. This does not mean that only nurses can provide case management intervention; other allied professionals have much to contribute. However, the typical cases referred to case management are high cost and medically complex, and nurses, in my opinion, are better prepared to handle the many responsibilities that are required.

Of course, not everyone licensed to practice as a nurse has the depth and diversification of educational and clinical background that supports good case management. Although the length of time that one has been a nurse is important, time and grade alone are not sufficient. Perhaps a nurse has been on a spinal cord unit for 8 years or has worked for 10 years in pediatrics; the scope of these practice settings is relatively narrow and would ill-prepare the nurse to work in most case management departments or companies. Only in very large companies might a case manager only be assigned pediatric cases or patients with spinal cord injuries. It is more often that nurses are assigned a wide range of cases. A typical caseload may include a post-CVA patient who needs placement in a rehabilitation facility; a chronic emphysema patient who has become severely compromised; a noncompliant diabetic adolescent; a woman with breast cancer who now, despite aggressive treatment, is a hospice candidate; and a newly diagnosed end-stage renal disease patient who will be on home dialysis. It is evident that a case manager needs a range of skills and expertise in order to manage this kind of caseload.

Although clinical experience is important, so too is the setting in which the knowledge is gained. Because case management is involved in arranging alternate care settings for patients, direct knowledge of nontraditional settings is highly desirable. It affords an understanding of what actually happens beyond the walls of the acute care hospital.

Educational Background

Educational background needs to be considered as well. Nurses can be graduates of diploma schools or have associate or bachelor's degrees. Should only those with bachelor's degrees be allowed to be case managers? The answer for now is no. Many nurses who have graduated from associate and diploma programs have continued to broaden their education. They attend workshops and conferences; subscribe to nursing journals, magazines, and newsletters; and may have also taken college courses in pursuit of a bachelor of science. On the other hand, there are also nurses who, once they get their degree, virtually shut down their education. This illustrates the importance of going beyond what appears on an application or résumé, making no assumptions or exclusions based solely upon schooling and degree(s) held.

Life Experience

Professional experience and educational background most assuredly need to be considered when hiring case managers. Another factor that deserves attention, however, often is not mentioned—the learning one derives from living. When an individual loses a child, spouse, or other family member to illness and goes through the stages of caring, letting go, and grieving, the entire process can be a sobering and, in many ways, enriching occurrence. Coping with life's travails, surprises, and challenges helps one in ways that education and work alone cannot. Adjusting to divorce, job changes, career hurdles, and family problems while maintaining one's sanity (or a reasonable facsimile thereof) actually prepares one very well for the position of case manager.

Because the kinds of cases usually referred for intervention are typically complex and chronic or catastrophic, patients and families will likely have deeply felt and highly personal responses to their illnesses or disabilities. These responses can, if recognition and intervention are lacking, destroy family structures, members, and, on occasion, the individual himself. A case manager's own life experiences can help her detect and deflect dangerous patient and family responses.

One source of stress for case managers is the interaction that occurs between patients and families, physicians, other healthcare team members, multiple providers, employer groups, and claims staff. Everyone has his or her own needs, priorities, and personality. Taking on the role of "director" of this drama is not easy, not even for experienced case managers. Novice case managers should probably not even attempt this role. To be credible, a case management professional needs sufficient life experience to strike the delicate balance between empathy and efficiency, negotiating and standing fast, providing support and pushing patients to draw on their own inner strength.

Other Intangibles

When I consider what it really takes to be a good case manager, I am still amazed at how many of the qualities are intangible, including the following:

- A sense of humor
- A strong work ethic
- Anger at the system (but not enough to be a hindrance to action)
- A belief in one's ability to make a difference (but not a need for personal power)
- Approachability
- Optimism
- An ability to look at the positives and build on them, tempered by the right amount of reality to prevent "pie in the sky" plans and goals
- An awareness of the business/financial aspects of healthcare
- A sense of objectivity
- Keenly developed ethical principles
- Energy and creativity
- A commitment to professionalism

The interview process should explore a candidate's personal characteristics, although they are admittedly more difficult to uncover and assess than the candidate's professional experience and educational background.

Much of the discovery of these personal qualities depends upon the level of skill of the interviewer and, of course, the structure, philosophy, and goals of the company or department. We always look to use the strengths of each individual, providing our company with a broader skill base.

We have an advantage when conducting interviews, as each candidate is interviewed by a case manager at one stage. Larger corporations might screen potential case managers through the human resources department. Would an HR employee know that a nurse would not say "black and blue" to describe a wound, but rather hematoma or ecchymoses?

The "intangibles" noted previously are important qualities I seek in case manager candidates. To incorporate these areas into interviews, we give all potential case managers five or six scenarios followed by questions that help us understand their approach to issues that might arise (see Table 13–1). In their answers to the questions posed by these scenarios, candidates tell us a bit about their attitude, aptitude, ethics, leadership skills, creativity in strategic planning, and personality.

Table 13–1 Scenarios for Potential Case Managers

To assess compassion and the ability to collaborate:

While monitoring the home care plan of a client with AIDS, you find that inadequate pain relief has been achieved and he is at risk of rehospitalization. The home health nurse appears to have limited experience with pain management strategies. What would you do?

To assess consensus building and empowerment:

In attending a rehabilitation team meeting, you find that the rehab team and client's family have differing opinions regarding a discharge plan. How would you approach this to achieve consensus?

To assess planning and organization:

To complete an assessment on a client who is in a rehabilitation hospital, you need to interview the client, family, physician, and the treatment team. You also need to review medical records. How would you approach this efficiently and collaboratively?

To assess advocacy and assertiveness:

In your assessment, you find that the client is not receiving counseling in the hospital as needed because of the counselor's vacation. Would you intervene, and if so, how?

Source: Courtesy of Options Unlimited, Case Management Services Division, © 2003, Huntington, New York.

In addition, we ask candidates to read through case briefs that center on different situations (see Tables 13–2 and 13–3) and then report back to us the issues they perceive as problematic, and steps they might take to move forward with the case. Responses can provide insight into their thought processes and problem-solving abilities.

Table 13–2 Case Situation Assessment—Pregnancy

Kim W. is a 37-year-old pregnant female who recently emigrated from Russia and is single. She is in her first trimester and recently had a blood glucose test with a result of 187. She is gravida 3 para 1. Her PMH (prior medical history) includes one miscarriage and a 2 1/2-year-old daughter. The physician at the clinic where she has been receiving prenatal care suggests home glucose testing with glucometer. She is scheduled for a three-hour glucose tolerance test. Her first pregnancy was a C-section due to infant size and claimant's condition at that time. She did not have the same OB/GYN at that time.

1. What risk factors and/or problems do you see in this case?
2. What additional information would you like to obtain?
3. Who would you ask to obtain this information and why?

Source: Courtesy of Options Unlimited, Case Management Services Division, © 2003, Huntington, New York.

Table 13–3 Case Situation Assessment—Asthma

Walkirya H. is a 16-year-old female admitted to Bronx Lebanon Hospital with a diagnosis of asthma. She has a PMH of recurrent hospital admits, three for asthma. She lives with her non-English speaking mother. Her parents are divorced. Her PMD is Dr. Diaz, internal medicine. He was not the admitting physician as claimant was admitted through the emergency room. Claimant is currently receiving IV steroids, nebulizer treatments, and ABGs, with peak flow and oxygen saturation monitoring. She was admitted 3 days prior to Options Unlimited being informed of hospitalization.

1. What do you see as problematic in this case?
2. What additional information would you like to obtain?
3. What would you anticipate as the patient's need at the time of discharge?

Source: Courtesy of Options Unlimited, Case Management Services Division, © 2003, Huntington, New York.

A tool to assist interviewers in identifying a potential candidate's knowledge areas and deficits was created by Sandra Lowery, BSN, RN, CCM, CRRN (see Figure 13–2). Offering a starting point, this checklist of care venues, funding sources, resources, and clinical categories can be modified by a case management department or agency, with alternative specialty areas added to address the needs of the group's patient base.

Lowery also offers lines of questioning to assess various skills and traits. For example, to assess assertiveness and problem solving, she suggests asking the candidate, "You find that the patient desires palliative care but is too intimidated by his physician to discuss the physician's plan for further chemotherapy. How would you address this situation?" Another line of questioning to judge resource knowledge, creativity, and planning might be, "You find that your client has a vital need for daily speech therapy. The attending physician agrees but reports that the closest speech therapist is over 75 miles away. What would you do to help this client?"[1]

At the end of this chapter are three additional forms that can be used to ascertain the strengths of potential and staff case managers. They are Appendix 13–D, Interview Evaluation Form, to be used during the first interview; Appendix 13–E, Summary Evaluation Scale, for the second or call-back interview: and Appendix 13–F, Competencies for Unit-Based Nurse Case Manager.

THE SEARCH FOR CASE MANAGERS

Before candidates can be interviewed and evaluated, they need to be located and be made interested enough to apply for a job. The usual search methods include posting jobs, running classified ads, and contracting with personnel agencies. There are, however, other viable ways of attracting prospective case managers, some of which require only a minimal financial outlay.

For example, writing an article for a professional magazine or local newspaper that gives an overview of the field helps likely candidates envision themselves in the case management role. Organizations, schools, employer groups, insurance carriers, and healthcare companies and clinics are always looking for speakers. Although the audience may enter the hall expecting to learn about how to work with case managers, an inspirational presentation may lead some listeners to pursue case management as a career. And sometimes merely "spreading the word" about employment openings will attract candidates, as will asking colleagues whether they know of individuals who might be looking to make a move.

Figure 13–2 Candidate's Knowledge Assessment Tool.

KNOWLEDGE ASSESSMENT

Rate your knowledge/familiarity of the following by using a scale of 1 to 5, with 1 indicating the highest level:

	1	2	3	4	5
Levels of Care					
—Acute hospital	[ ]	[ ]	[ ]	[ ]	[ ]
—Rehabilitation	[ ]	[ ]	[ ]	[ ]	[ ]
—Post hospital	[ ]	[ ]	[ ]	[ ]	[ ]
Funding Sources					
—Private insurance	[ ]	[ ]	[ ]	[ ]	[ ]
—Public insurance	[ ]	[ ]	[ ]	[ ]	[ ]
—Other	[ ]	[ ]	[ ]	[ ]	[ ]
Services/Resources					
—Home health	[ ]	[ ]	[ ]	[ ]	[ ]
—Home infusion therapy	[ ]	[ ]	[ ]	[ ]	[ ]
—Medical equip./supp.	[ ]	[ ]	[ ]	[ ]	[ ]
—Transportation	[ ]	[ ]	[ ]	[ ]	[ ]
—Outpatient	[ ]	[ ]	[ ]	[ ]	[ ]
—Residential	[ ]	[ ]	[ ]	[ ]	[ ]
—Hospice	[ ]	[ ]	[ ]	[ ]	[ ]
Service Costs					
—Acute hospital	[ ]	[ ]	[ ]	[ ]	[ ]
—Outpatient	[ ]	[ ]	[ ]	[ ]	[ ]
—Residential	[ ]	[ ]	[ ]	[ ]	[ ]
—Outpatient	[ ]	[ ]	[ ]	[ ]	[ ]
—Home health	[ ]	[ ]	[ ]	[ ]	[ ]

CLINICAL TREATMENT/OUTCOMES

Rehabilitation

	1	2	3	4	5
—Treatment	[ ]	[ ]	[ ]	[ ]	[ ]
—Resources	[ ]	[ ]	[ ]	[ ]	[ ]

Figure 13–2 continued

Neonates	1	2	3	4	5
—Treatment	[ ]	[ ]	[ ]	[ ]	[ ]
—Resources	[ ]	[ ]	[ ]	[ ]	[ ]

Pediatrics					
—Treatment	[ ]	[ ]	[ ]	[ ]	[ ]
—Resources	[ ]	[ ]	[ ]	[ ]	[ ]

Obstetrics					
—Treatment	[ ]	[ ]	[ ]	[ ]	[ ]
—Resources	[ ]	[ ]	[ ]	[ ]	[ ]

HIV Disease/AIDS					
—Treatment	[ ]	[ ]	[ ]	[ ]	[ ]
—Resources	[ ]	[ ]	[ ]	[ ]	[ ]

Oncology					
—Treatment	[ ]	[ ]	[ ]	[ ]	[ ]
—Resources	[ ]	[ ]	[ ]	[ ]	[ ]

Psychiatric Illness/CD					
—Treatment	[ ]	[ ]	[ ]	[ ]	[ ]
—Resources	[ ]	[ ]	[ ]	[ ]	[ ]

Transplants					
—Treatment	[ ]	[ ]	[ ]	[ ]	[ ]
—Resources	[ ]	[ ]	[ ]	[ ]	[ ]

Source: Reprinted from *The Case Manager,* Vol. 3, S. Lowery, "Qualifications for the Successful Case Manager," p. 74, © 1992, with permission from Elsevier.

Although more costly in dollars and time, attending job fairs and other conferences can be a fruitful method of finding candidates. At a recent CMSA conference, I posted a recruitment form when looking to

Figure 13–3 Recruitment Form Used at Job Fair.

CASE MANAGEMENT DEPARTMENT

NURSE CASE MANAGERS, MEDICAL/PEDIATRIC (FULL TIME/PART TIME); LONG ISLAND, NEW YORK METRO

Position Description:

Care Coordination of High Cost or Complex Cases. Develop and Implement (with treating physician, patient and other medical personnel) treatment plans to maximize patient outcomes while containing costs. Advocate for patients and families. Monitor treatment plans, assess ongoing needs. Patient and family support.

Qualifications:

Professional: RNs (degree preferred) - with minimum 5–10 years experience in hospital, home care, infusion care, discharge planning, Insurance Company or Employer selling.

Personal: Caring, high energy, independent, creative, good communication (verbal and written), problem solver, critical analytical skills.

Business: Financial awareness of health care or willingness to get involved in this area, computer skills a plus, bilingual a plus.

Training and supervision is provided, competitive salary, patient contact and case responsibility, small challenging case loads. On-site visits (in patient's home or hospital), car and travel required. Rewarding, challenging dynamic career for the accomplished, confident professional. Professional office, growing corporate environment. **FOR INFORMATION ON POSITIONS AVAILABLE CALL 1-XXX-XXX-XXXX OR FAX RESUME TO (XXX) XXX-XXXX.**

CATHERINE M. MULLAHY, PRESIDENT • 76 EAST MAIN STREET, HUNTINGTON, NEW YORK 11743 • (631) 673-1150 • FAX (631) 673-8369

Source: Courtesy of Options Unlimited, Case Manaagement Services Division, © 2003, Huntington, New York.

expand our office's nationwide network of case managers. The posting drew a fair response, and some good contacts were initiated. Attending conferences may actually serve several purposes besides recruitment, such as advertising services, developing a marketing image, garnering insight into needs of the industry, and generating more business through networking.

I've also used regional and local job fairs as opportunities to post similar recruitment forms for our headquarters office in New York (see Figure 13–3).

To fill a key position, such as manager or director, it may make sense to use a recruiting firm (also known as an executive search firm or "head-hunter"). Recruiting firms are highly specialized, and there are several that focus entirely on recruitment for the healthcare and managed care industries. Although the fees can be substantial (often 25 to 30% of a candidate's first-year salary), such firms can make the hiring process almost painless, and most will refund a fee (at least partially) should the candidate not prove suitable once hired.

Case management is already a proven if not yet integral element of the U.S. healthcare system. To my mind, this is an exciting time to be a case manager, whether employed by a provider or payer or running an independent company. Being independent just gives one that much more visibility and opportunity to shape and build this young industry.

NOTES

1. Lowery S, "Qualifications for the Successful Case Manager," *The Case Manager* 3, no. 4 (1992): 73.

APPENDIX 13–A

Sample Nurse Reviewer for Prenotification Department Position Description

Options Unlimited

Position Description: Nurse Reviewer for Prenotification Department

Primary Claimants Served:
This position requires that the employee be able to demonstrate the knowledge and skills necessary to provide all aspects of care based on physical, psychological, educational, safety, support systems, and related criteria, appropriate to the claimant served. The skill and knowledge base need to address age-specific issues, cultural diversity, socioeconomic factors, language differences, cultural traditions, spiritual belief systems/practices of the claimant and family members or supportive others. These issues are significant to the Nurse Reviewer's relationship with the claimant and will directly impact on the healthcare outcome.

Purpose of the Position:
The purpose of the Nurse Reviewer is to assess the medical appropriateness, quality, and cost-effectiveness of proposed hospital, medical, and surgical services in accordance with established criteria. This review activity may be conducted prospectively, concurrently, or retrospectively and in collaboration with claimants, physicians, and other professionals. Through this review process, the Nurse Reviewer will identify those individuals and circumstances that would benefit from the intervention of the case management professional. This position is critical in the maintenance of uniformity, quality, and consistency of benefit determination, administration, and application of the managed care programs. The Nurse Reviewer will provide telephonic case management intervention on behalf of claimants with short-term needs, by monitoring and evaluating options and services to effect an appropriate, individualized plan for the claimant across the continuum of care.

Specific Responsibilities and Duties:
The Nurse Reviewer at Options Unlimited must be able to demonstrate and be accountable for the standards of practice, policies and procedures, quality assurance, and the goals of the organization.

Healthcare Management:

1. Manages care of claimants through the healthcare system based on the individual's needs. Appropriately integrates the individual into the healthcare continuum, including procurement of services, health promotion and counseling, disease prevention, health education and screening, and community resources linkage. Responsibilities include, but are not limited to, the following:

   a. Advocates for the claimant and family throughout the entire episode of care. Maintains availability to the claimant/family as a resource to facilitate communication among providers and to monitor services rendered. Remains involved until the claimant achieves the planned level of functional health or closure criteria are met.

   b. Using independent judgment and discretion, in addition to consideration of standards outlined by M & R, Interqual, and others, identifies and plans strategies to reduce inpatient length of stay and resource consumption. Works in collaboration with physicians and appropriate healthcare providers regarding treatment plans required. Provides claimant/family or significant other with information about such issues as nursing visits, home care services, appropriate providers, etc.

   c. Coordinates/facilitates the claimant's progression throughout the continuum.

   d. Works collaboratively and maintains active communication with physicians, nurses, social workers, utilization review staff, and other members of the multidisciplinary care team to effect timely appropriate claimant management through the continuum.

   e. Makes initial contact with the claimant/family and multidisciplinary team based on identified needs.

   f. Applies knowledge of age-specific, cultural diversity, psycho/social, and developmental issues during the interview process, documentation, and intervention with the claimant, their family, or significant others.

   g. Remains in communication with claimants and the physicians and other members of the healthcare team to identify and resolve variances concurrently, and to assist the claimant in attaining the appropriate care with positive outcomes.

   h. Discusses and educates claimant/family on case management services. Confirms claimant's understanding of case management intervention and obtains case management approval when necessary and appropriate.

i. Knowledgeable on new regulations on the federal, state, and local level.

Process and Relationships:

2. Performs Nurse Review by applying clinical criteria to monitor appropriateness of admissions, level of care, and continued stays, and documents findings based on standards. Responsibilities include, but are not limited to the following:

a. Collaborates with the physician and the multidisciplinary team to facilitate the plan of care and assist in identification and concurrent resolution of variances.

b. Uses independent judgment and discretion to address, resolve, and process problems impeding the diagnostic or treatment progress. Proactively identifies and resolves delays and obstacles.

c. Seeks consultation from physicians, clinical, and other disciplines and departments as required to expedite care, monitor length of inpatient stay, and facilitate discharge.

d. Collaborates and communicates with all members of the multidisciplinary team to validate information.

e. Identifies potential risk factors.

Service Delivery:

3. Manages aspects of the planning process in anticipation of claimant variances or transitions. Responsibilities include, but are not limited to the following:

a. Collaborates and communicates with the physician and the rest of the care management multidisciplinary team to facilitate planning for variances or transitions.

b. Initiates and facilitates referrals for home healthcare, infusion therapy, hospice, other care facilities, medical equipment, and supplies.

c. Facilitates transfers to other facilities.

d. Identifies "at risk" individuals and develops and implements a comprehensive plan of care that addresses the specific need.

e. Maintains current and appropriate documentation.

f. Follows department guidelines for utilization of time.

Quality and Performance Improvement:

4. Appropriately identifies potential issues or "at risk" populations and anticipates the need for providing care.

5. Actively participates in clinical performance improvement process.
6. With respect to the individual claimant, analyzes and evaluates the effects of nurse reviewer on quality outcomes, fiscal parameters, customer satisfaction, and systems operations and develops strategies to improve performance.
7. Utilizing problem-solving techniques and conflict resolution skills, develops the plan to provide consistent quality to the claimant and the payer.

Managed Care Regulatory Knowledge:

8. Collaborates with the multidisciplinary team to assist claimant with benefits/resource management to include negotiations with out-of-network providers; with resolution of payment issues; with developing a more cost-effective plan of care; and with evaluating the appropriateness of the level of care or the use of services. Responsibilities include, but are not limited to the following:
   a. Communicates, as required, with claimants to provide understanding of plan language and/or payer guidelines. Discusses issues for treatment and/or discharge needs with the physicians and relevant staff to provide for appropriate, timely treatment or a safe discharge.
   b. Assists physicians, care providers, and claimant/family in understanding the plan language and benefits as required.

Communication:

9. Maintains open communication with all appropriate parties.
   a. Utilizes problem-solving skills and negotiating techniques to resolve conflict issues.
   b. Identifies, plans, and coordinates aspects of care for the claimant, their family, or significant other.
   c. Communicates with supervisory personnel for problem solving, direction, and planning as well as knowledge issues.
   d. Initiates required forms and/or letters to comply with organizational guidelines.
   e. Completes timely and appropriate assessments, documentation, reports, and cost-benefit analysis.
   f. Interacts with the physicians and members of the entire healthcare team in appropriate time frames.
10. Maintains strict standards for claimant confidentiality and claimant-related information in addition to security of electronic information; complies with organizational, federal, and state regulations and policy on confidentiality.

Professional Development:

11. Maintains current knowledge of plan language and benefit issues and requirements as it relates to potential denial (whether contractual or utilization related).
12. Attends educational training program to expand job knowledge.
13. Performs other duties as related to case management functions to support and foster an effective, quality case management program.
14. Maintains current knowledge of URAC's standard of practice.

Position Requirements and Qualifications:

Education and Experience:

1. Graduated from an accredited School of Nursing or College: current New York state RN license required, AAS, BSN, Bachelor of Science in Nursing or health-related field preferred.
2. Graduated from an accredited college with a degree and licensure as a Certified Social Worker.
3. Minimum of 3–5 years of relevant clinical medical surgical or specialty experience required as applicable to the position needs.
4. Required to pursue ongoing education, certification, and self-development to remain current with industry standards and business objectives related to case management.

Skills:

1. Basic knowledge of personal computer and software for word processing and/or good keyboard skills preferred, or the ability to enter and retrieve data from relevant computer systems.
2. Ability to effectively communicate with all levels of claimants, TPA, physicians, healthcare personnel, supervisory staff, and peers.
3. Demonstrates the ability to be organized and efficient in prioritizing and managing assignments with minimal oversight and direction.
4. Demonstrates the willingness to research, learn, and to obtain knowledge for the performance of the position.
5. Demonstrates a courteous, professional demeanor and team spirit and the ability to work in a collaborative, effective manner.
6. Ability to utilize critical thinking and apply sound clinical judgment and assessment skills for decision-making.

Knowledge:

1. Knowledge of JCAHO/CARF (as appropriate) standards and federal and state regulations.
2. Knowledge of acute care, home care, subacute care, long-term care, hospice interventions, and rehabilitation options and requirements.
3. Maintains knowledge of requirement to Third Party Administrators, regulatory agencies, and managed care entities concerning levels of care, continuity of benefits, and medical necessity guidelines.
4. Maintains knowledge of the quality assurance process and determination of positive outcomes.
5. Uses clinical experience, knowledge of managed care and the current standards and trends in healthcare, best practices, management tools, and familiarity with related resources and literature.

Signature: _____

Date: _____

Director's Signature: _____

Source: Courtesy of Options Unlimited, Case Management Services Division, © 2003, Huntington, New York.

APPENDIX 13–B

Sample Medical Case Manager Position Description

Options Unlimited

Position Description: Medical Case Manager

Primary Claimants Served:
This position requires that the employee be able to demonstrate the knowledge and skills necessary to provide care based on physical, psychological, educational, safety, support systems and related criteria, appropriate to the claimant served. The skill and knowledge needs to be able to address age-specific issues, cultural diversity, socioeconomic factors, language differences, cultural traditions, and spiritual belief systems/practices of the claimant, family members, or supportive others. These issues are significant to the case manager's relationship with the claimant and will directly impact on the healthcare outcome.

Purpose of the Position:
The purpose of the medical case manager is to assess, plan, implement, monitor and evaluate options and services to effect an appropriate, individualized plan for the claimant across the continuum of care. Using independent judgment and discretion, the continuum must be reassessed as an ongoing process for the individual being served by the case manager. This is applied to multiple environments and interactive with the relative components of the claimant's healthcare system. The process addresses the individual's broad spectrum of needs. The medical case manager utilizes clinical knowledge and competence, positive communication skills, problem solving and conflict resolution techniques, ability to effect change, strong skills in assessment, organization, and time management. The case management process requires a focus on customer service skills, knowledge of setting appropriate goals and measuring outcomes to effectively ensure optimal client outcomes with consideration to payer requirements.

Specific Responsibilities and Duties:
The Medical Case Manager at Options Unlimited must be able to demonstrate and be accountable for the standards of practice policies and procedures, quality assurance, and the goals of the organization.

Healthcare Management:

1. Manages care of claimants through the healthcare system based on the individual's needs. Appropriately integrates the individual into the healthcare continuum including procuring of services, health promotion and counseling, disease prevention, health education and screening, and community resources linkage. Responsibilities include, but are not limited to the following:

   a. Uses independent judgment and discretion, identifies and plans strategies to reduce in-patient length of stay and resource consumption. Works in collaboration with physicians and appropriate healthcare providers for changes in plans as required. Provides claimant/family or significant other with information about nursing visits, home care, and appropriate providers.

   b. Advocates for the claimant and family throughout the entire episode of care. Maintains availability to the claimant/family as a resource to facilitate communication among providers and to monitor services rendered. Remains involved until the claimant achieves the planned level of functional health or closure criteria are met.

   c. Coordinates/facilitates the claimant's progression throughout the continuum.

   d. Works collaboratively and maintains active communication with physicians, nurses, social workers, utilization review staff, and other members of the multidisciplinary care team to effect timely, appropriate claimant management through the continuum.

   e. As appropriate, meets directly with the claimant/family and multidisciplinary team based on identified needs.

   f. Applies knowledge of age-specific, cultural diversity, psycho/social, and developmental issues during the interview process, documentation and intervention with the claimant, their family, or significant others.

   g. Remains in communication with claimants and the physicians and other members of the healthcare team to identify and resolve variances concurrently, and to assist the claimant in attaining the appropriate care with positive outcomes.

   h. Knowledgeable of new regulations on the federal, state and local level.

Process and Relationships:

2. Case managers will maintain the integrity of the Code of Professional Conduct for Case Managers. Performs case management by

applying clinical criteria to monitor appropriateness of admissions, level of care, and continued stays; and documents findings based on standards. Responsibilities include but are not limited to the following:

a. Collaborates with the physician and the multidisciplinary team to facilitate the plan of care and assist in identification and concurrent resolution of variances.

b. Uses independent judgment and discretion to address, resolve, and process problems impeding the diagnostic or treatment progress. Proactively identifies and resolves delays and obstacles.

c. Seeks consultation from physicians, clinical, and other disciplines and departments as required to expedite care, monitor length of in-patient stay, and facilitate discharge.

d. Collaborates and communicates with all members of the multidisciplinary team to validate information.

e. Identifies potential risk factors.

Service Delivery:

3. Manages aspects of the planning process in anticipation of claimant variances or transitions. Responsibilities include but are not limited to the following:

a. Collaborates and communicates with the physician and the rest of the care management multidisciplinary team to facilitate planning for variances or transitions.

b. When appropriate, meets directly with the claimant/family based on identified needs. Develops an individualized comprehensive plan of care in collaboration with the physicians and multidisciplinary team.

c. Initiates and facilitates referrals for home healthcare, infusion therapy, hospice, other care facilities, and medical equipment and supplies.

d. Facilitates transfers to other facilities.

e. Identifies "at risk" individuals and develop and implement a comprehensive plan of care that addresses the specific need.

f. Completes reports on time.

g. Remains current on case management documentation.

h. Writes Cost-Benefit Analysis report and submits by the due date.

Quality and Performance Improvement:

4. Appropriately identifies potential issues or "at risk" populations and anticipates the need to provide care.

5. Actively participates in clinical performance improvement process.

6. With respect to the individual claimant, analyzes and evaluates the effects of case management on quality outcomes, fiscal parameters, customer satisfaction, and systems operations; and develops strategies to improve performance.

7. Utilizes problem-solving techniques and conflict resolution skills, develops the plan to provide consistent quality to the claimant and the payer.

Managed Care and Regulatory Knowledge:

8. Collaborates with the multidisciplinary team to assist claimant with benefits/resource management to include negotiations with out-of-network providers, for resolution of payment issues, to develop a more cost-effective plan of care, and evaluate the appropriateness of the level of care or the use of services. Responsibilities include but are not limited to the following:

   a. Communicates, as required, with claimants to provide understanding of plan language and/or payer guidelines. When it is identified that clients are out of network, discuss issues for treatment and/or discharge needs with the physicians and relevant staff to provide for appropriate, timely treatment or a safe discharge.

   b. Assists physicians, care providers, and claimant/family in understanding the plan language and benefits as required.

Communication:

9. Maintains open communication with all appropriate parties.

   a. Utilizes problem-solving skills and negotiating techniques to resolve conflict issues.

   b. Identifies, plans, and coordinates aspects of care for the claimant, their family, or significant other.

   c. Communicates with supervisory personnel for problem solving, direction, and planning as well as knowledge issues.

   d. Initiates required forms and/or letters to comply with organizational guidelines.

   e. Completes timely and appropriate assessments, documentation, reports, and cost benefit analysis.

   f. Interacts with the physicians and members of the entire healthcare team in appropriate time frames.

10. Maintains strict standards for claimant confidentially and claimant-related information in addition to security of electronic information; complies with organizational, federal, and state regulations and policy on confidentiality.

Professional Development:

11. Maintains current knowledge of plan language and benefit issues and requirements as it relates to potential denial (whether contractual or utilization related).
12. Attends educational training program to expand job knowledge.
13. Performs other duties as related to case management functions to support and foster an effective, quality case management program.
14. Maintains current knowledge of URAC's standards of practice.

Position Requirements and Qualifications:

Education and Experience:

1. Graduated from an accredited School of Nursing or college: current New York state RN license required, BSN, Bachelor of Science in Nursing or health-related field preferred.
2. Graduated from an accredited college with a degree and licensure as a Certified Social Worker.
3. Minimum of 3–5 years of relevant clinical medical surgical or specialty experience required as applicable to the position needs.
4. Required to pursue ongoing education, certification, and self-development to remain current with industry standards and business objectives related to case management.

Skills:

1. Basic knowledge of personal computer and software for word processing and/or good keyboard skills preferred, or the ability to enter and retrieve data from relevant computer systems.
2. Ability to effectively communicate with all levels of claimants, TPA, physicians, healthcare personnel, supervisory staff, and peers.
3. Demonstrates the ability to be organized and efficient in prioritizing and managing assignments with minimal oversight and direction.
4. Demonstrates the willingness to research, learn, and obtain knowledge for the performance of the position.
5. Demonstrates a courteous, professional demeanor and team spirit and the ability to work in a collaborative, effective manner.
6. Utilizes critical thinking, and applies sound clinical judgment and assessment skills for decision making.

Knowledge:

1. Knowledge of JCAHO/CARF (as appropriate) standards and federal and state regulations.
2. Knowledge of acute care, home care, subacute care, long-term care, hospice interventions, and rehabilitation options and requirements.
3. Maintains knowledge of requirement to Third Party Administrators, regulatory agencies, and managed care entities concerning levels of care, continuity of benefits, and medical necessity guidelines.
4. Maintains knowledge of the quality assurance process and determination of positive outcomes.
5. Uses clinical experience, knowledge of managed care and the current standards and trends in healthcare, best practices, management tools, and familiarity with related resources and literature.

SIGNATURE: _____

DATE: _____

DIRECTOR'S SIGNATURE: _____

COB:ja

Source: Courtesy of Options Unlimited, Case Management Services Division, © 2003, Huntington, New York.

APPENDIX 13–C

Sample Director of Case Management Services Position Description

Options Unlimited

Position Description: Director of Case Management Services

Primary Claimants Served:
This position requires that the individual is able to demonstrate the ability to monitor, educate, and support the knowledge, skills, and performance of the case management staff. The individual must be able to educate case managers so they remain current to provide comprehensive care based on physical, psychological, educational, safety, support systems, and related criteria, appropriate to the claimants. The Director of Case Management must be able to elevate the knowledge and the recognition to address age-specific issues, cultural diversity, socioeconomic factors, language differences, cultural differences, cultural traditions, and spiritual belief systems/practices of the claimant, family members, or supportive others.

The Director of Case Management supports and implements the CMSA Standards of Practice, URAC guidelines, Code of Professional Conduct for Case Managers, the Federal regulations on confidentiality, and the Options Unlimited policies, procedures, and organizational goals.

The Quality Management Program is developed and implemented by the Director of Case Management Services. It is the role of the Director to assist with the process of identifying the areas of concern within the case management structure and to support the corporate drive toward excellence.

Purpose of the Position:
The Director of Case Management orients, guides, and oversees the case managers within Options Unlimited. The role is to plan, develop, implement, evaluate, and refine case management intervention. This individual supervises the case management personnel; contributes to the hiring and termination decisions; develops job descriptions, competency and performance standards, and schedules; monitors assignments; and assesses activity levels to meet budgetary guidelines. The role provides counseling and training, addresses disciplinary problems, and appraises performance.

The Director of Case Management Services ensures that the case managers assess, plan, and deliver care appropriate to the age specifics of every claimant. The individual must demonstrate sensitivity to the special needs of the claimants, payers, case managers, Options Unlimited personnel, and to all others involved within the job structure.

The individual implements and supports a culture of continuous quality improvement, supports the CMSA standard of practice, URAC guidelines, code of professional conduct, and the federal regulations on confidentiality; all of these are implemented into the philosophy, framework, policy, and procedures of Options Unlimited. The individual in this role contributes to the team objectives and goals with support to the organization and departmental strategic plans.

Specific Responsibilities and Duties:
The Director of Case Management at Options Unlimited must be able to support and empower the case managers in performance of their position description and within the regulations of their licensure. The role fosters and supports accountability for the CMSA Standards of Practice; URAC Guidelines; Code of Case Manager's Conduct; regulations on confidentiality, policy, and procedures; quality management; and the goals of the organization.

Healthcare Management:
1. Supervises the case managers in performance of their role and position description.
2. Assists the case managers in the coordination of care and service of a selected client population across the continuum of illness.
3. Empowers the case managers in promoting effective utilization and monitoring of healthcare resources.
4. Provides leadership for the case management personnel to achieve optimal clinical and resource outcomes.
5. Formulates, implements, and evaluates the knowledge base of the case managers in the performance of their position description.
6. Analyzes the case management goals for the claimants, reviews the plan for its appropriateness, and reviews and identifies anticipated outcomes.
7. Recognizes that all plans of care for the individuals are not successful and the outcomes are not as anticipated; identifies and makes recommendations for a corrective plan.
8. Demonstrates skill and proficiency in applying highly technical principles and concepts.
9. Supports a climate for research and expansion of skill and knowledge.

Process and Relationships:

1. Develops and maintains a positive work climate that supports the overall staff efforts at Options Unlimited.
2. Assists in developing the philosophy, goals, and objectives for concurrent case management performance that meets clinical and financial requirements.
3. Implements the Standards of Practice for Case Management, URAC Guidelines, ethical performance, and functions relevant to the coordination of quality case management.
4. Anticipates, recommends, implements, and evaluates policies and procedures related to the Options Unlimited case management system.
5. Demonstrates knowledge in regard to the case management functions and recommends changes as needed to maintain and upgrade the standards of practice.
6. Demonstrates the ability to work within a team structure.
7. Contributes to the organization's goals and objectives; supports the organizational strategic plans.
8. Actively participates in the consensus building among the Options Unlimited personnel.
9. Empowers the case managers to strive for greater knowledge and promotes professional and personal growth.
10. Maintains strict confidentiality, as written by federal law, in regard to claimants and Options Unlimited personnel.
11. Demonstrates the ability to interact with a wide variety of individuals and to handle complex situations simultaneously.
12. Performs other duties as requested.

Service Delivery:

1. Provides orientation, continuing education, and training on case management.
2. Actively participates in the development of clinician guidelines and incorporates the process into the role of the case managers.
3. Interfaces with external agencies and provides appropriate information, consultation, and recommendations.
4. Supervises case management performance and the implementation of their role.
5. Contributes to the hiring process.
6. Develops job descriptions and performance standards.
7. Monitors the acuity level of the case managers.

8. Provides counseling and training.
9. Addresses disciplinary concerns.
10. Appraises performance.

Quality and Performance Improvement

1. Works within a team environment to manage the functions of the Options Unlimited Case Management Quality Management Committee.
2. Supports a culture of continuous quality improvement.
3. Uses quality improvement tools and strategies in problem-solving activities.
4. Prepares quality, screening abstracts according to current policy and procedure.
5. Identifies patterns or trends in case management that have or had the potential for adverse impact on claimant interventions.
6. Develops corrective action plans and reevaluation of outcomes.
7. Provides reports, summaries, trends, and statistical analysis to the President and Vice President and shares the data with the staff at Options Unlimited.

Managed Care and Regulatory Knowledge:

Collaborates, as required, with the multidisciplinary team to assist the case manager with benefit and resource management, to mentor those who need to negotiate services that are out of network, to resolve payment issues, to institute a more cost-effective plan of care, to evaluate the appropriateness of the level of care or the use of services. Responsibilities include but are not limited to the following:

1. Communicates with the case managers to provide an understanding of Plan language and/or payer guidelines.
2. When identification is made that the claimant is out of network, discusses the issues for treatment/discharge needs with the healthcare team to provide for an appropriate, timely treatment or a safe discharge.
3. Assists the case manager in assisting the physicians, care providers, and claimant/family in understanding the Plan language and benefits as required.
4. Shares the knowledge of the interventional time factors that impact case management services.

Communication:

1. Maintains open communication with all appropriate individuals.
2. Communicates within and outside Options Unlimited in a timely manner in regard to significant, relevant issues, and follows through with requests.
3. Written communication is clear, concise, well-organized, and follows the approved format of Options Unlimited.
4. Maintains a professional, courteous manner when communicating.
5. Utilizes problem-solving skills to resolve conflict.
6. Identifies, plans, coordinates, and implements the sharing of knowledge.
7. Maintains strict standards for confidentiality and the appropriate dissemination of information.
8. Knowledge of securing electronic information.
9. Complies with organizational, federal, and state regulations, and with policies regarding confidentiality.

Professional Development:

1. Knowledge of legislation that affects the case management process.
2. Attends educational and training programs to expand job knowledge.
3. Performs other duties as related to case management functions to support and implement an effective, quality case management program.

Position Requirements and Qualifications:

Education and Experience:

1. Graduated from an accredited School of Nursing or college.
2. Current New York state license as a Registered Professional Nurse.
3. Bachelor of Science in Nursing or Health Related field. (Preferred)
4. Minimum of 5–7 years of relevant clinical medical-surgical or specialty experience required. Supervisory experience preferred.
5. Required to pursue ongoing education, certification, and self-development to remain current with industry standards and business objectives related to case management.

Skills:

1. Knowledgeable in the use of personal computers and software for work processing and good keyboard skills.
2. Demonstrates the ability to efficiently enter and retrieve data from relevant computer systems.

3. Demonstrates the ability to communicate effectively.
4. Demonstrates organizational skills and is efficient in prioritizing and managing the case managers and other assignments.
5. Demonstrates the willingness and ability to research, learn, and obtain knowledge for the performance of the position.
6. Demonstrates courteous, professional demeanor and cooperative spirit.
7. Demonstrates the ability to work in a collaborative, effective manner.
8. Demonstrates the ability to utilize critical thinking and apply sound clinical judgment and assessment skills for decision making.

Knowledge:

1. Knowledge of CMSA Standards of Practice for Case Management.
2. Knowledge of URAC Guidelines.
3. Knowledge of the Code of Professional Conduct for Case Managers.
4. Knowledge of the different levels of claimant care and the qualifications required for each level.
5. Knowledge of ERISA regulations and time factors.
6. Knowledge of the plans and their language with the skill to gain interpretation of the specific dialogue.
7. Maintains knowledge of the quality assurance process and the ability to effect positive outcomes.
8. Maintains knowledge of regulatory agencies and managed care entities concerning levels of care, continuity of benefits, and medical necessity guidelines.
9. Uses clinical experience, knowledge of managed care, and the current standards and trends in healthcare, best practices, management tools, and familiarity with related resources and literature.

Signature: _____
Date: _____
President's/Vice President's Signature: _____

Source: Courtesy of Options Unlimited, Case Management Services Division, © 2003, Huntington, New York.

APPENDIX 13–D

Interview Evaluation Form

Employment Selection and Compliance System

Interview Evaluation Form

(Fill Out Immediately After Each Interview)

Name: _____ College: _____

Degree: _____ Major _____ Position Applied For_____

	Appraisal of Candidate				
	Excellent	Good	Average	Below Average	Poor
General First Impression (greeting, self expression, etc.)					
Personal Appearance					
Apparent Drive					
Initiative in Conversation					
Apparent Aggressiveness					
Apparent Ability to Get Along with People					
Attitude					
Speech					
Potential					
ASPIRATIONS - Extent to which the goals and aspirations of the applicant are consistent with available opportunity.					
TRAINING - Extent to which level of educational skills and relevant on-the-job training will enable applicant to cope with the demands of the job.					
WORK HISTORY - Extent to which the applicant's work experience applies to the performance of applicant's duties.					
MANNERS AND APPEARANCE - Extent to which the applicant is able to present and communicate his/her ideas to others.					
COOPERATION - Degree to which the applicant will be able to get along with others in the work environment. Is applicant a team player?					
RESPONSIBILITY - Extent to which applicant will exercise judgment in getting the job done, takes initiative when appropriate, and seeks assistance when required.					
OVERALL FINAL IMPRESSION					

ADDITIONAL COMMENTS

_____

_____

_____

Recommended for Further Interview: ⊕YES ⊕NO

Recommended for Hire: ⊕YES ⊕NO

Date: _____ Interviewed By: _____

The First Interview

Source: Reprinted from *Employment Selection and Compliance System*, p. 12, Profiles International Inc., © 2001.

APPENDIX 13–E

Summary Evaluation Scale

Employment Selection and Compliance System

Summary Evaluation Scale

APPLICANT: _____ DATE: _____ JOB: _____

EVALUATION FACTORS	Not Applicable	Unknown	QUALIFICATIONS						
			UNDER QUALIFIED Low Enough To Disqualify The Applicant	POOR Extremely Low But Other Factors Could Compensate	FAIR Low But Acceptable For The Job	AVERAGE The Typical Applicant On This Factor	GOOD Definitely A Cut Above The Average	OUTSTANDING Compares Favorably With Top Applicants	OVER QUALIFIED Interference With Success Is Probable
GENERAL EDUCATION									
SPECIALIZED KNOWLEDGE									
WORK EXPERIENCE									
JOB STABILITY									
GROWTH & DEVELOPMENT									
GENERAL INTELLIGENCE									
PRACTICAL JUDGMENT									
SPECIAL APTITUDES									
MANUAL DEXTERITY									
LEADERSHIP SKILLS									
COMMUNICATION SKILLS									
MOTIVATION									
MANAGEMENT OF TIME									
CHARACTER									
EMOTIONAL MATURITY									
INITIATIVE AND DRIVE									
DEPENDABILITY									
COOPERATIVENESS									
HUMAN RELATIONS									
INTERESTS									
APPEARANCE									
OVERALL QUALIFICATION FOR THE JOB									
JOB SUITABILITY %									

RECOMMENDATIONS:

EVALUATOR _____

The Second Interview

Source: Reprinted from *Employment Selection and Compliance System,* p. 3, Profiles International Inc., © 2001.

APPENDIX 13–F

Competencies for Unit-Based Nurse Case Manager

COMPETENCIES FOR UNIT-BASED NURSE CASE MANAGER

UNIT-BASED NURSE CASE MANAGER'S NAME: _____

COMPETENCIES	COMPETENT BY SELF-ASSESSMENT	EXPLANATION, DEMONSTRATION, OR REVIEW NEEDED	DATE AND INITIAL OF EXPLANATION, DEMONSTRATION, OR REVIEW	DATE AND INITIAL OF OBSERVATION OR DEMONSTRATION OF SKILLS
1. Collaborates with the attending physician to discuss patient progress and achievement of expected day-to-day outcomes defined by the MAP.				
2. Anticipates and identifies variances in the care process related to the patient's individual needs. Makes plans to resolve unexpected care requirements to facilitate returning the patient to the usual progress tract.				
3. Participates in the development and review of case management tools (i.e., MAPs, collaborative case management plans, patient education materials, and discharge instructions for designated patient populations).				
4. Coordinates with other clinical disciplines to facilitate the patient's receiving the required care within the expected time frame.				
5. Participates in nurse case management seminars:				
• Attends				
• Presents				
• Coordinates				
6. Initiates individualized MAP to meet patient needs.				
7. Discusses the collaborative plan of care with physician, associates, and staff from other disciplines.				
8. Initiates patient care conferences when indicated.				

continues

Competencies continued

COMPETENCIES	COMPETENT BY SELF-ASSESSMENT	EXPLANATION, DEMONSTRATION, OR REVIEW NEEDED	DATE AND INITIAL OF EXPLANATION, DEMONSTRATION, OR REVIEW	DATE AND INITIAL OF OBSERVATION OR DEMONSTRATION OF SKILLS
9. Directs and participates in care delivery.				
10. Attends case management workshop.				
11. Initiates or directs teaching plan.				
12. Facilitates posthospitalization follow-up contact. This may include the physician, office staff, and referral agencies when appropriate.				
13. Participates in professional growth and development through publications, seminars, workshops, conferences, and professional affiliations.				
14. Actively serves on case management committee including task force involvement when appropriate.				
15. Actively participates in quality management/ quality improvement activities.				

Source: Reprinted from F. Snowden, ed., *Medical Case Management: Forms Checklists and Guidelines, second edition,* pp. 2:33, 2:34, Aspen Publishers, Inc., © 2003.

Part IV

Emerging Trends and Opportunities

Chapter 14

Obesity: The New Epidemic

Affecting nearly two-thirds of adults and a distressing number of children and adolescents, overweight and obesity are two of the most significant public health threats facing the United States. As case managers, we are seeing first-hand the resulting secondary problems. Of course, there are the obvious ones that are routinely associated with obesity, including hypertension, type 2 diabetes, and stroke, but people living years with overweight or obesity are also increasing the incidence of joint-replacement surgery, back surgeries, and a host of other medical conditions that researchers are studying for possible correlation or its predisposition for other conditions. Conditions that previously affected primarily middle-aged sedentary adults are now being seen in youngsters! One can only wonder what *their* future will be like and how they will cope with a *lifetime* of conditions resulting from obesity.

Although science has certainly demonstrated the links between overweight and obesity and these life-threatening conditions, there is no real consensus today among patients, providers, and researchers on what constitutes successful weight loss. Healthcare professionals are not separate from society, and many of us are also dealing with obesity. Nurses in particular, I believe, have a more difficult time accepting that illness, including obesity and its related diagnoses, can strike them too. We somehow think, or possibly hope, that we will be able to know when we're in trouble, and *then* we'll do the "right thing." We often ignore what we know is sound medical advice given to our patients, feeling that it's for them and not us. It's almost akin to the feelings of invincibility that adolescents experience when they recklessly drive a car or, worse, drink and drive—the accident will happen to somebody else, not them. Although a good number of our colleagues are affected by obesity, somehow the expectations for health professionals, rightly or wrongly, are different. We are expected to be role models, individuals who lead healthy lifestyles, and educators who will help others.

Because case managers are absolutely on the front line, I wondered how case managers who might be overweight or obese might be able to work with patients who have the same diagnoses. I also wondered how their slimmer counterparts might be responding to patients who were obese. Additionally, I became increasingly concerned about the stigmatization of obese individuals and their ability to obtain competent care from compassionate professionals. As editor of *The Case Manager*, I seized the opportunity to bring the condition of obesity to the forefront in a "Special Focus" issue in November/December 2004. As the fourth edition of this book was being created, once again, it seemed appropriate that a separate chapter should address this complex problem. Removing barriers to care are certainly central to the role of the case manager and there are so many within the system itself, among the providers and payers, and of course with our patients that case managers will need to utilize the very best of their skills and expertise. Although expertise is important, so too is the caring heart of the case manager, which can surely make a difference, one patient at a time. In this chapter, we examine the issues that have resulted in obesity becoming the new epidemic, explore the treatment alternatives, consider the economic implications, provide some insight into the psychosocial issues, consider the ethical issues, and present just *some* of the opportunities where case managers can contribute and improve the outcomes for those who need their assistance.

OBESITY: A SIMPLE DEFINITION, A COMPLEX PROBLEM

The American Medical Association has defined obesity as a condition in which excess body fat may compromise the health of an individual. It is considered a complex disease that originates from a combination and interaction of social, environmental, genetic, physiologic, behavioral, lifestyle, cultural, and metabolic factors. It is an epidemic and a condition with so many contributing factors that a one-size-fits-all standard of care has not been developed. That's not to say that there are no solutions or strategies; however, it is and will continue to be one of the more challenging conditions for case managers now and in the foreseeable future.

The prevalence of overweight and obesity is increasing rapidly in the United States and worldwide and is already reaching epidemic proportions. An estimated 250 million people in the world are obese, and the number is projected to reach 300 million by the year 2025.[1] In the United States, 64% of those older than the age of 20 are overweight; 30% of adults are obese.[2] Although these figures certainly are of concern to those of us in healthcare, of more alarm is that on the basis of data for the National Health and Nutrition Examination Survey (NHANES), the prevalence of overweight in children between the ages of 6 and 11 years increased from 4.0% from 1971 to 1974 to 17.5% during 2001 to 2004; the prevalence in adolescents between 12 and 19 years increased from 6.1% to 17.0%.[3]

The incidence of obesity involves both genders, all age groups, all classes, and all income and educational levels. In the last decade, the percentage of obese children has doubled to almost 27% and overweight teenagers have an 80% chance of being overweight adults.[4] Dr. David S. Ludwig, Director of the Obesity Program at Children's Hospital in Boston, observes: "Obesity is such that this generation of children could be the first basically in the history of the United States to live less healthful and shorter lives than their parents."[5]

The Centers for Disease Control and Prevention (www.cdc.gov) and other organizations note that obesity greatly increases the risk of many diseases and conditions, including the following:

- Coronary heart disease
- Type 2 diabetes
- Cancers (endometrial, breast, prostate, and colon)
- Hypertension
- Dyslipidemia
- Stroke
- Liver and gallbladder disease
- Sleep apnea and respiratory problems
- Osteoarthritis
- Gynecological problems (abnormal menses, infertility)[6]

Obesity affects essentially every organ system in the body. In addition, quality of life is significantly decreased by increasing weight and is improved by losing weight. Obesity also affects mortality; additionally, the relative risk of death and disease increases disproportionately as weight increases. According to the American Obesity Association, "Obesity is associated with more than 30 medical conditions, and scientific evidence has established a strong relationship with at least 15 of those conditions."[7]

"The concept of obesity and obesity with associated co-morbidities as manageable, chronic conditions is emerging," advises the Disease Management Association of America Care Continuum Alliance (DMAA; www.dmaa.org).[8] In 2008, DMAA launched a website of information and tools (free!) for health plans, employers, physicians, consumers, and others. This obviously is good news for case managers who are already seeing increased numbers of patients with these complex conditions in their case loads.

Economic Impact

According to the Centers for Disease Control and Prevention, the economic consequences for obesity are considerable: Obesity accounts for 9% of national healthcare expenditures, or about $93 billion in 2002 dollars. The estimated annual direct cost of medical conditions related to overweight and obesity are $8.8 billion for heart disease, $98 billion for type 2 diabetes, and $4.1 billion for hypertension.[9] Many of us in case management are also involved in return to work and disability management programs, and we see that the costs related to absenteeism and *presenteeism*, a newer term used by human resource professionals, are significant. ("Presenteeism is defined as lost productivity that occurs when employees come to work but perform below par due to any kind of illness. While the costs associated with the absenteeism of employees have been long studied, the cost of presenteeism is newly being studied."[10])

Although health insurers, private and public, certainly bear the larger economic burden from conditions related to obesity, other insurers are experiencing the consequences as well. Disability insurer UnumProvident Corporation has acknowledged that claims from certain weight-related problems have *doubled* since 1996, and the National Institutes of Health estimates that healthcare costs attributable to obese and overweight people are $123 *billion* a year.[11]

Impact on Staff, Facilities, and Equipment

With a marked increase in the incidence of obesity, hospitals are seeing more patients who weigh 50, 100, and 200 pounds over the ideal. Because these facilities are staffed with professionals and paraprofessionals who may not be adequately trained or prepared to treat the obese, many are taking a closer look to improve outcomes and create safe environments for patients *and* staff. The American Nurses Association estimates that 12% of nurses leave the profession because of back injuries each year and more than 52% complain of chronic back pain.[12] Nurses (and their designated staff members) are called upon to examine and maintain skin integrity of hospitalized patients, and this requires frequent turning and repositioning. (*Note*: In 2007, the Centers for Medicare and Medicaid

Services [CMS] announced that effective October 2008, it will curtail payments to hospitals for specific conditions that a patient acquires while an inpatient and that can be "reasonably prevented" by following established evidence-based guidelines. These hospital-acquired conditions (HAC) include but are not limited to pressure ulcers (decubiti) stages III and IV, complications from extended use of catheters, and injuries caused by falls.[13]) Nurses must also transfer patients from bed to chair, lift them to bathe, dress, and feed them as well as position them during aspects of certain procedures. Obviously, more than one person, often several, is needed to perform these tasks for obese patients. This concentration of staff may result in neglect or delay in meeting other patients' needs.

Although hands-on care requires some reallocation of resources, the usual equipment and materials found in hospitals, physician offices, and other sites of care delivery are also lacking in many circumstances. As case managers who are involved in the coordination of care across the continuum in multiple settings, we need to keep height and weight of our patients in mind. As our patients move from hospital to extended care to home, the options for care need to be evaluated. Some but not all transport companies can accommodate obese individuals and also those considered supermorbidly obese; some but not all facilities have beds with automatic controls that convert the bed into a chair/recliner, and if the patient is ambulatory, this allows the patient to step out of the chair to an upright position; some hospitals are creating bariatric wings in their facilities; others are evaluating bariatric equipment including operating tables, beds, and wheelchairs, and plus-size accommodations are becoming standard in many healthcare facilities. Obviously, although we certainly want to create user-friendly environments for all of our patients, this is not without still yet another economic impact. Managing an obese patient adds additional challenges to the patient management process, our facilities, and providers. Case managers once again are right at the center!

METRICS TO DETERMINE OBESITY

In case management and disease management programs, it's always advantageous to be able to identify and appropriately target those individuals who would most benefit from our intervention as early as possible. Unfortunately, although it is also preferable to be proactive and early in our approach, patients who begin to show the symptoms of the complications from obesity often do not present themselves until damage has already occurred, resulting in not only one condition to assist with, but perhaps several. Thankfully, we now have some tools to utilize during risk assessments or wellness promotion programs that will assist us in the earlier identification of persons who could benefit from lifestyle modification, healthy living programs, or other earlier interventions that can prevent or at least minimize complications and the condition of obesity.

Height and weight tables that provide general guidelines for normal weight for height cannot predict disease associated with obesity. The body mass index (BMI) is a newer metric, was developed in the mid-1800s by a Belgian mathematician, and became popular in the 1950s and 1960s as concerns about obesity were increasing. BMI is a strong predictor of obesity and related comorbidities: The higher a person's BMI, the higher his or her risk for developing certain diseases. Waist circumference and waist-to-hip ratio are other measurements that can identify obese patients.

BMI

Obesity is determined by an individual's body mass index (BMI) and can be calculated easily by using the readily available BMI calculator at www.cdc.gov or other commercial sites on the Internet. BMI is defined as weight in kilograms divided by the square of the height in meters. Fortunately, for the mathematically challenged, the BMI calculator is amazingly easy and fast to use. Following are the ranges of BMI and classifications defined by the World Health Organization (WHO) in 1995:

- 18.5–25.0 = Normal
- 25.1–30.0 = Overweight
- 30.1+ = Obese (mild)
- 35 = Moderate obesity
- 40 = Severe obesity[14]

Waist Circumference

The National Heart, Lung, and Blood Institute, part of the National Institutes of Health (NIH), defines *waist circumference* as "the presence of excess fat in the abdomen out of proportion to total body fat [that] is an independent predictor of risk factors and morbidity."[15] For men, a waist measurement of 40 inches or more indicates a health risk; for women, that measurement is 35 inches.[16]

Although BMI and waist circumference are of assistance in identifying individuals that may be at risk, obviously medical history, family history, and other factors need to be considered as well.

Waist-to-Hip Ratio (WHR)

Research shows that people with "apple-shaped" bodies (more weight around the waist) face more health risks than those with "pear-shaped" bodies, who carry more weight around the hips. The calculator to determine body shape can be found at www.bmi-calculator.net/waist-to-hip-ratio-calculator/.

ETIOLOGY

Research continues to demonstrate that obesity is a multifactorial disease. Obesity, as noted in an article titled "The Epidemic of Obesity" in the *Western Journal of Medicine*, is a chronic disease that is caused by eating more calories than are expended. Obese people, therefore, are stigmatized and as a result are often extremely reluctant to seek treatment, especially with professionals who may be less than kind in their relationships with them. In addition to the calories in, calories out rationale, there are other considerations that may contribute to this condition. Cortisol, the stress hormone, has its influence; so too do genetic factors that include the inherent factors that may predispose a person to weight challenges. Physiologic factors include bone structure and body shape. Behavioral factors may include habits or patterns that people follow such as a low level of activity or high intake of certain foods. Because we have such a diverse culture, some of the preferred foods by a particular ethnic group may result in a higher incidence of obesity for that group. Another condition, depression, is getting closer attention today as a contributing factor for the development of certain diseases, including depression. Some research suggests that depressed people are more likely to develop the metabolic syndrome that often accompanies excess weight.

Although no one factor can be blamed for the fattening of America, there certainly seems to be a potent mix of less exercise, changes in work–life balance, more meals eaten outside the home, bigger portions, more fats and sugars in prepared foods, and a strong reluctance to consider any kind of moderation, especially with favorite foods, fueling this problem. In an article "Supersizing America—Obesity Becomes an Epidemic," Martha Coventry observes: "We have become so used to being fat, that we may have accepted it as our new national identity. A women's size 14 in the 1940s is a size 10 today. The average airline passenger now weighs almost 21 pounds more than in 1995 . . . and the extra-wide coffin business is taking off."[17] When companies discovered that it costs only a little more to produce large versus medium servings, the "supersize me" craze took off and waistlines increased.

In 1960, 18.6% of women with children younger than 6 years old were working outside the home; by 1993, that percentage had climbed to 59.6 (as one of these working women, there is no blame assigned!). Working women don't *cause* obesity, but the lifestyle adjustments that families make to accommodate this reality exacerbate the problem. Today, nearly half of all meals are eaten outside the house, many of them at fast-food restaurants, where food is loaded with fats and carbohydrates.[18]

As food intake increases and the *kinds* of food eaten are less healthy, another factor compounds and absolutely contributes to obesity: exercise, or rather a lack of exercise. We, our families, children, co-workers, and colleagues are spending more time in front of computers, at our desks, attending meetings, traveling, playing video games, and surfing the Net (but *never* at work) and return home after many hours of work/school to have a quick dinner, collapse in front of the TV, and then go to bed. Clearly, although we may be burning *some* calories with this stress-filled lifestyle, for some, the stress may drive us to eat more (people may console themselves with "comfort food," usually high in fat, sugar, and calories). Lack of exercise is absolutely problematic for all of us.

TREATMENT OVERVIEW

Several treatment approaches have proved successful, and some individuals must use a combination of these strategies. Treatment techniques include dietary monitoring, exercise at levels appropriate to the ability and risk factors of the individual, behavior therapy, pharmacology, and surgery. We live in a world where many of us demand instant results, a magic pill, or even approaches that promise weight loss: "Lose weight while you sleep, no exercise or dieting needed!" Unfortunately, because the weight gain that led to obesity likely occurred over months and possibly years, the resolution of this condition cannot come overnight. Currently, a vicious cycle is perpetuated by the lack of effective treatments for people with moderate obesity until the obesity becomes severe and refractory to nonsurgical treatment as well as associated with significant and costly comorbidities.[19]

Perceptions of Treatment

A perception or assumption that has become a major hurdle in the treatment of obesity is that nothing works. Because there really isn't consensus on how to define "clinically significant" or "meaningful" weight loss, the perception most surely becomes reality. With the lack of an agreed upon definition of success, there is widespread belief among physicians that the current array of treatment modalities including medications, lifestyle modifications, exercise, and counseling doesn't produce meaningful or sustained weight loss. It's no wonder, then, that so many treating physicians fail to address obesity with their patients—what physician would want to confront their patients with this diagnosis when they believe "nothing works"? Additionally, because obesity is a multifactorial condition, interventions are perceived as time-intensive and costly. So, when time and cost are weighed against results that are viewed as modest, treatment doesn't seem worth the effort.

Perceptions Among Health Professionals

Physicians and many other healthcare professionals are more comfortable when traditional surgery or medicines are used to treat medical conditions; this in fact is considered the practice of medicine. Although many chronic diseases can be partially treated or symptoms alleviated with medication, they often also require sustained behavior change. The practice of medicine has not fully embraced this still evolving science.

A 2003 survey of 620 physicians confirmed the sense of futility many physicians feel in treating obesity.[20] Respondents described a lack of confidence in treating obesity; expected patients to be unmotivated and noncompliant; believed patients did not want to discuss their weight; preferred avoidance of the topic themselves and apparently waited until the condition was severe before addressing it.

Perceptions Among People Who are Overweight or Obese

People who are overweight or obese recognize that doctors do not often adequately address obesity. They describe wanting more intensive treatments than physicians typically offer and as a result turn to nonmedical sources for help with weight management.[21] Americans spend about $60 billion on weight-loss products; at least two-thirds of obese people are actively trying to lose weight, with an average of three attempts to diet per year.[22] Obviously, there is a difference in perceptions between patients who are overweight or obese and their healthcare providers: Patients don't believe that trying to lose weight is completely futile as compared to their healthcare providers, who are certainly much less optimistic.

The Stigma of Obesity

Perhaps the most emotionally charged obstacle that affects patients and challenges the healthcare professionals who interact with them is the stigma of obesity. This is not exactly a new problem, but surely one that has become more pervasive and reflects the change not only in our population but the attitudes assumed by others, including healthcare professionals regarding those perceived as different. Charged with the role of advocate, it is increasingly important for case managers to shine a spotlight on the stigma of obesity for these individuals to feel comfortable and safe as they deal with the issues and medical problems arising from their condition.

Stigma is easy to define, but much more challenging to address and resolve. As it relates specifically to obesity, stigma is a set of negative attitudes directed toward people with obesity simply and solely based on their weight. The stigma against people with obesity has been called the "last socially acceptable form of prejudice." As a society we are ambivalent about stigmatizing obesity. Many individuals, including people who are obese themselves, think obesity happens because of lack of motivation, willpower, or self-discipline and is a matter of individual, not societal, responsibility.[23] Most people with obesity fear the social and psychological consequences even more than the risks to their health. Does the stigma, therefore, in some way serve as a motivator for people to want to lose weight? Would decreasing the stigma improve the *quality* of life for them, and therefore lessen the motivation to lose weight?

It is not considered stigmatizing for one not to want to be obese or to think that someone who is obese is at greater risk for health conditions compared to someone who is of normal weight. It is, however, stigmatizing to assume a person with obesity is lazy or slow, or to believe that he or she is less competent or productive simply because of the excess weight. Bias and prejudice are somewhat similar. It isn't biased or prejudiced to believe that an obese person is at risk for developing diabetes, but it is biased to assume that they are depressed or jolly. Because of the growing prevalence of obesity in adults and children, several television shows have attempted to shine a spotlight on this. Sometimes a reporter or normal-weight person will put on "fat suits" so that he or she can experience how obese individuals are treated differently. From coping with stares and looks ranging from curiosity to repulsion all the way through experiencing unkind acts and admonishments from total strangers, individuals who are obese have become victims in a society that is becoming less tolerant of them.

Stigma in Health Settings

The healthcare setting has not shown itself to be a haven from stigmatizing attitudes and behaviors against people with obesity. On the contrary, health professionals often view their obese patients negatively.[24] In surveys, health professionals specializing in obesity revealed a lesser degree of stigmatizing attitudes, yet bias was still present nevertheless.[25] Obese women are screened less often for breast and cervical cancer than are nonobese women, despite being at higher risk.[26]

It's important to gain some insight as to why we might stigmatize and, as healthcare professionals, to assess our own feelings carefully. As case managers, if we are obese, are we possibly rationalizing our own condition, and therefore not addressing obesity and its health risks with patients who are similarly afflicted? If we are of normal weight, are we perhaps overly critical, judgmental? Are we more compassionate when patients have conditions that were not influenced by their behavior, such as cancer, multiple sclerosis, or cerebral palsy, and less understanding when they have a condition that we judge to be influenced by unwise behavior, such as AIDS, chronic obstructive pulmonary disease (COPD), or obesity?

When patients perceive that the very individuals who could be of assistance in their efforts to lose weight or provide treatment for the complications that years of obesity may induce are, in fact, dismissive or judgmental, they delay seeking intervention. As obesity becomes more widespread, has it become more acceptable and therefore less stigmatizing than before? Research shows that the opposite may be true, as obesity increases in prevalence, so does the stigma of the obese. One study in children showed that, compared to 40 years ago, disliking an obese child had increased by about 40%.[27]

An Ethicist Weighs In

Case managers have been fortunate to gain the insight and perspective of other professionals as our own professional practice settings were evolving. Healthcare attorneys, physicians, pharmacists, behavioral medicine specialists, and ethicists have been among the valued colleagues we look to as we grapple with problems that we might not have encountered in our more traditional roles. John Banja, PhD, is an Associate Professor at the Center for Ethics at Emory University and was a columnist for *The Case Manager* for many years as well as a commissioner for the Commission for Case Manager Certification (CCMC). He examined the dilemmas and challenges of obesity in the Special Focus issue of *The Case Manager* mentioned earlier (for a more expansive discussion, please see that issue).

Banja writes: "If our contemporary media are responsible sources as to what Americans prefer in body size today, the esthetics of our age are nicely captured by the Duchess of Windsor's humorous quip, 'You can never be too rich or too thin.' " He notes further, "The signal ethical problem that occurs over whether we are justified in our moral criticisms of people with obesity (i.e., our contention that they are costing the health-care system money . . . our response being, '. . . how can they be so irresponsible . . . why can't they just exercise a little self-restraint . . . why are they so selfish with my money?') is that we lack the prerequisite science to persuade us that obesity is largely the result of freely willed, voluntary choice."[28]

Case managers must examine and understand their feelings about certain issues, especially the "hot" ones, such as race, religion, and dying, so that they can more effectively work with patients objectively and compassionately. This kind of insight and understanding helps us to accept ourselves for what we are (or as mentioned earlier, it creates opportunities to rationalize), but we frequently do not extend this empathy to other people. Why does this occur, and how can we change this?

Banja wonders about this as well and suggests the following:

> Instead of trying to understand why they are the way that they are, we succumb to the way we experience them. We infer their motivations or reasons as to why they are obese on the basis of how they affect us. And because many people experience the obese individual's appearance as revolting or grotesque, we proceed to think that they could not be concerned with anything except his stomach. We experience their appearance as a personal insult, which in turn encourages us to assault their character.[29]

There are many examples that could be provided that so clearly demonstrate the vicious cycle in this kind of thinking, but suffice it to say that we need some guidance in moving in a more positive direction. Banja recommends that rather than feeling anger or revulsion, "the first obligation is to understand him or her: to gain an insight into what it must be like to be him or her; to imagine and to interpret the world from his or her perspective experience; to engage in as the brilliant psychiatrist Heinz Kohut said, 'vicarious introspection.' In a word, I need to be empathetic, because the dividends from doing so are immense." He concludes: "As with the management of all 'difficult' patients, the healthcare professional must continually interrogate and evaluate his or her own anxieties and psychologic defenses because it is precisely this baggage that we bring to every encounter."[30]

As the condition of obesity continues to become more prevalent, and as more obese individuals become part of our caseloads, we obviously must apply a continual process of self-evaluation so that these individuals receive the care and compassion they so rightly deserve.

Treatment Availability and Funding

Although healthcare services do exist for obesity, they tend to be located in cities (often in specialty hospitals, medical practices, etc.), and many individuals will have to pay for their treatment out of pocket. This limits services to more affluent people, depriving those in rural areas, people with lower socioeconomic status, and those belonging to ethnic minorities, where the incidence of obesity is higher.[31] Although some insurance companies, self-funded employer groups, union health and welfare, and other payers will pay for obesity-related care and services, others have severely restricted language in their plans that specifically cites what will be covered and strictly enforced criteria that must be met before coverage will be granted. Still others deny coverage, especially for those individuals classified as overweight, but not yet obese. Once again, one wonders about the advisability of waiting until someone is at the more advanced stages of a condition such as obesity when clearly the costs of providing early intervention, education, and medical care would be less.

Because treatment outcomes are not predictable, the health plan industry is trying to learn from government, academic, and provider groups. There is ongoing collaboration with the CDC with the intent of bringing together these communities to develop strategies to identify and then to create the most cost-effective and best way(s) to treat this complex condition.

The U.S. Preventive Services Task Force recommends that healthcare professionals offer incentive lifestyle intervention to their patients or refer them to providers who can. An expert panel convened by the National Heart, Lung, and Blood Institute proposed a treatment algorithm in which lifestyle modification (diet, exercise, and behavioral therapy) is the cornerstone of treatment. Although there is an obvious need and a call out to clinicians to address obesity, and several successful strategies can be employed, a specific barrier exists for actual implementation: reimbursement. Anecdotal evidence exists, and from my years in case management, I find that physicians and providers are rarely reimbursed for the costs of weight management services for preobese individuals. The American Obesity Association, together with other organizations, campaigned for Internal Revenue Service (IRS) recognition of weight loss treatment. In 2002, the IRS announced that anti-obesity treatment could be claimed as a tax deduction. This ruling also allows participants to contribute pretax dollars to a flexible spending account for weight loss treatment. Specific language in many benefit plans precludes diet, nutritional counseling, and behavioral intervention whether at the community hospital, a physician's office, or in another provider setting.

There *is* some good news to report; however, it is with regard to obesity, not overweight. In 2004, Tommy Thompson, Health and Human Services Secretary, announced that there was a "new Medicare coverage policy that would remove barriers to covering anti-obesity interventions if scientific and medical evidence demonstrated their effectiveness in improving Medicare beneficiaries' health outcomes."[32] The new policy removes language stating that obesity is not an illness. Because Medicare pays only for illnesses, the older language allowed the denial of treatments for obesity. There remains a considerable problem, however, because Medicare/Medicaid will not provide coverage for obesity *unless* another disease related to obesity exists. (See Medicare Coverage *Issues Manual* Section 35-26, which states: *"obesity itself cannot be considered an illness."*) This language is being removed as a result of the recent decision by the Secretary of Health and Human Services. However, the change in the *Issues Manual* language will not directly affect current Medicare coverage of obesity treatment. Treatment for obesity alone remains noncovered, and treatment of diseases resulting in or exacerbated by obesity remain unchanged, and the following language applies:

> Services performed in connection with the treatment of obesity are covered by Medicare only when such services are an integral and necessary part of a course of treatment for diseases such as hypothyroidism, Cushing's disease, hypothalamic lesions, cardiovascular diseases, respiratory diseases, diabetes, and hypertension. . . . Therefore, services in connection with the treatment of obesity are covered services when such services are an integral and necessary part of a course of treatment for one of these illnesses.[33]

This change made by the Centers for Medicare and Medicaid Services (CMS) may facilitate payment for obesity treatments by more health plans because private insurers often follow the lead of public payers regarding covered services. CMS and health carriers will continue to review scientific evidence to determine which of the treatments warrant coverage and will publish these; *however*, patients, physicians, and others have to know to request them, and unfortunately, many do not know.

Quite clearly, more funding is needed on the front lines in disease management, wellness promotion programs, and broad scale educational initiatives, especially those directed toward children.

Treatment Strategies

Diet

Many diet regimens are available and recommended by medical professionals, and of course marketed directly to consumers in reputable and not so reputable publications, on websites, and in the media. Diets are generally divided into four categories: low fat, low carbohydrate, low calorie, and very low calorie. Several of these diet regimens offer heath education and support groups as well. These dietary approaches, however, often fall short in addressing the multifactorial issues associated with obesity. To optimize success and to realize significant and permanent changes individuals need to understand why they eat the way they do.

The National Institutes for Health (NIH) has published specific guidelines in *The Practical Guide: Identification, Evaluation, and Treatment of Overweight and Obese Adults* (www.nhlbi.nih.gov/guidelines/obesity/practgde.htm) and recommends the following:

- Low-calorie diets, creating a deficit of 500–1,000 kcal/day to produce a weight loss of 1–2 pounds per week
- Reduced fat intake as part of the low-calorie diet
- Physical activity that ideally is done at a moderate level of intensity most, if not all, days of the week
- Behavior therapy
- More frequent contacts over a longer period of time between client and provider

Behavior Therapy

Behavior therapy focuses on changing the eating habits and physical therapy, and is provided by many different professionals including psychologists, therapists, nutritionists/dietitians, physicians, nurses, social workers, and of course, case managers. Additionally, support groups, both formal and naturally occurring in workplaces and community groups, can provide peer-to-peer counseling, support, and encouragement.

Inpatient and Outpatient (Day Treatment) Programs

These programs exist for patients who may need more intensive, supervised, and structured healthcare to lose weight. Many of these programs are costly and frequently denied by insurers, so are reserved for more affluent individuals.

Pharmaceuticals

Medication for treating obesity, prescribed and monitored by a physician, may be beneficial for some obese patients and their weight-loss regimen when combined with lifestyle, behavior, and dietary modifications. There are currently two drug types that are approved by the Food and Drug Administration (FDA) for the long-term treatment of obesity:

- *Sympathomimetic drugs: Sympathomimetic* weight loss drugs help treat obesity by suppressing one's appetite through restricting nerve endings' ability to pick up norepinephrine and serotonin. Sibutramine, the generic marketed as Meridia, is marketed in the United States and worldwide under a different name.
- *Lipase inhibitors:* This class of weight loss drugs prevents the action of lipases—the enzymes that break down fat—produced in the pancreas. Orlistat, the generic marketed as Xenical, is the only weight loss drug approved to alter the way the body responds to fat intake. In February 2004, the FDA approved Xenical's use for the treatment of obesity among adolescents, thereby making Xenical the first approved weight loss treatment for children and adolescents in the United States.

Other FDA-approved weight loss prescription formulations for short-term use include phendimetrazine tatrate (Bontril), diethylpropion (Tenuate), benzphetamine (Didrex), and phentermine (Lonamin, Oby-Cap, Fastin, and Adipex-P). People with obesity who also have chronic conditions including heart disease, high blood pressure (including hypertension), or thyroid problems (thyroid disease, hypothyroidism) should not use these weight loss drugs.

Future Treatments

Clinical trials for several weight loss drugs that are not yet approved for the treatment of obesity are currently being conducted. For instance, metformin was recently found to produce a 1- to 3-kilogram weight loss over an average of 2.8 years in the randomized, double-blind Diabetes Prevention Program (DPP). Bupropion, which is marketed as Amfebutamone, Wellbutrin, and Zyban, is an antidepressant and antismoking drug that produced significantly more weight loss in a randomized clinical trial than placebo during a 1-year examination. Although it was found effective for significant weight loss, topiramate, a drug approved for treatment of epilepsy, also produced significant side effects during several trials of 6 to 12 months duration. Zonisamide, an anti-epileptic drug, also produced significant weight loss in a 4-month randomized clinical trial.

Over-the-Counter (OTC) Weight Loss Treatments

Many OTC weight loss pills contain ephedrine, a compound that encourages weight loss by reducing the patient's appetite while stimulating the body to produce more heat. One form of this weight loss drug is found in the Chinese plant ma huang and is sold in the United States without a doctor's prescription. There are many other herbal weight loss treatments containing ephedrine marketed to promote weight loss. Ephedrine is not proven safe for the treatment of obesity. Although some preliminary studies showed that taking supplements containing ephedrine was, at times, associated with weight loss, it is important to note that there are serious side effects associated with this weight loss treatment. On February 6, 2004, the FDA published a regulation prohibiting the sale of weight loss supplements containing ephedrine. This prohibition took affect April 12, 2004. The Endocrine Society supports this regulation: Individuals are *strongly* advised to consult with a physician before taking any OTC product for weight loss.[34]

Other OTC weight loss pills, including Dexatrim and Acutrim, are now ephedrine free. Although these products could be used in the treatment of obesity and claim to help weight loss by boosting energy levels and stimulating metabolism, there are no published peer-reviewed data to support these weight loss claims.

Genetics

The genetics industry is closely linked with pharmaceutical companies. Now that the human genome is in the spotlight, these highly specialized companies are working to provide solutions for weight control. This kind of technology may have the potential to create *specific* drugs to combat obesity and may just be the magic bullet so many are seeking.

Note: Because we are seeing many more patients in our caseloads with obesity and with comorbid conditions, case managers should *routinely* assess for the use of any of these medications (prescribed or OTC) during assessments and monitor the use of these throughout the intervention process.

Bariatric Surgery

Bariatric surgery is the use of surgical procedures specifically targeted to reduce obesity by modifying the gastrointestinal tract. These procedures are increasingly utilized, and in fact, I am concerned that they are being viewed by some as the magic bullet for weight loss and a quick solution to a long-term and lifestyle problem. Evidence of this was revealed over several years as my case management company saw the frequency increase in a few of the employer groups with whom we worked. We would receive calls in our prenotification program where employees would share with coworkers their experiences regarding a bariatric procedure, and then the coworkers would decide bariatric surgery was "perfect" for them; occasionally, they would try to schedule it quickly so that they'd look great for an upcoming wedding or other event!

Overall, these procedures are viewed—and should be—as a last resort for extremely obese patients who have been unsuccessful in attempts to lose weight through weight loss diets, prescription medications, and group support. In fact, many insurers require specific and detailed documentation of the weight loss efforts and results for a 2- to 3-year period of time before the requested surgery. Specific criteria define candidates for this kind of surgery, and each of the procedures has complications, but those complications are considered to be less important than the obesity itself. Centers of Excellence exist for the care of obese patients and specifically for surgical intervention; these centers have considerable expertise not only in the appropriate selection and preoperative evaluations of patients but in the extremely important follow-up care that is required.

Several procedures are performed for obesity:

- Some procedures are generally approved by most major carriers.
- Other procedures are approved only if the patient is at increased risk for complications resulting from the existence of an existing comorbid condition.
- And still other procedures are denied because peer-reviewed literature shows them to be unsafe or inadequately studied.

Because the literature and studies are ongoing, most of these procedures require preapproval by payer sources.

Generally, the following criteria are applied:

1. Body mass index (BMI) exceeding 40; *or*
2. BMI greater than 35 in conjunction with any of the following severe comorbidities:

  - Coronary heart disease; *or*
  - Type 2 diabetes; *or*
  - Clinically significant obstructive sleep apnea; *or*
  - Medically refractory hypertension

Additionally, most carriers and Centers of Excellence require that the following criteria to be fulfilled:

- Patient has completed growth, that is, has reached the age of 18 or bone growth has been documented.
- Patient has attempted weight loss (documented) in the past without success.

- Patient participates in a physician-supervised nutrition and exercise program.
- Patient participates in a multidisciplinary surgical preparatory regimen.

Related Procedures and Considerations

In addition to the bariatric surgical procedures that are directly related and address and treat obesity, there are others (panniculectomy, liposuction, and reduction mammoplasty) that are or may be indirectly related to treat obesity. Unfortunately, one of them, the reduction mammoplasty, is being used far too frequently, in my professional opinion.

Our company had as one of its client groups a very large university medical center that self-funded its medical plan. We provided prenotification, concurrent review, utilization review, case management, and disease management services. As we began working with this group, including the professional members of the staff, we became increasingly concerned with the number of procedures being requested that were directly related to obesity, and then we noted that many women who were obese were requesting breast reduction procedures.

Clearly, although health was most definitely the "business" of this client group, the overall health of many of their employees was somewhat worse than most of our other groups. The medical director of the plan, who was also the director of employee health, shared our concerns. All requests for gastric bypass were reviewed and approved based upon the criteria as described previously. We also reviewed several requests for reduction mammoplasty, and then brought these to the attention of the medical director (and, as per Health Insurance Portability and Accountability Act [HIPAA], preserved confidentiality). Together we determined that the vast majority of these requests were from women who were obese, many morbidly obese. It seemed that although they may have technically met the criteria for the procedure, they were *still* going to be obese after the surgery.

Much discussion and research took place, and a decision was reached. The medical director, and our management team who also served as consultants to this group, determined that those individuals who were obese would have to enroll in the disease management's obesity program, attain weight loss that would place them within a certain percentage of their desired weight, and then be reevaluated for the mammoplasty procedure. They were assured that the procedure wasn't being denied, but rather deferred.

Although met with considerable resistance from these individuals initially, this decision and the support these women received from our case managers resulted in considerable success. We were able to enroll more individuals in the disease management program and actually avoided many of the procedures. Once the women had reached their ideal weight, their breasts were no longer problematic. Additionally, cholesterol levels decreased, triglycerides and glucose levels were reduced, and those with hypertension saw an improvement in their numbers as well. Clearly, this was a win-win, and certainly was focusing attention on the problem of obesity and its core issues rather than treating the symptoms with reduction procedures!

Intervention Opportunities for Case Managers

The condition of obesity is one that certainly affords case managers so many opportunities truly to make a difference. By providing advocacy, education, and emotional support, we can create a more positive continuum of care. So many obese patients follow well-established patterns of attempted weight management programs followed by some success, and then regression followed by periods of discouragement and difficult-to-manage comorbid conditions. Case managers can be invaluable in identifying core areas of intervention that are appropriate based on the client's readiness to change and can collaborate with the client and members of the healthcare team to determine a goal-directed plan of care. Acting as the coordinator, the case manager can bring the multiple providers *and* the patient together. Providing encouragement, information, and reinforcement of attained goals (often difficult for patients to appreciate when the end goal seems so very far away) provides the invaluable contribution that is at the core of case management. It's the *relationship*, the trust and caring that we can communicate, that enables our patients to feel valued and that paves the way for the patient to move toward a healthier lifestyle.

GOING FORWARD

The topic of weight and body size is, as has been discussed, an emotionally charged one. Many individuals, including health professionals, view obesity as a character flaw; many others seek to gain more widespread acceptance of it as a disease. Although most certainly recognize that obesity is indeed a multifactorial condition needing better treatment, there are still others who promote the celebration of overweight people fighting for their right to be overweight and happy. The National Association to Advance Fat Acceptance is a staunch supporter of obese people and stands firmly against obesity surgeries and other forms of treatment.[35] Overweight and obesity, as is the case with other volatile subjects, has extremes at both ends of the spectrum. Case managers, at the heart and center, can be part of the solution. Through involvement with our families, workplaces, communities, and professional associations we can help to create an environment (and perhaps policies) that would end discrimination against obese persons, while at the same time promote practices that would result in improved health outcomes and hopefully the prevention of this condition in future years.

NOTES

1. Bray G and Macdiarmid E, "The Epidemic of Obesity," *Western Journal of Medicine* 172, no. 2 (February 2000): 78–79.

2. NCHS Fast Facts, Health-E Stats, http://www.cdc.gov/nchs.fastats/overwt.htm.

3. National Center for Health Statistics, *Health, United States, 2007*, http://www.cdc.gov/nchs/hus.htm.

4. Coventry M, "Supersizing America—Obesity Becomes an Epidemic," *UM NEWS*, Winter 2004, http://www1.umn.edu/umnnews/Feature_Stories/Supersizing_America.html.

5. Belluck P, "Children's Life Expectancy Being Cut Short by Obesity," *New York Times*, March 17, 2005, http://query.nytimes.com/gst/fullpage.html?res=9F01E3D7133CF934A25750C0A9639C8B63&sec=health.

6. Centers for Disease Control and Prevention, "Overweight and Obesity: Introduction," http://www.cdc.gov/nccdphp/dnpa/obesity.

7. DMAA: The Care Continuum Alliance, "Obesity with Co-Morbid Conditions: Definition," http://www.dmaa.org/pdf/Obesity_Definition.pdf.

8. http://www.medicalnewstoday.com/articles/43556.

9. DMAA: The Care Continuum Alliance, "DMAA Launches Online Obesity Resource Center for Professionals, Consumers," October 14, 2008, http://www.dmaa.org/news_releases/2008/pressrelease_101408.asp.

10. Levin-Epstein J, *Presenteeism and Paid Sick Days* (Washington, D.C.: CLASP Center for Law and Social Policy, 2005), http://www.clasp.org/publications/presenteeism.pdf (accessed November 15, 2005).

11. Jung J, "Obesity—The New Majority," *The Case Manager*, November/December 2004, 51–53.

12. Jung, "Obesity," 51–53.

13. Centers for Medicare and Medicaid Services, http://www.cms.hhs.gov.

14. World Health Organization Global Strategy on Diet, Physical Activity and Health, "Obesity and Overweight," 2003, http://www.who.int/hpr/NPH/docs/gs_obesity.pdf.

15. Heart, Lung and Blood Institute, NIH, http://www.hih.gov.

16. Chalk M, "Obesity: Addressing a Multifactorial Disease," *The Case Manager*, November/December 2004, 47–50.

17. Coventry, "Supersizing America."

18. Coventry, "Supersizing America."

19. Jain A, Ferguson C, Mauery D, et al., "Revisioning Success: How Stigma, Perceptions of Treatment, and Definitions of Success Impact Obesity and Weight Management in America," *A Research Report for the Strategies to Overcome and Prevent (STOP) Obesity Alliance*, George Washington University School of Public Health and Health Services, Department of Health Policy, November 2, 2007.

20. Foster GD, Wadden TA, Vogt RA, and Brewer G, "What Is a Reasonable Weight Loss? Patients' Expectations and Evaluations of Obesity Treatment Outcomes," *Journal of Consulting and Clinical Psychology* 65, no. 1 (February 1997): 79–85.

21. Waddenm TA, Anderson DA, Foster GD, et al., "Obese Women's Perceptions of Their Physicians' Weight Management Attitudes and Practices," *Archives of Family Medicine* 9, no. 9 (September–October 2000): 854–860.

22. Wing PR and Phelan S, "Long-Term Weight Loss Maintenance," *American Journal of Clinical Nutrition* 82, no. 1 (July 2005): 222S–225S.

23. Fuemmeler BF, Baffi C, Masse LC, et al., "Employer and Healthcare Policy Intervention Aimed at Adult Obesity," *American Journal of Preventative Medicine* 32, no. 1 (January 2007): 44–51.

24. Faulkner NH, French SA, Jeffrey RW, et al., "Mistreatment Due to Weight Prevalence and Sources of Perceived Mistreatment in Men and Women," *Obesity Review* 2, no. 3 (August 2001): 173–182.

25. Puhl RM and Brownell KD, "Bias, Discrimination and Obesity," *Obesity* 9, no. 12 (December 2001): 788–805.

26. Olson CL, Schumaker HD, and Yawn BP, "Overweight Women Delay Medical Care," *Archives of Family Medicine* 3, no. 10 (October 1994): 888–892.

27. Latner JD, Stunkard AJ, and Wilson GT, "Stigmatized Students: Age, Sex and Ethnicity Effects in the Stigmatization of Obesity," *Obesity* 13, no. 7 (July 2005): 1226–1231.

28. Banja J, "Obesity, Responsibility and Empathy," *The Case Manager*, November/December 2004, 43–46.

29. Banja, "Obesity, Responsibility and Empathy," 43–46.

30. Banja, "Obesity, Responsibility and Empathy," 43–46.

31. Bray and Macdiarmid, "The Epidemic of Obesity," 78–79.

32. Department of Health and Human Services, News Release—July 2004, http://www.hhs.gov/news/press/2004/pres/20040715.html.

33. *Medicare Coverage Issues Manual*, Section 35-26, May 2001, http://www.dmerc.com/manual/Medical%20Procedures.htm#_1_32.

34. ObesityInAmerica.org, "Medications—Issues and Options," http://www.obesityinamerica.org/medications.html.

35. Stokes D, "The Impact of Obesity on Healthcare Delivery," *For the Record* 16, no. 2 (January 26, 2004): 34.

Chapter 15

Our Nation's Multiculturalism and Challenges to Case Managers

Based on the latest census figures, our nation's melting pot is increasingly more multicultural. If you are a case manager in one of the country's more homogeneous and rural settings, you may not have noticed the changes that have been occurring over time, especially in the last 10 years. Suffice it to say, the world is changing along with our nation's demographics. Patients caught in the convolutions of our healthcare delivery system certainly have enough stress as they try to navigate. For patients from cultures different from mainstream America, or perhaps representing America as it used to be, the experience can be particularly stressful and challenging.

The increasing multiculturalism is not just confined to patients and families. Our healthcare colleagues and those with whom we interact are more diverse as well. So, although we hear about the increase in medication errors, lack of adherence to treatment plans, fragmentation and disconnects in care, and a plethora of other problems that directly affect patient outcomes, we truly have to shine a larger spotlight on the particular challenges of cultural diversity.

CHANGING DEMOGRAPHICS

The United States has 150 different ethnic cultures (estimated in 2008) among 301,621,177 million people, and, because immigration is likely to increase, so too will the number of ethnic groups. According to the latest statistics from the U.S. Census Bureau in 2000, there are 311 languages spoken; 162 are noted to be indigenous to the various regions and another 149 are immigrant languages. There are more than 14 million households today in which a language other than English is spoken. Even within these many languages, there are dialects that further increase the nuances. Each one of these variations exacerbates the challenges we all face as we endeavor to improve the communication among us.

In its figures of the U.S. population's distribution by race and ethnicity in 2006, the U.S. Census Bureau noted a total population of 299 million of which 74% were white alone, 66% were white, Hispanic and Latino American, 14.8% were Hispanic or Latino of any race, 13.4% were black or African American, 6.5% were some other race alone, 4.4% were Asian alone, 2.0% were two or more races, 0.68% were American Indian or Alaska Native alone, and 0.14% were Native Hawaiian or Pacific Islander alone. A report in August 2008 from the U.S. Census Bureau projects that by 2042, non-Hispanic whites will no longer represent the nation's majority. This projection is further confirmed by a report from the Pew Research Center in 2008 that projects that by 2050, non-Hispanic whites will make up 47% of the population; a decrease from the 67% level in 2005. The Pew Research Center's report also projects that the Hispanic population will increase from 14% to 29% in 2050 and that the percentage of Asian Americans will almost double by 2050.[1]

Additional data from the 2000 Census, for instance, shows that more than 26% of Californians were born outside the United States, and that more than one language is spoken in 40% of California households. Nationwide, one in five children enters school speaking a language other than English. Unfortunately, the youngsters lose most of their native language in the process of learning English, and typically, the heritage language virtually disappears within three generations. This process, in fact, is encouraged in our schools and becomes a part of natural assimilation. When we as case managers look to family members to assist with interpreting on behalf of some of our non–English-speaking patients, we may not be able to utilize these abilities and will have to rely upon other resources.

In another look toward the future, the Agency for Healthcare Research and Quality (AHRQ) determined that minority Americans are expected to make up more than 40% of the U.S. population by 2035.[2]

It is important to discuss acculturation and assimilation because these directly affect an individual's ability to access the best that our healthcare delivery system has to offer. Some ethnic groups acculturate or adopt the culture, values, and norms of the dominant population. This was very typical of those immigrants who came to the United States in the late 1800s. These immigrants felt that to succeed in their new home they needed to learn the language and immerse themselves and their family in all things American. This is the process referred to as *assimilation*. Individuals abandon their native culture, beliefs, norms, and traditions and replace them with those of the dominant group. That's not to say that they forget or abandon their homeland, but early immigrants really did believe that holding on to their past traditions and values would somehow impede their ability to be successful in their new country and that, after all, was usually their primary reason for coming to the United States.

In the past, it was assumed that immigrants either acculturated or did not. It is more likely that individuals fluctuate between one or the other extreme, and in other circumstances land somewhere in between. In more recent years, we have witnessed somewhat of a departure from this. We now see generations of immigrants come to the United States and steadfastly retain their language, customs, lifestyles, and beliefs. An example in my own town is a woman from Korea. She has been here for more than 15 years, owns and operates a very busy and successful nail salon, hires as employees members of her extended family and others from the community of Korean immigrants, and yet has extreme difficulty speaking English and conducting some of the more simple business transactions required of her. I have assisted her in communicating with a credit card company. She would use hand gestures and very limited English to explain her plight to me, and then I would assist her in getting it resolved. Frequently, I wondered just how she had managed so many transactions over these years to open and expand her successful business. One day, I saw a business-to-business yellow page directory that was written all in Korean. She was able to conduct most all of her business with other Korean-owned businesses. I then saw the community where she lived. Thirty years ago, there were perhaps several blocks of businesses in this small Asian community. Today, the area is several miles! She and other members of the Korean community operate within a very well planned network of businesses—auto dealers, insurance brokers, banks, clothing and furniture stores, churches, attorneys, physicians—and other entities serving the needs of this continually expanding community. As with so many other things in our society, there is an unending number of variations on this ethnic diversity. It is important for us to recognize this as we strive to obtain appropriate care for our diverse populations.

Obviously, those individuals who come to the United States and immerse themselves in American culture, language, and so forth soon become comfortable and, in fact, deliberately make a decision to embrace what the country has to offer, including healthcare. Of course, there are also those who, for a variety of reasons, cannot or do not develop this comfort level, yet still need to use that same healthcare system. We as case managers need to be prepared to meet the needs of all of our patients and their families and not just those who look like us, speak like us, and share our values and customs.

As case management continues to expand into more and more practice settings, from corporate health and managed care, hospitals, home care, and workers' compensation and disability management and into newer models in physician practices and direct-to-consumer community-based practice, opportunities will present themselves for us to improve access to and quality of care. We certainly can ensure that our patient assessments go beyond the essential elements of medical, behavioral, and so forth and include cultural, religious, and language needs. As patient/client advocates and professionals who, more times than not, have ongoing relationships across the continuum of care, we can bring to the forefront the more specific cultural issues and concerns and ensure that these are incorporated into treatment plans. An excellent illustration of an effective initial assessment form and plan of care form (Figure 15–1 and 15–2) incorporates cultural information, not only about the patient, but about the case manager as well. It is advisable for case managers and others involved in the creation of software and case management tools to ensure that cultural issues are integrated in the system, which moves us closer to actually providing culturally competent care.

The Differences

With each culture come different beliefs and sensitivities relating to how members of a particular ethnic group view and respond to illness, medical treatment, medical technologies, and medical professionals. Healthcare consumption patterns also vary among ethnic groups. In its *2008 Survey of Health Care Consumers*, the Deloitte Center for Health Solutions, part of Deloitte LLP, found that the 3,000 survey respondents, age 18–75, clearly fell into six segments of healthcare consumers: "Content & Compliant" (29%), "Sick & Savvy" (24%), "Online & Onboard" (8%), "Shop & Save" (2%), "Out & About" (9%), and "Casual & Cautious" (28%). Many interesting findings of this survey reveal the differences in how consumers regard healthcare and related aspects of care (e.g., health insurance, healthcare providers, pharmaceuticals, treatment modalities). For example, based on the survey, only 52% of consumers say they understand their insurance coverage, 84% prefer generics to name-brand drugs, 1 in 3 want more holistic/alternative therapies, 3 in 4 want expanded use of in-home monitoring devices and online tools that would reduce the need for visits and allow individuals to be more active in their care,

60% want physicians to provide online access to medical records, test results, and online appointment scheduling, and 1 in 4 say they would pay more for this service.[3] Add to these healthcare consumption traits culturally driven attitudes, and it is evident that case managers must begin to drill down into their patients' (and their patients' families') total psyches regarding their medical care.

Let's look at some of the cultural nuances that influence the way individuals consider healthcare. According to a report commissioned by the National Hispanic Medical Association (NHMA) titled *Model Hispanic Health Programs: Prevention, Treatment, Training and Research*, and presented at the NHMA's 7th annual conference in 2003, Hispanic men's health was being negatively affected by their poor health literacy and

Figure 15–1 Initial Assessment Form.

continues

Figure 15–1 continued

Educational Level: Home Country: _____ Years   In the U.S.: _____ Years

Interpreter Need: ❑ Yes ❑ No

Interpreter Availability: ❑ Yes   If yes, who would it be? _____
                            ❑ No

Place (Country) of Birth: ❑ U.S.A. ❑ Other   If other, which country? _____
                            Year when client moved to the U.S.: _____
                            Age when client immigrated to the U.S.: _____ years old
                            Reasons of immigration: _____

Cultural Needs: _____

Food Preferences (including Ethnic Food): _____

Dietary Needs: _____

Religious Preferences: _____

Emergency Contact Name: _____   Relationship: _____
Address: _____   Phone: ( ) _____
City: _____   State: _____   Zip: _____

Emergency Contact Name: _____   Relationship: _____
Address: _____   Phone: ( ) _____
City: _____   State: _____   Zip: _____

Caregiver Name: _____   Relationship: _____
Address: _____   Phone: ( ) _____
City: _____   State: _____   Zip: _____

Financial Resources: ❑ Social security   ❑ Supplementary security income (SSI)
                        ❑ Pension   ❑ Help from family members
                        ❑ Other

Insurance: ❑ Medicare   Policy #: _____
                        ❑ Private Health Insurance Policy #: _____
                        ❑ Private Dental Insurance Policy #: _____
                        ❑ Long-term Care Insurance Policy #: _____
                        ❑ Other   Policy #: _____

Hobbies: Currently enjoy doing: _____
                        Used to enjoy doing: _____
                        Family activities: _____

Reasons for the initial contact:
_____
_____
_____
_____
_____

Source: Cress, 2007.

Figure 15–2 Plan of Care Form.

Date: _____

Name of Client: _____

Name of Care Manager: _____

Name of Agency: _____

Address: _____

Phone Number: (   ) _____   Cell Number: (   ) _____

Fax Number: (   ) _____   E-mail: _____

Ethnicity/Race of Care Manager: _____

Linguistic competency besides English: _____
                                                                    (Name of Language)
                                    ❑ Speak   ❑ Read   ❑ Write

Name of Social Worker: _____

Name of Agency: _____

Address: _____

Phone Number: (   ) _____   Cell Number: (   ) _____

Fax Number: (   ) _____   E-mail: _____

Ethnicity/Race of Social Worker: _____

Linguistic competency besides English: _____
                                                                    (Name of Language)
                                    ❑ Speak   ❑ Read   ❑ Write

Client - Personal Information

Client Name: First: _____   Middle: _____   Last: _____

How does the client prefer to be addressed? _____

How does the client's family address him/her? _____

DOB: _____   Sex: ❑ Male   ❑ Female

Ethnicity/Race: _____

Street Address: _____

City: _____   State: _____   Zip: _____

Phone Numbers: Home: (   ) _____   Cell: (   ) _____

Former Occupation: U.S.A. _____   Other than U.S.A. _____

Live Alone: ❑ Yes   ❑ No   Marital Status: _____

Other Living Arrangement: _____
_____
_____
_____

continues

Figure 15–2 continued

Has the client had any change in residence in the past year?   ❑ Yes   ❑ No

If yes, how and why? _____

Does the client wish to remain at home?   ❑ Yes   ❑ No

Has the client had any life event or traumatic experience
in the past year (hospitalization, move, etc.)?   ❑ Yes   ❑ No

If yes, what, when and why? _____

Names, Addresses, and Phone Numbers of Children:

Name: _____	Relationship: _____
Address: _____	Phone: ( ) _____
City: _____ State: _____	Zip: _____
Name: _____	Relationship: _____
Address: _____	Phone: ( ) _____
City: _____ State: _____	Zip: _____
Name: _____	Relationship: _____
Address: _____	Phone: ( ) _____
City: _____ State: _____	Zip: _____

Current Care Arrangements among Family Members: _____
_____
_____
_____

Preferable Language: _____

Interpreter needed: ❑ Yes   ❑ No

Names of Interpreters: _____

Cultural Needs: _____

Food Preferences (including Ethnic Food): _____

Dietary Needs: _____

Religious Preferences: _____

Emergency Contact Name: _____	Relationship: _____
Address: _____	Phone: ( ) _____
City: _____ State: _____	Zip: _____
Emergency Contact Name: _____	Relationship: _____
Address: _____	Phone: ( ) _____
City: _____ State: _____	Zip: _____
Caregiver Name: _____	Relationship: _____
Address: _____	Phone: ( ) _____
City: _____ State: _____	Zip: _____

Figure 15–2 continued

Medical Information

Primary Physician: _____ Phone: ( ) _____

Hospital: _____ Phone: ( ) _____

Interpreter Available: ❏ Yes ❏ No

Dentist: _____ Phone: ( ) _____

Interpreter Available: ❏ Yes ❏ No

Pharmacy: _____ Phone: ( ) _____

Interpreter Available: ❏ Yes ❏ No

Name of Health Insurance: _____

Address: _____

Phone Number: ( ) _____ Fax Number: ( ) _____

Policy #: _____

Name of Dental Insurance: _____

Address: _____

Phone Number: ( ) _____ Fax Number: ( ) _____

Policy #: _____

Name of Long-term Care Insurance: _____

Address: _____

Phone Number: ( ) _____ Fax Number: ( ) _____

Policy #: _____

Physical Health Symptoms: _____

_____

_____

Mental/Cognitive Symptoms: _____

_____

_____

Scheduled Medication

Name of Medication	Dosage	Time of Day	Instruction

continues

Figure 15–2 continued

Does the client have a Durable Power of Attorney for Health Care? ❑ Yes ❑ No

    Name of the person/agent: ———————————— Relationship: ————————

    Address: ————————————————————————————————

    Phone Number: ( ) ———————— Fax Number: ( ) ————————

If no, who will make the client's health care decisions?

    Name of the person: ———————————— Relationship: ————————

    Address: ————————————————————————————————

    Phone Number: ( ) ————————

    Name of the person: ———————————— Relationship: ————————

    Address: ————————————————————————————————

    Phone Number: ( ) ————————

Does the client have a Do-Not-Resuscitate Order (DNR)? ❑ Yes ❑ No

If no, who will make decisions on behalf of the client?

    Name of the person: ———————————— Relationship: ————————

    Address: ————————————————————————————————

    Phone Number: ( ) ————————

    Name of the person: ———————————— Relationship: ————————

    Address: ————————————————————————————————

    Phone Number: ( ) ————————

Personal Care

	Needs Assist	Devices
Ambulation		
Bathing		
Dressing		
Feeding		
Foot Care		
Grooming		
Medication		
Oral Care		
Skin Care		
Toileting		
Transfers		
Vision Care		
Other Care		

Figure 15–2 continued

Meal Preparation

Food Preferences (including ethnic food): _____

_____

Dietary Needs: _____

_____

Breakfast: _____

       Time: _____

       Eating Arrangements: _____

Lunch: _____

       Time: _____

       Eating Arrangements: _____

Dinner: _____

       Time: _____

       Eating Arrangements: _____

Snacks: _____

       Time: _____

       Eating Arrangements: _____

Meals-on-Wheels (MOW) requested? ❑ Yes ❑ No

    MOW: ❑ Yes ❑ No Which days? _____

    Ethnic MOW: ❑ Yes ❑ No Which days? _____

Is the client able to receive MOW without assistance? ❑ Yes ❑ No

Time of MOW delivery: MOW: _____ Ethnic MOW: _____

Additional Meal Instructions:_____

Housework

	Need Assist	Frequency/Instructions
Dishwashing		
Dusting		
Kitchen cleaning		
Bathroom cleaning		
Floor cleaning		
Laundry		
Vacuuming		
Other Housework		
Other Housework		

continues

Figure 15–2 continued

Schedule of Activities

Daily Activities:

     Morning: _____

     Afternoon: _____

Hobbies: _____

Outside Group Activities: _____

Religious Activities: _____

Exercises: _____

Additional Arrangements (such as ethnic video, mobile book programs, etc.):

_____

_____

_____

Finances

Is the client able to manage his/her finances without assistance?   ❑ Yes   ❑ No

Does the client have agents (representative payee, conservator, power of attorney for finances, etc.)

    Finances?   ❑ Yes   ❑ No

    Name of the person/agent: _____   Relationship: _____

    Address: _____

    Phone Number: (   ) _____   Fax Number: (   ) _____

If no, who makes financial decisions for the client?

    Name of the person: _____   Relationship: _____

    Address: _____

    Phone Number: (   ) _____

    Name of the person: _____   Relationship: _____

    Address: _____

    Phone Number: (   ) _____

  Source: Cress, 2007.

---

machismo. The report found that many Hispanic men don't go to a doctor because of their machismo attitude even when care is readily accessible. It also found that this attitude was contributing to their higher percentages of illness in certain areas. For instance, 37% of Hispanic men versus 21% of non-Hispanic whites die prematurely of diabetes. Within the Hispanic male category, 4% of Mexican American men versus 2.5% of non-Hispanic whites die prematurely of this disease.[4]

Mexican American men and women share a common belief that health is derived from one's spiritually; a belief they share with older, rural African Americans as well as older Filipinos. Different ethnic groups also view end-of-life care and directives differently. African Americans seek out all possible life-sustaining measures and tend to distrust advance directives as giving license to provide inferior care based on their race or socioeconomic position. Korean Americans may lean toward having a natural death absent of any life-prolonging technology, but do want their children to request lifesaving measures.[5]

The influence of spirituality on healthcare also can be demonstrated within other culturally driven traditions, for example:

- Within the Latino culture, religious healing, praying to certain saints, and the use of religious symbols to maintain health
- Within the Asian culture, the need for a balance between yin and yang to preserve health achieved by using certain foods and herbs, as well as the unblocking of the free flow of *qi* (chi) or energy through the use of acupuncture
- Within the African culture, the belief that harmony with nature provides power and energy, and belief in the healing power of religion[6]

In the Vietnamese and Armenia Health Attitudes Survey by Denise Jamin, published in the *Journal of Multicultural Nursing and Health* Winter 1999 edition, it was found that individuals of Vietnamese descent most often seek out healthcare from physicians of their own ethnicity, but one-third does visit Western doctors. Compare this to Armenians who most typically receive healthcare from a Western doctor, but 50% of whom also visit physicians of their own ethnic background. The problems for which medical care was frequently sought also varied among these two groups. Whereas the Vietnamese survey respondents most frequently sought help in the areas of dentistry, medications, eye care, pediatric, stomach/intestinal (for infections), and blood pressure, the Armenians most frequently used health services for dental, medications, and eye care. These two groups also varied as to their attitudes regarding waiting in various healthcare settings. The Armenians were found to be more tolerant of county health facilities and the bureaucracy associated with them, whereas the Vietnamese held that it was degrading to be seen waiting in a county facility and that they would rather pay more for more courteous and prompt treatment in a physician's office.

Their perceptions regarding the safety of various treatments and screening devices also differed. Of the Vietnamese respondents, 60% were willing to take pills, 30% were willing to take injections (24% were not), 46% thought that surgery was generally safe (24% believed surgery was unsafe), and 46% thought X-rays were safe (18% believed they were unsafe). Of the Armenian respondents, 75% were willing to take pills, more than 60% were willing to receive injections, 75% believed that surgery was safe, and 35% believed that X-rays were safe (35% also believed they were unsafe).[7]

Family Values

Each family whether born in this country or from a different ethnic culture has values unique to their background. Americans are encouraged and raised to be independent, assertive, autonomous, and in control of our lives from birth to death. Of course, that doesn't mean that we each are successful in these areas, but it is the culture of our country. We are encouraged to communicate and even question authority figures, including physicians, and to demand individual rights. Interestingly, over the past several years, consumers have had more and more direction to take charge of their own healthcare.

The U.S. healthcare system places a great deal of emphasis on patient autonomy and the patient's right to know. We have legislation, the Patient's Bill of Rights, that ensures this. This belief, however, is not shared by all cultures. The custom in many cultures, including Mexican, Filipino, Chinese, and Iranian, is for a patient's family to be the first to hear about a poor prognosis, after which the family decides whether the patient should be told and, if so, just what should be told. These families may believe that full information takes hope away, possibly hastening the death of their loved one.

The study titled "Ethnicity and Attitudes Toward Patient Autonomy," published in the September 13, 1995, issue of the *Journal of the American Medical Association*, found that "Korean-American and Mexican-American subjects were more likely to hold a family-centered model of medical decision making than the patient autonomy model favored by most of the African-American and European-American subjects." The survey involved 200 subjects aged 65 years and older representing four ethnic groups (i.e., European American, African American, Korean American, and Mexican American). The study also revealed cultural preferences regarding whether patients should be informed of a terminal illness (i.e., 88% of African Americans and 87% of European Americans agreed, whereas 65% of Mexican Americans and 47% of Korean Americans agreed).[8]

Other families may have stronger religious beliefs. They may believe that only God really knows when an individual will die and that telling the patient anything related to the possibility of death is of little consequence.

In other cultures, the focus may not be as much on the individual but greater emphasis may be placed on the immediate or extended family, the village, or the tribe. Children are warned not to bring shame on their families, and some cultures stress nonconfrontational behaviors and encourage deference to authority.

Communication

The ways that individuals communicate their feelings, concerns, symptoms, and pain are as different as the individuals themselves. Even when the language is the same, gender, age, religion, and ethnicity may obscure some of the important considerations surrounding the elements of a patient's medical condition. For example, in some cultures, direct eye contact is perceived as threatening; for the healthcare professional who is trying to communicate with an individual from such an ethnic culture, the patient's avoidance of eye contact may be mistakenly interpreted as resistance to the information being given, embarrassment, or even depression. If the patient is Chinese, he may be showing respect; if female from a Muslim country, and the physician is male, she may be trying to avoid sexual impropriety.

Many healthcare professionals, especially nurses who are the largest group of professionals in case management, are taught the importance of touch and instinctively offer comfort or reassurance to a patient using a physical gesture. If that patient is of the opposite sex and an Orthodox Jew, it is important to know that for the Orthodox religion contact outside of hands-on care is prohibited.

From these few illustrations, one can readily appreciate that gaining knowledge of the customs and beliefs of particular cultures can be an additional challenge for case managers. We need to distinguish between generalizations and stereotypes. Certain cultures may indeed have beliefs and even fears; however, this is not to be deemed as factual for all within the culture. The knowledge about a particular ethnic group should serve as a *beginning*, not a conclusion, advises Geri-Ann Galanti, PhD, in her article titled "An Introduction to Cultural Differences."[9] In another article, "The Challenge of Serving and Working with Diverse Populations in American Hospitals," Dr. Galanti discusses this further, noting that although we do look for similarities among groups, we then need to see whether a particular individual fits the pattern. She sees that the generalization is the starting point and that "making the appropriate generalization in healthcare situations can be a useful tool that narrows the field of thinking and sometimes can help save a life or prevent complications." On the other hand, Galanti cautions that a stereotype as an end point can be dangerous. In this form of thinking, Galanti notes that "we develop conventional, formulaic and oversimplified conceptions and opinions. . . . It then becomes easy to categorize a patient as being a certain way and make no further effort to learn whether the individual in question fits the conception."[10]

Galanti offers more than 200 different case studies that underscore the challenges that case managers and our colleagues in healthcare may face; however, the core issues of generalizing and stereotyping are wonderfully illustrated by the following:

Take the statement: "Mexican women often express their pain loudly." If there is a Mexican female patient who is moaning about her pain and she is ignored with the thought: "Don't worry, Mexican women express their pain loudly," then this is stereotyping, and certainly not helpful. If, on the other hand, knowing that female Mexican patients often express their pain loudly, the case manager checks with a family member to see whether this particular woman is vocal when in pain, and then follows up by checking the woman's complaint, this is a generalization and in this example is a first step in the resolution of this woman's discomfort.[11]

Where You're From *Does* Matter

There are significant differences among racial and ethnic groups in our country and throughout the world. The underlying reasons for this vary but certainly are influenced by the complex factors that affect health for all: socioeconomic status, family history, behavioral risk factors (e.g., smoking, alcohol, exercise), stress, and so forth. When individuals are from minority or disadvantaged groups or groups of a different ethnic culture and/or who speak another language, other factors influence their health. Some of these factors include the cost and availability of healthcare, lack of culturally competent care, cumulative prejudice, and discrimination.

Culture and language may influence health, healing, and wellness belief systems; how illness, disease, and their causes are perceived by patients; the behaviors of those seeking healthcare and the attitudes they may have toward their providers; and of course, the actual delivery of these services by providers who tend to see the world through their own values and experiences.

Each society presents its own challenges in providing healthcare delivery services. According to Nancy Davis, RN, PhD, FACMT, Director (retired), Office of Managed Care, Indian Health Services, Aberdeen, South Dakota, privacy and client confidentiality are big concerns for case managers working among American Indian populations. "The entire community knows everything about the patient almost before the door shuts." American Indians conceive of individual wellness as harmony and balance among mind, body, and spirit. The same belief that gives him spiritual strength can present a dilemma for a diabetic patient requiring leg amputation. How can he be whole in his afterlife if he is buried without his leg?

Indian medicine incorporates consultations with medicine men, a high degree of family involvement, and the Native American concept of individual wellness as harmony and balance among mind, body, and spirit. These elements of care are acknowledged, supported, and initiated by patients and their families. The beautiful spiritual rooms at the Pine Ridge and Rosebud hospitals are used often.

Profiled by Jane Gross in the *New York Times*, Chief of Obstetrics and Gynecology at New York University Downtown Hospital, Dr. Iffath Abbasi Hoskins has created a welcoming atmosphere to serve the 65% of the obstetrics patients in the hospital who are Chinese. The staff is bilingual and there are Chinese-language videos for expectant mothers. Sensitivity training for staff members teaches that the cultural resistance to breast-feeding stems from new immigrants feeling that using formula indicates assimilation into the American culture. The suggestion to sooth a sore bottom with an ice pack often is rejected because it goes against the rules of yin and yang.

During a visit to China, Kathleen Moreo, cofounder of Professional Resources in Management Education, observed that the Chinese do not say "no" because it is associated with disrespect. When they disagree, they are silent. An American greeted with silence usually assumes there is a misunderstanding and reiterates the question, position, or statement. Moreo cautions that this is the worst thing a case manager can do when speaking with a Chinese American. The case manager immediately breaks any developing trust because the patient has made a decision and believes the case manager is trying to force her to change her mind.[12]

Michael J. Demoratz, COO of CareMedical Systems, cites a number of ways in which cultural diversity affects pain management. He notes that patients from Hispanic, Middle Eastern, or Mediterranean backgrounds generally express pain openly, whereas those from Asian or northern European lineage tend to underreport pain. In certain cultures, among them Asian and Christian African American populations, pain and suffering are believed to redeem or purify. Individuals may present a stoic front or refuse medication.[13] For such reasons, a patient might not be able to give to the case manager an accurate assessment of pain.

Honoring one's elders is integral to the Japanese, Chinese, and Korean cultures. Turning over a loved one's care to a professional, rather than to family members, can be unthinkable to the family. Italian, Greek, French, South-Central American, Middle Eastern, and some Asian societies consider it inhumane to reveal a terminal diagnosis to a patient. Among the Japanese, discussing gastrointestinal conditions is shunned.[14] Most Americans fear death to the point of refusing to consider end-of-life planning.

Guidance

To further illustrate the significance of the differences among the cultures, it is helpful to examine some of the specific concepts and preferences in a few groups. The University of Washington Medical Center (http://depts.washington.edu/pfes) has developed a number of educational tools that address these disparities (Appendices 15–A through 15–D) among several ethnic cultures (African American, Albanian, American Indian/Alaska Native, Chinese, Korean, Latino, Russian, Somali, and Vietnamese). These "tip sheets" are focused on improving the communication between patients and healthcare professionals. *Culture Clues* examines the perception of illness, patterns of kinship and decision making, and comfort with touch and provides extremely useful insight and guidance to enhance relationships with diverse cultures.

The Office of Minority Health at the U.S. Department of Health and Human Services (www.omhrc.org) provides assistance and guidance to improve care for those in minority groups. OMS developed the National Culturally and Linguistically Appropriate Standards (CLAS) in healthcare tool, which contains training modules for healthcare professionals in regard to cultural awareness. In an interview with *Case in Point* (official magazine of the Case Management Society of America), Garth N. Graham, MD, MPH, deputy Assistant for Minority Health, specifically mentions CLAS guideline 11 as one that could greatly benefit case managers:

"Healthcare organizations should maintain a current demographic, cultural, and epidemiological profile of the community as well as a needs assessment to accurately plan for and implement services that respond to the cultural and linguistic characteristics of the service area."[15] He comments: "Case managers get to interact with patients in a unique way . . . right at the nexus point in terms of understanding the full spectrum of the patient . . . they understand not just the clinical scenario, but the social and cultural scenarios too . . . from the provider perspective, there are many times that case managers know more about patients than physicians do."[16]

This branch of the federal government, which was established in 1985, works closely with accrediting bodies and other organizations that are seeking to improve culturally appropriate care. OMH offers a comprehensive continuing education program, Culturally Competent Nursing Modules (CCNMs), which is based on the CLAS standards and which is divided into three categories: culturally competent care, language access services, and organizational support. Because URAC's Case Management Standards strongly urge development and education in cultural diversity, this resource is an important one and can be accessed at www.thinkculturalhealth.org.

CULTURAL COMPETENCY

Culture refers to integrated patterns of human behavior that include language, customs, beliefs, values, and institutions of racial, ethnic, religious, or social groups; *competence* implies having the capacity to function effectively as an individual or organization within the beliefs, behaviors, and needs presented by consumers and their communities.[17] Cultural and linguistic competency, as noted on the Office of Minority Health Web site (www.omhrc.gov), is a set of congruent behaviors, attitudes, and policies that come together in a system, agency, or among professionals that enables effective work in cross-cultural situations.

Cultural competency is essential to close the widening gaps of disparities in healthcare. For patients and healthcare providers, including case managers, to come together and explore and resolve healthcare concerns, cultural differences should not be a hindrance to the conversation, but rather something that hopefully enhances the discussion. When it is known that providers are knowledgeable, respectful, and responsive to the issues surrounding cultural diversity, positive outcomes are much more likely to occur.

Achieving cultural competency is no easy matter for many organizations as they become filled with diverse patient *and* provider populations.

This most assuredly is the ideal breeding ground for conflict and misunderstandings. By understanding that virtually every organization is concerned about costs, that pressures to achieve more with less are the norm, and that education is among the last resource surrounding patient care to obtain funding, we each need, once again, to assume some responsibility for cultural competence ourselves. Case managers and other healthcare professionals cannot always depend on their employing organization to provide them with ongoing educational preparation. Fortunately, much of this information is just a "mouse click" away. Some organizations, however, do see cultural education as a necessary part of their business and part of their responsibility as part of the business community, and have created wonderful programs for staff and patients.

Blue Cross and Blue Shield of Minnesota provides literacy and motivational interviewing for its case management staff. Jane Cavanaugh, RN, CCM, CPHQ, interviewed for an article in the *Case Management Advisor*, commented that traditional approaches that are fine with American-born members won't necessarily work with those from other cultures. She provides an example of managing a Vietnamese woman diagnosed with lung cancer who needed transportation for appointments. Cavanaugh learned that the woman would ride in a car only with her husband, so Cavanaugh had to arrange the woman's appointments around the husband's work schedule—somewhat more complicated a process to be sure, but certainly a meaningful gesture made by the case manager and understood by the woman.

The same article (for which I was also interviewed) described how care coordinators with UCare Minnesota's Senior Health Options visit homes of clients from other cultures with a staff member from the client's same culture. This obviously communicates acceptance and a real desire to understand and meet unique needs of diverse cultures.

CASE MANAGERS MAKE A DIFFERENCE

As with other challenges that we face, case managers once again are at the forefront and right in the middle of the swirling issues surrounding cultural diversity. It's not just because we are caring professionals who want the best for our patients, though that certainly is true, but many of the individuals who come from diverse cultures possess some of the other characteristics (e.g., chronic illnesses, financial issues) that become red flags that signal a need for case management. Once again, we don't need to *look* . . . they are there in our midst, just waiting for someone to reach out.

Just as we look within our organizations for assistance in medical, nursing, and therapeutic domains, we must once again step outside of our comfort zone to find solutions to some of these other problems. In well-established cultures, there is often a wealth of information and resources available to assist the members of that particular group.

CMSA in its yearly conferences, as well as in many of the chapters across the country, has responded to requests from its members and provides ongoing workshops addressing the broad issues of cultural diversity as well as more specifically the dominant cultures in various regions. Several case management publications have also focused attention on this subject as well, and this is likely to continue as our population continues to evolve.

DEVELOPING CULTURAL COMPETENCY

Taking the First Step

Various techniques are used for developing cultural sensitivity. A good place to start is to understand how your own cultural heritage has influenced your attitudes toward illness and healthcare. Looking back on your own experiences with individuals from different cultural, socioeconomic, and religious backgrounds is also helpful in raising your own awareness.

In its "Techniques to Develop Cultural Sensitivity,"[18] the Geriatric Interdisciplinary Team Training Resource Center of New York University recommends such steps as follows:

> engaging trainees in exercises designed to uncover their cultural heritage (i.e., describe the community in which they grew up, name two or three important values they learned from their family, indicate the ethnic/racial/cultural/spiritual groups they identify with, . . . describe how they know and learned what to do when they have a headache, describe how they know and learned what to do when they have abdominal pain); engage trainees in exercises to assess their level of cultural competence (i.e., explore advantages/disadvantages of being this person in team setting, explore advantages/disadvantages of being this person in majority community, explore advantages/disadvantages of being this person in minority community, . . . explore a rewarding and difficult experience had in working with people from different socioeconomic, ethnic, religious, age groups); introduce a framework for understanding the cultural influences brought by another to the

caring interaction between provider, patient and family (i.e., determine the person's age and birth locale, define the person's ethnic background, clarify the person's religion, . . .); introduce the explanatory model for understanding illness in the context of culture (i.e., ask person what they think caused their problem, ask them why they think it started when it did, ask them what they think their sickness does to them, . . .); and apply learning mnemonic to ensure a culturally sensitive response (i.e., listen—to person's explanation of what's wrong and what caused it, explain—what you think may have caused the problem, acknowledge—areas of agreement and disagreement, recommend—your treatment or course of action, negotiate—for what is most important, involve—person in the interaction, never negate—other person's beliefs or views, gather—the family or decision makers whenever necessary).

In addition to participating in cultural sensitivity training programs such as the aforementioned one, case managers should seek out reading materials by which to self-learn about different cultures and their attitudes regarding healthcare. An online search at any time will uncover enlightening articles on the topic. In addition, some medical schools are now beginning to offer cultural sensitivity and competency courses for both matriculated and nonmatriculated students. It is a good idea to contact schools in your area to determine whether they offer these programs.

Local medical societies in states with legislation enacted or pending that mandates requirements relating to cultural and/or linguistic competency on the parts of physicians, medical professionals, and/or healthcare providers in their jurisdiction also offer educational programs or continuing education courses. Among the states with this legislation are New Jersey, which requires physician cultural competency training as a condition of licensure (Bill S144); California (AB 810 Chapter 510 and AB 1195); Washington (ESB 6194); New Mexico (SB 600); Arizona (SB 1468); Illinois (SB0522); Ohio (SB 160); Maryland (HB883, HB 1455, HB 1127); and New York (AO3751).[19] Case managers should also continue to take advantage of the programs offered by the Case Managers Society of America.

In addition to these organizations, the American Medical Association offers a *Cultural Competence Compendium* as a guide to assist physicians and other health professionals in their communications with patients. Sections of the book are accessible on the AMA's website at www.ama-assn.org/.

The Web sites of the Center for Cross-Cultural Health (www.crosshealth .com) and DiversityRx (www.diversityrx.org) are also good resources for information that is helpful in guiding individuals, communities, and healthcare providers toward providing culturally sensitive and competent healthcare.

Beyond gaining knowledge of the subject, case managers should also strive to know themselves and whether or not they can effectively serve a multicultural population. It is common for people to be more comfortable with the familiar. For case managers who find it difficult or uncomfortable relating to or understanding a patient's cultural differences, it may be best to consider a healthcare setting where there is lesser exposure to patients of multiple cultures and beliefs. Conversely, for case managers who are excited to become further integrated into our nation's increasingly diverse population, becoming more competent in the beliefs of various ethnic and multicultural patient groups is likely to be a very fulfilling and rewarding experience.

To determine just where you might be on the cultural competency learning curve, take a few minutes to respond to the questions that appear in Table 15–1.

Table 15–1 A Cultural Competency Self-Test

---

1. Name two diseases/conditions that are influenced by racial/ethnic factors. Explain.
2. Describe two cultural values or beliefs that influence how a cultural group, different from your own, responds to being sick.
3. Do you respect differences in health behaviors practiced by your client?
4. Name two ways in which your practice is responsive to the needs of diverse groups.
5. Do you take culture, gender, and race into consideration when examining risk factors faced by your clients?
6. Do you involve your clients in the decision-making process when considering a course of treatment?
7. What is a question you commonly ask to learn about your clients' ethnic or sociocultural background? How is this information relevant to your practice?

Add up your score. Give yourself one point for each item named on questions 1, 2, 4, and 7. Give yourself one point for a yes on questions 3, 5, and 6.

Score 9–10: Good work, keep it up! Cultural competency is a continuous quality improvement process.
Score 2–8: Keep working, you have a way to go.
Score 0–1: It is time to start developing your competency skills.

Source: Reprinted with permission, *CareManagement* © 2003 Mason Medical Communications, Inc.

Table 15–2 Twelve Steps to Cultural Competency

1. Find out about the family's internal dynamics, as well as family members' beliefs and what those beliefs mean to them and to the patient.
2. Look at the length of time the family has been in the United States.
3. Don't make an assumption based solely on the country of origin.
4. Don't make assumptions about why people act the way they do.
5. Don't be afraid to ask questions in a respectful manner.
6. If you need an interpreter, find someone who is not a family member, if possible.
7. Compile a list of available translators and have it at your fingertips.
8. Go out of your way as a clinician to learn basic language skills for members of the predominant patient groups you are likely to encounter.
9. Develop a "cheat sheet" of cultural issues that affect case management.
10. List the cultures you may be coming in contact with and do some basic research on their beliefs.
11. Find the resources you need to educate yourself.
12. Above all, treat the families with respect and let them know you care.

Source: Courtesy of *Case Management Advisor* 12, no. 10 (2001): 147. Providing culturally appropriate care abd services

And a 12-Step Program

Thankfully, several outstanding professionals in the field of cultural competency have partnered with case managers and have shared their insight and expertise with us. In addition to those cited earlier in this chapter, Dr. Josepha Campinha-Bacote, president of Transcultural C.A.R.E. Associates (www.transculturalcare.net), created a model to assist healthcare professionals in providing culturally appropriate care and services. See Table 15–2.

Lessons Learned

Clearly, there is much to learn . . . and never enough time. Following are some quick lessons about cross-cultural communication adapted from Craig Storti's *Cross Cultural Dialogues*:

1. Don't assume sameness.
2. What you think of as normal behavior may only be cultural.

3. Familiar behaviors may have different meanings.
4. Don't assume that what you meant was what was understood.
5. Don't assume that what you understood was what was meant.
6. You don't have to like or accept "different" behavior, but you should try to understand where it comes from.
7. Most people do behave rationally; you just have to discover the rationale.[20]

CONCLUSION

Although some of our colleagues in case management may feel uncomfortable among different ethnic groups, and may inadvertently convey this discomfort to others, still others will see this as yet another adventure, another chapter to be explored. Where will you be?

NOTES

1. Wikipedia, "Demographics of the United States," http://en.wikipedia.org/wiki/Demographics_of_the_United_States.
2. AHRQ, "Reports on Needs Assessment," http://www.ahrq.gov.
3. Deloitte, "Survey Reveals U.S. Health Care Consumers Are Not Homogeneous," February 2008, http://www.deloitte.com/dtt/article/0,1002,cid%253D192722,00.html.
4. Hispanic PR Wire, "Machismo Attitudes Keep Hispanic Men from Going to the Doctor," March 17, 2003, http://www.hispanicprwire.com/news.php?l=in&cha=9&id=149.
5. Topic 5: Multiculturalism, compiled from Kramer BJ, "Cultural Assessment," in *Encyclopedia of Elder Care*, ed. M. Mezey, B. J. Berkman, C. M. Callahan, and E. L. Mitty (New York: Prometheus Books, 2004); C. Fasser, *Interdisciplinary Team Training Curriculum Resource Document* (New York: Geriatric Interdisciplinary Team Training Resource Center of New York University, 1999).
6. Topic 5: Multiculturalism, compiled from Kramer BJ, "Cultural Assessment."
7. Denise Jamin, Jin-Hui Yoo, Mariea Modoveanu, Lou Tran, "Vietnamese and Armenian Health Attitudes Survey," *Journal of Multicultural Nursing & Health*, Winter 1999.
8. Agency for Healthcare Research and Quality, "AHCPR Announces First Evidence Report Topics," http://www.ahrq.gov/news/press/epctoppr.htm.
9. Geri-Ann Galanti, "An Introduction to Cultural Differences," *Culture and Medicine* 172 (May 2000).
10. Geri-Ann Galanti, "The Challenge of Serving and Working with Diverse Populations in American Hospitals," *Diversity Factor*, Spring 2001.
11. Galanti, "The Challenge of Serving."
12. Thomas MB, *Case Management Advisor* 12, no. 3 (2001): 147.
13. Demoratz MJ, "Managing Pain Across Diverse Cultures," *Disease Management Digest* 7, no. 3 (2003): 3.

14. Demoratz, "Managing Pain," 3.

15. Office of Minority Health, http://www.hhs.gov/culturalcompetency.

16. Hagemann J and Llewellyn A, "Working Together Toward Cultural Competency," *Case in Point*, 2008, http://www.caseinpointmagazine.com.

17. Office of Minority Health, "What Is Cultural Competency?" October 19, 2005, http://www.omhrc.gov/templates/browse.aspx?lvl=2&lvlid=11.

18. Fasser C, *Interdisciplinary Team Training Curriculum Resource Document* (New York: The Geriatric Interdisciplinary Team Training Resource Center of New York University, 1999).

19. U.S. Department of Health and Human Service OPHS, Office of Minority Health, *National Standards for Culturally and Linguistically Appropriate Services in Health Care* (Washington, D.C.: U.S. Department of Health and Human Service OPHS, Office of Minority Health, March 2001), http://www.omhrc.gov/assets/pdf/checked/executive.pdf.

20. Storti C, *Cross-Cultural Dialogues* (Intercultural Press, 1994), http://uiowa.edu/hr/administration/linguistics.

APPENDIX 15–A

Culture Clues™   **Patient and Family Education Services**

Communicating with Your Chinese Patient

Perception of Illness • Patterns of Kinship and Decision Making • Comfort with Touch

Culture Clues™ is designed to increase awareness about concepts and preferences of patients from the diverse cultures served by University of Washington Medical Center. **Every person is unique; always consider the individual's beliefs, needs, and concerns.** Use *Culture Clues*™ and information from the patient and family to guide your communication and your patient care.

How does the Chinese culture deal with illness?

Helping Your Patient Feel Comfortable with UWMC
- Remember to find out if this is your patient's first visit to University of Washington Medical Center.
  - **Keep in mind that patients who are new to the system may not be aware of the role of the Primary Care Team or the process for getting a referral to a specialist.**

Explaining the Cause of Illness and Disease
- Your patient may have specific cultural beliefs, for example they may view illness and death as a natural part of life.
- Health may be viewed as finding harmony between complementary energies such as cold and hot, dark and light. These forces are called *yin* and *yang*. Most Chinese actually are very comfortable with duality between western and traditional Chinese health beliefs.

Building Bridges Between Traditional Remedies and Western Health Care
- Your patient may use foods and herbs to restore *yin/yang* balance. In addition to special foods, your patient may use other traditional Chinese remedies as an initial approach for healing, especially during the early stages of illness. Some traditional Chinese therapies, including massage, acupuncture, and moxibuxtion are commonly used as an adjunct to western medicine.
- Your patient may prefer to drink only hot liquids (water or tea) when sick or postpartum.
- Patients may try traditional approaches first, and will seek western medical care if these treatments fail. Patients may occasionally delay seeking care out of concern for communication barriers, costs, etc. As a result, patients may present at the medical center acutely ill.
  - **Ask your patient, "What do you call your problem? When did it start? What do you think caused the problem? Have you taken any medicines or herbs? What results have you had from the medicines or herbs? Do you believe the illness is serious? How can I help you?"**
  - **Build bridges between traditional medicine and western care: when considering traditional practices, determine when the remedies are beneficial, neutral, or harmful. Incorporate beneficial and neutral remedies into the plan of care, such as dietary advice. Consider potential drug interactions.**

Helping Your Patient Understand Medicines
- Your patient may believe that western medicine is too strong and may not take the full dose or complete the course of treatment. Your patient may cut the dose in half or stop taking the medicine whether he/she feels better or not.
  - **Explain that the dose is customized for your patient's height, weight and metabolic needs. Describe the need to take the full dose whether your patient feels better right away or not. Talk about side effects. Share your plan in dealing with side effects. Ask open-ended questions to ensure understanding.**
  - <u>Alert</u>: **Be aware that your patient may have enzyme deficiencies that may require a change in medication or dosage. Contact the pharmacy if the patient does not appear to be responding to medications or if he/she appears to be especially sensitive to medications' effects.**

How are medical decisions made in the Chinese culture?

Understanding Relationships
- The Chinese culture emphasizes loyalty to family and devotion to traditions and puts less emphasis on individual feelings. Assess your patient's kinship relationships and determine which family members are most influential in decision making. When possible, engage the whole family in discussions that involve decisions and education about care.
  - **Be aware of the importance of family members serving in caregiver roles and consider extending visiting hours. Explain the visitation policy before admission or surgery so that the family knows what to expect.**

- Bad medical news is often shielded from the patient by the family in the belief that telling the patient will only make the patient's condition worse.
  - **Ask your patient whom they want included in medical decisions. If patients do not want to make medical decisions for themselves, let them know they need to prepare a Durable Power of Attorney for health care.**

Customs that Influence Decision Making

- In addition to religious beliefs, there are many cultural and traditional beliefs that your patient may subscribe to that will influence decisions about health care treatment. For example, your patient may seem hesitant to make a decision about surgery because of preference to retain full complement of body parts (eg., uterus, gall bladder, etc.).
- Whenever possible, allow time for the patient to gain perspective and make decisions. Schedule a follow-up appointment or set up a scheduled phone call to allow for needed time. Offer time limits that are acceptable to patient and medical necessity. Patients tend to rely heavily on doctor's advice, so they may have trouble deciding between different options.

Understanding Communication About Health Care and Treatments

- Your patient may nod, smile, and/or say "yes" or "ya" to acknowledge he/she heard you, rather than that he/she understands or approves. Your patient may be reluctant to say "no" to a doctor or health care provider because it may be considered disrespectful or cause disharmony.
  - **Ask your patients open-ended questions to verify understanding and encourage them to ask questions.**
  - **Ask them to repeat what they understand in their own words.**

What are the Chinese culture's norms about touch?

Understanding Norms About Eye Contact and Body Language

- Respect is shown to authority figures by giving a gentle bow and avoiding eye contact.
- Nonverbal cues are an important part of communication. For example, smiles when appropriate may be one way to build rapport.
- Your patient may highly value emotional self-control, appearing stoic. Be aware that your patient may not show pain or ask for pain medications.
  - **Instead of asking your patient about pain, ask, "May I get you something for pain?"**
  - **Be respectful of your patient's desire to keep emotions in control when asked about upsetting subject matters.**

Understanding Norms About Modesty

- Consider the modesty of women and girls when giving a pelvic exam. Many young women are modest about having an exam and may prefer a female doctor to do it. In some cases, your patient may refuse a gynecological exam from a provider of either gender.
  - **Before you begin a gynecological exam, it is important to ask your patient, "May I examine you?" Ask your patient if she prefers a female doctor, attendant, or interpreter to remain in the room during the exam.**

What is unique about this patient and family that you will not learn from culture tips or information?

There is a wide range of cultural differences based on age, ethnic group, country of origin, religious beliefs, generation, migration wave, and length of time away from China.

Check Out These Resources to Learn More About Health Care and Chinese Culture

- ✓ *Culture and Nursing Care, A Pocket Guide*, J.G. Lipson, S.L. Sibble, P.A. Minarik, 1997, pp. 280-290*.
- ✓ *Explaining Illness Research, Theory, and Strategies*, Whaley, Bryan B., Lawrence Erlbaum Associates, 2000, pp. 283-297*. (*Available at UWMC's Learning Resource Center – Room cc420.)
- ✓ Culture Clues and End-of-Life Care Sheets: *http://depts.washington.edu/pfes/cultureclues.html*

Culture Clues™ is a project of the Staff Development Workgroup, Patient and Family Education Committee
Contact: 206-598-7498/Box 358126/pfes@u.washington.edu

The Chinese *Culture Clues*™ was developed with thanks to Eddie Brolley, Annie Tu, and Emily Wong.

UNIVERSITY OF WASHINGTON
MEDICAL CENTER
UW Medicine

APPENDIX 15–B

Culture Clues™   ***Patient and Family Education Services***

Communicating with
Your American Indian/Alaska Native Patient

Perception of Illness • *Patterns of Kinship and Decision Making* • *Comfort with Touch*

Culture Clues™ *is designed to increase awareness about concepts and preferences of patients from the diverse cultures served by University of Washington Medical Center.* **Every person is unique; always consider the individual's beliefs, needs, and concerns.** *Use Culture Clues™ and information from the patient and family to guide your communication and your patient care.*

American Indians (AI) and Alaska Natives (AN) are terms identifying the indigenous peoples of North America. In the 2000 Census, four million people identified themselves as American Indian or Alaska Native. About ¾ of this population live near urban areas; about ¼ live in non-urban areas, including reservations. There are more than 500 federally-recognized tribes and over 245 tribes without this federal designation, which may have state recognition. Be aware that there is variability between tribes in their health care seeking and health promotion behaviors. The AI/AN culture varies considerably by age, place, or residence (urban, rural, reservation), education, socioeconomic factors, and awareness and utilization of community resources.

In the AI/AN culture, there is historical mistrust of mainstream institutions due to centuries of abuses such as broken treaties and forced relocations. In addition, only the small percent of American Indians who are affiliated with registered tribes receive treaty-granted health care benefits. Acknowledging this history is an important step in building trust with your patient and their family and understanding that at times this lack of access to health care can lead to frustration.

While it is important to have a basic knowledge and respect for this culture, remember that all, some, or none of these beliefs may be associated with each patient and their family.

How does your AI/AN patient perceive illness?

Cause of Illness

- Your patient may have a holistic view in which people, community, nature, and spirituality are interconnected and interrelated. This perspective views physical, spiritual, mental, and emotional health in unity, instead of in discrete categories. Sickness may be viewed as the result of disharmony between the sources of life.
  - **Consider this holistic view when assessing, diagnosing, and treating an illness.**
- Your patient may seek western medicine for treatment of symptoms of illness. However, patients may also seek traditional healers to address the disharmony that caused the illness. Traditional practices may include different rituals and ceremonies as well as herbal remedies. The sweat lodge is an example of a health practice American Indian patients may apply.
  - **Ask your patient if he/she is using traditional healings or practices. Acknowledge the value of traditional practices and whenever possible incorporate beneficial and neutral remedies into the plan of care. Consider potential drug/herb interactions.**

Understanding Time Orientation

- Time orientation may be perceived as cyclical, present-oriented, and "in-the-moment" as compared to linear, future-oriented, and "time-by-the-clock" in western culture. As a result, patients may be late or miss appointments.
- Transportation issues and unfamiliarity with the city and the medical center neighborhood may also impact your patient's time of arrival for their appointment.
  - **Schedule appointments within a window of time to allow for more flexibility.**
  - **Whenever possible, use natural events such as sunset or meal times to schedule prescribed medications.**

How are medical decisions made in the AI/AN culture?

Concept of Family/Community

- The concept of family may include immediate family, extended family, and community and tribal members.
- Your patient's medical decisions may depend on how the family is affected because of the importance of group orientation. As a result, your patient may include the entire family when making important medical decisions.

Culture Clues™: Communicating with Your American Indian/Alaska Native Patient   *page 2*

- Urban AI/AN may not have family living nearby, and AI/AN who live on reservations may be receiving care far away from home. Lack of family support during medical decision making may be a source of stress for your patient.
  - **Ask your patient about who they would like to have included in their medical decisions. Give your patient time to process and consult with family, community, and tribal members as desired, before making health care decisions. Be aware that a large family contingent may be present.**

Informed Consent
- Due to a history of misuse of signed documents, some patients may be unwilling to sign informed consent, advance directives, and durable power of attorney forms. Your patient may perceive verbal agreement as sufficient.
  - **If it is your patient's first experience with informed consent, explain its purpose. You may want to consider a Social Work consult. Every care area has available the UWMC publication, "Information About Your Health Care" (UH2056) to support this discussion.**

How can I reduce the communication barriers with my AI/AN patient?

Nonverbal Communication
- Direct eye contact may be avoided out of respect or concern for soul loss or theft.
- Traditionally, AI/AN have been taught to resist any expression of pain. Your patient may not express pain directly and instead report feeling uncomfortable or use storytelling.
  - **Ask your patient, "May I get you something for your pain?" Respect their wishes if they decline.**
- Time and silence may be used to maintain harmony, be non-confrontational, and as a way to prepare to listen to your patient.
  - **Listen for at least 2 minutes without saying a word. Let patients talk or let them be silent. Be aware that it may take 3 or 4 encounters before trust and dialogue emerge.**

Verbal Communication
- Storytelling and circular conversation may be used to build trust or describe symptoms. For example, a personal story about an ill neighbor may be a metaphor for the patient having the same symptoms.
  - **Listen for signs of symptoms that your patient may not be expressing directly. Sharing a personal experience may be a way to build trust with your patient.**

Explaining Touch
- Touch may be very personal for your patient. The head and hair may be considered particularly sacred.
  - **Before touching, always explain what will be done and why.**
- Hair, jewelry, ornaments, or other regalia may have a spiritual meaning.
  - **Ask your patient if they have any spiritual objects with them. If it is necessary to remove an object from the patient's body, have the patient or family member remove the item, and if possible keep it close to the patient until it is reattached. The item can be placed in a plastic bag and kept with the chart during surgery. Whenever possible, return the item to the patient in the recovery room.**

Check Out These Resources to Learn More About Health Care and AI/AN Culture
- ✓ *Culture and Nursing Care, A Pocket Guide,* J.G. Lipson, S.L. Dibble, P.A. Minarik, 1996, pp. 11-12 (available at the Learning Resource Center cc420).
- ✓ **Urban Indian Health Institute:** *http://www.uihi.org*
- ✓ **NLM American Indian Health:** *http://americanindianhealth.nlm.nih.gov/tribes.html*
- ✓ **Culture Clues and End-of-Life Care Sheets:** *http://depts.washington.edu/pfes/cultureclues.html*

Culture Clues™ is a project of the Staff Development Workgroup, Patient and Family Education Committee. Contact: 206-598-7498/ Box 358126/pfes@u.washington.edu
The *AI/AN Culture Clue™* was developed with thanks to Polly Olson, Native American Center for Excellence, Maile Taualii, Urban Indian Health Institute, and UW School of Public Health Students: Longondo Eteni, Roberto Orellana, Nadia Nijim, Michael Sanchez, and Lesley Steinman.

UNIVERSITY OF WASHINGTON
MEDICAL CENTER
UW Medicine

APPENDIX 15–C

Culture Clues™   **Patient and Family Education Services**

Communicating with Your Latino Patient

Perception of Illness • *Patterns of Kinship and Decision Making* • *Comfort with Touch*

Culture Clues™ is designed to increase awareness about concepts and preferences of patients from the diverse cultures served by University of Washington Medical Center. **Every person is unique; always consider the individual's beliefs, needs, and concerns.** Use *Culture Clues*™ and information from the patient and family to guide your communication and your patient care.

How does the Latino culture deal with illness?

Explaining the Causes of Illness and Disease

- Your patient may see illness as an imbalance. The imbalance may be between internal and external sources (for example, hot and cold, natural vs. supernatural, the soul is separate from the body).
  - **Ask your patient, "Can you tell me what caused your illness?"**
- There are folk-defined diseases such as *empacho* (stomach ailment) and standard western medically defined diseases such as measles, asthma, and TB.
- Many patients seek medical care from *curanderos* or other folk healers.
  - **Ask about use of pharmaceuticals or home therapies such as herbal remedies or certain foods. Screen for possible patient use of injectables, especially antibiotics or vitamins. Ask if you can see the home treatment if your patient cannot identify the substance.**

Helping Your Patient Take an Active Role in Care and Recovery

- Your patient may believe that God determines the outcome of illness.
  - **Consider the impact religion will have in your patient's active participation in health care recovery. You can validate your patient's belief by asking, "Will God be served by taking the best care of yourself?"**
- The patient is seen as an innocent victim, and will be expected to be passive when ill.
  - **Help your patient take an active role in her or her recovery.**

Helping Your Patient Feel Comfortable with UWMC

- Remember to find out if this is your patient's first visit to University of Washington Medical Center.
  - **Keep in mind that patients who are new to the system may not be aware of the role of the Primary Care Team or the process for getting a referral to a specialist.**

Understanding Concerns About Depression

- Depression may not be seen as an illness. It is often seen as a weakness and an embarrassment to family.
  - **Treat these issues with respect. You may want to also offer the services of a clergy member.**

How are medical decisions made in the Latino culture?

Making Decisions About Health Care

- The mother determines when a family member requires medical care; the male head of the household gives permission to go to the medical center.
- Head of household, often oldest adult male, is the decision-maker, but important decisions often involve the whole family. The family spokesperson is usually the father or oldest male.
  - **Ask your patient about whom they want to be included in medical decisions. If the patient does not want to make medical decisions for themselves, let them know they need to prepare a Durable Power of Attorney for health care.**
  - **When possible, engage the whole family in discussions that involve decisions about care.**

Managing Medical News

- The family would prefer to hear about bad medical news before the patient is informed. The family spokesperson usually delivers information about the severity of illness. The family may want to shield the patient from the bad news.
  - **If your patient consents, meet with the identified persons to strategize how to communicate medical news.**

Gaining Family Support

- *La familia* – the family – is an important source of emotional support during recovery. Patients like to be able to see and embrace their family members.
  - **Be aware of the importance of this and consider extending visiting hours. Explain the visitation policy at the time the patient is admitted or before a surgery, so that the family knows what to expect.**
- The family may want to allow the patient to remain passive during recovery while they provide complete support for activities of daily living.
  - **Educate family members about the importance of the patient's active participation during recovery.**

What are the Latino culture's norms about touch?

Understanding Relationships

- Your patients value relationships. They prefer a polite and friendly encounter before a therapeutic relation.
  - **Take time to develop relationships. Shake hands and greet your patient by name, or ask the patient what they prefer to be called. An older patient may prefer to be called Señor (Mr.) or Señora (Mrs.).**

Understanding Norms About Eye Contact and Body Language

- Eye contact with health care professionals or people of authority may be avoided as a sign of respect.
- For some patients, eye contact may be related to evil spirits. An illness may be attributed to receiving an "evil eye" or *mal ojo*.
- Another example of evil eye is the belief that if you admire a child by looking without actually touching him or her, the child can become very ill.
- When your patient nods his or her head, it does not necessarily signify agreement, but that he or she is listening to you. Silence is more likely a sign of not understanding or disagreement.
  - **To ensure understanding, ask open-ended questions and encourage the patient to ask questions.**

Understanding Norms About Touch, Modesty, and Body Language

- Consider the modesty of women and girls; having a female provider may be helpful.
  - **Ask your patient about her gender preference for providers. Consider having a female attendant present when a male provider is examining a female patient.**

What is unique about this patient and family that you will not learn from tips or information about their culture?

Country of origin, education, and income level make a difference about how your patient perceives illness and makes health decisions. What are the questions you want to ask to learn more about this patient and their family?

Check Out These Resources to Learn More About Health Care and Latino Culture

- ✓ **Culture and Nursing Care, A Pocket Guide,** J.G. Lipson, S.L. Dibble, P.A. Minarik, 1997, pp. 203-215 (available at the Learning Resource Center cc420).
- ✓ **Culture Clues and End-of-Life Care Sheets:** *http://depts.washington.edu/pfes/cultureclues.html*

Culture Clues™ is a project of the Staff Development Workgroup, Patient and Family Education Committee
Contact: 206-598-7498/Box 358126/pfes@u.washington.edu

UNIVERSITY OF WASHINGTON
MEDICAL CENTER
UW Medicine

APPENDIX 15–D

Culture Clues^{TM}   *Patient and Family Education Services*

Communicating with Your Russian Patient

Perception of Illness • Patterns of Kinship and Decision Making • Comfort with Touch

Culture Clues™ is designed to increase awareness about concepts and preferences of patients from the diverse cultures served by University of Washington Medical Center. **Every person is unique; always consider the individual's beliefs, needs, and concerns.** Use *Culture Clues™* and information from the patient and family to guide your communication and your patient care.

How does the Russian culture deal with illness?

Helping Your Patient Feel Comfortable with UWMC

- Remember to find out if this is your patient's first visit to University of Washington Medical Center.
  - **If it is your patient's first visit to UWMC, take a few moments for orientation.**
  - **Keep in mind that patients who are new to the system may not be aware of the role of the Primary Care Team or the process for getting a referral to a specialist.**

Explaining the Causes of Illness and Disease

- Your patient and his or her family may believe that illness is caused by weather or social experiences, such as stress from the living situation or because of arguing with the family.
  - **Ask your patient if they have experienced stresses or strains recently.**
- Your patient may not like to take excessive medications. When an option, ask your patients if they prefer over-the-counter or homeopathic medicine.
- Spend time with the patient to show that the patient is cared for.

Communicating with the Patient Experiencing Depression

- Mental health does not receive due respect in the former Soviet Union. Even the word "mental" has negative connotations because it is connected with "mental illness."
  - **Use the term depression, not mental health or mental illness.**
  - **The social worker in your clinical area is a resource to help with referrals and other ways of addressing mental health issues.**

How are medical decisions made in the Russian culture?

Making Decisions About Health Care

- Often the extended family – a working-age couple, their children and parents – have immigrated together. They may have other family members who might have immigrated to the United States at other times.
- There are strong kinship bonds and everyone in the family provides support and service during a crisis.
- Decisions are made by the parents or the oldest child.
- The elders are respected.
- There are no major gender issues; decisions could be made by the mother, father, or eldest son or daughter.
  - **Ask your patient about whom they want to be included in medical decisions. Then meet with the identified family members to strategize how to communicate the medical news. If the patients do not want to make medical decisions for themselves, let them know they need to prepare a Durable Power of Attorney for health care.**

Managing Medical News

- Bad medical news is often shielded from the patient by the family in the belief that telling the patient will only make the patient's condition worse.
  - **If the patient consents, meet with the designated persons to strategize how to communicate medical news so that you are sure of the patient's informed consent for treatment.**

What are the Russian culture's norms about touch?

Understanding Norms About Touch and Body Issues
- **Direct eye contact with your patient is acceptable.**
- **A handshake is welcome from the health care provider.**

Explaining Touching

- Before touching your patient, always explain what will be done and why.

- Your gender as the health care provider is not likely to be an issue for your patient when doing peri-care or assessing urinary catheters.

- Your patient may prefer that opposite gender family members leave the room.
  - **Find out if this is the case for your patient.**

- Female patients may prefer a female OB Gyn.
  - **Ask your patient to learn about her preference.**

Understanding Concerns About Hygiene and Health

- When sick, your patient may prefer sponge baths to daily baths or showers.

- Your patient may not wash hair as frequently when sick, especially when in the hospital, for fear of catching a cold or headache.
  - **Your patient may prefer to keep the room warm and the window shut.**

- Hygiene may be performed by the patient, family, or with the help of a nurse or aide.
  - **Maintain modesty and privacy issues with patient's opposite-gender family members present.**

What is unique about this patient and family that you will not learn from tips or information about their culture?

Birth region, education, and income level make a difference about how your patient perceives illness and makes health decisions. What questions do you want to ask to learn more about this patient and their family?

Check Out These Resources to Learn More About Health Care and the Russian Culture

- ✓ **Ethnomed:** *http://ethnomed.org*
- ✓ **Culture and Nursing Care, A Pocket Guide,** J.G. Lipson, S.L. Dibble, P.A. Minarik, 1997, pp. 239-249 (available at the Learning Resource Center cc420).
- ✓ **Culture Clues and End-of-Life Care Sheets:** *http://depts.washington.edu/pfes/cultureclues.html*

Culture Clues™ is a project of the Staff Development Workgroup, Patient and Family Education Committee
Contact: 206-598-7498/Box 358126/pfes@u.washington.edu

UNIVERSITY OF WASHINGTON
MEDICAL CENTER
UW Medicine

Chapter 16

Health Literacy and Adherence Issues

As a case manager, I have certainly witnessed the impact when individuals lack the understanding necessary to be active participants in their own treatment. All too often, we are tempted to perpetuate the perceptions of our colleagues in healthcare, that this or that patient is nonadherent (or in previous years, noncompliant). It has been my long-held belief that *most* patients do not freely decide to cause harm to themselves, to deliberately cause deterioration in the quality or quantity of their life, or as care providers, in the lives of their loved ones. The issue of nonadherence is more in my opinion a matter of health literacy than anything else.

Those of us who are charged not only with improving the outcomes for our patients but with cost containment as well are well advised to explore and understand the issues surrounding health literacy more completely.

INCREASED NEED FOR HEALTH LITERACY

Medical care has grown increasingly complex as technology and advances have made the treatment of very complex conditions possible. Surgical innovation, pharmaceutical discoveries including biologics, and other innovations result in a seemingly unending array of treatment alternatives. Although the education of the professionals involved in *providing* treatment is ongoing and demanding, the education of the patients *receiving* the treatment is seriously lagging behind. The need for patients to become more actively involved in their care is growing, yet we have not adequately prepared them for their "new" role.

Years ago, patients with congestive heart failure may have been treated with digoxin and diuretics and would have been advised to "watch" their diet. Today, patients with that same condition are likely to receive beta blockers and angiotensin-converting enzyme inhibitors in addition to digoxin and diuretics, and we expect them to know the names of these meds, the dose, frequency, and possible side effects of each. Because it is highly likely that these patients are also hypertensive and have high cholesterol levels, they are prescribed meds for these conditions as well. Because monitoring of early signs of impending heart failure is important, patients are frequently advised to do daily weights, take waist circumference measurements, know which foods are low in sodium and cholesterol, and keep accurate records and report back to their clinicians any noted changes. The aforementioned is just *one* diagnostic condition for which the standard of care and evidence-based guidelines have changed the protocols and prescribed treatment regimens; there are countless others, as we well know.

ECONOMIC IMPACT OF HEALTH LITERACY

Medication errors, excess hospitalizations, longer hospital stays, increased use of emergency rooms, and a generally higher level of illness are all attributable to limited health literacy. These factors are estimated to result in excess costs to the U.S. healthcare system of between $50 billion and $73 billion per year.[1]

LITERACY AND HEALTH LITERACY

In our work with patients, especially as we conduct initial assessments, provide discharge planning assistance, and offer direction for medical and community resources, it is important for us to determine patients' literacy competency. By acknowledging that all patients will be involved in their own care, we then need to ascertain which tools are appropriate to convey the necessary information that will keep them safe and empower them to be active participants. In Chapter 14, we discussed cultural diversity and its impact on patient care. Within the confines of cultural diversity is that of literacy and health literacy. It is important for us to understand the relationships that each of these have in the development of our case management plans.

Categories of Literacy

In an open conference call addressing the issues outlined in *Health Literacy: A Prescription to End Confusion*, Dharma Cortes, PhD, a noted researcher, cited the three categories of literacy and provided examples of each. In the first, *prose*, the individual needs to be able to identify a sentence in a text; the second, *document*, is a person's ability to identify portions of a text, for example, looking at a license and picking out the expiration date; the last, *quantitative,* is the determination of an individual's ability to differentiate between numerical values, for example, in a grocery flyer to decide which price is less expensive for cereal.[2]

Levels of Health Literacy

Every 10 years, the U.S. Department of Education conducts a national survey called the National Assessment of Health Literacy (NAAL) to document the state of literacy of the American public. The most recent survey was conducted in 2003. Although the main purpose of this assessment is to measure general literacy, specific items and situations were incorporated to assess health literacy. The results were divided into four levels: proficient, intermediate, basic, and below basic.[3]

Most doctoral-level clinicians fall into the proficient level, whereas 36% of American adults, 78 million people, have only basic or below-basic skills. Five percent of individuals couldn't be tested at all because they lacked the skills needed to participate, which results in more than 89 million adults with limited health literacy.[4] A cover article in *Fortune* magazine told the stories of several *billionaire* executives who had limited literacy skills.[5] As with nearly all poor readers, they had developed coping mechanisms that apparently served them well in their business and social lives, but that may not work for them at all in an urgent healthcare situation.

Healthy People 2010 defines health literacy as "the degree to which individuals have the capacity to obtain, process, and understand basic health information and services needed to make appropriate health decisions."[6] These are the skills that all people need, for instance, to find their way to the right place in a hospital, fill out medical and insurance forms, and communicate with healthcare providers. When individuals are deficient in health literacy, they often take medications on an erratic schedule, miss appointments, and do not understand or act on instructions regarding treatment.

According to the American Medical Association, poor health literacy is "a stronger predictor of a person's health than age, income, employment status, educational level and race."[7] In *Health Literacy: A Prescription to End Confusion*, the Institute of Medicine (IOM) reports that "nearly ninety million people in the United States have difficulty understanding and then using health information,"[8] and this number is expanding.

Health literacy varies by context and setting and is not necessarily related to years of education or general reading ability. A person who functions adequately at home or work may have inadequate health literacy. With the growing emphasis on a consumer-centric healthcare system to improve quality of care and decrease costs, patients will need strong information skills. Health literacy requires a complex group of reading, listening, analytical, and decision-making skills *and* the ability to apply these skills to health situations.

Just as there are categories and competency assessments in literacy, so too are there indicators to guide us in determining an individual's competency in health literacy. At the below-basic level, an individual should be able to circle the address on the appointment slip; at basic level, a patient should be able to state two important lifestyle changes after reading a pamphlet about diabetes; at the intermediate level, an individual should be able to find health information on a chart such as his body weight versus ideal BMI. Those at the proficient health literacy level are able to obtain treatment options in a complex document for breast cancer.

Although the majority of adults perform at an intermediate level of health literacy, unfortunately, most health documents are prepared at the proficient level. Because women are the majority of individuals involved in healthcare matters for their family members, and they interact with the healthcare system more frequently, they have a higher than average competency.

It's important for us to realize that limited understanding of health concepts and information is not solely a problem of persons with low literacy skills. Highly literate, well-educated, and extremely successful individuals report difficulty in understanding information provided to them by clinicians—often because some of the professionals *assumed* understanding by these executives, which was far from accurate. We always need to create "safe" environments for *all* individuals, regardless of their state in life, whether it be as an attorney, CEO, or other respected occupation; we need to acknowledge that they may *not* understand. Occasionally, the more prominent the individual is, the more unrealistic are his or her expectations and embarrassment in admitting to the lack of understanding.

DAY-TO-DAY CONSIDERATIONS

Every profession has its own jargon. In healthcare, one's proficiency in pronouncing and using the litany of terms and acronyms allows entry into the inner sanctum. When we use medical jargon terms with individuals who have limited or severely deficient health literacy skills, the consequences can be substantial. One study of patients with low health literacy found that many did not really understand the meanings of words that clinicians regularly used in their discussions with patients, terms like *bowel, colon, screening test,* or *blood in the stool.*[9] In another study, one out of four women who said they knew what a mammogram was turned out not to know.

When I was a very much younger nurse, my mom told me that she was to have a hysterectomy. She was explaining what had occurred during the preoperative visit with her doctor, and then shared with me: "Well I'm not too pleased that she's removing my uterus, but at least I'll still have my womb." These conversations and misperceptions occur far more often than we would like to acknowledge.

Contributing Factors

When examining the issue of health literacy we also need to be aware of some of the factors that might contribute to this problem. Some of those problems can be easily remedied, while others might call out for more systemic solutions. Certainly, groups of individuals in this country are more vulnerable to a deficiency in health literacy than others; these groups may include the following:

- *Older adults.* As individuals age, some of their cognitive and physical functionality (e.g., vision, hearing) may decline, so the usual or previous skills employed to learn or understand new information may place them at risk.
- *Minority populations.*
- *Immigrant populations.*
- *Low-income populations.** Approximately half of Medicare/Medicaid recipients read below the 5th-grade level.
- *People with chronic medical and/or physical health conditions.*

*Note: With the evolution of managed care as a dominant force in the healthcare marketplace, managed care organizations (MCOs) compete for Medicare/Medicaid contracts and face filling the needs of a clientele that they may never have seen before. Many of these contracts specify and require language and cultural accessibility. Recognizing that some of this can be provided only with face-to-face contact, some contracts are also requiring "feet in the street" (case managers onsite in communities with culturally diverse or minority populations).

Other Factors

Stress

Stress can play a role in an individual's ability to process health-related information. Even those of us who are healthcare professionals respond quite differently when we or a member of our family becomes the patient. Just hearing the word *cancer*—despite the fact that many oncological conditions are chronic conditions rather than a death sentence—may cause an individual to go into shutdown or panic mode. Patients are nervous about information they will be given, concerned that something is "wrong" with them, self-conscious about being in an uncomfortable environment, and of course may be hearing their diagnosis in a possibly matter-of-fact rather than an empathetic manner.

Stigma

Those patients with heavily stigmatized diseases such as HIV/AIDS, tuberculosis, and mental illness may experience social isolation and labeling. Although treatment for these conditions is readily available and successful, patients may be reluctant to seek them out or to have their conditions become known by others. In the early to mid-1980s, when HIV/AIDS was at its peak, I vividly recall individuals paying for treatment themselves rather than submitting their claims and seeking out providers in other communities so as not to be recognized.

Time

The most precious commodity for everyone today is time. Unfortunately, especially with more complex and/or comorbid conditions, giving and receiving information regarding treatment regimes require significant expenditures of time. Providers may want (and patients may require) several opportunities to repeat and revisit education that has been given, especially concerning medications. For those who are health literate, the lack of time may present a level of inconvenience or annoyance, and they will seek out health information themselves or assert their needs with providers more directly. For those who lack competency in this area, the consequences of time-limited health discussions may be very damaging. A recent study at Case Western Reserve University demonstrates that the average time a medical doctor spends with a patient is 13.3 minutes;[10] the time for an interpreter-assisted visit would need to be considerably longer because each line of information would need to be passed through a third party. Obviously, if the expanded time isn't available, the patient is placed at risk.

Gender

Many patients are more comfortable in a healthcare setting when they are cared for by a member of their own gender. Especially in matters of reproductive health, or in circumstances that might involve discussion of sexual abuse or dysfunction, feelings of embarrassment may result in incomplete medical assessments, diagnosis, and treatment. Additionally, people tend to be more at ease with the intimate aspects of the physical examination and diagnostic procedures when the care provider is of the same gender. With care providers of the same gender, it is easier for patients to establish rapport, ask questions, and attain a comfort level that is so important, especially when prolonged treatment is likely.

Trust and Communication

Although technology, care, and expertise are certainly important, the relationship that a patient develops with the physician is no less important in health literacy matters. When individuals do not trust the relationship or feel accepted and valued, they may be reluctant to admit to a lack of knowledge or understanding. For example, a patient may be embarrassed to reveal that she didn't take medications because of religious fasting, or she didn't adhere to the prescribed diet for similar reasons. Because we recognize that patients often decide to ignore or alter the treatment recommended by a treating physician, it becomes increasingly important to explore what might be the obstacles that can prevent an open exchange of information, even if that information might reveal a certain level of disrespect or disagreement by either party. Disclosing and then understanding the issues bring us closer to obtaining the kind of results that patients need and deserve.

HEALTH LITERACY MANIFESTATIONS

Although the core components and activities involved in case management are crucial to achieving the expected outcomes, unfortunately many case managers apply these principles at the outset of a case but may not continue the process across the continuum.

Most of us can cite examples of how we became aware of some of the instances when our patients, for whatever reason, did not follow directions from their physicians; in fact, some of these individuals may be us. Patients don't always follow medical advice; treatment may deviate from the prescribed medication regimen and may go undetected for many weeks or months until a complication or problem arises that possibly results in a hospital admission or worse.

When a patient has low health literacy, he or she may do any or all of the following:

- Discontinue using prescribed medication (without notifying anyone) when symptoms subside; the patient may think it is okay to stop taking the medication(s).

- Change dosage amount, frequency, or time of day the medication is taken (this situation may result in a physician prescribing a stronger dose or different medication).
- Modify restrictions and special instructions.
- Initiate taking someone else's medications for a perceived common symptom.
- Consider treatments such as follows:
  - Old prescriptions
  - Medications prescribed by different providers
  - Over-the-counter remedies
  - Herbal or other traditional medications acquired from abroad
  - Black market remedies as drugs

We must understand that this happens far more often than we may like to admit and that it might be misinterpreted as nonadherence. It may be helpful for us to consider some of the thinking, beliefs, or health literacy deficits that result in nonadherence. Some individuals, especially those in more vulnerable population groups, visit the doctor only when they have symptoms. If they have chronic conditions such as asthma or hypertension, the visit may be precipitated by an exacerbation in symptoms or symptoms that indicate an unmanaged condition. When the prescribed medication results in an alleviation of these symptoms, these individuals may believe that they are cured and may stop taking the medication. People with severe economic concerns may "save" the unused meds for a time when the symptoms reappear.

I recall visiting with a patient in her home. I had asked her in advance to have available all of her medications for us to review. When I arrived, she had 2 shopping bags filled with meds, some older than 10 years! The woman's diagnosis was coronary heart failure (CHF), hypertension, and diabetes (type 2). She had multiple medications for each condition that were prescribed by different physicians and filled at different pharmacies (which precludes a pharmacist at one location from knowing about any potential interactions or problems with other prescriptions that had been filled elsewhere by other pharmacists). As I reviewed the medications that she acknowledged to be taking, I noted that despite the fact that some were to be taken everyday it was obvious that most of them were not being taken. When I commented about this, she explained: "Oh, yes, that's my water pill. I only take that when my wedding ring is tight." When I asked her about her metformin, noting the same evidence of nonadherence, she answered: "Yes, I do have a touch of sugar, so I take this when I've been a bad girl and have had too many sweets." Obviously, I had much work to do!

Although sometimes patients create their own rules, occasionally the system contributes to problems as well. This past summer I visited with an 84-year-old man who has known my husband since my husband was a teen. We were on our way to vacation in New Hampshire; we heard that his wife had passed away, so we stopped to see him. Carl had been having "some . . . problems with my heart." When I saw him, I noted him to be tired, and when I commented on this, he declared that he was exhausted, stating: "I can barely do anything without feeling like I need a nap. I think it's the Nitro they gave me." I asked Carl to show me *all* the medications he was taking, and he took out four prescription bottles. First, there was digoxin, and then Toprol (metoprolol succinate) 100 mgm once/day (prescribed June 15, 2008), and then another for Toprol 50 mgm once/day (prescribed June 22, 2008), and then Lasix (furosemide) 40 mgm once/day. I asked Carl: "Which of these are you taking?" He replied: "All of them, just like it says: one of each of them every day." I showed Carl that two of the meds (Toprol) were the same. We then realized that when he saw his MD the week following the original prescription for 100 mgm of Toprol and mentioned feeling very tired, the physician had adjusted and reduced the dosage to 50 mgm—but Carl did *not* know or realize this. (Perhaps he was not told very clearly and precisely: "Do *not* take the 100 mgm Toprol anymore. *Just* take the 50 mgm tablets.") Because Carl obviously was unaware of some important information, he was taking *150 mgm* instead of 50 mgm! I asked Carl whether his physician or the pharmacist had mentioned anything about not taking the 100-mgm tablets anymore, but he said no. I looked closely at the two bottles of Toprol, and on the side of the 50 mgm one was a tiny yellow label that read: *"THIS IS THE SAME MEDICATION AS ONE ALREADY PRESCRIBED . . . YOU MAY WANT TO CHECK WITH YOUR MD"* in *very* small print. I contacted the pharmacy and explained the situation and advised of this apparent overdose problem. When I asked if anyone had called the physician or discussed the change in medication with the patient, the pharmacist replied: "No, we didn't. Didn't his doctor tell him to stop the 100 mgm?" I advised Carl of what he needed to do, removed the 100 mgm bottle, placed it away from the others, and wrote a note to the physician explaining what had occurred. I suggested to Carl that he could read what I wrote to the physician when he called. Carl said: "No, I'm going to take your note to him." Later, Carl told us that the people at the physician's office were very apologetic: "Told me it will take a while for me to feel better," he said.

My husband, who has never really understood what case managers do, that day saw it up close and personal. He saw that what we do each and every day does make a difference!

Sharing Is Caring

Families and friends often share advice . . . and sometimes prescribed treatments, which may include medications. When symptoms appear to be the same between two people, patients sometimes offer their own medications to the other person, who, they believe, may have the same diagnosis. (Oh, yes, patients diagnose themselves as well!) When patients are no longer taking a specific medication (either by their own decision or when it has been discontinued by the physician), an individual may decide to save the medication for use at another time or to share with another. One can only begin to imagine what may occur when several different medications are stored in one container, leaving indications and dosages to the individual's recollection, and then this same individual assumes the role of physician and pharmacist either for himself or another!

Perceptions and Values

We have examined in Chapter 15 that those from diverse backgrounds have different perceptions of illness and different values regarding what they view as acceptable treatment. In the United States, people of diverse backgrounds may retain some of their traditional curative and healing practices, and they may be reluctant to share this information with health-care providers because they expect or fear disapproval. As case managers, we need to be able to advocate for these patients and create the kind of environment that promotes full disclosure and sharing of this kind of information. Fortunately, it is often possible that Western therapies and traditional healing practices can be safely combined.

THE CASE MANAGER'S VITAL ROLE

Perhaps the most valuable contribution case managers make is the empowerment of individuals with necessary information and education so that they can more fully participate in their own care. Although there is an unending amount of information available, regrettably, as we have examined, much of it is unusable by the very individuals who need it most. Poor communication between patients and clinicians is a contributing factor resulting in malpractice lawsuits. Attorneys, in fact, estimate this to be the major factor in nearly 75% of malpractice suits.[11] Case managers can become the intermediary agent and facilitator of the kind of information that will keep patients safe and promote quality care and cost-effective outcomes.

General consensus exists among health literacy experts that there are six basic methods for improving communication with patients.[12] These methods, while seemingly simplistic in nature, are incredibly valuable. These strategies were initially recommended based upon expert opinion, but now research is proving that they work:

1. *Slow down.* Communication is enhanced by speaking slowly and distinctly, and by spending just a small amount of additional time with each patient. When you have the opportunity for face-to-face interaction, certain other behaviors can convey true caring, concern, and a desire to hear the patient's concerns. Sitting, rather than standing, listening more than speaking, and encouraging patients to ask questions create a more favorable impression and an environment more conducive to a patient-centered visit. Obviously, we need to employ somewhat different strategies when our intervention is provided telephonically. When case loads are high and there never seems to be enough time, and when we come from parts of the country where rapid-fire speech is the norm (I am, unfortunately, guilty) this may be more challenging; however, the results are so worthwhile that we should try to explore, at least for some of our patients, ways to slow down the process of communication.

2. *Use plain, nonmedical language.* As stated previously, healthcare professionals frequently use professional jargon, which certainly does communicate one's expertise and membership in the "club" of other professionals; however, this practice only serves to create an uncomfortable distance between patients and providers. A good approach is to use the same language and illustrations that you might use to explain something to your grandmother, a neighbor, or a friend. Conversational language is certainly less intimidating than clinical dissertations or monologues and conveys to patients that you really want them to understand the issues at hand.

3. *Show or draw pictures.* Every individual learns differently. For some, a picture is truly worth a thousand words. Although patients may have difficulty understanding medical conditions especially when they also must understand the organ that is involved, pictures or very simple diagrams can be extremely helpful. Videos or anatomic models may also be useful in enhancing the necessary comprehension but should never be substitutes for written or verbal communication. Again, if you are a case manager working telephonically, you may be somewhat disadvantaged, but many patient education resources to enhance health literacy are available. (See the Resources at the end of this chapter.)

4. *Limit the amount of information given at each visit, and repeat it.* Information is best remembered when given in small amounts and when it is relevant to the patient's current needs or situation. After discussing the initial information with a patient, review this information and repeat it; it most certainly can and should be repeated by other members of the healthcare team, too. Reinforcing information with patient-friendly handouts can serve as additional education and can be helpful in that patients can read the handout in a less stressful environment. Whether your involvement is face to face or telephonic, follow-up telephone calls can be particularly helpful. Phone calls are opportunities for case managers to ascertain knowledge, clarify any misunderstandings, and determine the patient's ability and desire to adhere to the recommended treatment plan.

5. *Use the "teach-back" technique.* It is often easier and certainly quicker to ask patients the kinds of questions that elicit simple "yes" or "no" responses. Are you taking your medications? "Yes." Have you been checking your blood glucose levels three times a day? "Yes." Do you have any questions? "No." However, we need to ask questions in such a way that we elicit responses that demonstrate that the patient has adequate knowledge (and therefore is a safe and hopefully adherent patient) or that indicate that additional information is still needed. Occasionally, in my years of practice, I have heard from physicians or members of their staff that patients have been given information, shown how to use a glucometer, for example, were given educational materials, and so on, and they are *"still* not compliant." Upon further exploration, I've discovered that the patient really didn't understand what he or she needed to understand to be appropriately engaged. Some individuals *need* periodic assessments of their knowledge or refresher courses. By allowing patients the time to explain back to you step-by-step instructions or to repeat what you've just told them will assure both of you that they really *do* understand.

6. *Create a shame-free environment; encourage questions.* Each of us needs to feel safe in a learning environment. I think this is important for all communication and learning opportunities, but especially so when the student is a patient. A simple method that I have used successfully is to advise individuals something like this: "Many patients have difficulty reading and understanding medical information, so please feel comfortable asking as many questions as you need," or "Occasionally, patients feel embarrassed or that they're using too much of the doctor's time by asking so many questions.

Or they feel stupid because the doctor seems to be so much smarter. But I want and need you to understand this information so that you can be well, so let's go over some of this information again, okay?" Offering patients the opportunity to bring a family member with them for a visit or to have a trusted friend obtain information by speaking to you on their behalf may also be helpful; obviously, you must obtain appropriate consents and document this in your records. Another, more formal strategy, the Ask-Me-Three program, is sponsored by the Partnership for Clear Health Communication and encourages patients to ask and physicians to answer three basic questions during every medical encounter:

1. What is my main problem?
2. What do I need to do (about the problem)?
3. Why is it important for me to do this?[13]

This program is getting widespread attention for obvious reasons, and case managers can certainly encourage their patients to ask these basic questions of their providers. Additional information and materials are available through the organization's website at www.askme3.org.

CONCLUSION

Assessing and then addressing the health literacy of our patients is an extremely important element in the case management process. We understand that knowledge, communication, and a safe patient-centered environment are essential components that affect the health and wellness of our patients. We can be the leaders in our organizations or practice settings to promote improved outcomes for patients who will have the skills and knowledge necessary to be active and confident collaborators in their own care.

RESOURCES

Health Literacy Organizations and Programs

American Medical Society Foundation
515 North State Street
Chicago, IL 60610
www.ama-assn.org/ama/pub/category/8115.html

Ask Me 3
www.npsf.org/askme3/

Harvard School of Public Health
Department of Society, Human Development and Health
677 Huntington Avenue, 7th Floor
Boston, MA 02115
www.hsph.harvard.edu/healthliteracy/overview.html

National Institute for Literacy
1775 I Street N.W., Suite 730
Washington, DC 20006-2401
www.nifl.gov

Office of Minority Health
P.O. Box 37337
Washington, DC 20013
www.omhrc.gov

Pfizer Clear Health Communication Initiative
www.pfizerhealthliteracy.com

World Education, Literacy and Health Initiative
44 Farnsworth Street
Boston, MA 02111-1211
www.worlded.org

Bibliographies, Webliographies, and Web Resources

National Library of Medicine, *Understanding Health Literacy and Its Barriers*
www.nlm.nih.gov/pubs/cbm/healthliteracybarriers.html

National Library of Medicine, MEDLINE/PubMed Search and Literacy Information Resources
www.nlm.nih.gov/services/health_literacy.html

NOTES

1. Weiss BD, *Health Literacy and Patient Safety: Help Patients Understand*, 2nd ed. (Chicago: American Medical Association, 2007).
2. Nielsen-Bohlman LN, Panzer AM, and Kindig DA, eds., *Health Literacy: A Prescription to End Confusion* (Washington, DC: National Academies Press, 2004).
3. Kutner M, Greenberg E, Jin Y, and Paulsen C, *The Health Literacy of America's Adults: Results from the 2003 National Assessment of Adult Literacy*. National Center for Education

Statistics (NCES) Publication No. 2006-483 (Washington, DC: U.S. Department of Education, September 2006).

4. Kutner et al., *Health Literacy of America's Adults.*

5. Morris B, "Overcoming Dyslexia," *Fortune*, May 13, 2002, 55–70.

6. U.S. Department of Health and Human Services, *Healthy People 2010: Understanding and Improving Health*, 2nd ed. (Washington, DC: U.S. Government Printing Office, November 2000), http://www.health.gov/healthypeople.

7. Ad Hoc Committee on Health Literacy for the Council on Scientific Affairs, American Medical Association, "Health Literacy: Report of the Council on Scientific Affairs," *Journal of the American Medical Association* 281, no. 6 (February 10, 1999), http://jama.ama-assn.org/cgi/content/abstract/281/6/552.

8. Nielsen-Bohlman et al., *Health Literacy.*

9. Davis TC, Dolan NC, Ferreira MR, et al., "The Role of Inadequate Health Literacy Skills in Colorectal Cancer Screening," *Cancer Investigation* 19 (2001): 193–200.

10. Gottschalk A and Flocke S, "Time Spent in Face-to-Face Patient Care and Work Outside the Examination Room," *Annals of Family Medicine* 3 (2005): 488–493.

11. Beckman HB, Markakis KM, Suchman AL, and Frankel RM, "The Doctor–Patient Relationship and Malpractice: Lessons from Plaintiff Depositions," *Archives of Internal Medicine* 154 (1994): 1365–1370.

12. Williams MV, Davis T, Parker RM, and Weiss BD, "The Role of Health Literacy in Patient–Physician Communication," *Family Medicine* 34 (2002): 383–389.

13. Partnership for Clear Health Communication, "Ask-Me-Three," http://www.askme3.org.

Chapter 17

Pharmaceuticals: The Ever-Evolving World

While our nation's healthcare system continues to strain under an infrastructure in dire need of revision, one segment, the pharmaceutical industry, is taking measures to change. For many years, the world of pharmaceuticals has been very dynamic, with new drugs being developed at unprecedented rates and clinical trials following close behind. However, many factors have converged to influence some significant changes. High-profile lawsuits stemming from drug-related deaths, direct-to-consumer advertising, the troubled economy, and new demands by payers for clinical proof that branded products are worth more than generics have all made the pharmaceutical companies sit up, take notice, and more important, take action to change.

A white paper published by Regent Atlantic Capital, LLC (Chatham, New Jersey) titled "The Continuing Evolution of the Pharmaceutical Industry: Career Challenges and Opportunities" conveys the results of an 11-month study conducted by a 14-person research team who interviewed more than 100 pharmaceutical industry experts. Interviewees included current and former CEOs and executives of pharmaceutical and biotech firms, academics, recruitment and outplacement firms, attorneys, and consultants. Among the conclusions of this major study is the fact that the pharmaceutical industry will transition to a more decentralized business model wherein there will be fewer large companies and thousands of smaller drug companies along with many independent contractors. Furthermore, the survey concludes that pharmaceutical companies will be more focused on late-stage drug development, marketing, and distribution.[1]

The finding regarding the pharmaceutical companies' focus on late-stage drug development is further validated by a September 30, 2008, news article published in the *International Herald Tribune*. In "Big Pharma Prunes R&D as Times Get Tough," Reuters reporters Ben Hirschler and Lewis Krauskopf note that "the world's top drugmakers are taking the knife to research and development." They cite GlaxoSmithKline's plans to reduce its R&D team by 850 jobs, which follows 350 R&D cuts in June 2008. The combined cuts comprise 6% of its former R&D workforce. Also noted in the article is Pfizer Inc.'s decision to stop developing drugs for heart disease, obesity, and bone health. Other examples of a more focused pharmaceutical industry cited in the Hirschler and Krauskopf article include Merck & Company's decision to focus R&D on nine therapeutic areas and the spinning off of certain R&D activities into new companies (e.g., AstraZeneca's spinoff of research on gastrointestinal disease drugs into the new company Albireo, and Sanofi-Aventis SA's spinoff of its bone health research into the ProStrakan Group).[2]

Not everyone is pleased about the R&D cutbacks. At least one blogger on the World of DTC Marketing.com website, commenting on both the R&D cutbacks and the large drug companies' practice of instituting major staff cutbacks once a top-selling drug comes off its patent, writes, "Big pharma is its own worst enemy and it seems that most CEOs are only looking to keep the boat afloat rather than acknowledge that the river is too narrow to turn the boat around quickly."[3]

The direct-to-consumer (DTC) movement, although adding yet another layer of bureaucracy and costs to pharmaceutical marketing, also has introduced a new element of change. Now consumers, exposed to television, radio, magazine, and newspaper drug advertisements, are asking their physicians about various drugs and in doing so are taking a more active role in their own treatment plans. For some critics of DTC drug marketing, there may be a safety concern in this trend. Most, however, believe that the more informed consumers are about their choices, the better the healthcare system will be.

For case managers, the evolving world of pharmaceuticals requires the great need to stay abreast of how all these factors influence our role as intermediaries between patients, their family members, physicians, and providers.

WHEN DRUGS BECOME DEADLY

Over the past several years, we have witnessed deaths attributed to side effects from Food and Drug Administration–approved pharmaceuticals that were used as prescribed and according to the manufacturer's protocol. Some of these deaths have resulted in lawsuits against the manufacturers. Among the more publicized pharmaceuticals associated with these outcomes have been tPA, a clot-buster drug prescribed for stroke victims; the popular statin drug Lipitor (atorvastatin calcium), prescribed to treat high cholesterol; and painkillers known as COX-2 inhibitors (e.g., Vioxx [rofecoxib] and Bextra [valdecoxib]). However, many more drugs deliver adverse reactions that kill tens of thousands of people yearly.

In her article for *Discover* magazine, titled "Wonder Drugs That Can Kill," Jeanne Lenzer describes the dilemma facing physicians when prescribing drugs.

> Doctors have to navigate a tangle of administrative and medical concerns, one physician noting that if you have a patient in your office, you can't say, 'Oh, I'm going to look at the drug company's online database about Zyprexia.' Most doctors don't even know the databases exist. But even if they did, the next thing you know, three or four hours have gone by and you've missed all the patients waiting to see you.[4]

This scenario is also one to which case managers can relate. Although we do not prescribe medicines, our role does place us in a position to field questions from patients about medicines and to report on patients' conditions while using various medications.

The fact is that being vigilant is important for all medical professionals but is no assurance that patients still won't be adversely affected by their prescription drugs. Regardless of whether drugs are FDA approved, many believe medical studies on drugs are flawed. One individual with a high profile for his role in criticizing drug studies is Curt Furberg, a well-respected cardiovascular epidemiologist and the former chief of the clinical trials branch at the National Heart, Lung, and Blood Institute (Bethesda, Maryland). He holds that many of the studies are industry-sponsored and are therefore biased in interpreting the findings. This belief is supported by an analysis of the studies. One study performed by Yale School of Medicine Associate Professor of Medicine Cary P. Gross and published by the *Journal of the American Medical Association* finds that "industry-sponsored research was positive 87% of the time compared with 65% positive for research that was not industry-sponsored" and "industry sponsorship was likely to yield pro-industry results."[5] Other studies have come to the same conclusion.

In addition to unintended consequences of prescribed drugs, there are the risks associated with accidental drug overdoses. A study titled "Patterns of Abuse Among Unintentional Pharmaceutical Overdose Fatalities," published in the December 10, 2006, issue of the *Journal of the American Medical Association*, found that in 2006, there were 295 deaths associated with accidental overdoses of which 67.1% were men, 63.1% used painkillers including methadone, Oxycontin (oxycodone), and Vicodin (hydrocodone bitartrate and acetaminophen) for which they did not have a prescription, and 21.5% had prescriptions from at least separate doctors.[6] The concerns are not only about the risks of overdose, but also that there are so many doctors writing prescriptions for pain medications and that patients are not being counseled thoroughly. The Centers for Disease Control and Prevention places drug overdoses in the United States as the second leading cause of unintended deaths, right behind motor vehicle deaths.[7]

Here are a few more sobering statistics:

- At least 2 million older Americans are taking a combination of drugs or supplements that pose great risk to their health, based on a study funded by the National Institutes of Health and the University of Chicago. The same study found that 91% of Americans (more than 50 million people) aged 57–85 take at least one medication and that more than half of them use at least five remedies including prescription drugs, over-the-counter medications, and/or supplements.[8]
- Based on federal data, almost 7 million Americans abused prescription drugs in 2007; this number is up by 80% since 2000, and the number of Americans treated for abuse of painkillers increased by 321% from 1995 to 2005.[9]
- According to a Florida Medical Examiners Commission report, prescription drug–related deaths have surpassed deaths caused by illegal drugs. The report also notes that an analysis of 168,900 autopsies performed in Florida in 2007 revealed that three times as many deaths were caused by legal drugs over all the deaths caused by cocaine, heroin, and all methamphetamines: 2,328 people were killed by opioid painkillers including Vicodin and Oxycontin, 743 were killed by drugs containing benzodiazepine including the depressants Valium (diazepam) and Xanax (alprazolam), 843 deaths were caused by cocaine, 121 deaths were caused by heroin, 25 deaths were caused by methamphetamines, and 0 deaths were caused by marijuana.[10]

Case managers have the opportunity to assume a greater role in advocating and caring for their patients by becoming more proactive and informed regarding prescription medications, their side effects, and the potential for overdoses associated with certain medications, in particular, pain medicines. Especially when patients have comorbid conditions requiring interventions and prescriptions to be made by several physicians from a variety of settings (office, clinic, hospital, walk-in urgent care centers, to name a few) and specialties, the role of the case manager becomes even more important. All too often, the side effects from all of the medications some individuals take result in symptoms and *other* conditions that necessitate additional treatment and regrettably additional prescriptions.

Case managers often play the role of detective and spreadsheet analyst as they try to determine just what may be resulting in an increase of symptoms and/or worsening of the patient's status. You can probably recall instances when you have tallied the long list of medications a patient takes, looking them all up in a reference source, and thought: "No *wonder* these problems are occurring! The adverse and side effects from some of these are *exactly* what my patient is experiencing. I wonder if all of the physicians actually *know* what this patient is taking?" The next challenge, and often the most difficult one, is getting *one* of the physicians to serve as the coordinator of care and central prescriber. This is especially crucial when there is evidence of abuse or increasing dependency on some of the medications.

MARKETING DRUGS DIRECT TO CONSUMERS

Although U.S. drug companies were allowed to advertise their products direct to consumers in the early 1980s, it wasn't until a loosening of regulations in the late 1990s that direct-to-consumer (DTC) drug advertising really took off. In 1983, the FDA issued a voluntary moratorium following a promotional campaign by the Oraflex manufacturer Lilly. Five months after the product was introduced, it was withdrawn when it was found to cause risks of liver failure.[11] However, the moratorium was lifted in 1985,[12] and since that time, DTC advertising has been growing.

In 1990, pharmaceutical manufacturers spent $100 million in DTC advertising.[13] By 2000, the figure had grown to $2.5 billion.[14] In 2003, DTC drug advertising spending had climbed to $3.7 billion, and then to $4.1 billion in 2004.[15] In 2004, the largest expenditures for DTC advertising were made for five drugs: Nexium (esomeprazole magnesium; $226 million), Crestor (rosuvastatin calcium; $193 million), Cialis (tadalafil; $152 million), Levitra (vardenafil; $142 million), and Zelnorm (tegaserod maleate; $122 million).[16]

According to a U.S. Government Accountability Office report dated November 2006, drug companies spent $4.2 billion in DTC advertising in 2005 compared to $7.2 billion that same year marketing drugs to physicians.[17]

Consumer Safety

So, exactly what do all of these figures represent to consumers? Dr. John Abramson reported in his book *Overdosed America* that the "1997 change [in DTCA law] unleashed an unprecedented onslaught of commercials. By 1999, the average American was exposed to nine prescription drug advertisements on television every day. The number of television ads increased 40-fold between 1994 and 2000."[18]

As of this writing, it is apparent that prescription drug advertising direct to consumers has not subsided. The broadcast and cable networks are filled with advertisements for pharmaceutical companies as are the pages of news, women's, men's, and health magazines and newspapers. Still, concerns abound regarding the ramifications of DTC advertising on drug safety and related risks. To address these concerns, the pharmaceutical industry introduced some guidelines for DTC advertising; namely, the Pharmaceutical Research and Manufacturers of America established voluntary DTC guidelines in 2005.[19] Members of the industry are calling for better analysis of clinical trial data and drug studies.

In her interview with Next Generation Pharmaceutical's Leslie Knudson, Judith Sills, Vice President of Medical Safety Operations in the Integrated Medical Safety Department of Novartis Pharmaceuticals, says, "All the companies are posting trial results in clinical trial registries, thereby ensuring this data is available. Health authorities are also increasing their transparency through their websites, posting decisions and data so that it's available to the public."[20]

She also notes, "Probably the most important (tangible result) is the awareness of the importance of drug safety and proactive safety risk management throughout the pharma organization. The implementation of Safety Management Teams and the Medical Safety Review Board has led to a more streamlined, rigorous, and consistent process for evaluating safety information on an ongoing basis through product development and post marketing." In her comments, she notes that the linking of public, private, and commercial databases via medical claims and electronic health records would also help advance the safety factor.[21]

STAYING ABREAST OF PHARMACEUTICALS

Case managers must stay abreast of the DTC drug advertising trend and related developments, particularly those pertaining to consumer safety. Seeking out continuing education courses on pharmaceuticals is, of course, valuable, as is establishing best practices to manage patients' compliance with prescribed drug regimens. This is especially important for patients with complex medical conditions that require multiple medications that could cause side effects and/or could lead to abuse situations.

In our role as intermediaries between physicians and patients, case managers could also play a vital role in reinforcing with patients the importance of having regular dialogues with their physicians regarding medications, proper usage, side effects, and the need to be cautious both of manufacturers' drug warnings and claims. Case managers can also serve as physicians' watchful eyes, raising red flags when troublesome patient behaviors that can be a result of a drug-related problem are observed.

Economic and Ethical Considerations

Thankfully, through research, it is now possible for many conditions to be managed through pharmaceutical intervention. With the direct-to-consumer marketing and chat rooms especially for those with certain conditions, patients are often more quickly informed about the "latest and greatest" drugs long before case managers can access journals, newsletters, online programs, or other educational formats. This means that patients are chatting in real time with others who have been part of some off-label use of certain medications for conditions previously untreated with this medication. Patients may also decide that, rather than be treated with routinely prescribed and effective (and often less costly) medication for specific conditions, they now want the latest and greatest drug available. Oftentimes, patients discover results that are amazingly wonderful, convincing, and encouraging, and they now want the same treatment. Regardless of the fact that clinical trials may only be at phase I and that evidence-based practice guidelines and protocols for use have not been completed, patients want what they want—and they want it yesterday.

In these circumstances, case managers must be the voice of reason, advising and counseling to ensure that patients are fully informed about the potential for risks and complications as well as benefits. Additionally, case managers also bear the additional responsibility to be stewards of resources. When cost-effective, safe, and often generic alternatives are available and successful in the treatment of certain conditions, we must advise patients and encourage them to use their pharmaceutical benefits wisely and to perhaps consider a tiered approach to treatment. We can encourage patients to pursue typical treatment at the outset of a diagnosis, and then gradually to move to more aggressive, cutting-edge, and, usually, more costly treatment when the usual treatment fails to result in improvement, when the condition progresses rapidly and potentially threatens survival, or when the patient has certain other problems and contraindications that preclude the use of routinely prescribed medications.

Health plans, including Medicare Part D for prescription coverage, usually have definite requirements for use of certain classifications of medications and often mandate precertification as well as capitations (yearly limits), co-payments, and mail-order requirements for certain prescription medications, including biologics, intravenous medications, and certain chemotherapy agents. These measures ensure patient safety, the appropriate use of medications, and of course the efficient use of fund dollars. Many plans include language that expressly forbids the use of medication for off-label use or for uses that would be considered experimental or investigational.

Case managers, unfortunately, occasionally are in the position of knowing that medication is being used off-label, but because we see ourselves as patient advocates, we are reluctant to report the matter. This is truly a discomforting position to be in, and case managers who are also employees of the health plan have additional responsibilities to uphold the language of the plan. The conflicting loyalties described here are vexing and the reason why organizations need to establish ethical guidelines and committees to address such matters. Regrettably, employers and health plans, private and public, are often viewed as the bad guys when treatment, especially medications, is denied.

If federal regulations change—they are being reviewed by the FDA and the courts—the drugs that have not yet been approved for use will be made available to patients. As the regulations currently stand, a physician can prescribe a drug that shows potential even though it has not received FDA approval if certain of the following conditions are met:

- The patient's condition must be serious or immediately life-threatening.
- Comparable approved and experimental treatment options must not be readily available to the patient for some reason.
- The drug must have some potential to save the patient's life as shown in preliminary, ongoing clinical trials.
- The FDA—this is the center of the current debate—must approve the use of the drug in the patient. This is done on a case-by-case basis for what is known as "compassionate use" or "investigational new drug treatment" use.[22]

In those instances when approval from a payer source is lacking, when there are financial limitations for pharmaceutical coverage, when co-payments are unaffordable, or when coverage is simply unavailable, many pharmaceutical companies provide financial assistance for patients. Additionally, many states have programs for underinsured patients or uninsured individuals, and case managers should explore these options on behalf of patients to uncover potential resources and assistance.

CONCLUSION

The role of case manager is a demanding and ever-expanding one. Keeping abreast of the many resources, including those of the pharmaceutical industry, is getting to be more complicated but is an extremely important component of the work that we do. The valuable contributions to healthcare of the pharmaceutical companies cannot be underestimated, and I encourage organizations and individuals to take advantage of the many educational opportunities they make available to professionals and patients. From sponsorships and symposia at our local and regional conferences; contributed articles in professional journals, magazines, and newsletters; online educational presentations on corporate websites as well as those that they make available to hospitals, managed care organizations, and others; and on-site programs for case management chapters and organizations employing case managers across the country, our colleagues in the pharmaceutical industry are truly partners in care.

NOTES

1. Michael Steiner et al., "The Continuing Evolution of the Pharmaceutical Industry: Career Challenges and Opportunities," December 2007, http://www.fiercebiotech.com/whitepapers/continuing-evolution-pharmaceutical-industry-career-challenges-and-opportunities.

2. Ben Hirschler and Lewis Krauskopf, "Big Pharma Prunes R&D as Times Get Tough," *International Herald Tribune*, September 30, 2008, http://www.iht.com/articles/reuters/2008/09/30/business/OUKBS-UK-GLAXO-JOBS.php.

3. World of DTC Marketing, blog, October 2, 2008, http://www.worldofdtcmarketing.com/files/b5edd83854e70dc1cc3fe8ae8b5d281f-462.html.

4. Jeanne Lenzer, "Wonder Drugs That Can Kill," *Discover*, June 20, 2008, http://discovermagazine.com/2008/jul/20-wonder-drugs-that-can-kill/article_print.

5. Ibid.

6. Aron Hall et al., "Patterns of Abuse Among Unintentional Pharmaceutical Overdose Fatalities," *Journal of the American Medical Association* 300, no. 22 (December 10, 2008): 2613–2620, http://jama.ama-assn.org/cgi/content/full/300/22/2613.

7. Hall et al., "Patterns of Abuse," 2613–2620.

8. http://www.wtopnews.com/?nid=106&sid=1558153.

9. RedOrbit, "More Americans Addicted to Prescription Drugs," July 30, 2008, http://www.redorbit.com/news/health/1502234/more_americans_addicted_to_prescription_drugs/index.html.

10. Free Internet Press, "Prescription Drugs Kill 300 Percent More Americans Than Illegal Drugs," November 14, 2008, http://freeinternetpress.com/story.php?sid=19132.

11. Basra LR, "Direct-to-Consumer Advertising: Today's Issues and Tomorrow's Outlook," *Journal of Drug Issues* 22, no. 2 (1992): 317–330.

12. Feather KR, "Direct to the Consumer Advertising—How Close Can We Come?" *Journal of Pharmaceutical Marketing and Management* 2, no. 1 (1986): 67–71.

13. Mertens G, "Direct to Consumer Advertising: Global Drug Promotion," *Financial Times Healthcare (London)* (1998).

14. Rosenthal MB, Berndt ER, Donohue JM, Frank RG, and Epstein AM, "Promotion of Prescription Drugs to Consumers," *New England Journal of Medicine* 346 (2002): 498–505.

15. Arnold M, "Changing Channels," *Medical Marketing and Media* 401, no. 4 (2005): 34–39.

16. Arnold, "Changing Channels," 34–39.

17. http://www.sourcewatch.org/index.php?title=Direct-to-consumer_advertising_in_the_United_States.

18. SourceWatch, "Direct-to-Consumer Advertising in the United States," May 2008, http://www.sourcewatch.org/index.php?title=Direct-to-consumer_advertising_in_the_United_States.

19. http://www.sourcewatch.org/index.php?title=Direct-to-consumer_advertising_in_the_United_States.

20. Next Generation Pharmaceutical, "The Evolution of Drug Safety," http://www.ngpharma.com/currentissue/article.asp?art=273240&issue=246.

21. Next Generation Pharmaceutical, "The Evolution of Drug Safety."

22. http://www.hhs.gov/fda/clinicaltrials.

Chapter 18

The Aging Population, Medical Advancements, and New Case Management Considerations

OUR GRAYING POPULATION

America is getting older. According to the latest U.S. Census statistics, on July 1, 2004, there were 36.3 million older adults age 65 and older in the United States, 12% of the total population. By 2050, this number is expected to increase to 86.7 million, or 21% of the total population. To present the graying of America in perspective, from year 2000 to 2050, the U.S. population of adults 65 years and older is expected to grow 147% while the overall population of the United States is projected to increase by just 49%. The United States is not only getting grayer, but the gray is lasting longer. According to the U.S. Census data, the estimated number of centenarians (individuals age 100 years or older) on November 1, 2005, was 67,473. By 2040, that number is projected to be 580,605.[1]

With the graying of America comes increased incidence in certain medical conditions associated with aging. Among the more serious of these conditions are Alzheimer's and Huntington's diseases. Regarding Alzheimer's, although unconfirmed, it is believed that approximately 10% of Americans age 65 and older suffer from some degree of Alzheimer's disease. By 2050, it is projected that 14 million Americans will have the disease. Other common age-related changes are losses in vision and hearing, diminished muscle mass and strength, decreased efficiency of the nervous system, and a weakened immune system.[2]

NEW CHALLENGES

The increased longevity of older adults in the United States and around the world poses new challenges for healthcare systems and for case managers. The Centers for Disease Control and Prevention's report "Healthy Aging for Older Adults" notes that "critical knowledge gaps exist for responding to the health needs of older adults. For chronic diseases and conditions such as Alzheimer's disease, arthritis, depression, psychiatric disorders, osteoporosis, Parkinson's disease, and urinary incontinence, much remains to be learned about their distribution in the population, associated risk factors, and effective measures to prevent or delay their onset."[3]

The State of Aging and Health in America 2007, a joint report by the Centers for Disease Control and Prevention and the Merck Company Foundation, notes that an estimated 80% of older Americans are living with at lease one chronic condition and that the cost of providing healthcare for an older American (65 years or older) is three to five times greater than the cost for caring for Americans younger than 65 years of age. By 2030, U.S. healthcare spending is expected to increase by 25% owing to the older age demographics. This projection should be an incentive for those comprising our nation's healthcare system to engage in best practices in caring for older adults.[4]

The challenge for case managers is to create efficient systems for managing complex patients who often are elderly and have multiple medical conditions. These systems must address physician communications and reporting procedures, patient communications and monitoring policies, communications with patients' family members, and interfacing with health insurance companies, Medicare, Medicaid, and Medicare Part D prescription benefit plan administrators.

Case managers' best practices must place a greater emphasis on interface and communications with home care providers, and the administrators, medical staff including physicians, nurses, medical social workers, nutritionists, physical and occupational therapists, speech-language therapists, psychologists, and other counselors at nursing homes, assisted living communities, and hospices. It will be increasingly important for case managers serving the elderly population to really understand the intricacies and obstacles to providing the best medical care presented by these various healthcare settings and the different professionals who collectively provide care for older adults. Additionally, case managers must gain a heightened expertise relating to the financial aspects of caring for a complex elderly patient. This includes understanding the healthcare delivery philosophy of each setting and associated financial payment formula, including Medicare's payment structure, hospice financing, and costs for routine and continuous home care services.

Geriatric care managers have been working with older adults and their families for many years. Through conversations with many of them over the last several years, I have come to readily appreciate the growing challenges that all case managers and healthcare professionals encounter now and in future years. Because case management evolved as a direct response to the need to better manage diminishing resources, there is an ever-increasing need today to balance resource allocation with safe, quality care and improved outcomes for older adults.

Although technology and advances in medical research have resulted in individuals living longer lives, these lives often are incredibly difficult ones. Managing complex conditions, medications, and care requirements isn't an easy matter even for those who are in their prime and free from the many problems that many of older adults experience. When spouses die or become chronically ill and/or incapacitated; when friends pass away; when adult children relocate for employment or other reasons; when finances no longer meet day-to-day needs; when physical, mental, and emotional resources are diminished, individuals can become compromised. As with other issues in U.S. society, the needs of this growing group of people are far greater than our ability to provide for them.

Communities and various organizations are attempting to respond to this predicament, and several have implemented very creative and strategically important programs and services. As with other need-based programs, federal, state, and local organizations depend upon governmental funding and charitable contributions that have become seriously jeopardized over the last few years. Because programs lose funding and mergers and acquisitions occur, among other things, case managers must continually keep abreast of just what is available for their elderly patients. The Internet is a good source of information for available resources, as are courses, books, and organizations who are dedicated to serving older adults. (Several resources appear in the appendices at the end of this book, including another Jones and Bartlett publication to which I contributed a chapter: *Care Managers Working with the Aging Family* by Cathy Jo Cress, MSW.)

Although some professionals engage exclusively in geriatric care management, many more of us work with older adults in virtually all other practice settings in case management. Case managers who work with employer-sponsored health plans or workers' compensation used to think that there was no need for them to become involved in issues related to older adults. Changing economics, however, has created an absolute increase in the number of individuals actively employed beyond the age of 65. These employees and their health problems, whether occupationally related or lifestyle related, present challenges that need to be addressed. Virtually every healthcare setting will provide services for older adults. Case managers can be at the center and lead the way to ensure that there will be caring case managers to provide assistance.

NEW OPPORTUNITIES

With these new challenges come many opportunities for case managers whose patients include older adults. For one thing, case managers can return to their roots and really exercise their "caring" role in serving elderly patients. Very often, geriatric patients' family members elevate case managers to a higher stature because they truly value the case manager's ability to manage effectively and stay abreast of the many overlapping elements in the elderly patient's care and treatment plan. Case managers also can realize greater fulfillment and job satisfaction by taking an active role in helping to address key "Calls to Action" as indicated in *The State of Aging and Health in America 2007*, such as the following:

- Address health disparities among older adults, particularly in racial and ethnic minority populations
- Encourage people to communicate their wishes about end-of-life care
- Improve oral health of older adults and increase physical activity among older adults by promoting environmental changes
- Increase adult immunizations, particularly in racial and ethnic minority populations
- Increase screening for colorectal cancer
- Prevent falls, a leading cause of hospitalization and injury deaths among older adults[5]

The steadily increasing senior market in the United States coupled with the increased need for medical case management resulting from the longevity factor and the medical conditions associated with aging make this an ideal time for case managers to consider blazing a new career path by starting a direct-to-consumer community-based case management business. This subject is discussed more fully in later chapters of this book.

NOTES

1. Sharon O'Brien, "Fun Facts About the Senior Population: Demographics," About.com: Senior Living, http://seniorliving.about.com/od/lawpolitics/a/senior_pop_demo.htm.

2. "Aging and Death: Disease Associated with Aging," http://science.jrank.org/pages/124/Aging-Death-Diseases-associated-with-aging.html.

3. Centers for Disease Control and Prevention and the Merck Company Foundation, *The State of Aging and Health in America 2007* (Whitehouse Station, NJ: Merck Company Foundation, 2007).

4. Centers for Disease Control and Prevention and the Merck Company Foundation, *The State of Aging.*

5. Centers for Disease Control and Prevention and the Merck Company Foundation, *The State of Aging.*

Chapter 19

Dying in America

A PERSONAL STORY

From the time of my dad's diagnosis of Alzheimer's disease and over the course of the following 5 years, I tried to prepare him, our family, and myself for the inevitable event, his death. Of course, as a nurse, case manager, and daughter, I experienced the wide range of emotions that one would expect. When I first saw the changes in my dad, the subtle symptoms, I denied their presence. I reasoned that he was disinterested in some conversations or not paying attention because of a hearing loss caused by his years of sirens and bells experienced with the New York City Fire Department. His inability to remember what certain tools were used for, this man who spent so many spare hours tinkering, repairing, crafting wood cabinets and a fiddle to play his beloved Irish music, surely these were just innocent memory lapses. I was having these, too. This man who kept meticulous checkbooks, never needing a calculator, this strong, active, humorous man who was endlessly challenging his mind through daily crossword puzzles and his own inventions, he couldn't possibly have this dreaded disease. He didn't fit the "profile," and of course, as the symptoms grew more pronounced, I refused to accept what I most feared.

At long last, after the diagnostic tests and consultation with a variety of specialists, the diagnosis was made. Because the diagnostic phase spanned a few months, I had a chance to start coming to terms with the reality of the situation. This time also gave me an opportunity to make some plans.

As a case manager, I witness all too many instances of individuals who experience what could only be described as miserable deaths. Their last days are spent in hospitals away from family and friends. They are being probed, tested, and aggressively treated with painful procedures, medications that cause horrendous side effects, and management that only prolongs their suffering.

I wanted to ensure that my dad lived each of his days in a way and manner that was of his choosing and that his final days were peaceful,

657

comfortable, and as dignified and gentle as he was. My experience and knowledge of the workings of the healthcare system would, I believed confidently, help make that happen. We had many conversations over the years about his end-of-life wishes. Still, death always seemed far removed and these discussions merely hypothetical. To bring the "what ifs" into reality while my dad was highly functional and cognitively capable, I scheduled an appointment for us with a dear friend who was a nurse and elder care attorney. In a thoroughly professional and caring manner, the appropriate advance directives were prepared and executed for my parents. They had very definite and sometimes differing opinions and preferences. Finally, with their three children present, their wishes and directives were notarized. Copies of these documents were provided to their treating physicians, and to us.

The first years of this diagnosis were relatively uneventful and happy as I researched and secured optimum treatment for him and respite for my mom, who became the 24/7 care provider. Eventually, it became evident that he was in the final stages of Alzheimer's. The pivotal event occurred while I was on a business trip one March. My dad appeared to have suffered a CVA. The rescue squad was called and he was admitted to a university hospital on Long Island. After several days at the acute care level and with acknowledgment that he could not return home just yet, he was transferred to a subacute rehabilitation unit. The goal was to optimize his functional capabilities so he could return home.

I realized during this episode of several weeks that each member of my family had quite different perceptions. Some were very realistic, and some were in absolute denial of the reality. Despite the fact that throughout the 5-year duration of this disease I had patiently explained the probable course of Alzheimer's, there were family members who viewed this as a totally unrelated, sudden event, and one that my dad would recover from. Because he was now considerably cognitively and physically impaired, he was unable to actively participate in his rehabilitation and, as per Medicare criteria, would need to be discharged. Now, I would face the challenge of trying to understand and meet everyone's needs on an almost daily basis.

My mom could no longer be a care provider because of her own fragile medical status and emotional state as she watched her loving partner and best friend disappear. He did not know who she was, and she felt rejected and very alone. We had endless discussions and explored a reasonable and safe discharge plan, and brought in round-the-clock home care. None of our planning could prevent my mom's devastation at the painful process of witnessing her husband's continuing deterioration in their home. She felt caring for him at home was her only ethical choice because, "He would never want me to put him in a nursing home."

My brother reinforced her guilt continuously as he became more entrenched in his own feelings of denial. Realizing that his support and acceptance would be key, I had arranged for us to tour a local assisted living facility that offers a wonderful Alzheimer's program. He refused to go, had hurtful conversations with all of us, and made known his strong oppositions to "putting my dad away." Whereas he continued his daily visits with my dad, he cut off all communication with my mom, sister, and me. This most unfortunate action was so stressful for my mom that she was admitted to the hospital on Mother's Day with chest pain and acute anxiety/depression. How did all of this happen, what did I do wrong? What was the best solution or, in this case, the least horrible one?

The emergency admission of my mom had one good outcome. It helped her understand, with reinforcement from her doctor and daughters, that her husband would never want her to suffer any more than she already had, and that his 24/7 care at home was both physically and emotionally exhausting and totally unrealistic for her. My dad was becoming more combative, further heightening the difficulty of securing willing care providers. I, too, realized I had to give up my idea of my home as a possible care setting option.

With tears and regrets, I took my mom and dad for his admission evaluation for the Alzheimer inpatient program. He was deemed a candidate and we planned for his admission within the week. Because life does go on, I tried to resume a limited business schedule. I was in Philadelphia on an appointment when my office contacted me. My dad had suffered a massive GI bleed and was taken from the Skilled Nursing Facility back to the acute care hospital. I rushed home, and my sister arrived soon after from Washington, D.C.

Going straight to the emergency room, I was met by the surgeon-on-call, who explained that they needed to find a location of the bleed and were prepping him for colonoscopy and then the O.R. They had already done a type and cross match and had administered one unit of packed cells. In disbelief, I asked this physician if he was aware or had seen my dad's advance directive, and, if so, why was he being scheduled for surgery? The physician acknowledged that no one had advised him of this (despite the fact that from the very first admit to acute care, then to rehabilitation, then to the SNF unit, I ensured that these documents were part of each record).

In a manner that I had utilized before, I asked the doctor, "If this were your dad, what would you do?" He quite rightly and kindly responded,

"Oh no, now you know better. I cannot tell you that. This needs to be your decision." But, I thought, my dad long before had made his decision very clear and no one on staff in this hospital was paying attention to his choice.

Patiently, I reviewed the more pertinent facts with the surgeon; my dad was in the last stages of Alzheimer's, had experienced a CVA, lost more than 40 pounds, did not know anyone, and surely would be an incredible operative risk, to say nothing of potential post-op complications, pain, and his continued suffering. The doctor acknowledged my right to make a decision for my dad and added, "What do you want to do?" Why, I wondered, couldn't he simply admit that surgical procedures were not going to improve my dad's condition or lifestyle, and that it was time to consult his advance directive, prepared for this exact situation. Ah, well, it seems there are those legal issues, so I became my father's voice. I was certain he would not want this procedure, and in fact, it was specifically against his wishes.

My dad was transferred out of the E.R. to a medical unit where, after completing the admission process, I was met by a nurse and another physician exiting my dad's room. They told me they had just hung another unit of packed cells and that they would be checking his hemoglobin/hematocrit to see if he would need more, because "you decided against surgery." I asked why they would be continuing to give him more blood, knowing his situation. The nurse looked me in the eye and said, "You mean you are going to let him bleed to death?"

Feeling as if I had been slapped in the face, I explained to these professionals that rather than viewing it from that perspective, I considered that *not* giving him more blood would result in a gradual decrease in his hgb/hct to a point that would be incompatible with life, and he would peacefully expire. They looked at me, shrugged, and said, "Obviously, you can do what you want," and walked away. They made it clear that they felt I was denying my dad treatment. I wondered why they ignored my dad's directives and virtually accused me of causing his death.

Within a few days, my dad's condition had stabilized enough for him to be transferred back to the SNF unit within the hospital. Fortunately for my dad and for me, I met with a physician assistant within an hour of the admission. Her genuine concern for my obvious distress was evident, and as she kindly put her hand out to pat my shoulder, the weeks and months of inner turmoil were unleashed. Through tears, I related to her the previous events. This woman seemed to instinctively understand my anguish, which now infiltrated so many of my emotions: sadness, confusion, exhaustion, and a powerful feeling of abandonment by my professional colleagues. I found myself protecting my father from a system that disregarded his wishes and was blind to the painful experiences of his last months of life. Somehow, I had believed that they would understand and help me through this incredibly difficult time, as they would wish to be helped in a similar circumstance. Why didn't they? Why did this new professional in her first assignment actively reach out to me and allow me the opportunity to share my frustration, anger, and feelings of guilt and helplessness? With her assistance and at my request, a hospice program for my dad was finally implemented. Despite the fact that Alzheimer's is a terminal illness, not once did any professional ever suggest hospice or even explore our feelings about it. If I had not requested it, I'm certain it would never have been offered.

Creating a hospice program within the SNF was one hurdle. Making certain the facility adhered to the program was another challenge. During the very last weeks of my dad's illness, it was clear that he was experiencing significant pain. His body movements and facial grimaces indicated to me that his pain medications were not being administered every 3 to 4 hours as needed. I would arrive and find him obviously uncomfortable, and suggest that he needed his medication. A nurse would come in, call his name, and ask if he was in pain or if he wanted his pain medication. This to a man who no longer knew his name and was, for the most part, in a semicomatose state.

Continued intervention with the nursing staff was needed as they cautioned me, "We don't want to overmedicate him," or "We don't want to depress his respirations" at the same time my dad was having more frequent episodes of discomfort. I discussed this very odd and upsetting scenario with the hospice physician, and a decision was made for my dad to be medicated every three hours around the clock.

My dad wasn't the only family member who needed assistance. I was on call to help comfort my mother, sister, and brother through these last days. My brother tracked my dad's progress. If our father's temperature was elevated, he wanted him on antibiotics. If dad rejected ice chips, my brother thought his intravenous fluids should be increased. He was clearly unable to come to terms with reality. My mom visited less and less, each time saying good-bye for what she believed would be the last time. The next day my brother would report, "Dad is looking better today."

Throughout the process, I longed for a case manager to lend support and help guide me and my family through this emotionally charged event. I wanted to be a daughter, not the nurse, and definitely not the case manager. Yet, I know that my intervention gave my dad the kind of death he had hoped for, one that was far better than it would have been without my presence. Two months following his admission, he quietly and comfortably passed away.

A peaceful, pain-free death, with final days spent on one's own terms is a wonderful and measurable outcome of individual case management. Advocacy in life and especially in death is at the very heart, or should be, of case management.

DEATH IS NOT AN OPTION

Despite the overwhelming evidence that death is inevitable, most Americans choose to ignore the natural human process that will profoundly affect them and their families. Our nurses and physicians-to-be are not trained on a universal basis as part of their baccalaureate, undergraduate, or graduate studies to address end-of-life (EOL) issues. People feel free to discuss their colonoscopies, but not their feelings about death. Typically, much more research, preparation, and discussion occurs prior to a sweet 16 birthday party than before the final days of one's life. A 1999 National Hospice Foundation survey of Americans age 45 years or older found that more than 50% never discussed their thoughts or feelings about death with family members even when they, or a family member, were terminally ill with less than 6 months to live.[1] The goal of hospice is to keep individuals comfortable and in their own homes. The statistics show that although most people hope to die at home, approximately 50% of the general population dies in the acute care setting.[2]

Although the goals of offering hospice care seem obvious, almost every hospice provider has heard a loved one's lament: "If only we'd known about hospice sooner!" Case managers hear this as well. So, why isn't hospice embraced more eagerly? As stated earlier, Americans do have a cultural aversion to death. From families to physicians, Americans choose to add days to their lives rather than adding life to days, rather than the quality of life rather than quantity argument that we try to encourage. In fact, more than 20% of Medicare patients who have advanced cancer start a new chemotherapy regimen 2 weeks before they die.[3]

Moliere said, "We die only once—and for so long!" Yes, we do, and case managers, as patient advocates with clinical expertise, are in a good position to help individuals and their loved ones replace misinformation with education, fear with calm resolution, and pain with peace.

Studies conducted on end-of-life issues report that patients are most concerned about being mentally aware, not placing a burden on their family, and feeling at peace with God. A majority of terminally ill patients said that euthanasia and physician-assisted suicide should be available, but very few felt they would ever consider these options themselves.[4]

Passed in 1990 and instituted in December 1991, the Patient Self-Determination Act (PSDA) indirectly encourages individuals to make decisions now about the type and scope of medical care they will want when they are no longer able to make that decision themselves due to incapacitation. Under PSDA, all healthcare agencies and facilities that receive Medicare and Medicaid funding must recognize living wills and power of attorney for healthcare as advance directives. In addition, the Act requires healthcare agencies (hospitals, long-term care facilities, and home health agencies) to ask patients if they have advance directives, and provides them with educational materials about their rights under state law.

Case managers should note that each state has its own definitions and practices regarding how individual rights to determine one's own healthcare treatment are guaranteed. For example, a doctor in New York is not required to follow a family's wishes for the patient if they do not have an advance directive naming a healthcare proxy.[5]

Jeanne Boling, MSN, CRRN, CDMS, CCM, and executive director of CMSA, notes that "case managers enjoy an advantage not shared by any other healthcare professional; that of working directly with each element impacting the patient over multiple treatment settings and payment sources. Case managers are as vital to insuring a good outcome during a patient's final illness as at any other life stage. The challenge case managers face when it comes to EOL issues is to help healthcare professionals, patients, and families recognize that a peaceful, dignified death is a good outcome."[6]

EXAMINING YOUR OWN FEELINGS

Patient advocacy is a core function for case managers. Advocating for patients in life and as death approaches is an ethical responsibility. We, as healthcare professionals, must examine our own feelings, as well as our willingness to allow patients to die and to represent their interests in a proactive and ethical manner. This entails approaching the issues surrounding death straightforwardly, honestly, and kindly.

First, be honest and straightforward with yourself. Do you fear death? Do you feel that requesting pain medication indicates a weakness? You might be the healthcare professional who needs to tell parents that their child is nearing death. Can you do that and remain objective and strong enough to advocate for and support the family? Are you willing to object to a physician's reluctance to follow a patient's DNR order?

Case management is a demanding role in the healthcare field. You will need respite, too. You will need to remove yourself from the center of family discussions to retain your ability to assist them effectively. Remember to be as kind to yourself as you are to your patients.

ADDRESSING THE ISSUE OF DEATH

Death and dying present singular problems. This is true whether a spouse is caring for an ill partner, a parent is at the bedside of a child, or an adult is nursing a parent. Sometimes, the patient has accepted the situation and is comfortable with dying but the family cannot let go. Often, the patient and family do not communicate honestly and frankly, especially when death seems imminent. Such dishonesty is not deliberate; it is caused by reluctance to address the issue. In a grim situation (as when a patient has cancer that is metastasizing and may spread to the brain), the case manager might be the person most able to introduce the subject by asking, "Have you thought about a living will? Perhaps you want to discuss this with your physician or your attorney?"

The case manager can make the patient and family aware of support services; help the patient and family come to grips with the reality of the prognosis; and assist in the completion of an estate will, a living will (Table 19–1), a do-not-resuscitate (DNR) order, or a healthcare proxy (also

Table 19–1 Living Will

I, *, residing at *, County of Suffolk and State of New York, do hereby make, publish and declare this is my *Living Will* in manner as follows:

First: I willfully and voluntarily make known my desire that no life-sustaining procedures be used to prolong my dying. If at any time I have a terminal condition certified to be such by two physicians who have personally examined me, one of whom is my attending physician, have determined that my condition is irreversible and that my death will occur within a relatively short period of time without the use of life-sustaining procedures which would serve only to prolong the dying process, then in that event, I direct that the procedures be withheld or withdrawn, and that I be permitted to die naturally. These procedures shall specifically include but shall not be limited to mechanical respiration, cardiac resuscitation, blood transfusion, feeding and hydration tubes, or organ transplant. I direct that this advanced directive be liberally construed.

I further direct my physicians to take the same action with the same responsibilities and consequences as set forth above in the event that I should become irreversibly senile. To help my physicians to make such determination, I direct that I be deemed senile if I am unable to communicate my name, the place where I am, or the names of my immediate family members.

In addition, I make the same directions and relieve the same persons from any responsibility in the event that I am afflicted by an incurable, fatal, or debilitating disease, and have been judicially declared incompetent.

Table 19–1 continued

Second: This *Living Will* is intended to include but is not limited to such life-sustaining procedures as machines that act as substitutes for organs, blood transfusions, feeding tubes and surgical operations. It does not include such procedures or medication that would make me more comfortable and relieve my physical pain.

Third: In the absence of my ability to give directions regarding the use of life-sustaining procedures, it is my intention that this Declaration be honored by my family and physicians and any health facility in which I may be a patient as the final expression of my legal right to refuse medical or surgical treatment and I accept the consequences from the refusal. In this event, I hereby appoint my wife *, as my irrevocable attorney-in-fact, to communicate to the fullest extent possible all of my directions and intentions declared in this my LIVING WILL, to all necessary persons, including but not limited to my physicians, all other healthcare providers and all members of my family. This power of attorney shall not be affected by my subsequent disability or incompetence. In addition, I hereby nominate my said designated agent as Conservator of my property and Committee of my person and property upon the happening of any of the events named herein. In the event my wife predeceases me, fails to qualify, or ceases to act as my said agent, then I hereby appoint my *, *, to act in her place and stead.

Fourth: I hereby relieve physicians, any hospital or other institution and my designated agents of any liability for damage or death resulting therefrom, directly or indirectly, including any claim of malpractice by me or my Estate.

Fifth: I direct that if my physician, or my hospital or other institution refuse to obey my wishes in this matter, that my designated agent herein nominated commence suit against such physician and/or hospital or other institution, for all of the hospital costs, drugs, medical expenses, and all other damages flowing from such refusal, and I direct further that neither their bills for subsequent services be paid nor the bills of any other doctors substituted therefore.

Sixth: This *Living Will* may be revoked only by personal service of a revocation executed by me upon all persons in possession of the original or to whom any certified copy hereof has been delivered, or known to be in possession thereof, and is otherwise irrevocable. I understand that the Court of Appeals has held that my family or designated agent(s) must show that "as far as is humanly possible" I have not had a change of mind, and I intend that any change of mind must be shown as directed in this paragraph only, and without such written revocation, it is my direction that it must be permitted that I have not had a change of mind, no matter how long a

continues

Table 19–1 continued

---

time has elapsed between the execution of this document and the enforcement of this Living Will. An affidavit by the attorney in possession of the original with regard to the issuance and location of certified copies hereof shall be deemed sufficient.

Seventh: This document must be executed in the same manner as a Will.

Subscribed, this * day of *, 2 .

Living Testator

We, whose names are hereto subscribed, *Do Certify and Attest* that on the date stated above, the Living Testator subscribed his name to this instrument, in our presence and in the presence of each of us and at the same time in our presence and hearing declared the same to be his *Living Will* and requested us and each of us to sign our names thereto as witnesses to the execution thereof, which we hereby do in the presence of the Living Testator and of each other on the said date, and write opposite our names and respective places of residence. We do further attest and affirm that at the time of the execution of this instrument by said Living Testator, it appeared to us that he was a person of sound mind and memory.

_____ residing at _____

_____ residing at _____

Source: Courtesy of Davidow, Davidow, Seigel & Stern, © 2003, Islandia, New York.

---

known as medical directive, a document that clearly states the patient's wishes regarding life-prolonging measures; see Table 19–2). The case manager can also help arrange for a healthcare surrogate (a person named by the patient to make healthcare decisions for him in the event of his incapacitation), cremation, a grave plot, or donation of organs. Information on living wills and healthcare surrogates is accessible through the media, hospitals, attorneys, healthcare organizations, and lay publications. Many hospitals distribute information on the healthcare proxy, DNR order, and living will in a printed piece titled, "Advance Directive Information."

Advance directives enable patients and families to confront issues and make decisions prior to a crisis situation, before the stress of an illness weighs heavily on all concerned, making clear thinking more difficult

Table 19–2 Healthcare Proxy

---

(1) I, _____ hereby appoint _____
(name, home address and telephone number) _____

_____ as my healthcare agent to make any and all healthcare decisions for me, except to the extent that I state otherwise. This proxy shall take effect when and if I become unable to make my own healthcare decisions.

(2) Optional instructions: I direct my agent to make healthcare decisions in accord with my wishes and limitations as stated below, or as he or she otherwise knows. (Attach additional pages if necessary.)

This Healthcare Proxy contains no limitations. I have discussed with my Agent, and my Agent knows my wishes concerning artificial nutrition and hydration. (Unless your agent knows your wishes about artificial nutrition and hydration [feeding tubes], your agent will not be allowed to make decisions about artificial nutrition and hydration.)

(3) Name of substitute or fill-in agent if the person I appoint above is unable, unwilling or unavailable to act as my healthcare agent.

_____ (name, home address and telephone number)

(4) Unless I revoke it, this proxy shall remain in effect indefinitely, or until the date or conditions stated below. This proxy shall expire (specific dates or conditions, if desired):

_____

_____

_____

(5) Signature
   Address _____
   Date _____

Statement by Witnesses (must be 18 or older)

I declare that the person who signed this document is personally known to me and appears to be of sound mind and acting of his or her own free will. He or she signed (or asked another to sign for him or her) this document in my presence.

Witness 1 _____

Address _____

Witness 2 _____

Address _____

Source: Courtesy of Davidow, Davidow, Seigel & Stern, © 2003, Islandia, New York. Prepared by: Lawrence Eric Davidow, Esq.

(see Table 19–3). The case manager can assist families by asking questions about treatments and illnesses. Are there medical procedures the patient does not want to undergo? Are there lifesaving measures that the patient deems unnecessary or excessive? She can also answer a patient's questions not fully covered by the provider and serve as a strong advocate should the patient wish to decline continued treatment.

DNR ORDERS

In an emergency, it is assumed that all patients would consent to cardiopulmonary resuscitation (CPR). However, this is not the case for some seriously or terminally ill people or for those who are now healthy but prefer not to have CPR should their heart or breathing stop. Case managers can help make patients aware of the processes included in CPR (mouth-to-mouth resuscitation, external chest compression, electric shock, intubation, injection of medication into the heart, heart massage), when and how it is administered, and its benefits and drawbacks.

Table 19–3 The Choice in Dying Patient's Advance Directive Checklist

---

✔ Discuss your wishes regarding end-of-life care with your family, friends and healthcare providers.

✔ Obtain copies of advance directives (a living will and a medical power of attorney) for your state. These are available through Choice In Dying, your state's department of health and sometimes your local hospital.

✔ Choose a trusted family member or close friend who is willing to accept the responsibility to advocate for you if you cannot speak for yourself. Appoint this person as your agent in your medical power of attorney form.

✔ Complete the living will and medical power of attorney forms following your state's law.

✔ Keep the forms in a safe, yet accessible place. Give copies to your agent, physician, family, and friends.

✔ If you enter a hospital or nursing home, have photocopies of your advance directives placed in your medical chart.

✔ Be sure to talk with your agent, physician, family and friends about your wishes regarding medical treatment. Discuss these wishes often, particularly if your medical condition changes.

Source: Reprinted by permission of Choice in Dying, 200 Varick Street, New York, NY 10014-4810. 212/366-5540.

Appendix 19–A shows a guide for patients and their families that is used in a New York teaching hospital.

The importance of making, documenting, and aggressively communicating end-of-life decisions was illustrated earlier by my own experience as my father neared death. The terms of the PSDA were in effect, but ignored in the facility my father entered. The 1995 Study to Understand Prognosis and Preferences for Outcomes and Risks of Treatment (SUPPORT) study, still one of the most far-ranging surveys conducted among terminally ill patients, showed that fewer than half the physicians whose patients had prepared a DNR order stating they did not want cardiopulmonary resuscitation were aware of the DNR order. Further, a *New England Journal of Medicine* study reported that a third of Medicare payments are for care delivered to patients in their last year of life, and that much of this care was for high-tech, high-cost, unwanted interventions.[7] Clear communications and patient-centered care are lacking for those in the last stages of life. Case managers can help patients prepare explicit advance directives and make certain physicians are aware of patients' directives and their contents.

Some of the national groups that can provide assistance to providers, employers, and individuals facing the complexities of advance directives, funeral planning, helping employees manage their grief, and end-of-life care issues include the American Hospice Foundation, Choice in Dying, Funeral and Memorial Societies of America, Grief Encounters Inc., and the National Hospice Foundation. Addresses and phone numbers for these organizations appear in the book's Appendix A.

Case managers not only face the issue of death, but they also face issues of continued "living." How many drugs, unproved treatments, or severe pain will a patient and family endure? Some patients desire treatment even when there is only a 1% chance of success, whereas others with a 75% chance of remaining alive but facing a different way of life choose to forgo treatment. In these difficult situations, the case manager must provide the objective viewpoint.

It is important to impress on the patient and family that decisions should be made in a timely manner; it is too late when the patient is in and out of a coma and family members start arguing over what to do. It might be appropriate to suggest a family meeting early on, especially if there are several adult children and a dying elderly parent. Families need to be told that patients almost always want to be involved in decision making about their care and their future. The case manager should ensure that the patient knows he or she does not have to consent to all forms of treatment. Everyone should be clear about the arrangements that the patient wants and the family is going to be comfortable with. Perhaps a father says he wants to be cremated and have his ashes spread on the ocean. His youngest son objects because he would prefer his father's ashes to remain at a specific site he can visit over the years after his dad's passing. This is an issue to bring into the open.

PAIN MANAGEMENT

According to John Cloud in his 2000 *Time* magazine article, "A Kinder, Gentler Death," nearly one half of Americans die in pain, surrounded and treated by people they do not know. Dr. Diane Meier, head of the Hertzberg Palliative Care Institute at Mount Sinai Medical Center in Manhattan, and her colleagues conducted a nationwide survey of 1,900 physicians regarding their experiences with end-of-life patients, reported in the July 29, 2003 *Newsday*. They found that one in five doctors had been asked by a terminally ill patient to help hasten death. The reason cited most often was unbearable pain. They also noted that doctors were 2.5 times more likely to medicate a patient in severe pain and 4 times more likely if the patient had less than 1 month to live. (And we wonder, what of the cancer pain when they had 2 months to live?) Further, doctors were significantly less likely to help if there was any evidence of depression. (This begs the question: Only happy terminally ill patients are eligible for pain medication?)

In April 2003, legislation was introduced to recognize pain as a priority health problem in the United States. The National Pain Care Policy Act, H.R. 1863, calls for the development of a National Center for Pain and Palliative Care Research at the National Institutes of Health. If passed, the bill would provide for a White House conference on pain care, education and training programs for healthcare professionals, and the creation of a national outreach campaign to educate consumers.[8]

Caring Connections (www.caringinfo.org) is a program of the National Hospice and Palliative Care Organization whose mission is to promote understanding and guidance to consumers to improve care at the end of life. Caring Connections developed a "Pain Care Bill of Rights" and asserts that although not always required by law, the following are the rights that patients should expect:

- The right to have your report of pain taken seriously and to be treated with dignity and respect by doctors, nurses, pharmacists, and other healthcare professionals.
- The right to have your pain thoroughly assessed and promptly treated.
- The right to be informed by your doctor about what may be causing your pain, possible treatments, and the benefits, risks, and costs of each.

- The right to participate actively in decisions about how to manage your pain.
- The right to have your pain reassessed regularly and your treatment adjusted if your pain has not been eased.
- The right to be referred to a pain specialist if your pain persists.
- The right to get clear and prompt answers to your questions takes time to make decisions, and refuse a particular type of treatment if you choose.[9]

HOSPICE CARE

Hospice care centers on caring, not curing. Care is provided in the patient's home, in freestanding hospice centers, hospitals, nursing homes, and other long-term care facilities. Hospice services are available to patients of any age, religion, race, or illness and are covered under Medicare, Medicaid, most private insurance plans, HMOs, and other managed care organizations. (The National Hospice Foundation survey noted earlier in this chapter revealed that 90% of Americans were unaware that hospice care is a covered Medicare service.[10])

In her own experience, Anne Llewellyn, RNC, BHSA, CCM, CRRN, CEAC, 2003–2004 president of the CMSA board of directors, and whose parents both received hospice care during their final illnesses, has found that it was not the patients who had difficulty "letting go," but the health-care professionals who were treating them. "Physicians many times do not want to 'give up'. This means that patients and their families often are left without adequate time to prepare for death. My mother was afraid of dying, and I asked her physician about hospice because I thought it would help her address her fears. Her physician was not supportive. He said, 'Hospice? Why not a psychiatrist?'"[11]

There remains a fear of hospice care in the population at large. "Hospice" is a name, not a place. It is a service that improves the comfort level of people during their final months of life. Pain is treated, and the quality of life is maintained.

PALLIATIVE CARE

Palliative care extends the principles of hospice care to a broader population that could benefit from receiving this service earlier in their illness or disease process. No specific therapy is excluded from consideration. An individual's needs must be continually assessed, and treatment options should be explored and evaluated in the context of the individual's values and symptoms. Palliative care, ideally, would segue into hospice care as the illness progresses.

One problem in creating a strong palliative/hospice care program is the way hospital discharges occur. Under managed care, hospitals feel more pressured to discharge patients promptly. This becomes more complicated when the patient suffers from a chronic condition that will cause his death. Does any discharge planner really want to release a patient 2 or 3 days before his death? To a nursing home far from family members? To a home hospice program if there is no live-in caregiver at home and the patient is very close to death? No one model for hospice care is workable at all hospitals, which adds to the difficulty of assembling model programs and teams.[12]

The obstacles patients and families face in benefiting from hospice care are mirrored in finding and utilizing palliative care. Patients and families are not comfortable discussing death among themselves and with healthcare professionals, patients are often too close to death to fully utilize the palliative service, and healthcare professionals are not fully informed regarding the presence and use of palliative care. Again, education in and the creation of palliative care services will offer another option to patients, families, physicians, and the discharge planners who struggle with finding appropriate EOL settings and facilities for terminally ill patients.

It is estimated that approximately 1,000 hospitals nationwide have palliative care teams. This figure leaves us with plenty of room for growth in this area.

CMSA'S 2002 "DYING IN AMERICA" SURVEY

In a 2002 online survey on end-of-life issues conducted by CMSA, case managers reported that 92% of their patients had their advance directives ignored or delayed more than 50% of the time. Ninety-one percent of their clients suffered as their DNR orders were ignored or delayed more than 50% of the time. Similarly, wishes for hospice care were ignored or delayed 50% of the time for 92% of the patients. Roughly 75% of patients received 30 days or less of the 6 months of hospice care available to the terminally ill, and more than 50% spend 14 days or less in hospice.

When asked to expand on their checked responses, anonymously if they preferred, the 142 respondents revealed their frustration and their clients' pain and confusion during the last months of life. Among the pressing challenges they noted:

- "I work in a long-term care setting with a subacute unit. I frequently see patients admitted from the hospital setting with rehabilitation/therapy orders when it is clear that the patient is actively dying. It then becomes my job to discuss the realistic nature of the patient's condition. We frequently hear from families that the hospital/doctor never told them their loved one is dying."

- "Symptom management in end-of-life care has been dismal at best, particularly for pain."
- "I have had patients/families labor over their decision before asking their physicians to withdraw or not pursue further treatment, only to have their physician imply they were making a bad decision."
- "MDs are not willing to refer to hospice early enough for members to get the benefits of hospice care. They are often admitted just days to two to three weeks prior to death and are actively dying at the time of admissions."
- "Oncologists don't seem able to say the word terminal . . . patients get sent to aggressive rehabilitation hospital rather than hospice . . . where they fail and have the additional disappointment of expectations being dashed. I work in the rehab hospital and have witnessed firsthand the poor transmission of 'bad news'."
- "More often I find that the clients are not realistic about their disease and cling to any thread of hope the specialist gives them. There also continues to be a fear surrounding hospice."
- "Individual wishes to not be resuscitated are overridden by family members."
- "I believe American society needs much education in end-of-life issues. I work hard with patients and families to get them to understand what resuscitation *really* means and what we do with end-stage patients *after* we save them. Many patients who end up in the nursing home tell me they wish they had never asked for life support if this is the outcome. I make sure that patients and families know this in their decision-making."[13]

The case managers responding to the CMSA survey reiterate what many of us have found in our personal experience; there is a great need for more complete EOL education for providers, patients, and families, and a gaping discrepancy between a patient's wishes for end-of-life care and his actual treatment. This is a clarion call to all case managers, who are in a powerful position to make a significant impact to improve quality of care, one patient at a time.

"It is an inspiring and rewarding experience to see a person die peacefully," notes Llewellyn. "As a case manager, it is important to be the person who gives the family encouragement and 'permission' to talk to the physician about EOL issues such as stopping treatment or providing more pain medication."[14]

CULTURAL DIVERSITY AND END-OF-LIFE ISSUES

Ethnic minorities currently comprise approximately one-third of the population of the United States. Our model of healthcare values and promotes autonomy in medical decision making; however, this is not easily applied to some racial and ethnic groups. Although there is an expansive discussion of the issues surrounding multiculturalism and the challenges that it presents to case managers and other healthcare professionals in Chapter 15, it may be helpful to include some additional information in this chapter as well.

Research has identified three basic dimensions in end-of-life treatment that vary culturally: communication of bad news, locus of decision making, concealment from patients of serious diagnoses because disclosure may be viewed as disrespectful, impolite, or harmful to the patient. When faced with the U.S. model of healthcare, patients from diverse backgrounds may react in ways that support their traditional health beliefs and behaviors, especially when facing end-of-life situations. On the other hand, physicians from diverse backgrounds may also revert to *their* comfort zone and preferences when discussing certain conditions with patients. For example, many African and Japanese physicians, when discussing cancer with patients or family members, choose terms such as *growth*, *mass*, *blood disease*, and *unclean tissue* rather than specifically describing a potentially terminal condition.[15] In Hispanic, Chinese, and Pakistani communities, family members actively protect terminally ill patients from knowledge of their condition, including not translating the "bad news" to their loved one. (For these reasons the use of a translator is encouraged for people of diverse backgrounds involved in the U.S. model of healthcare.[16]) Recent immigrants to the United States described Bosnian physicians as "going around" the diagnosis and being insulted by the directness of American physicians whose communication style they described as "hurtful."[17]

Chapter 15 provides several resources and Web sites on cultural issues and guidelines for healthcare professionals for caring for diverse patients. Most of these resources also contained specific information that can be utilized for end-of-life care planning. The University of Washington Medical Center (http://depts.washington.edu/pfes) developed a number of educational tools that address the disparities between cultural and ethnic groups; a few are included here in Appendices 19–B, 19–C, and 19–D. These illustrate the differences among several ethnic cultures. These "tip sheets" are focused on improving communication between patients and healthcare professionals. Culture Clues examines the perception of illness (including end of life), patterns of kinship and decision making, and comfort with touch and provides extremely useful insight and guidance to enhance relationships with patients of diverse cultures.

Whether we or our patients represent a different ethnic group, we must ask ourselves some of the following questions:

1. How do I/they feel about dying and death?
2. What are the cultural formulations for these feelings?
3. What are the cultural or religious biases?
4. What is my/their predominant worldview?
5. What stage of dying is the client experiencing?
6. Where can I go for additional assistance and understanding so that the needs of my patient can be better met?[18]

CONCLUSION

Case managers have chosen a gutsy career. How many others opt for a role in an industry with skyrocketing costs, limited and federally regulated funding, life-and-death responsibilities, high accountability, and a frequent lack of authorization to carry out our compassionate mandate? Despite all its challenges and uncertainties, case management has many rewards, and one of the greatest roles a case manager can play occurs when a client approaches death, a time certain to come to every human being. End-of-life situations entail formidable need, emotion, understanding, and advocacy. Clearly, case managers are uniquely positioned within the healthcare delivery system to take a leading role in making this most difficult time more compassionate, peaceful, and dignified.

ENDNOTE

I began this chapter with a personal story about the death of my father, who passed away in 1999, and my experiences as his nurse case manager daughter. Since the last edition of this book was printed, my mom has passed away, in 2005. Sadly, not much had changed during those 6 years—death was still not an easy experience. The following appeared in my editorial column for *The Case Manager* and is reprinted here, with permission:

> In the last issue of *The Case Manager,* I wrote that I was welcoming a new addition to our family, and now, just a short time later, I bid farewell to another. My mom passed away on May 12, and once again I needed to confront a system that continues to have difficulty letting people die.
>
> My mom was 84 years old, fiercely independent, and had definite ideas about what she wanted—and didn't want. As the oldest child and the only nurse and case manager in the family, I was her healthcare proxy. Although appropriate advance directives were prepared and shared with the team caring for her, I was startled and saddened to find that, in the 6 years since my father's death from his long battle with Alzheimer's disease, not much has changed in many healthcare professionals' attitudes and actions concerning the process of dying. As with my dad, all too often I had to intervene to ensure that my mom's suffering was not made more protracted by the treatment of this symptom or that abnormal laboratory value.
>
> She had a long and complicated medical history, and this was her 12th hospital admission within 10 years. Her diagnoses included diabetes, coronary disease, and peripheral vascular disease, and her surgical interventions included coronary bypass, cataracts, femoral popliteal bypass, and intestinal obstruction. In the last few days of her life, intubated and nonresponsive, my mom's blood glucose was elevated to 300 mg/dL. The protocol was an insulin drip with finger sticks *every hour* (previous to this, they were testing her every 4 hours). The MD and I discussed this situation, and I asked if we could just continue to cover her with insulin, rather than a continuous infusion, and with testing as before, rather than every hour. He responded, "Well, how about we'll just do the insulin drip and test her every 2 to 3 hours? I just *feel* weird *not* treating this." Yes, I thought, but what about my *mom's* feelings?
>
> The day before my mom died, a rapid ventricular fibrillation developed. Before the nurse assigned to her that day could get to her bedside from the other patient she was caring for, a resident was at my mom's bedside with the defibrillator, paddles in hand, all set to act. The nurse intervened and advised him of the do-not-resuscitate (DNR) order. Yes, even when a DNR order is

in place, there is no guarantee that it is communicated to every professional in the ICU. Medication was administered instead, and my mom's heart was converted to a slower but still irregular rhythm.

The very next morning (which became the day of her passing), just hours after this episode, I received a call from the nephrologist. He acknowledged that he was aware of the severity of my mom's condition, the advanced directives and DNR order, and that he understood and accepted this, but he wanted to advise me that now her kidneys were shutting down but there *was* treatment for this called hemodialysis. Did I want to consider this? I took a deep breath and, once again, explained that my mom wouldn't have wanted this, that it would only prolong her suffering, and that, no, I did *not* wish this treatment.

Not all of this experience was a dreadful struggle for my mom and me. She was on lorazepam and morphine infusions and was as comfortable as one could be with tubes, lines, and monitors in place. Her children and grandchildren had all visited. The nurses were caring and supportive of me; they *allowed* me to be both a grieving daughter and a nurse.

After another consultation with the hospice team and my siblings, I made the request for my mom to be extubated, and we would wait the hours or days for this struggle to conclude. In less than 10 minutes, she was gone. The "suddenness" of this overwhelmed me and made me realize just *how* artificial all of the readings I had been looking at on the monitor during *all* of these final days actually were. In fact, the nurse assigned to my mom that morning had joined me as I arrived and commented, "Her vitals look good, her O_2 sat is much better, BP and pulse look great. . . ." Although she perhaps meant to be reassuring, the reality of the situation was vastly different. The ventilator was functioning; my mom was not!

As we tearfully left the hospital, my sister asked me, "How do other families do this *without* a case manager?" How do they, indeed? Although there is an emptiness and sadness in my heart, I am glad that as a nurse, as a case manager, I was able to advocate for my mom one more time.

We as case managers have much work to do to assist other patients, other families, as they cope with end-of-life issues. Our colleagues in medicine and nursing need to be educated in alternatives when a miracle is unlikely to occur and encouraged and supported as they embrace this change to more empathetic and realistic care as patients move from curing to palliative and hospice care. This all needs to be a seamless process rather than the absolute, defined, until-the-last-second lines that now exist; the legal and reimbursement systems unfortunately add still more complexity.

Our role with other professionals needs to be expanded as well. Through ongoing conversations, we can make a difference. Start with yourself, then your family and friends. Have discussions and then document your wishes concerning life and death.

Source: Reprinted with permission *The Case Manager* – Elsevier 2009.

RESOURCES

Aging with Dignity: www.agingwithdignity.org
Americans for Better Care of the Dying: www.abcd.org
Last Acts: www.lastacts.org
National Hospice and Palliative Care Organization: 1-800-989-9455, www.caringinfo.org
Suzanne Salimbene, *What Language Does Your Patient Hurt In? A Practical Guide to Culturally Competent Care,* 2nd ed. (Amherst, MA: Diversity Resources, 2005).

NOTES

1. Hoffmann LF, "CMSA Finds American Families and Physicians Need Help Addressing End-of-Life Issues," Case Management Society of America press release, June 7, 2002, Little Rock, AR.

2. Teno JM, *The Brown Atlas of Dying* (Providence, RI: Brown University Center for Gerontology and Health Care Research, 2004), http://www.chcr.brown.edu/dying.

3. Szabo L, "End of Life Patients Need Big Picture," USA Today, June 11, 2008.

4. Associated Press, "Study Shows Priorities at Death," *Newsday* 61, no. 74 (2000): A21.

5. Mercer TA, "Do Not Resuscitate Orders," *Advance for Nurses* 4, no. 2 (2002): 7.

6. Hoffmann, "CMSA Finds."

7. Ziegler J, "How Corporations Cope When Death Intrudes," *Business & Health* 14, no. 11 (1996): 40.

8. Burness Communications, *The Last Acts Policy Newsletter* (Bethesda, MD: 2003)

9. Caring Connections, http://www.caringinfo.org/LivingWithAnIllness/TheTruthAbout Pain/PainCareBillOfRights.

10. Hoffmann, "CMSA Finds."

11. Hoffmann, "CMSA Finds."

12. Mercer TA, "Shining Light on Death," *Advance for Nurses* 4, no. 2 (2002): 25.

13. Case Management Society of America, *Dying in America—Preliminary Survey Report* (Little Rock, AR: CMSA, 2002).

14. Hoffmann, "CMSA Finds."

15. Searight HR and Gafford J, "Cultural Diversity at the End of Life: Issues and Guidelines for Family Physicians," *American Family Physician* 71 (2005): 515–522, http://www .aafp.org/afp/20050201/515.html.

16. Searight and Gafford, "Cultural Diversity at the End of Life," 515–522.

17. Searight and Gafford, "Cultural Diversity at the End of Life," 515–522.

18. Warren B, "The Cultural Expression of Death and Dying," *The Case Manager*, January/ February 2005, 45–47.

APPENDIX 19–A

Deciding about CPR: Do-Not-Resuscitate Orders (DNR): A Guide for Patients and Families

What do CPR and DNR orders mean?

CPR (cardiopulmonary resuscitation) refers to the medical procedures used to restart a patient's heart and breathing when the patient suffers heart failure. CPR may involve simple efforts such as mouth-to-mouth resuscitation and external chest compression. Advanced CPR may involve electric shock, insertion of a tube to open the patient's airway, injection of medication into the heart and, in extreme cases, open-chest heart massage.

A do-not-resuscitate (DNR) order tells medical professionals not to perform CPR. This means that doctors, nurses, and emergency medical personnel will not attempt emergency CPR if the patient's breathing or heartbeat stops.

DNR orders may be written for patients in a hospital or nursing home, or for patients at home. Hospital DNR orders tell the medical staff not to revive the patient if cardiac arrest occurs. If the patient is in a nursing home, a DNR order tells the staff and emergency medical personnel not to perform emergency resuscitation and not to transfer the patient to a hospital for CPR.

Why are DNR orders issued?

CPR, when successful, restores heartbeat and breathing and allows patients to resume their previous lifestyle. The success of CPR depends on the patient's overall medical condition. Age alone does not determine whether CPR will be successful, although illness and frailties that go along with age often make CPR less successful.

When patients are seriously or terminally ill, CPR may not work or may only partially work, leaving the patient brain-damaged or in a worse medical state than before the heart stopped. In these cases, some patients prefer to be cared for without aggressive efforts at resuscitation upon their death.

Can I request a DNR order?

Yes. All adult patients can request a DNR order. If you are sick and unable to tell your doctor that you want a DNR order written, a family member or close friend can decide for you.

Is my right to request or receive other treatment affected by a DNR order?

No. A DNR order is only a decision about CPR and does not relate to any other treatment.

Are DNR orders ethically acceptable?

It is widely recognized by healthcare professionals, clergy, lawyers, and others that DNR orders are medically and ethically appropriate under certain circumstances. For some patients, CPR offers more burdens than benefits, and may be against the patient's wishes.

Is my consent required for a DNR order?

Your doctor must speak to you before entering a DNR order if you are unable to decide, unless your doctor believes that discussing CPR with you would cause you severe harm. In an emergency, it is assumed that patients would consent to CPR. However, if a doctor decides that CPR will not work, it is not provided.

How can I make my wishes about CPR known?

An adult patient may consent to a DNR order orally by informing a physician, or in writing, such as a living will, if two witnesses are present. In addition, the Healthcare Proxy Law allows you to appoint someone you trust to make decisions about CPR and other treatments if you become unable to decide for yourself.

Before deciding about CPR, you should speak with your doctor about your overall health and the benefits and burdens CPR would provide for you. A full and early discussion between you and your doctor will assure that your wishes will be known.

If I request a DNR order, must my doctor honor my wishes?

If you don't want CPR and you request a DNR order, your doctor must follow your wishes or:

- Transfer your care to another doctor who will follow your wishes; or
- Begin a process to settle the dispute if you are in a hospital or nursing home.

If the dispute is not resolved within 72 hours, your doctor must enter the order or transfer you to the care of another doctor.

If I am not able to decide about CPR for myself, who will decide?

First, two doctors must determine that you are unable to decide about CPR. You will be told of this determination and have the right to object. If you become unable to decide about CPR, and you did not tell your doctor or others about your wishes in advance, a DNR order can be written with the consent of someone chosen by you, by a family member or by a close friend. The person highest on the following list will decide about CPR for you:

- The person chosen by you to make healthcare decisions under New York's Healthcare Proxy Law
- A court appointed guardian (if there is one)
- Your closest relative (spouse, child, parent, sibling)
- A close friend

How can I select someone to decide for me?

The Healthcare Proxy Law allows adults to select someone they trust to make all healthcare decisions for them when they are no longer able to do so themselves, including decisions about CPR. You can name someone by filling out a healthcare proxy form, which you can get from your physician or other healthcare professionals.

Under what circumstances can a family member or a close friend decide that a DNR order should be written?

A family member or close friend can consent to a DNR order only when you are unable to decide for yourself and you have not appointed someone to decide for you. Your family member or friend can consent to a DNR order when:

- You are terminally ill; or
- You are permanently unconscious; or
- CPR will not work (would be medically futile); or
- CPR would impose an extraordinary burden on you given your medical condition and the expected outcome of CPR.

Anyone deciding for you must base the decision on your wishes, including your religious and moral beliefs, or if your wishes are not known, on your best interests.

What if members of my family disagree?

In a hospital or nursing home, your family can ask that the disagreement be mediated. Your doctor can request mediation if he or she is aware of any disagreement among your family members.

What if I lose the ability to make decisions about CPR and do not have anyone who can decide for me?

A DNR order can be written if two doctors decide that CPR would not work or if a court approves of the DNR order. It would be best if you discussed your wishes about CPR with your doctor in advance.

Who can consent to a DNR order for children?

A DNR order can be entered for a child with consent of the child's parent or guardian. If the child is old enough to understand and decide about CPR, the child's consent is also required for a DNR order.

What happens if I change my mind after a DNR order has been written?

You or anyone who consents to a DNR order for you can remove the order by telling your doctor, nurses, or others of the decision.

What happens to a DNR order if I am transferred from a nursing home to a hospital or vice versa?

The DNR order will continue until a doctor examines you and decides whether the order should remain or be cancelled. If the doctor decides to cancel the DNR order, you or anyone who decided for you will be told and can ask that the DNR order be entered again.

If I am at home with a DNR order, what happens if a family member or friend panics and calls an ambulance to resuscitate me?

If you have a DNR order and family members show it to emergency personnel, they will not try to resuscitate you or take you to a hospital emergency room for CPR.

What happens to my DNR order if I am transferred from a hospital or nursing home to home care?

The order issued for you in a hospital or nursing home will not apply at home. You, your healthcare agent, or family member must specifically consent to a home DNR order. If you leave a hospital or nursing home without a home DNR order, a DNR order can be issued by a doctor for you at home only with your consent or the consent of someone you appointed as a healthcare agent.

Source: Courtesy of Winthrop University Hospital, 2003, Mineola, New York.

APPENDIX 19–B

 Culture Clues™   **Patient and Family Education Services**

End-of-Life Care: The Latino Culture

Dying is one of life's unique experiences. Clinicians are privileged to meet people at a time of crisis in their lives and provide expert assistance. A person's attitude toward death and bereavement is shaped to a large extent by their cultural heritage, religious practices, and family unit. Always remember that there are nuances within each cultural grouping, which can be addressed through comprehensive communication with the patient and family.

Birth region, education, and income level also influence how your patient perceives illness and makes health decisions.

What are the patterns of kinship and decision-making when caring for your terminally ill Latino patient?

In the Latino culture, there is a complex relationship between health and illness, as well as the physical, mental, and spiritual parts of a person's life.

- Family involvement is very important. The family-centered model of decision making is highly valued and may be more important than patient autonomy. In the Latino culture, this is called *familismo,* which is characterized by interdependence, affiliation, and cooperation.

- Relatives participate in the spiritual and physical care of their ill family member. The family may be apprehensive about giving technical care without receiving education and training.
  - *When involving family members in the care of their loved one, ask about preferences for their involvement. Provide the necessary education to prepare the family members for any technical care they may need to give.*

- The family may prefer to hear about medical news before the patient is informed so that they can shield the patient or deliver the news gradually.
  - *If your patient consents, meet the family members first to strategize how to communicate news about the illness. If your patient does not want to make his or her own medical decisions, let them know a Durable Power of Attorney for health care needs to be prepared.*

- Your patient and family may prefer to be at home at the end of life. The patient may believe that the hospital setting is impersonal or that the routine disrupts the family's ability to take care of their loved one.
  - *Explore the patient and family's understanding about treatment choices including the option for care at home at the end of life. Enlist the aid of Social Services to explore available options and feelings about hospice care.*

- Your patient and family may believe that God determines the outcome of illness and that death is a natural part of the life process. Because of this acceptance of the sick role, the patient and family may not seek health care until the condition worsens significantly. This outlook may also allow your patient to tolerate a high level of pain because pain is perceived as something that you live with. This belief can also serve a protective role by preparing the patient and family for grief and death.

How to communicate with your terminally ill Latino patient and his/her relatives

- When talking to your patient and family about terminal illness do not use euphemisms. They do not translate well, and it makes it difficult for the interpreter to communicate. Use of clear and specific language will help the patient and family better understand the prognosis and make decisions about palliative care.

- Your patient and family members may not be assertive or aggressive when communicating with doctors and clinical staff. They may not want to have any direct disagreement. As a result, important issues and problems may not be discussed, unless you initiate a dialogue.
  - *Ask your patient to voice opinion about issues concerning end-of-life care to provide opportunity for discussion. Make sure your patient is clear about risks and benefits of life-extending measures.*
  - *Ask, "How do you feel about what is going on?" Explore options for care, including the patient's desire to be at home at the end of life. Educate the patient and family about hospice. Ask how the clinical team can support end-of-life decisions. Ask, "How can we help make things better for you?"*

Useful tips to increase trust with your terminally ill Latino patient

- Be aware that there are a variety of Latino cultures. In addition, there is diversity in the religions practiced by Latinos. *Catholicism, Magico,* or *Cristiana* (Protestant Evangelical practices) may provide religious means of dealing with life and death for your patient.
    - *Ask your patients and family members about their preferences and rituals to better understand their needs.*
- A good strategy to learn more about your patient is to have informal conversations with the extended family. Extended family members may be more available and approachable than the immediate family during time of grief.
- *Respeto* (respect) is an important concept in the Latino culture. Respect implies that relationships are based in common humanity, where one is required to establish respect – it is not assumed. Older patients may prefer to be called *Señor* (Mr.) or *Señora* (Mrs.). Ask your patients how they prefer to be called. To develop an effective therapeutic relationship, the doctor and other health care providers need to be brought into the extended family circle. This is accomplished by gaining trust and showing respect.
- Grieving is considered a natural part of the life process. Your patient's family may not feel comfortable with consultations from psychologists or psychiatrists to assist with the grief process because there is an expectation that these services are used for mental illness.

Rituals

- Prayer and ritual may be a part of the end-of-life process for your patient and the family members. Family members may use prayer or bring special amulets and rosaries (prayer beads) while visiting a dying patient.
- The family members may request that they keep candles burning 24 hours a day as a way of sustaining worship. Electric candles are available for patients and families. Call Interpreter Services at 598-4663.
- Your patient and the family may display pictures of saints. Saints have specialized and general meanings for Catholics. For example, St. Peregrine is associated with cancer, St. Joseph with dying, and Our Lady of Lourdes with body ills.
- Some families may want to honor their deceased relative by cleansing the body.
- There may be a belief that a person's spirit is lost if they die in the hospital rather than the home setting.
- The last rites are important for people who are Catholic. A priest or lay visitor may be asked to perform these rituals when a person is close to death.
    - *If your patient is Catholic, ask about their preference and plans for this ritual.*
- Wailing and the demonstration of strong emotions at the time of death may be considered a sign of respect. While patients and family members may exhibit stoicism during an illness, the stoicism may not be maintained when a death has occurred. Organ donation and autopsy may not be an acceptable practice. It may be allowed but many families prefer not to donate organs nor have autopsies of their loved one.
    - *Be respectful when asking about autopsy or organ donation.*

Refer to Culture Clues: Communicating with Your Latino Patient for additional information and references. Culture Clues™ is on the Web.

Visit http://depts.washington.edu/pfes/cultureclues.html *to learn about other cultures.*

There are Spanish language tools available to assess physical and psychosocial issues, such as the Rotterdam Symptom Checklist to assess quality of life, and the Visual Analogue Scale (VAS) and Face Scale (FS) to assess pain. (See Journal of Hospice and Palliative Nursing, Vol. 3, No.1 Jan-Mar, 2001 for references.)

Culture Clues™ is a project of the Staff Development Workgroup,
Patient and Family Education Committee
Contact information: pfes@u.washington.edu / 206-598-7498

This End-of-Life Care: The Latino Culture was developed with thanks to
Diana Cardenas, M.D., Christina Garces, Deborah Johnson,
Karen Montes and Lorane West

UNIVERSITY OF WASHINGTON
MEDICAL CENTER
UW Medicine

APPENDIX 19–C

 Culture Clues™   **Patient and Family Education Services**

End-of-Life Care: The Russian Culture

Dying is one of life's unique experiences. Clinicians are privileged to meet people at a time of crisis in their lives and provide expert assistance. A person's attitude toward death and bereavement is shaped to a large extent by their cultural heritage, religious practices and family unit. Always remember that there are nuances within each cultural grouping, which can be addressed through comprehensive communication with the patient and family.

Birth region, education and income level make a difference about how your patient perceives illness and makes health decisions.

What is unique about this patient and family that you will not learn from tips or information about their culture?

What are the patterns of kinship and decision-making when caring for your terminally ill Russian patient?

- Health care information is shared with family members. Try to include family members when telling the patient that their illness is terminal. One family member or friend may be designated to serve as a lead in this role.
  - *Include family members in the decision about the time and the way that "telling of the truth" about the illness will take place. To identify the closest lead family member; ask, "Who is the person that speaks for the family?"*
- Patient problems are family problems and are discussed by the entire family. The entire family makes decisions, with the patient and the person closest to the patient having the most influence.

How to communicate with your terminally ill Russian patient and his/her relatives

- The doctor, not the nurse, is expected to transmit the medical news to the family or to the patient.
  - *The news that an illness is terminal preferably comes from the doctor to the family. If possible, inform the patient gradually. Consider giving details in small parts over time.*
- There are expressions of grief; however, efforts are made to not openly grieve in front of the dying person. The dying patient is allowed to freely express grief.
- Your patient or the family members may be demonstrative or expressive when discussing quality of care issues as a way to draw attention and get the best from the health care system.
  - *Assure the patient that you are giving the best care, the same care given to all patients regardless of nationality or financial status.*

Useful tips to increase trust with your terminally ill Russian patient and his/her family

- The doctor is typically regarded as the ultimate authority in all medical matters. The doctor is expected to orchestrate the work of the health care team.
  - *Whenever possible the doctor should introduce each member of the care team to the patient and to the closest relatives, stressing their credentials. If another team member is the designated lead for care management, this should be explained and assurances given that the doctor is kept informed.*
- Patients and family members appreciate talking with clinicians as long as possible. Your patient or the family member may prefer that the conversation occur in a private setting such as a doctor's office or consult room.
- Gifts may be offered to members of the health care team, such as flowers, candy, traditional food, liquor, etc. Clinician acceptance helps to remove embarrassment for the family and establishes a better reciprocal understanding.
- In general, your patients want to understand the etiology of their disease and they have a strong tendency for self-diagnosis using medical books and other sources.
  - *Try to explain the possible causes of their condition and how the treatment affects them. Encourage self-directed learning, however, encourage the use of credible sources of information and welcome opportunities to discuss their findings and conclusions.*
- Administration of morphine may be misinterpreted as a sign of a hopeless situation and abandonment.
  - *Try to explain carefully first to the relatives then to the dying patient that morphine is a painkiller and not a last resort. Express that the patient's comfort is of primary concern and the team is committed to delivering excellent care.*

End-of-Life Care: The Russian Culture

- Autopsy is accepted if a doctor orders it, but organ donation, withholding or withdrawing treatment and signing of Durable Power of Attorney are usually declined.
  - *Try to explain to your patient the community benefits of organ donation. Explain that the highest standards and safeguards are used to ensure organ donations are treated with respect and honor. It is preferable to wait until after the death to discuss this.*
  - *Explain the benefits and risks of withholding and withdrawing treatment to help your patient and family make decisions. Allow time for the family to make the decision.*
  - *Provide detailed information on Durable Power of Attorney and take the time to address all concerns.*

Rituals about death

Don't be surprised if you come across the following rituals related to death and dying:
This list includes some of the rituals that your patients <u>may</u> practice. Always ask your patients and family members about their customs, as there are variations among individuals, ethnic/religious groups, urban and rural practices, and socio-economic status.

- Russians tend to be cheerful with the dying person to avoid distressing the patient.
- Family plays a major role in supporting the sick person. Usually there is a family member nursing day and night at the bedside. Continuous death watching is a widespread phenomenon in Russia.
- Relatives and friends are all expected to visit the patient. Usually people bring food and may include gifts for the clinicians. Often visitors sit for hours visiting with the patient and one another to catch up with all the news. Prayer may or may not be part of the visit.
- Patients who practice their religion may consider prayer as an important and powerful healing tool.
- For Russians in general, and in particular for Russian Jews, nutrition is the primary determinant of health. The family may be happy when the patient is able to eat.
- For some families it is customary for the dying person to offer a blessing by laying hands on their family members' heads.
- Religious icons may be brought in the room depending on the religion and the level of practice of the people involved.
- The earth is considered sacred. Even today, people who have left Russia sometimes keep pots of Russian soil in their adopted homes.
- Depending on the denomination, it may be desired by the family to have a pastor, priest, or rabbi present at the moment of death.
- The patient and family may want all mirrors covered during the time of death.
- You may see the Orthodox priest say a prayer and light a candle right after the death.
- The family may close the eyes and mouth of the deceased; otherwise, it is considered a bad omen. The family may want to place coins on the eyelids and a roll of cloth under the deceased's chin.
- The family may desire that the coffin be taken to the patient's home on the way to the funeral service, so that the deceased can visit their home for the last time.
- Wailing and other displays of grief may be reserved primarily for expression in the home.
- The family may have some specific practices for washing the body after the death. Ask about preferences and try to accommodate.
- Your Russian Orthodox patients and their family members may decline cremation.
- In accordance with the Jewish tradition, Russian Jews want to bury the dead within 24 hours, except when the death occurs on Friday after sundown, on Saturday, on a Jewish holiday, or when waiting for family members to arrive.

Refer to Culture Clues: Communicating with Your Russian Patient for additional information and references.
http://depts.washington.edu/pfes/pdf/cclue-russian.pdf and
http://depts.washington.edu/pallcare/training/curriculum_pdfs/CultureModule.pdf

Culture Clues™ is a project of the Staff Development Workgroup,
Patient and Family Education Committee
Contact information: pfes@u.washington.edu / 206-598-7498
This End-of-Life Care: The Russian Culture was developed with thanks to
Yuliya Milshteyn and Olga Petrov

UNIVERSITY OF WASHINGTON
MEDICAL CENTER
UW Medicine

APPENDIX 19–D

 Culture Clues™   ***Patient and Family Education Services***

End-of-Life Care: The Vietnamese Culture

Dying is one of life's unique experiences. Clinicians are privileged to meet people at a time of crisis in their lives and provide expert assistance. A person's attitude toward death and bereavement is shaped to a large extent by their cultural heritage, religious practices, and family unit. Always remember that there are nuances within each cultural grouping, which can be addressed through comprehensive communication with the patient and family.

Birth region, education, and income level also influence how your patient perceives illness and makes health decisions.

What are the patterns of kinship and decision-making when caring for your terminally ill Vietnamese patient?

- Family has a central role in the Vietnamese culture. The extended family includes children, parents, grandparents, and ancestors.
- Consult with the family in cases of serious or terminal illness. The family may want to make the health care decisions to avoid worrying the patient. The health care provider can build trust and promote the therapeutic relationship by including the family in health care decisions.
- Decisions are often the responsibility of the eldest male. Older women may also have significant influence. Traditionally, the eldest male is the family spokesman; often the person with the best English assumes this role.
  - *If your patient consents, meet the family members first to strategize how to communicate news about the illness. If your patient does not want to make his or her own medical decisions, let them know a Durable Power of Attorney for health care needs to be prepared. Ask your patient whom he/she wants included in medical decisions.*
  - *Be aware that your patient may not have the extended family living nearby, adding to the stress of the illness.*
- Removal of life support may require extensive family discussion, placing the responsibility for the decision on the entire family rather than on one individual.
- Your patient and family may prefer to be at home at the end of life with family members around them.
  - *Explore the patient and family's understanding about treatment choices including the option for care at home at the end of life. Enlist the aid of Social Services to explore available options and feelings about hospice care.*

How to communicate with your terminally ill Vietnamese patient and his/her relatives

- Language difficulties may provide significant barriers to communicating about personal issues. Use clear and specific language to help your patient and family understand the prognosis and make informed decisions about care.
- Your patient may have a deep respect for elders and for people with authority. Your patient may be reluctant to say "no" to a doctor or health care provider because it may be considered disrespectful or cause disharmony.
- Ask your patient to voice opinions about issues concerning end-of-life care to provide opportunity for discussion. Make sure your patient is clear about risks and benefits of life-extending measures.
  - *Ask, "How do you feel about what is going on?" Explore options for care, including the patient's desire to be at home at the end of life. Educate the patient and family about hospice. Ask how the clinical team can support end-of-life decisions. Ask, "How can we help make things better for you?"*

- It is valuable and welcome to ask both the patient and the family about "Do Not Resuscitate" orders. Documenting these wishes gives the patient and family a sense of security that their wishes will be followed.
  - *Ask, "Would you want us to resuscitate you if your heart stopped, or if your breathing stopped?" Explain that their wishes will be documented to ensure that they are followed.*

Useful tips to increase trust with your terminally ill Vietnamese patient

- Older patients, or patients who you do not know well, may prefer to be called Mr. or Mrs. Ask your patient how he or she prefers to be addressed.
- Your patient may accept pain and illness in a stoic manner; motivated by a strong desire to go home, your patient may mask his or her pain. Watch for changes in facial expressions, vocalizations, physical movements, or changes in blood pressure and/or pulse, that suggest pain is present. Build trust over time to increase your patient's comfort with discussing symptoms and pain.
- As a result of the high regard your patient may have for the doctor, he or she may anticipate that a diagnosis will be made in one visit, and may not understand the need for follow-up visits and extensive testing.
  - *Explain your assessment plan to your patient and family. Use open-ended questions to increase opportunity for understanding.*
- Your patient and family may not have a cultural concept of mental illness, attributing somatic symptoms for psychological problems. As a result, your patient or his or her family members may not feel comfortable with consultations from psychologists or psychiatrists to assist with the grief process.
- Your patient and family members may believe that surgery is a treatment of last resort. They may also believe that blood loss, including blood drawn for lab tests, could make them sicker.
  - *Be aware of this concern and explain the reason for any procedures and lab tests that are performed as part of palliative care.*
- Upon death, organ transplant and/or autopsies may be accepted with very careful explanation.

Rituals

- Be aware that there are a variety of Vietnamese cultures and religious practices. Most Vietnamese are Buddhist; other religious preferences include Catholic, Evangelical Protestant, and Chinese Confucianism.
  - *Ask your patients and family members about their preferences and rituals to better understand their needs.*
- Patients who practice the Buddhist faith may call a monk to give blessings. Buddhist patients may chant and may also create an altar for prayer.
- Patients who are Catholic may ask for a priest for last rites at end of life.
- Food is considered important for health in the Vietnamese culture. It is common for family members to force food on patients when they are ill.
- White is the color for mourning in the Vietnamese culture.
- The family may express grief with a stoic response or they may respond with crying and weeping.
- The bereavement process has a positive impact on family health. At first, there is an intensive and extensive community involvement with frequent visits from family and friends; visits are slowly weaned off over a 2- to 3-year period.

Refer to Culture Clues: Communicating with Your Vietnamese Patient for additional information and references. Culture Clues™ is on the Web. Visit http://depts.washington.edu/pfes/cultureclues.html *to learn about other cultures.*

Culture Clues™ is a project of the Staff Development Workgroup, Patient and Family Education Committee
Contact information: pfes@u.washington.edu / 206-598-7498
This End-of-Life Care: The Vietnamese Culture was developed with thanks to Stephanie Lee, Lanchi Le Phan, and Judy Tran.

UNIVERSITY OF WASHINGTON
MEDICAL CENTER
UW Medicine

Chapter 20

The Growing Need for Direct-to-Consumer, Community-Based Case Managers: Our Changing Times

As Bob Dylan wrote, "The times, they are a-changin.'" The time has never been better for a new breed of case managers—the direct-to-consumer, community-based case manager. The convergence of consumer-driven healthcare, wherein consumers take a more active role in decisions regarding their healthcare, coupled with an overburdened healthcare system has made the need for accessible, dedicated patient advocates more critical than ever. The rising costs of healthcare are further driving the need for professionals who are more directly involved and accountable to patients, and patients alone. That is not to say that direct-to-consumer case managers do not continue to foster positive, cooperative relationships with their patients' physicians, healthcare providers, and payer groups. To be effective, collaborative interfaces are essential. However, direct-to-consumer case managers are not hindered by other masters to serve that can hinder their ability to put their patients' interests first.

Not every case manager is a candidate for a direct-to-consumer role. Definite traits and requirements must be met.

INDEPENDENT, DISCIPLINED, PROACTIVE

Self-realization is a powerful tool and extremely useful in determining whether you have what it takes to be a direct-to-consumer case manager.

By asking yourself the following questions, you can perform your own self-assessment, an important first step:

1. Can I envision myself as my own boss and an entrepreneur providing case management services to members of my local community?
2. Do I have the self-discipline, self-motivation, confidence, and organizational skills to manage my own business?
3. Am I prepared to make the necessary investments in my business (i.e., computer and phone systems, marketing materials, patient file system, and communications/reporting forms) as well as in my professional training and development (i.e., professional certification, continuing education, "Best in Class" seminars, professional conferences)?
4. Can I develop a strong, effective voice to advocate on behalf of my patients within the traditional hierarchy of the healthcare system (i.e., with physicians, providers, payer groups, government agencies), and if so, can I balance this advocacy with open, cooperative, and collaborative communications to be effective working within the system?

For case managers (or those aspiring to be case managers) who answer "yes" to these questions, our country needs you now, and your future as a direct-to-consumer case manager is entirely up to you. You will need to be fully committed to your dual role as patient advocate and change agent in a new and improved healthcare model.

THE CASE MANAGER AS CHANGE AGENT

Case managers existed as far back as the early 1900s when they served as care coordinators for patients requiring integrated, multidisciplinary healthcare services. At that time, they were employed by public health service providers. Soon, they entered another venue wherein their services were used in cases involving certain types of patients (i.e., lower income patients, those with mental illness, older adults). The case manager's role then evolved to include vocational rehabilitation and workers' compensation cases.

By the mid-1970s, the first generation of case management developed in the context of rehabilitation management. From there, case managers gained the attention of certain insurance companies that saw rehabilitation case management as a means to manage their cases more effectively *and* generate a new revenue stream. In the years that followed, the insurance carriers expanded their application of case management to include certain categories of medical claims.

The advent of AIDS in the 1980s ushered in the next phase of case management. This disease, with its high cost of treatment and multidisciplinary requirements, was viewed as particularly well suited for case management and the associated risk management designed to contain costs. It was during this period that the role of case managers was primarily linked to cost containment, with patient advocacy relegated to the background. That was unfortunate and has been one of the reasons underlying our declining healthcare system.

All of the blame, however, cannot be placed on the shoulders of the carriers, the providers, and "the system." Case managers, too, must assume some responsibility because they did little to articulate and highlight their intrinsic value. Now, within the parameters of the 21st-century healthcare system and its dire need for change, there is a tremendous opportunity for case managers to be that agent of change and make a real difference.

As case management advances beyond its adolescence, its greatest growth is yet to come. Although the majority of professionals now in this advanced practice setting are employees of organizations, the personal and professional challenges they face are causing many of them to question if this is indeed the role for them. Too many have high case loads, making it difficult if not impossible to provide the kind of intervention that patients with complex conditions require. Still others are burdened by so many systems, forms, authorizations, and data entry requirements that it's increasingly difficult to remember that the patient is at the center of what we do.

Whereas earlier models of case management were community based, case management today, especially in managed care organizations, is telephonically based, eliminating the person-to person relationship that is so important. Further hindering the role of case managers today are factors such as practicing across state lines without appropriate licensure (see Chapter 5 for further discussion of this issue) and lack of proper educational preparation and training. It's no wonder that there is such a high turnover rate for case managers, that few are entering the profession, and that those who remain are facing enormous challenges and frustrations. The good news here is that the *process* of case management is not broken—it works wonderfully well!

Over the past several years, the healthcare pendulum has swung completely in the opposite direction from where it has been. Previously, treating physicians directed all healthcare and consumers were given little or no choice in their treatment plans. Now, treating physicians allow patients more control. Unfortunately, the majority of consumers did not go to medical school and do not have the time or the expertise to understand and then act upon the never-ending supply of medical information that is available. Every case manager can become a catalyst in advancing this contemporary, consumer-oriented and physician-aligned format.

For those experienced case managers who have become discouraged, there *is* another career path! Instead of serving patients telephonically, or working at a computer station or in a hospital where you expedite the discharge and reduce the length of stay only to see many of your patients readmitted, or wondering how a specific family is coping with their catastrophically ill child, there is another door to be opened. You can be in the field seeing patients and interacting with them, their families, and their physicians. You can become an entrepreneur in your own business with your patients as your customers. You can decide your fees and exactly what you wanted your caseload to be. You can make your own hours (great for working moms, those who are not quite ready to retire, and those in the sandwich generation that take care of their own families and their parents).

To serve effectively as change agents, direct-to-consumer, community-based case managers must do the following:

- Advocate for their role in the community with patients and their families, physicians, employers, insurance companies, managed care companies, businesses and government entities.
- Embrace an entrepreneurial, can-do attitude; be willing to take risks and refuse to take no for an answer when advocating for their patients.
- Adopt new "Best in Class" practices that foster effective communications and cooperation between all parties along the continuum of healthcare, and help integrate the services of each silo in this continuum (i.e., healthcare providers, home care providers, employers, health plans).
- Gain greater financial awareness about the costs associated with healthcare including a better understanding of the cost-to-benefit analyses pertaining to various healthcare treatments, procedures, and settings.
- Assume the role of "go-to" person with each of their patients and family members, as well as with other individuals involved in their patients' treatment plans and healthcare services.
- Think globally while acting locally and staying connected to providers, employers, trusted advisors (i.e., accountants, estate attorneys, financial planners), healthcare advocacy groups, and nonprofit organizations serving patients with various diseases and medical

conditions (e.g., American Heart Association, American Cancer Society, American Diabetes Foundation). All can be valuable marketing sources for referrals to you.

By participating actively as a central figure in healthcare and patient services, direct-to-consumer case managers are in position to influence changes and improvements in our healthcare system.

Opportunities are Waiting, Are You Ready?

For the right individual, at the right moment, this Help Wanted ad may have your name on it. If you're an experienced case manager, you've already survived the challenges, demonstrated your clinical expertise, and may be ready. It won't happen overnight, you'll need some additional skills and, yes, once again a caring heart and passion to be at the center, to make a difference, for those just waiting for you to answer the call. That's where all the action is—just waiting for you to step up!

Assistance is already available in your community through business groups and organizations that work with entrepreneurs. Courses are available on-site and online (see www.mullahyassociates.com); professional associations and local colleges and universities are involved as well and a *new* handbook especially for this practice setting is being created . . . stay tuned!

Chapter 21

Behavioral Health

As the world in which we live becomes a much more stressful place, those case managers who work in behavioral health settings will be extremely busy. In a country dealing with continuing threats of terrorism, economic uncertainty, job insecurity, and the increasing anxiety and stress that all of this produces, medical problems also occur and a combination of medical and behavioral issues exacerbates the impact on already-struggling families.

Escalating healthcare costs attributed to high-risk populations have fueled a need for a more proactive approach to deal with people affected by complex mental health issues that coexist with medical conditions. In the past few years, there has been a definite increase in creative and in-home behavioral health case management programs.

In the United States, psychiatric disorders affect approximately 25% of the population in a given year. Fifty percent or more of all primary care physician visits are estimated to be due to underlying behavioral problems. Primary care physicians have become stand-ins for a true mental health system, writing more than 70% of all psychiatric prescriptions. Unfortunately, the quality of mental care provided is often inadequate.[1]

A patient struggling with complex medical problems or complex behavioral health issues faces a tough challenge. The patient with multiple diagnoses struggles with medical conditions that affect her mental health and with psychiatric problems that influence her recuperation and healing process. It is known that patients with chronic medical illness exhibit a higher rate of behavioral disorders than the general population, with up to 50% having a concurrent psychiatric diagnosis.[2] Obviously, there is an unmet need in our healthcare delivery system. Case managers are part of the solution.

To better manage a patient's healthcare treatment plan, a case manager needs to understand behavioral health issues. Too often, case managers view behavioral health as a concern separate from medical case management, and behavioral health case managers do the same. In the same way that there is often little or no communication among precertification, utilization review, case management, and disease management staff within the same organization, many of us focus on medical or psychiatric issues, but do not consider a case from both standpoints. Behavioral health case management is a special practice; still, no patient, from pediatric to eldercare clients, can adhere to a treatment plan when facing behavioral health problems. Substance abuse, anxiety disorders, incest, depression, schizophrenia, paranoia, delusions, and other behavioral challenges limit a patient's ability to care about her welfare, much less follow a rehabilitative exercise program or schedule and attend physician appointments. The training and background of a case manager make her uniquely prepared to bridge the gap between medical and psychiatric practices and contribute toward improved outcomes for patients.

Building partnerships between case managers and behavioral healthcare specialists in the United States is only one part of improving care for people with mental illness. Society and Congress are still struggling with the concept of parity in funding and insurance support for behavioral health treatments. There are far more (in number and in acceptable condition) medical facilities and clinics than sites for people with mental illness to receive treatment, find respite, and recover. The good news is that research is showing that illnesses such as depression are physiological and should be treated rather than an "attitude" that the patient should just "get over." Employers are more aware of lost work hours because of employees suffering from untreated behavioral health conditions and have put a spotlight on the problem. In fact, in the United States, the estimated cost of depression is $43 billion annually, including $17 billion in lost work days. Missing from these figures entirely is the phenomenon that's become known as "presenteeism," or the cost of lowered productivity of employees who still manage to get to work every day, but just don't get as much done.[3] These are, obviously, welcome signs of improvement not only for our patients, but for us as case managers.

CHRONIC DISEASE AND DEPRESSION

In regard to depression, Steven E. Locke, MD, President of Veritas Health Solutions, and a practicing psychiatrist, acknowledges that "among elderly patients, who often have three or four chronic conditions, the prevalence rises to as much as 40 to 50 percent . . . almost 60 percent go undetected . . . and those that are correctly diagnosed, only about one in five gets proper treatment."[4] The majority of the cases that we manage are patients with at least one condition. Some of us work with patients who have catastrophic injuries and exhibit symptoms of not only depression but other mental disorders and substance abuse problems as well. Because of this, it is important for us to expand our knowledge of the resources available.

Chronic Mental Illness

Chronic mental illness is often associated with various social problems such as child neglect, domestic abuse, imprisonment, and behavioral disturbances in children. Several socioeconomic factors become additional stressors and with a lack of resources for food, housing, communication, and transportation, patients then utilize physicians, emergency rooms, and hospitals as emergency rooms. These factors have become so problematic that many hospitals now have case managers assigned to their emergency rooms and teams of social workers to assist with the complex issues of those with chronic mental illness in the hopes that hospital admissions can be avoided.

In 2005, a Milwaukee-based mental health clinic addressed the social issues that were affecting healthcare costs by using a revolutionary program. Using the experiences of providing in-home psychotherapy, the clinic developed an in-home behavioral health case management program. Because the patients form trusting relationships with their case managers, often they call them (rather than going to the ER) before a crisis occurs. Situations are stabilized, coping skills are reinforced, and costs have decreased.[5]

Once again, the one-to-one relationship between case managers and their patients is key to achieving success. The removal of barriers to care, empowering patients, and providing advocacy for individuals are at the core of case management and are especially meaningful and essential when provided on behalf of those who may not be able to do this for themselves.

PARTNERING SUCCESSFULLY WITH BEHAVIORAL HEALTH PROFESSIONALS

Many medical case managers do not have a strong knowledge base in psychiatric and behavioral healthcare issues and treatments. The first steps in preparing for cases to come, and toward building collaborative relationships with behavioral health professionals, are to attend workshops, seminars, and conferences, read books and journals that address behavioral health topics, gather reference materials from associations and agencies that focus on specific mental disease states, and begin to network with colleagues experienced in psychosocial problems. Ask for their opinions on cases you might be working on, and offer to help with any clinical information you can if they have questions regarding a patient.

Social workers can be a valuable resource for insight into behaviors, area treatment facilities and options, and community programs. A number of case managers are social workers, and case managers in general interface with social workers often in the course of handling a medical case. It is beneficial to both practice areas when individuals discuss their various challenges and the solutions they have found.

Case managers can use the same techniques they apply when meeting medical physicians to begin a working association with psychiatrists (see Chapter 9). Introduce yourself as a patient advocate, reiterate that case managers increase patient compliance, and note that case managers intervene to help a patient move successfully through the healthcare system.

Following are several actions case managers can take to help obtain good outcomes in complex cases:

- Refresh your knowledge base on the behavioral issue or diagnosis the case presents. Update yourself on current treatments and medications, including dosages.
- Request a psychiatric consultation as soon as the patient is alert enough to communicate. Include the consulting psychiatrist and the outpatient psychiatrist after obtaining the appropriate consents.
- Speak with family members to obtain information on the patient's long-term psychological history, as well as her behavior just prior to the event that brought you to the case. This allows you to establish the rapport that will help smooth the case management intervention, discharge planning, and the patient's relocation to another care facility or home.
- Consider early on the possible patient needs following discharge, based on her psychiatric diagnosis. This affords you time to make plans.
- Establish a rapport with the outpatient psychiatrist, treating psychiatrist, and treating medical physician, reinforcing the case manager's role as a communicator, facilitator, and valuable partner in assuring patient adherence to the treatment plan and guiding transitions across the continuum of care.
- Be respectful of the patient as a human being, and be aware of her symptom level to maintain communications with her, as well.[6]

Other techniques a case manager can use to prepare for a medical/ behavioral health case include the following:

- Ask an associate who is employed by an outpatient clinic or psychiatric facility if you might, with appropriate permissions obtained, observe at her workplace. Being on the floor with patients or spending an hour at a colleague's side can provide insight on how staff collaborates and patient interaction techniques that work. It will also accustom you to the sometimes odd behavior you may encounter when working behavioral cases.
- Review a patient's insurance plans carefully and thoroughly for psychiatric coverage. As with medical coverage, a number of services may or may not be covered. Case managers should be well-versed in their options when planning for patient discharge or transfer.
- Join the National Alliance for the Mentally Ill organization in your area. Members pay a small fee and receive informative newsletters and insight into how people cope with mental disorders.[7]

BEHAVIORAL HEALTH DISEASE MANAGEMENT PROGRAMS

Behavioral health programs are being incorporated into some disease management programs. This is progress on the face of it, but can become a problem when treatment is provided as a carve-out as part of an EAP health program, and there is no integration with medical case managers. Opportunities for success are missed when case managers do not talk to disease managers or utilization managers. For example, a diabetes patient with multiple hospital admissions who is enrolled in a disease management program should also be referred to a medical case manager and the behavioral health staff. Case managers will assist with compliance issues and follow-through on the physician's treatment plan, and behavioral health specialists can offer support as the patient goes through his grieving process (loss of lifestyle, and, should it come to it, loss of eyesight or limbs).

RESOURCES

National Association of Psychiatric Health Systems
(202) 393-6700
www.naphs.org/

National Alliance for the Mentally Ill
(800) 950-6264
(703) 524-7600
www.nami.org

National Institute of Mental Health
(866) 615-6464 toll-free
(301) 443-4513
www.nimh.nih.gov

Anxiety Disorders Association of America
(204) 485-1001
www.adaa.org

Mental Health Infosource
Continuing Medical Education, Inc.
(800) 993-2632
www.mhsource.com

Health Enhancement Research Organization
www.the-hero.org/

World Health Organization
www.who.int

Medstat
(734) 913-3000
www.medstat.com

NOTES

1. Gray GV, "Case Managers and Behavioral Disease Management," *Inside Case Management* 8, no. 9 (2001): 8.
2. Gray, "Case Managers," 8.
3. Miller D, "Unmasking Depression," *Case in Point*, February/March 2007, 31–35.
4. Miller, "Unmasking Depression," 31–35.
5. Theis G, Kozlowski D, and Behrens J, "In-Home Behavioral Health Case Management," *Case in Point*, November/December 2006.
6. Happel R, "Do the Voices in My Head Bother You?" *The Case Manager* 14, no. 3 (2002): 66.
7. Happel, "Do the Voices in My Head Bother You?" 66.

Part V

Cases in Profile

Chapter 22

Care at Home

In most cases, home care not only benefits the patient and family, but also is less costly, which is reflected in the recent rapid growth of the home care industry. Over the past several years, there has been increasing recognition of the expense of treatment in the acute care setting. In 2007, spending on healthcare was projected to be 16.2% of the gross domestic product, and this figure has grown faster than the economy since the 1960s. $2.2 *trillion* is the total amount projected for healthcare expenses, with 30.8% of this for acute hospital care and 3.4%, or $57.6 billion, projected for home healthcare.[1]

Obviously, with the growing trend to decrease days in the hospital and increased use of alternate care settings including home care, the home care industry should continue to expand. Approximately 7.6 million individuals currently receive care from 83,000 providers because of acute illness, long-term health conditions, permanent disability, or terminal illness.[2] Several studies have compared inpatient care to home care costs for specific groups of patients and have found a statistically significant relationship, concluding that home care is a cost-effective substitute.[3]

Hospitals, employers, and insurance companies have made serious efforts at cost containment while finding ways to provide patients with the services they need in medically sound alternative settings. For the very ill, appropriate settings include rehabilitation centers with specialized programs and skilled nursing facilities. Although the latter are usually looked on, especially by consumers, as residences for the very old that provide long-term custodial care but no real hope of recovery or improvement, recently these facilities have begun to be perceived as appropriate centers for younger ill patients who need a higher level of care for a finite period of time.

Another alternative treatment location is the patient's home. There is strong evidence that recovery tends to occur more quickly and be more comprehensive when the patient is at home. Also, the patient's quality of life usually improves. Being able to participate in decisions about care imparts to the patient a sense of independence and well-being. Specific treatments and medication needs can be integrated into the family's schedule, minimizing disruption to routines and alleviating the patient's feeling of being a burden. An additional benefit of recuperating at home is the decreased risk of contracting a nosocomial illness (an illness from a hospital-borne infection).

The shift from hospital to home care became possible through advances in technology. Home care has become practical as more and more operations and treatments previously offered only in hospitals were provided on an outpatient basis. Dialysis, intravenous antibiotic therapy, blood transfusions, chemotherapy, HIV-related services, preterm labor infusion therapy, continuous positive airway pressure devices, and ventilator and pain management programs can all be safely administered in the home setting. The National Home Infusion Therapy Association estimates annual revenues for home infusion therapy to be $4.5 billion.

Although technology transfers very well from the hospital to the home, the patient's condition must be relatively stable prior to the switch to home-based care. A patient who is in an acute level ICU or is experiencing one crisis after another is not a candidate for home care. After the patient is transferred from the intensive care unit to a floor, home care may become an option, even if sophisticated equipment and services are required. However, there are some situations in which home care may end up costing as much as hospital care or even more, especially when 24-hour-a-day nursing care and very high-tech services are needed. In such situations, the benefits, expenses, and potential liability of home care must be very carefully weighed.

Home care is particularly appropriate in certain types of cases. Long-term, chronically ill patients—those with chronic neurological problems, such as MS or amyotrophic lateral sclerosis, and those recovering from a complex traumatic brain injury who may still need skilled nursing care while facing a prolonged recuperation—do very well in a home setting. Cancer patients who face the prospect of periodic readmission to the hospital are also home care candidates. Patients undergoing immune system-destroying chemotherapy and AIDS patients with compromised immune systems are highly susceptible to nosocomial infections and may benefit greatly by being transferred to a home setting. Those affected by hemophilia or genetic emphysema can receive replacement therapies at home. Younger children, regardless of the diagnosis, improve well at home, away from the high-tech, impersonal, and often overwhelming atmosphere of a hospital. Even in the case of very ill children, a home setting is preferable, all things being equal, because it supports the nurturing process and the continuing "childhood" of the child.

For these reasons, a movement evolved to keep each patient in the hospital only as long as a coordinated medical team approach is required, and then to explore all avenues of removing the patient from the hospital while still providing the quality and comprehensive services needed. Cited as potentially less expensive, home care was tested and proved to be effective for most, but by no means all, recuperating patients. Even so, what started as a cost-containment measure took on new dimensions— home care was thought to be a healthier and more humane alternative for those with critical or terminal illnesses.

CONSUMER DEMAND—AND AMBIVALENCE

At the same time that hospitals and insurance companies are demonstrating increased interest in home healthcare, consumers, often for different reasons, are demanding it more frequently. When an individual is hospitalized, it can be a very disruptive experience for the entire family. First, many patients and families feel intimidated by the hospital setting. Second, practical concerns, such as scheduling hospital visits or conferences with physicians, taking time off from work, and hiring babysitters, add tension to the worry experienced by the family members. Scheduling difficulties may be especially acute for two-income families with limited time and energy or in situations in which the patient is in a specialized facility distant from the home. Consequently, consumers have welcomed care alternatives, especially home care, which for many is the most attractive option.

There is, however, also some uneasiness among consumers about home care. All patients may not welcome it. The hospital environment provides a sense of security. The patient and family alike may well be heartened as recovery progresses and may look forward to the patient's return home, but there is also concern and fear, especially when a life-threatening problem—a stroke or heart attack, for example—is involved. "How am I going to cope? What happens if there is a problem? I can't push a buzzer and have nurses come running. Can I trust this person hired to give me injections?" Facing the loss of their safety net, patients and their families need to be convinced of the benefits and safety of home care through education and the correction of misconceptions.

Many patients still think of home care simply as consisting of periodic visits by a nurse or other healthcare provider. They do not perceive it as an ongoing process, a support system that can improve and speed their recovery. In considering and responding to patient reactions, it is important for case managers to remember that patients may receive mixed signals from their families and the medical community. The hospital staff may feel the patient requires a lengthier stay, the spouse may be dreading the responsibility of providing needed care "alone," and the physician might be concerned that he or she will not be kept appropriately informed of the patient's status.

Such fears and concerns are valid and must be recognized and addressed. Many patients, especially older ones, are absolutely bound to this thought: "If I'm sick, I will see the doctor and receive care in the hospital." They worry about the consequences if the doctor is not immediately available. Younger patients, after seeing nurse practitioners and nurse clinicians working with physicians as colleagues, are more willing to consider alternatives. Case managers can play a pivotal role in loosening the hold of long-held beliefs and stereotypes and explaining the benefits of home care.

THE CASE MANAGER AS A PIVOTAL LINK

A case manager must approach each case considered for home care very thoroughly and provide the link between the physician, the discharge plan, the patient, the family, at-home service providers, and the payer. The case manager's concerns lie where medical, nursing, and benefit payment issues dovetail.

First, a home discharge must be safe. Although the primary care physician, in cooperation with any other consulting physicians, has responsibility for discharging a patient, all those involved in the patient's treatment plan, including the nursing staff, the case manager, and home care company employees, share in the responsibility and liability for providing appropriate care. The physician writes the discharge orders stating what medications, services, and ongoing care are required. The nursing staff interprets those orders and their implications and develops a detailed discharge plan. The case manager then takes an active role in determining how the elements of the discharge plan can be best implemented. Is a visiting nurse needed twice a week or daily? Should a physical therapist or a respiratory therapist be requested? What equipment is required? What drugs must be administered and by whom? Using her knowledge of the clinical data included in the discharge orders and plan, the patient's status, area home healthcare providers, durable medical equipment suppliers, and other community resources, the case manager devises a home care plan that meets all stipulations of the discharge plan.

Often this calls for discretion and creativity. Most benefit policies and discharge plans automatically mention RNs as the most appropriate care support, even when other services from within the home care spectrum might provide more effective help. A home health aide, homemaker, or personal care assistant might tend to the patient's needs very well. Some case managers, for example, have revised plans to incorporate babysitting to tend to an older child and allow an expectant mother with a high-risk pregnancy to get off her feet and get the rest needed to carry the baby full term. For a small amount of dollars, a homemaker can do laundry, go grocery shopping, and prepare meals, enabling a patient to return home rather than remain in the hospital at a daily rate upward of $1,500 minimum. Instead of assuming that a benefits plan or a discharge plan is etched in stone, case managers need to argue for solutions not covered by the plan language to create a better answer. By working the system and then articulating the results in dollars and cents, case managers help promote progressive care and optimum outcomes.

Case managers also need to be able to distinguish cases in which home care is not the best option. Even if a patient is diagnostically suited for home care and medically stable, the family situation or home layout may preclude home care. Case managers need to be acutely aware of the vulnerability of families as they bring patients home. This is especially true when professional assistance is available only part-time. When the patient was in the hospital, the family could come to see the patient, perhaps endure a draining visit, but then leave and recharge. Now, the patient is home and the family must provide physical and emotional support. Suppose the presence of a home health aide for only a 2-, 3-, or 8-hour shift can be justified given the language of the policy, which means the family bears the bulk of the responsibility. When evaluating a patient for home care, the case manager should assess the ability of the family to absorb additional stress.

Another consideration is the geographic setting of the home to which the patient will be discharged. Is it a rural area, suburban neighborhood, or inner-city area? Each type of location has different levels of access to support and emergency services. Reviewing the setting is especially important for patients needing high-tech equipment and services. What are the rescue squad capabilities? What is the response time to a 911 call? Are emergency vehicles capable of reaching the home in 3 minutes or 45 minutes? If a power failure occurs, can the local electric utility provide backup generator support for an individual at home on a ventilator?

A personal visit to the home illuminates conditions that may affect the safety of the discharge. The family may have failed to mention that the home is an apartment five flights up with no elevator and is so small that there is no room for oxygen equipment. How many individuals live in the home; will the patient have any privacy? Are there cultural issues to consider? In a Muslim home, a male nurse or IV technician might be very unwelcome if the patient is female.

A visit also allows a case manager to pick up on the emotional state of the family member who will be the primary caregiver. Is he or she verbally expressing a willingness to care for the patient but also exhibiting fear, hesitation, or reluctance? In an underinsured or poor family, the person providing support might be facing social and financial issues that are more complex than the medical care plan. If the case manager is unable to see the patient and family at home due to her contracted role in a particular case, she should delegate someone on-site to be her eyes and ears and provide her with a mini-home assessment. The home care RN might be a candidate for this.

A case manager must approach each situation individually, evaluating the patient's condition and ongoing needs in consultation with the physician, the family, the family member who will be the main care provider, the availability of respite for the care provider, the range of community services, and so on. Home care may not be the best choice; it may be feasible but require ongoing support. Sometimes, a case manager can be put under pressure to move patients from the hospital into a home setting in order to reduce expenditures and establish credibility. It is important to remember that each case is unique and must be evaluated in light of the particular conditions that exist.

CASES IN PROFILE

Home Care is Not Always the Answer

As discussed, some medically stable patients may not be candidates for home care because of the family situation. The following case history illustrates this, as well as the problems of paying for needed services that don't appear in the benefit plan, and shows the crucial role a case manager can play in achieving an optimal outcome.

Janet Carr, a 59-year-old mail sorter for a self-funded employer group (an insurance company), was contacted by her employer's disability review program after she had been absent from work for 7 days without submitting a medical report. She explained she had been suffering from severe abdominal pain but had not wanted to "bother" her physician. The following day, the company nurse received a call from a precertification utilization review nurse notifying the disability review program that Mrs. Carr had been admitted to a hospital on an emergency basis for a ruptured bowel and acute peritonitis. Extremely ill, she required emergency surgery, which had high risk due to infection and dehydration. Because she was expected to be in the hospital at least 10 days and because a physician report cited longstanding emotional and psychiatric problems suffered by the patient and possibly her husband, the employer decided to refer Mrs. Carr for case management intervention.

In an initial brief visit with Mrs. Carr several days after her ileostomy and colostomy, the RN case manager noted her debilitated, critical condition and guarded prognosis. In a subsequent visit with Mr. Carr, she noted that he seemed developmentally impaired and, although able to answer certain questions, was tearful and fearful when talking about his wife, who "takes care of us." Seeking further information, the case manager met with Mrs. Carr's primary nurse and surgeon regarding the Carr's ability to comprehend the extent of Mrs. Carr's illness. The case manager was also able to contact Mrs. Carr's sister, who confirmed that both Mr. and Mrs. Carr suffered from longstanding comprehension problems as well as emotional and psychiatric problems.

During Mrs. Carr's recovery in the hospital, it became clear that Mr. Carr not only did not understand what type of surgery his wife had undergone or the care she would need, but also was unable to perform everyday household chores, such as bill paying and laundry, without his wife's help. He told the case manager that they had no washer or dryer, did not use a Laundromat, and that he had left the laundry "soaking in the bathtub so she can take care of it when she comes home." Prior to Mrs. Carr's illness, the couple had been able to manage without assistance from outside agencies. It was apparent that this would no longer be true. Mrs. Carr was unable, physically or mentally, to learn anything about ostomy care. Mr. Carr was insistent that his wife return home immediately but "with no outsiders."

Mrs. Carr became medically stable, and her treating physicians felt that continued hospitalization increased her risk for further infection. The consensus among her medical providers was that she would require continuing medical supervision regarding infection control, nutritional status, electrolyte imbalance, and depression for a prolonged period of time. The Carrs had no family physician. Given Mrs. Carr's need for medication administration, ostomy care, dressing changes, and monitoring, and Mr. Carr's inability to provide any support, she was a candidate for around-the-clock nursing care.

The case manager here was faced with several challenges. The first was Mr. Carr. After being shown his wife's incisions and ostomies and given a brief explanation of the care she needed, he became willing to consider assistance from outside professionals, although his ability to cooperate was minimal. The next difficulty was Mrs. Carr's medical coverage. She had an indemnity plan funded and administered by her employer, an insurance company, that provided for up to 365 days of hospitalization if required, for skilled nursing care in the home if certain criteria were met, for durable medical equipment and supplies, and for 30 days in a rehabilitation facility. There was no coverage for care in a nursing home or for home health aide or homemaker services. After reviewing discharge needs, alternative services, the family situation, the insurance coverage, and available community resources, the case manager proposed the following options to the benefits administrator:

1. Continued hospitalization, which could be justified because of the need for ongoing care, at a minimum cost of $1,500 a day.
2. Twenty-four-hour-a-day skilled nursing care at home at a negotiated cost of approximately $1,080 a day. This option lacked homemaker and housekeeping services assistance the couple needed. In addition, Mr. Carr strongly resisted this option.
3. A skilled nursing facility. This option would require demonstration of cost benefits and approval from the benefits administrator. Negotiated cost was $300 per day.

Following previous successful experiences with case management services, the employer group had instituted a large case management program that allowed modifications to the basic coverage, limiting exceptions to situations suitable for case management intervention and supported by medical and cost justification documentation. Through this program, the case manager received approval to accompany Mr. Carr to three skilled nursing facilities near the couple's home. Mrs. Carr was admitted to a facility within short walking distance, at an all-inclusive cost per day of $300. For a small additional charge, Mr. Carr was able to join Mrs. Carr for lunch and dinner. The insurance company covered the facility's fees under the large case management provision of its policy in lieu of acute hospitalization. Coordinating with the hospital physicians, the case manager arranged to have Mrs. Carr's medical care provided by the surgeon and then by an internist, who would be the couple's primary physician. Next, the case manager assisted in arranging for disability payments from the employer to the couple, contacted the couple's landlord and utility companies and apprised them of the situation, and helped Mr. Carr record and mail the necessary payments.

Mrs. Carr remained in the skilled nursing facility for 2 months, returned to the hospital for reversal of the ostomies, and recuperated at the skilled nursing facility for 2 weeks. She then went home, stronger and healthier and able to care for herself and her husband. This scenario provided the patient with the best care—in this case, not in the home but in an alternative care center—and also resulted in substantial cost savings for the payer. Continuous hospitalization for two months and two weeks would have cost $105,000; 24-hour-a-day nursing care for the same period would have cost $75,600 (at a negotiated $45 an hour; the nonnegotiated fee for this time period would have been $92,400 at the least). Care in the skilled nursing facility cost $21,000 and case management services cost $6,500 over a 7-month period. The savings were substantial, the actual amount being $84,000 less than hospitalization would have cost and $54,600 less than home nursing care would have cost. Unaccounted for are the savings resulting from prevention of complications likely to have occurred if the case manager had not intervened on behalf of the patient and her spouse.

A Home Care Case that Succeeded

James was born 6 weeks prematurely following a maternal infection and premature labor. He developed respiratory distress and was ventilator dependent for several months. After two abdominal surgeries for treatment of an intestinal obstruction and placement of a gastrostomy tube, his condition gradually stabilized, and his parents were given instruction in home care.

Discharged from the hospital at 5 months, James came home with respiratory equipment and medical supplies, including an apnea monitor, oxygen, an oximeter, suction machines, an ambu bag, and feeding and additional supplies. His home care program incorporated 4 hours per day of RN care.

Shortly after James returned home, the family called our case manager with a request for additional nursing hours. New to the case, the case manager conducted an initial home assessment and found the parents completely overwhelmed by the emotional and physical demands of caring for 6-month-old James, dependent on multiple pieces of sensitive medical equipment, as well as his two siblings, active 2- and 4-year-old preschoolers. The parents were attempting to maintain home care and keeping in contact by telephone with their primary physician, who was 75 miles away at the university hospital. They transported James those same 75 miles in heavy traffic to their hospital's emergency room (rather than their community hospital), even during episodes of respiratory distress. Although the parents were pleased with the quality of nursing care provided by an agency, they were dissatisfied with the service and equipment supplied by their home medical equipment dealer. The case manager determined that the care plan was putting James at risk for a respiratory crisis and rehospitalization.

Consulting with all concerned, she presented a number of recommendations. To avoid rehospitalization and to more properly attend the child at home, RN hours were increased to 16 hours per day. The home medical equipment contract was awarded to a dealer whose personnel were particularly adept at working closely with families and healthcare professionals. James's oxygen supply system was switched from indoor to outdoor tanks to remove his siblings' temptation to tamper—a potential hazard.

After talking with the family, with the primary treating physician, and with a local hospital, it was agreed that James would be brought to this nearby facility in an emergency, cutting 60 miles off the one-way commute. The case manager negotiated lower fees with the home medical equipment dealer and the nursing agency, and direct payment arrangements were made with the insurance carrier, avoiding co-payment terms for the family and resulting in a significant cost savings to both the carrier and the family.

Because there were limited healthcare dollars available for James over his lifetime for home nursing care and other services, the case manager referred the family to the Medicaid model waiver program. Participation in this community-based alternative to hospice or institutional care spread expenses between the family, the insurance carrier, and Medicaid. Funded by federal, state, and county sources, the waiver program for chronically ill children extended James's coverage over his lifetime and provided the family with access to other public funding programs.

Timely intervention by the case manager resulted in the stabilization of James's condition and shortened hospital stays (when they were necessary due to distress or infection). A reinforced emphasis on parent education and increased nursing and supportive services reduced the overall number of hospital admissions, and the use of a more accessible hospital helped prevent a catastrophic event such as respiratory arrest. Further, the case manager, who was on-site for regular assessments, was able to intervene in several crises and provide prompt care in situations in which the parents tended to delay medical attention.

Without case management, it is likely that James would have floundered in the medical system and experienced numerous and lengthy hospitalizations at great cost to the family and carrier. His frequent trips to a distant emergency room might well have resulted in respiratory arrest, potential brain damage, and ventilator dependency. Early intervention; referral to physical, speech, feeding, and educational therapies; and enrollment in the Medicaid model waiver program helped prevent developmental delay and mental retardation, optimizing the boy's chances of realizing his full potential. The care-at-home program has prolonged the life of the claims dollars available for James, and prompt case management is now saving his family, the insurer, and Medicaid upwards of $175,000 annually.

ONGOING SUPPORT AT HOME

When a patient is released to home care, the patient and family need ongoing support, and that requires free and frequent communication between all parties involved. After the various elements of home care are successfully established, the necessary medical equipment delivered and set up, the nursing hours arranged, the supplies ordered—regular monitoring and follow-up are essential. The case manager must be alert to the changing needs of the patient, the quality of the care provider service, and signs of family caregiver burnout. Perhaps a family member is providing the primary care with a weekly visit from a nurse to check a catheter. After a few weeks or months, the caregiver will need a respite. A case manager has a responsibility to see that the payer (employer group or insurance company) is convinced of the need, that extra help is temporarily provided, and that the primary caregiver is not punished for being willing and able to care for the patient. The problem of caregiver burnout and need for relief is often most acute in situations in which the parents are primary caregivers for a seriously ill child and are also trying to do the grocery shopping, get their other children to the dentist or to soccer practice, and continue working at their own jobs.

The case manager needs to be aware that the primary caregiver not only must be willing to provide care for the patient, but also must have the physical stamina as well—to get the patient in and out of bed or a wheelchair, for example. Does the caregiver have a chronic back problem or predisposition to back problems? A heart condition? Sometimes, the case manager may need to bring in additional support services so the caregiver is not overburdened. Perhaps a wife has agreed to be the primary caregiver for her husband but has a back condition and requires additional support equipment if she is to be able to care for him. It may be difficult to convince the payer, particularly if the husband and wife are on the same insurance policy, that the extra support is requisite. What has to be made clear to the payer in situations like this is that if the extra support is not provided, the caregiver may be the next casualty, and the payer will have a second claim to reimburse.

IMPORTANCE OF FEEDBACK AND COMMUNICATION

In her combined role as coordinator, troubleshooter, and problem solver, the case manager should actively pursue and receive feedback from all sources—the healthcare providers, the durable medical equipment suppliers, the patient (if possible), the family member providing the majority of care, and other family members. Specific parameters for communication must be set up: what to communicate, by whom, to whom, and how often. The case manager may request that the nursing service call in weekly reports or submit copies of weekly nursing notes. This regular feedback allows the case manager to follow the patient's condition and evaluate the need for services. It is unfortunate when a case manager learns from a payer that a patient discharged to home care 2 months earlier has been back in the hospital for a week because of a deterioration in his or her condition or the failure of the home care setup to function as planned. The case manager must make sure that she is contacted immediately if a change occurs—if the patient's condition worsens, the caregiver service switches personnel or hours, or any family arrangement that can affect the patient is altered. This is not to say that if a sudden emergency or need arises, the home healthcare provider or family caregiver should not react and do what is called for. If, for example, increased services are required on a weekend and the case manager cannot be reached, the services should be provided. The case manager should then be informed as soon as possible, at which point she can help decide how the patient's differing status can best be accommodated on a long-term basis—in a cost-effective manner appropriate for the patient, the family, and the payer.

What sometimes happens is that, after a discharge plan is devised and home services arranged for, the case manager may be told by the payer (especially if it has an in-house case management service) or the healthcare provider service, "We'll track patient progress now and contact you if a problem arises." If the case manager feels that her continuing on-site objective assessments are important, she must communicate that message. When turning a case over to a payer's in-house case management service, the case manager should relay all pertinent case information and acknowledge the ability of the payer's case manager to take on the case, but also make it clear that she is available for interim on-site assessments as needed. If a claims examiner decides to continue tracking a case, the case manager should make certain he or she understands the case manager's role in keeping services in place at the appropriate level. She should also suggest that the claims examiner call her if certain complications arise and leave a list of red flags for his or her reference. When a home care provider case management service offers to take over management of a case, the case manager must be diplomatic. Especially in determining the need to increase or decrease home care services, the case manager is likely to be more objective than the home care service provider. She might review her thoughts on the patient's needs with the home care service and make it clear that she is available for on-site assessments as needed should the patient's status change.

Decisions should not be made arbitrarily by one of the parties. A home healthcare service may not be the most objective judge of when a change in services is needed. Physicians might not be aware of all the details of the home care arrangement. Ideally, the case manager should be the one to adjust the level of services and then discuss all the ramifications of any changes with the provider services and the payer. For example, the healthcare service that is providing 8-hour-per-day nursing service at home should not arbitrarily increase the hours to 16 or 24 hours per day. The nursing service can report to the case manager that the patient's condition has worsened and an increase in hours is probably needed, the family caregiver may request additional help, or the physician in charge of the patient may deem more extensive services or medical equipment necessary. In all cases, the case manager should be the pivotal person involved in making the decision and then implementing it.

Follow-up on the use of durable medical equipment is also necessary. Only then will the case manager know whether equipment is actually being used and whether the patient or caregiver is satisfied with it and comfortable using it. There are cases in which equipment remains in the home unused yet is paid for month after month. Perhaps the equipment was part of a standard discharge package, the family caregiver never learned how to use it, the equipment broke, or it was used for a while but is no longer needed. In obtaining information about the use of durable medical equipment, the case manager should speak not only with the health provider, but also with the patients and family members.

The case manager must make it clear to the family that if there is a problem with equipment, if they are not satisfied with the healthcare provider, or if they are overwhelmed, they should call the case manager. A patient or family may be dissatisfied with the healthcare provider or with the durable medical equipment but be hesitant to complain simply because they do not know what to expect, feel unable to be assertive, or fear that the patient may not continue to get the best service if they mention a problem. It must be remembered that there may be certain things a healthcare provider would be reluctant to tell a case manager—that three shifts of care providers failed to show up for work one weekend, for instance. Families need to know that there is someone to turn to if a problem arises.

Although follow-up is often conducted over the phone, there are definite benefits to making personal visits. A visit to the home allows a case manager to pick up on emotional states and to see if there is equipment sitting unused in a corner. Are there signs that the patient is being well cared for by the professional healthcare service and by the family caregiver? Is the patient progressing? If not, why not?

The case manager should be more than an observer. She should be a catalyst for patient progress. This means giving feedback to all parties—not only recording it, but also troubleshooting and devising answers.

As the pivotal person involved in decisions about needed changes in service and their implementation, the case manager must see that everyone is in the loop—the physician, the home care provider, the therapists, the home medical equipment supplier, the patient (if possible), the primary family caregiver, other family members—and must maintain open communication channels between all involved to ensure that the patient, family, and payer are well served. Only with communication and feedback will come the support that is needed if home care is to be a successful care alternative.

PAYMENT CONCERNS

As stated at the beginning of this chapter, the original impetus for the growth of home care was cost containment. And, in most cases, home care is less expensive than hospital care. However, cost savings are not automatic. Expenses must be calculated, managed, and negotiated intensively.

First, the case manager must determine if and to what extent a benefit plan will allow home care. Today, a provision for home care is included in most benefit plans, but there may be specific limitations. Employers often fear that if too generous a home care benefit is in place, it will be abused and some employees will utilize unneeded home care on a regular basis. Therefore, plans include strict restrictions on home care benefits and tough plan language to eliminate the potential for abuse.

Over the last several years, studies have revealed an increased interest in benefit plan design and have demonstrated that a plan's structure can affect the experience of the employer. An employer or benefit manager can, for example, make the plan language so constrictive that individuals are forced to remain in a hospital or other high-cost facility for longer than is necessary if they are to be eligible for any benefits. Or, plan language can be flexible enough to allow an umbrella of coverage, with limits designed to prevent abuse.

For example, a plan may provide up to one million dollars in benefits per year but, although covering hospital care up to the limit, may allow only 52 four-hour home nursing visits per year. A patient requiring 24-hour care is out of luck. Someone who no longer needs acute care in a hospital but is facing a prolonged recuperation period (for example, 6 months) is going to need two to three visits by a nurse per week and numerous other support services. However, if the plan prohibits that option, the case manager may be forced to utilize the other option—in this case, keeping the patient in the high-cost hospital setting.

Or, perhaps the plan covers skilled nursing services at home but excludes home health aides or homemaker services. What happens if a patient needs a skilled nurse visit only once per week but cannot manage without the support of a home health aide or homemaker services a few hours each day? Is the patient to stay in the more costly and less desirable hospital setting because the plan will not allow needed ancillary services?

Unfortunately, situations like these arise frequently, and case managers are faced with trying to persuade and negotiate with the payers to allow the other services "out of contract" to make exceptions to the plan language that will meet the needs of patients and at the same time reduce costs. In this type of situation, a case manager should not feel intimidated but should argue the point with the plan administrators and explain that by allowing a full spectrum of services to be provided at home, they will enhance the outcome for the patient and also save money. By presenting concrete examples of improved care and verifiable savings, ideally including an example involving the employer's own plan, the case manager can strengthen her argument.

Sometimes, semantics lies at the crux of an employer's reluctance to permit exceptions. In allowing alternative arrangements, employers and benefit administrators often talk of "out-of-contract" benefits or "contract exceptions"—that is, benefits they are not required to provide. Employers need to learn—and case managers should be prepared to do the informing—that alternative arrangements should be viewed as something done to prevent greater contract exposure. The case manager needs to present the situation clearly, demonstrating that "if you do not allow for and pay for this, then your option is this—which is more costly and may not be the most beneficial step to take." A detailed cost-benefit analysis can be the case manager's most potent tool in presenting the figures.

In addition to investigating and pursuing all of the benefits obtainable through the patient's health plan, the case manager should utilize other resources for providing at-home services to help the patient and payer defray costs. There may be local, county, or state agencies and disease-specific organizations, foundations, or philanthropic groups that can provide services or guidance. The United Way, Meals on Wheels, and "I Can Cope" programs and loaner wheelchairs from the American Cancer Society are examples of available assistance. Food & Friends in Washington, D.C., provides three free meals a day to clients suffering from AIDS, cancer, Alzheimer's, and many other debilitating diseases. Easter Seals offers support services on a sliding scale for children and adults with crippling diseases. For help in seeking financing for home care, case managers can contact hospital social workers and discharge planners, city and county health departments, Social Security and public aid offices, community referral agencies such as United Way, senior citizen centers, local councils on aging, the Department for Aging, and the other social agencies listed in the Yellow Pages and community service directories (available at local libraries). In addition, Gale Research annually publishes the *Encyclopedia of Associations*, a comprehensive source of detailed information on over 135,000 nonprofit membership organizations worldwide, and a resource guide including those established to support individuals with certain diseases or injuries. (This guide is available at local libraries and online.) The Internet is an in-depth source for information, as well.

Even if a benefit plan allows for a particular service, community and other resources should be tapped. The case manager need not spend plan money just because it is there. A plan might allow for transportation assistance for an at-home patient to travel to and from necessary medical appointments; a local disease-specific society (e.g., the Multiple Sclerosis Society) might also provide transportation services for free. Or, a plan might provide for ambulance costs, yet the local volunteer fire department might offer such services for free. By making a one-time donation to an agency, a corporation might secure transportation or other services for an employee for an indefinite period of time. The key is to be cost-effective and not give away the store. This is especially true if there is a ceiling on overall home care expenses in the plan.

The case manager must also hone negotiating skills in order to deal with home healthcare providers more effectively. When arranging for a home health agency to provide two shifts of nurses for a patient for an expected 2-month period, some negotiation is in order. The case manager need not accept the usual per diem rate but should suggest an appropriate rate. Assuming services are satisfactory, the provider can look forward to a guaranteed income for a specific duration.

In an effort to make the hoped-for positive impact on patient care and cost management, a case manager often will accept responsibility for negotiating a better price on a care package when, in reality, her hands are tied by the Plan language or the timing of case receipt. Even with clear potential for appropriate care and savings, arrangements cannot always be made. When a case manager receives the case 3 months after hospitalization, medication, and DME equipment bills have been paid, she has lost her ability to negotiate on behalf of the client. There is a 2- to 3-day "framework of decision-making" that occurs as a treatment plan is put in place. If the case manager has not been involved from the beginning, thousands of dollars have already been lost. Hopefully, case managers will continue to empower themselves with the financial knowledge and "corporate" skills to become part of the decision-making managed care team. Toward this goal, it is encouraging to see that CEOs and CFOs are beginning to understand the role of case managers and allow it to work for them and their employees.

The growth in home care presents great opportunities for case managers. We provide that essential and pivotal link between patient and family, healthcare providers, and payers—or, in other words, we make sure that home care works.

NOTES

1. Kaiser Family Foundation, "Health Insurance/Costs," http://www.kff.org/insurance.

2. National Association for Home Care and Hospice, *Basic Statistics About Home Care 2008*, 2008, http://www.nahc.org/facts/08HC_Stats.pdf.

3. Pigott HE and Trott L, "Translating Research into Practice," *American Journal of Health Care Quality*, no. 3 (1993): 138–144.

Chapter 23

Managing a Long-Term Case

Long-term cases present special challenges to the case managers, to the payers, and, above all, to the patients and families. Among the personal, professional, and business issues for the case manager are explaining the benefits that case management can offer in terms of outcome and cost containment, clearly presenting findings to the referral source, demonstrating concretely how case management can improve the situation overall, and maintaining an objective and encouraging attitude with the patient and family. The single most important contribution the case manager can make is to identify a probable long-term case early on, before numerous services are put in place and before costs start to spiral.

A long-term case is diagnosis driven; long-term care is typically needed for patients with multiple sclerosis, amyotrophic lateral sclerosis, cerebral palsy, cancer, brain or spinal cord injury, multiple trauma (e.g., amputation or burns), and for premature babies. Services may be required for several months, for several years, or for life. To recognize a long-term case, a case manager refers to the diagnosis, all available medical data, and the prognosis. Through use of this information, supported by prior experience and knowledge of the usual length of time for particular types of cases, the case manager can judge how long a case is likely to be open. Educated speculation on the anticipated length and severity of the case is of interest to the client or payer.

The following are five red flags indicating cases that have potential to be long-term:

1. Lack of improvement or complications and setbacks in a seemingly short-term case
2. Terminal illness
3. Six months of treatment (no matter what the type)

4. Multiple medical conditions (e.g., diabetes and hypertension)
5. An increase in complications, indicating possible systemic involvement

INFORMING THE CLIENT

After she has identified a likely long-term case, the case manager should inform the client company as soon as possible. It is important to be frank and make the client aware that a patient will require care and services for an extended period of time and that, consequently, expenses on the case will be ongoing. Just as a claims administrator is responsible for "claims reserving" (determining, at the earliest opportunity, the potential for a claimant to require additional monies and earmarking dollars accordingly), a case manager must evaluate a patient's condition and offer an educated guess as to the care that will be required.

Long-term cases—those that require 6 or more months of case management intervention—are anathema to some clients and payers. A client's perceptions of a patient's probable needs may differ substantially from the case manager's. Therefore, it is very important to clarify the role of case management in long-term cases to the client. Even when the diagnosis identifies a case as long-term and the case manager feels that long-term involvement is necessary or advisable, the client may request that the case manager limit her role. To avoid confusion and unnecessary delays in the provision of care, the case manager must be able to spot potential misunderstandings before they occur and inform the client promptly of changing circumstances to prepare the client for the possibility of a long-term case as soon as that possibility becomes evident.

The case manager's role is often particularly difficult when a referral source has assigned a case that, based on its information, seems not to be problematic. Suppose that during an on-site visit the case manager discovers a situation that does not mesh with what has been relayed to the referral source over the telephone. The patient's condition or the home dynamics may be much more complex than the referral source realizes. Also, in some cases that at first appear to be short-term, unexpected complications or setbacks occur, requiring additional medical attention. A case manager who has established straightforward and forthright communications with the client company and payer will have a stronger foundation to work from when requesting additional funds due to unforeseen circumstances. Such requests become more crucial when specific dollar limits exist in the coverage language or if claims reserving suddenly becomes necessary, because then they have greater potential to negatively impact the case manager's working relationship and ability to put needed treatments in place.

Some case managers, especially those with less experience or those working with a new client or referral source, are reluctant to be totally honest. In an effort to maintain the client relationship, they knowingly overestimate anticipated progress in long-term cases or withhold especially stark information. This strategy can only backfire, diminishing the payer's confidence in case management. By sharing all the information and giving a studied professional opinion, the case manager can help clients appreciate issues of long-term care that they otherwise would not be able to appreciate.

LEVEL OF INVOLVEMENT

For a case manager, the type and level of involvement on a long-term case depends on several factors: the diagnosis, patient's age, prior medical history, current medical situation, treatment plan, and services required, among others. One especially important factor is the nature of the benefit plan. The provisions of the plan may severely limit the specific activities and functions that the case manager can offer, even though the case manager may be confronting a long-term problem in need of attention. The amount of family support may also influence a case manager's participation. Is the family willing and able to care for the patient at home? Will they accept use of an alternative setting—a skilled nursing facility, for example? If problems arise with the services as arranged, is there a family member who can handle the situation? As in home care, the patient's geographic setting and the community resources available are other factors that determine the level of case management needed or advisable.

The timing of a case manager's introduction to a case also affects her role. In general, case management involvement is more time-consuming and labor-intensive in the early stages of a probable long-term case, because on-site visits, telephone calls, numerous written reports (as requested by the client), and written agreements with service providers are required. General tasks include establishing a relationship with the patient, family, care providers, and client; gathering information (e.g., from the physician and hospital discharge plan); assessing patient needs and possible family participation; and arranging for medical care or other assistance.

After the case manager has put the treatment plan into action (i.e., services are in place and the care routine is established), her role usually becomes a less active one. The goal of case management is to enable the people most directly involved with a long-term illness such as the patient and family, to live as comfortably and normally as possible. Provided with the appropriate support and the knowledge and resources to manage minor crises (e.g., when a nursing shift fails to show up), the family has been empowered and has become, in effect, its own case manager. The case manager may call once a day in the beginning for purposes of monitoring. Later, she may touch base once a week. After the case manager becomes confident that the family is progressing well, she may only check in every other month, having established the conditions under which she should be called, such as when a minor problem threatens to turn into a major problem.

In a long-term case of 9 months or 2 years in which there are no major changes in the patient's condition or the care provisions, the need for frequent detailed reports to the client diminishes. This is especially true if follow-up at that point is largely telephonic. Then, reports can take the form of a status update letter or an addendum to a previous report, perhaps submitted monthly or quarterly. A telephone update noted in the client's file might be all that is necessary: "Patient's condition is unchanged since last report 3 months ago. Care services put into place remain the same and are still working effectively."

IMPORTANCE OF ONGOING INVOLVEMENT

In long-term cases, ongoing involvement is always advisable. It not only benefits the patient and family, but also benefits the client, providing increased cost containment because problems are addressed early. Continuing contact can be achieved in several ways, depending on the client group, its in-house capabilities, the funds available, and other factors. The contact link might be an in-house case manager. When an insurance company is the original referral source, it sometimes hires a field case manager to help set up services in coordination with its in-house case manager. After the patient's out-of-hospital routine is established, ongoing contact is often managed by the in-house case management service via telephone. The field case manager is only called back in if a problem occurs. Although this is not ideal because on-site visits reveal things not detected through telephone conversations, contact with the patient is maintained. Through experience, a case manager knows which questions will elicit information indicating how the patient's medication and treatment plan are working, whether symptoms are improving or worsening, how the family is coping, and whether there is increasing tension. Picking up on potential trouble spots during phone interviews, the case manager can go back into the field to determine exactly what is going on, what has changed from the original scenario, and what needs to be done to put it all back together before the care plan deteriorates. (Field case managers should make certain they tell in-house case management services that they be called promptly for a detailed in-the-field analysis of a situation if any hint of change is noted during telephonic contact.)

A case manager working with a self-funded employer group bears the responsibility of communicating to the group or the TPA the importance of keeping a case open. The case manager's contribution might be restricted to moving the patient from hospital to home with appropriate services, thereby "closing" the case. When this occurs, the case manager should carefully explain to the client that she will not be visiting every week or even every month and will not be sending unnecessary or overly detailed reports (and not billing for this level of work), but that regular contact will help keep any small difficulties from getting out of hand. What is important is maintaining a link. Case managers need to articulate this to their referral sources. Examples help to prove the point. The case manager can cite a case (preferably one handled by the same referral source) that was closed, seemingly with justification but prematurely, after which point the claims department suddenly discovered that the patient was back in the hospital. This high-cost situation could have been avoided and the problem handled in a more cost-effective manner if case management had been tracking the case.

As in any home-care case, ongoing case management contact also improves the relationship between the patient and family and the physician by keeping the physician "in the loop"—informed about the home situation, the patient's progress, and the patient's adherence to medical directives. And again, the case manager can maintain a liaison with service providers, as the need for particular equipment or support may increase or decrease with improvements or setbacks in the patient's condition. Regular on-site visits also enable the case manager to detect caregiver burnout and suggest temporary changes to handle the immediate situation, thus helping to make the long-term continuation of care feasible.

Premature closing of cases also jeopardizes the effectiveness of the case manager role. The case manager comes to be seen as a person whose function is merely to set up support services after a patient's discharge from a hospital; this view prevents the case manager from becoming an integral member of the care team and reduces the team's ability to provide needed care for the patient in a cost-effective manner.

CHANGES IN LONG-TERM CASES

Solutions that were once workable and cost-effective sometimes become ineffective over the course of a long-term care case. The case manager should expect to modify her plan or renegotiate prices due to staff changes at selected agencies, service that is no longer satisfactory, or a personality clash between a care provider and the patient or family. As mentioned, a change in service or cost often signals a change in the patient's medical condition. Complications occur. A cancer patient is undergoing chemotherapy and/or radiation, with the disease confined to one organ, the stomach. Unfortunately, the disease metastasizes to the liver and lungs and 2 months later to the brain. It might be as "simple" as a rise in body temperature to 101.4°, requiring that the patient be rehospitalized for antibiotic treatment because her chemotherapy has so deeply compromised her immune system. The patient who initially was compliant and cooperative develops breathing difficulties and other complications due to the upset of metabolic processes. She might be in pain, uncooperative, combative, hostile, and later comatose. Through these stages of the illness, the case manager must adjust services to fit the need.

In cases like traumatic brain injury or spinal cord injury, rapid gains and improvements in the beginning of treatment are often followed by long stretches of slower, less evident progress and plateaus. Plateaus present problems for the patient, family, and entire care team. They are disheartening and can be the root of both undue despair and false hope. The patient and primary caregiver feel that progress has halted, that they are stuck right where they were months ago. The claims examiner feels that "no news is good news" and that there are no problems. The referral source sees no need to call in a field case manager because the patient is stable. The case manager finds herself asking, "What can I offer here?"

Through phone contact or on-site visits, the case manager should explain what plateaus are, and provide encouragement and support. Because she does not see the individual daily, her perspective is key. Although progress might seem agonizingly slow to the family, the case manager can say, "Wow, since last month I can see such change in the strength of his movements, and now he can lift his arm 6 inches off the bed instead of stopping at 2 inches." By maintaining a journal herself and encouraging the family to jot down notes, the case manager helps lighten the dismay at the slowness of progress and focus attention on the progress being made. By making on-site visits, the case manager can also suggest ways in which the care situation might be changed (e.g., recommending equipment that will encourage more movement and giving the family tips on engaging the patient in his own care). This proactive involvement helps keep a family and its support system intact, provides tools and coping skills, and makes it less likely that more expensive services will be needed to correct a problem that went unnoticed.

Family situations also change. Initially, a family's ability to cope may be very good, and they will insist that they will do whatever it takes to care for the patient and keep him at home. And in the beginning, this is so; everyone is very energetic and involved. But then, the primary care provider gets burned out. The family then requires support, for example, a homemaker, home health aide, or RN.

Another red flag to watch for is financial difficulty. There is a myriad of ways in which monetary affairs can change during a long-term case and affect the long-term care situation and the family's stability. Insurance often pays part of the expenses involved in caring for the ill patient while the family funds the rest. The resulting financial strain can gradually become overwhelming. A number of factors are at play. The primary caregiver may have left a part-time job because of the need at home, diminishing family income. The primary wage earner in the family may become unemployed. The patient may be coming to the end of a period of salary replacement but still need several months of care. Continuing longer than expected, the case may hit a benefit ceiling. Throughout the course of care, the case manager must track financial resources and make the best use of them. The only way a case manager can monitor the patient and family situation and be able to prevent small, moderate, and major problems from becoming catastrophic is to maintain some degree of ongoing involvement in the case.

NEGOTIATING FOR LONG-TERM CARE

When negotiating for long-term services, case managers often overlook a cost-containment tactic available to them: Long-term cases provide a long-term guaranteed income for service providers. Therefore, case managers should address long-term cost issues with the providers upfront, stating frankly that because they will be billing for a set amount over a period of perhaps 5 or 6 months, negotiating costs is appropriate. This is true whether the provider is a skilled nursing care facility, home health aide service, or nutritional supplement manufacturer. The case manager's job is to get patients the level of service they need at the time they need it in the most cost-effective manner. This means negotiating based on need and fair market value and always holding out for the best price available. It is the case manager's responsibility to be familiar with competitive rates and comfortable with challenging costs and seeking deals while always leaving room to negotiate. For example, a vendor or facility representative should never be told the total amount available through a benefit plan; the release of this information would significantly reduce the case manager's bargaining power.

Intensive negotiation is particularly appropriate when a patient's needs and the required levels of services change during a prolonged period of care. An individual brain injury or multiple trauma patient may demand intense skilled nursing and ancillary services at the outset of treatment but will require less and less care during the later stages of recovery. In situations like this, renegotiation is key so that costs reflect the patient's improved condition and reduced need for many services. Further, other services may be requested. For instance, whereas skilled nursing care may be curtailed, physical or occupational therapy may be started. Overall, the case manager should see to it that changes in the levels and types of services being provided to a patient are reflected in changes in costs.

EMPLOYING ALL POSSIBLE RESOURCES

Financial resources for long-term care are always a concern, whether for a young, long-term patient or for the care of an elderly person. Long-term care insurance policies vary greatly in the type and extent of funding they provide and in the restrictions put on types of services. Resources and benefits may alter as the patient ages, and the family support system and finances may change. In addition to the patient's specific health plan (employer-funded plan, TPA, workers' compensation, or other), long-term care policy, or disease-specific policy, all other possible resources for funding and services should be investigated.

As with home care cases, many disease-specific organizations and groups provide or arrange for services. Further, recognizing the long-term needs of patients, disease-specific groups use a sliding scale, based on the patient's financial resources, for determining reimbursement. (A sliding scale arrangement is usually not available for acute, short-term care.) For example, there may be a dollar limit on a plan's psychological benefits. Depending on the need, arrangements can be made for payment on a sliding scale. In this way, a young person with an eating disorder may pay a minimum predetermined per-visit rate over a longer period of time. Case managers need to be aware of these types of resources and arrangements, including the funding available through grants, foundations, and other organizations, and use them to supplement and even protect the funding available from the insurance plan so it can be reserved for later use.

Again, community resources should also be tapped. Why pay for transportation to a doctor's appointment or for ambulance service if there are local community organizations providing the service free? Because long-term care is always a financial drain, case managers should make every effort to use whatever resources are available and to safeguard the insurance coverage the patient has at his or her disposal.

LONG-TERM CARE OF THE ELDERLY

Case management can also be applied to manage the long-term care of older adults who are not seriously ill but require support services. This is especially true now that long-term care insurance policies are available and companies are calling on case managers to evaluate the medical and emotional condition of elderly individuals. It is especially significant as the cost of the top 50 drugs prescribed to seniors rose 6.1% in the past year, 60% of drug errors come from physicians failing to monitor patients after prescribing a medication, and elderly patients are particularly inclined to skip doses to save money, or take a mix-and-match approach to their drug regimen.

Insurance companies are not the only clients seeking to use case management services in the care of the elderly. Adult sons and daughters of aging parents often recognize the need for help in locating community resources, daycare programs, and other services that address the needs of the elderly at minimal cost. These may include senior day activity programs with bus transportation, meal preparation and delivery, housekeeping services, and shopping services. Expanded professional services can be phased in later. Housing situations can also be assessed. For example, an elderly person may benefit from moving from a two-story domicile to a single-level apartment and possibly later to an adult residence at which services such as transportation, meal preparation, and housekeeping are available.

Gaining in popularity, geriatric networks or continuums mirror the best case management programs in that they move the elderly population away from fragmented, episodic care into an integrated model that is flexible and offers a range of services designed to meet the needs of the population. Multidisciplinary in nature, these eldercare programs maintain contact with participants. The elder enrollee is able to access available services through a case manager who coordinates communications among the providers, payers, patients, and community. Figure 23–1 is an example of one such continuum designed by Fowler Healthcare Affiliates.

Figure 23–1 The Geriatric Continuum.

At-Risk Geriatric Population—Levels of Case Management

Category	Low risk	Medium risk	High risk
Sample characteristics	• Lifeline or similar service participant • Minimal support system • Compromised financial status	• Newly diagnosed chronic illness • 2–3 comorbidities • New lifestyle change (e.g., loss of spouse) • No active support system • 3 or more medications • Active treatment by 2 or more physicians	• 75 years or older • In assisted living • 2–3 comorbidities and/or major functional limitations • 2 or more acute care admits within past 12 months • 1 or more ER or observ. admits within past 12 months • Multiple MD interventions • On dialysis • In day treatment • Using home health
Level of case management	Maintenance	Active	Intensive
Case management by:	Social worker (BS)	Social worker (MS) and/or RN	RN
Frequency of contact between case manager and enrollee	Approximately every 6 to 8 weeks	Approximately monthly	Approximately every 2 weeks or more as appropriate

Source: Reprinted with permission from F. J. Fowler and F. L. Machisko, The Geriatric Continuum, Continuing Care, Vol. 16, No. 4, p. 24, © 1997, Stevens Publishing Corporation.

IMPLICATIONS OF LONG-TERM CARE FOR THE FAMILY

Long-term care has numerous implications for the family, many of them resulting from the patient's illness and prognosis. It is much easier for the family and for the case manager when the long-term situation has improvement as an end goal. The more uncertain or grave the future, the more stressful the case becomes. In this type of situation, the case manager cannot say, "It's a bad day; things will get better." When the prognosis is not good, a family may accept the likely death of the patient or refuse to believe the physician's opinion. In most cases, the family sees someone who was once a healthy active member and contributor but is now irreversibly changed.

Attention must also be given to the primary caregiver. Just as the patient should be encouraged to find a disease-specific support group, so too should the caregiver be encouraged to arrange for periods of respite and to talk with people facing similar challenges. There are numerous associations for spouses, parents who have a child with a long-term illness, and for siblings or children of individuals suffering from a long-term illness. The benefits are multiple: for the caregiver, for the long-term patient, and, more practically, for the client who will continue to contain costs.

Quite often in long-term cases, whatever strains there were in the family before the illness become exacerbated and the whole situation seems beyond remedy. I call it the "fractured family syndrome." Divorce, alcoholism, emotional illness, overwhelming depression, adolescent rebelliousness, child abuse—case managers may see some and occasionally all of these issues in such situations. The combination of horrendous healthcare problems, personal or family stresses, and real or potential financial difficulties can cause unending emotional turmoil. Tension builds, especially in younger families. It is typical for a young mother to be the care provider for an aging and ill parent while fulfilling the roles of wife and parent. Her husband or children may feel neglected. What case managers sometimes see then is resentful and attention-seeking children who develop behavior problems or start experimenting with drugs. Or, a spouse may start drinking heavily or become totally involved in work, avoiding the home. In some cases, the family falls apart. The primary caregiver cannot manage it any more. There are many examples of the spouse of a person with multiple sclerosis simply leaving, after years of giving caring support and knowing that there are years to come of the same or worse.

What should the case manager do in situations such as these? Following are some tips on helping families through a crisis period:

- Suggest family counseling.
- Suggest the primary caregiver join an appropriate support group.
- Recommend books on coping, such as the *Family Guide to Stroke* (American Heart Association), *The Family Guide to Surviving Stroke and Communication Disorders* (Allyn & Bacon), *Taking Time: Support for People with Cancer and the People Who Care about Them* (National

Cancer Institute, National Institutes of Health, U.S. Department of Health and Human Services), *Right to Die* (Group for the Advancement of Psychiatry), *The AIDS Caregiver's Handbook* (St. Martin's Press), *The Caregiver's Journey* (HarperCollins), *The Forgetting Alzheimer's: Portrait of an Epidemic* (Anchor Books), *There's Still a Person in There: The Complete Guide to Treating and Coping with Alzheimer's* (Perigee), *The Lupus Book: A Guide for Patients and Their Families* (Oxford University Press), *New Hope for People with Lupus: Your Friendly, Authoritative Guide to the Latest in Traditional and Complementary Solutions* (Prima Publishing), and *Guarded Prognosis: A Doctor and His Patients Talk About Chronic Disease and How to Cope with It* (Hill & Wang). (For pertinent guides, check with national associations, which often put together recommended reading lists.)

- Direct families to resources that help them claim some of the billions in untapped public assistance dollars provided by state and federal assistance programs. The web site www.benefitscheckup.org includes information on Supplemental Security Income, Medicaid, state drug benefits, Meals on Wheels, food stamps, health insurance counseling, and veterans' medical care and transportation. The site offers addresses and phone numbers of local government offices, and screens candidates for property tax exemptions, utility bill relief, talking-book programs, an inexpensive lifetime pass to national parks, and home repair and renovation services. The web site www.homeinsteadsolutions.com provides access to a national network of eldercare products and services; Home Instead can also be reached toll-free at 1 (888) 405-4242.
- Remind family members to keep their own appointments and to take care of themselves. Encourage them to go to their gym regularly, or make an appointment for a massage, facial, or manicure.
- Help the family members communicate and achieve some level of comfort with feelings of fear, anxiety, and so on.

Case managers should also remember to get support for themselves through contact with peers. Some case managers try to relive their own experiences through other families, which is detrimental to all involved.

IMPLICATIONS OF A LONG-TERM CASE
FOR THE CASE MANAGER

It is important to note that long-term cases have many implications, often hidden at first, for case managers. Case managers react very differently when working on long-term cases than on shorter cases that frequently have positive outcomes. The more problematic the case and the more discouraged and overwhelmed the family becomes, the greater the burden placed on the case manager. Even though the patient's medical condition may become more stable, other long-term problems occur, and the case manager might feel like the only person who is truly attempting to face them. The family may want out and may dump their concerns on the case manager as a way of seeking relief. Frequently, case managers become disheartened and burn out.

Some case managers do a very good job of being compassionate and supportive while keeping themselves from becoming too personally involved. However, others cross the line, which is dangerous because they sacrifice their objective professionalism. There are many reasons or triggers that may lead a case manager to become too personally connected. A 34-year-old case manager, working a case in which a husband is caring for his 34-year-old wife dying of breast cancer, can become too connected. A transference of feelings occurs, and the case manager identifies with the patient. She loses her objectivity and, not realizing it, starts to make decisions based on how she would personally like things done if she were the patient.

There are other circumstances that may obstruct objectivity. Perhaps the husband–caregiver reminds a case manager of her ex-husband, with whom she is fighting for child support payments. Perhaps the patient is dying of Alzheimer's and the case manager's mother has just been diagnosed with Alzheimer's. There may be a personality conflict between the case manager and the caregiver, which can obstruct objectivity as much as feelings of empathy can.

There can also be situations in which the case manager has not lost objectivity but simply is no longer effective or useful on the case. At the beginning stages of the case, her energy level was high, she carefully analyzed all parameters, and she devised a workable and cost-effective plan that met the needs of the patient. After a while, changes occurred and everything she tried in response failed. Now the case manager is running out of ideas. The case begins to haunt her, and there is no end in sight. She is no longer a catalyst for improvement.

When no longer objective or effective, case managers need to be honest concerning their own feelings. They must recognize their worth and their contribution or lack of contribution. They need to have open communication with peers and supervisors.

In fact, I think long-term cases require periodic conferences between case managers and supervisors so that the value of the case management process can be continually assessed. Is the case manager making a difference? Is she just reporting to the client, almost like a journalist? Is she acting as a catalyst for change? Or, is she identifying the same problems month after month but not coming up with any new solutions? Such reevaluations can uncover the need for a fresh perspective on the case and perhaps that of a different case manager.

Confronting a lack of effectiveness can be very difficult for a case manager, particularly if she has a one-person business and substantial income may be lost if she gives up the case. But honesty is absolutely necessary, and if the case manager is not moving toward some positive results, for whatever reason, she does not belong on the case. A supervisor in a larger case management unit or company may have to make such decisions, but ideally each case manager will develop an ability to judge her own contributions accurately. Honesty must also extend to the family and client. If a case manager decides that she is no longer effective, she should discuss this with the client, explaining that although the case still requires case management services, she is not the right person for this particular case at this time. Difficult? Yes, but vital if the case manager is to remain effective and provide real help to patients and families in long-term cases.

FROM ACUTE CARE TO HOME CARE: A CASE HISTORY

Marge Reynolds, a 46-year-old mother of two teens, has a 27-year history of chronic colitis, which she apparently had under control using a combination of medication and diet. In April, she was admitted to the hospital for complaints of abdominal and gastrointestinal distress, vomiting, weight loss, and abdominal pain. Two-and-a-half years earlier, she had developed increasing and unremitting abdominal pains and had entered the hospital at that time for a diagnostic work up. She underwent a colectomy with anastomosis following the discovery of a partial bowel obstruction, but she elected to forgo a colostomy despite the warnings of her physicians. One week after the surgery, Mrs. Reynolds suffered acute abdominal bleeding. Additional surgery and a colostomy were performed. Her recovery progressed well, and she returned to her normal activities.

The next year, Mrs. Reynolds experienced prolonged vaginal bleeding and was diagnosed as having uterine cancer. Based on her medical history, a complete hysterectomy was done, with additional testing to rule out metastatic disease or ovarian cancer. Her chemotherapy treatments were completed just prior to the onset of the pains and vomiting that led to her hospital admission in April.

Twelve days after her admission and diagnostic work ups, which incorporated CAT scans and MRI testing, Mrs. Reynolds's surgeon performed exploratory surgery. The operations included a resection of the bowel and stoma, relocation of the stoma site, resection of the abdominal wall, and insertion of a Teflon mesh to replace an excised section of body wall necessitated by multiple tumors of metastatic origin.

Mrs. Reynolds's timely recovery was compromised by her generally weakened condition from previous chemotherapy treatments and further complicated by the need for the insertion of a Porta-Cath to provide nutritional support, as she was experiencing vomiting, diarrhea (related to short bowel syndrome), dehydration, and malnutrition. The hospital social worker recommended that Mrs. Reynolds be kept in the hospital based on the delay in her stabilization, the fact that she required highly sophisticated intravenous TPN 24 hours a day, and her determined resistance to hospice care.

When a hospital extension was first requested for patient stabilization, a preadmission-utilization review nurse red-flagged Mrs. Reynolds's file for case management. One of our independent case managers visited Mrs. Reynolds in the hospital. Finding her too ill to converse, the case manager consulted her chart and reviewed her progress with Mrs. Reynolds's husband, the treating physicians, the nursing staff, the utilization review nurse, and a hospital social worker. From the family physician and Mr. Reynolds, the case manager learned of Mrs. Reynolds's previous hospital admissions, her fight against colon and ovarian cancer, and her recent chemotherapy treatments.

In her initial report, sent to the insurer just short of 1 month after Mrs. Reynolds entered the hospital, the case manager noted the patient was in a generally weakened condition and was hampered by an under-functioning ileostomy and episodes of vomiting and frequent diarrhea. The assessment also included detailed descriptions of treatment and medication, the surgeon's planned insertion of a triple lumen, central venous catheter, or Porta-Cath, and the observation that Mrs. Reynolds was able to get out of bed only with assistance and required help with ambulating and hygiene.

During her on-site visit to the hospital, the case manager had been able to discuss the home environment and the potential for home care services with Mr. Reynolds, the hospital nurses, and the social worker. That home care seemed a possibility was welcome news, as Mrs. Reynolds had made it clear that she did not want to be admitted to a hospice. Due to the complexity of Mrs. Reynolds's treatment, the option of home care had not occurred to the treating physician, nurses, or social worker, but the case manager was able to assure the hospital staff and family that home care was a viable alternative for Mrs. Reynolds. In conversation, the case manager confirmed that the insurer would cover the cost of a home health aide, episodic RN attendance, and home IV therapy or hyperalimentation (which was then being considered by the treating physician). The case manager also received word from the treating physicians that home care was a perfectly acceptable medical alternative to hospice care. Discharge was delayed until Mrs. Reynolds's condition improved.

In mid-May, a Porta-Cath was inserted and TPN infusion begun in an effort to stabilize Mrs. Reynolds's condition. She responded well to the nutritional support and experienced less nausea, vomiting, and gastric distress. During the case manager's next visit, Mrs. Reynolds was eating several small meals a day. Working closely with the hospital staff, the case manager continued coordinating discharge planning and home care services.

Mrs. Reynolds's family supported the idea of home treatment, but were unable to be at home during the day to administer that care. Accepting bids from the most qualified suppliers and negotiating for the most cost-effective treatment, the case manager arranged for home nursing services (HNS), a home health aide, and TPN services. In early July, less than 7 weeks after she arrived at the hospital, Mrs. Reynolds was able to go home.

Instead of continuing her acute hospitalization, she was able to receive treatment at home, assisted by a home health aide who helped with bathing, dressing, meal preparation, and other personal activities. An HNS nurse taught Mr. and Mrs. Reynolds how to hang her intravenous fluids, how to perform tubing changes, how to monitor the electrolyte balance and glucose levels, and what to do in an emergency. From her office, the case manager pushed the insurer to allow her to make a home visit a few days after Mrs. Reynolds's discharge. She wanted to see the program in action and make sure her plan was effective. Her visit was timely.

The infusion company had overstocked the Reynolds's home with supplies, making it difficult to move through the house, and charged for unneeded equipment and fluids that could not possibly be used before their expiration date. Reviewing the invoices, the case manager also found that the firm had charged for a period of 28 days when Mrs. Reynolds was still in the hospital, and it was billing for pump rental and infusion nursing visits that it had previously agreed would be included in the per diem cost. The case manager arranged for immediate credits to the account.

She also noted that Mrs. Reynolds was receiving 24 hours of TPN, unusual for homebound patients because it eliminates any freedom of movement the individual might enjoy. Following conversations with the HNS nurse and family physician, approval was given for Mrs. Reynolds to receive her full prescribed volume of TPN Intralipids over a 20-hour period. The case manager's aim was to allow Mrs. Reynolds to move about her home, increasing her stamina and independence. To boost her mobility, the case manager got carrier approval for a rental wheelchair (no loaner wheelchairs were available from community loan closets). The allowed interruption in infusion therapy and the wheelchair enabled Mrs. Reynolds to attend her son's high school graduation later that month, an important emotional and physical outing that boosted her spirits and reinforced the family's sense of wholeness.

The case manager continued monitoring the home infusion therapy and TPN, Mrs. Reynolds's medical condition, and the need for nursing and home health aide services. In subsequent visits, the case manager noticed that Mrs. Reynolds appeared to have gained strength and a little weight and was pleased with her increased mobility. With her TPN and other infusions now being completed in 18 hours, she was able to take showers, sit outside during good weather, and attend family gatherings. Mrs. Reynolds was also independent in setting up her TPN solutions, tubing, and changing infusion bottles. Her daily life was a far stretch from the acute hospitalization she could well have been experiencing.

Unfortunately, due to the onset of severe back pain and other complications from previous battles with cancer, Mrs. Reynolds was subsequently readmitted to the hospital. With ongoing intervention by the case manager, her hospital stay was of short duration, and she was able to return home. The case manager's continued home visits proved invaluable when the case manager found Mrs. Reynolds in a medical crisis that the attending home health aide was unable to manage. After contacting the treating physician and conducting a reevaluation of Mrs. Reynolds's home situation in light of her deteriorating condition, the case manager arranged for additional RN support. She also suggested family counseling to help ease the stress felt by Mr. Reynolds and the two teenagers, who were trying unsuccessfully to cope with terminal illness and death.

Through the case manager's early involvement, Mrs. Reynolds was able to experience increased self-reliance and to live the last months of her life at home with her family. Although the wheelchair rental was a very small item in the whole home care picture, it gave Mrs. Reynolds and her family a highlight to remember. Because of the case manager's attention to detail and knowledge of the latest technologies, Mrs. Reynolds received a preferred alternative to hospital or hospice care, and the insurer paid fewer and less expensive claims.

The value of case management to Mrs. Reynolds and her family might be incalculable, but a review of one quarter's cost-benefit analysis report sent by our case manager to the insurer shows exactly what case management meant to the bottom-line. Under "avoidance of potential charges," there are 70 days in the hospital at $1,750 per day, plus pharmacy and physician charges totaling $132,500. Total actual charges for case management fees, reduced-rate TPN, and negotiated fees for home health aide and nursing services came to $54,500, for a net savings of $78,000. The case manager also discovered $12,500 in overcharges submitted by the TPN vendor; this amount would have boosted actual charges to $67,000.

Chapter 24

Public Sector Case Management

NEW DIRECTIONS IN PUBLIC SECTOR CASE MANAGEMENT

Just as the private sector of healthcare payers has realized the effects of increased costs, of a longer living population, and of a changing and more convoluted healthcare delivery system, so, too, has the public sector. As case management has become an integral part of efforts to promote quality of care, improve patient outcomes, and contain costs for the private payers, we are seeing a real growth of case management in the public sector.

FUNDING SOURCES FOR PUBLIC SECTOR HEALTH BENEFITS

In the United States, health insurance benefits are funded either in the private/commercial sector through employers, individuals, associations, and others or through the government at the federal (including military), state, or local levels. The U.S. government provides healthcare coverage to a variety of groups, including federal government employees, military (active and veterans), and Native Americans; Medicare and Medicaid, however, account for the largest number of enrollees: 83 million.[1]

The following sections provide a brief overview of the funding background for these programs.

Medicare

Medicare is an entitlement program that was created in 1965 and that is funded entirely at the federal level. It is a health insurance program for people age 65 or older, people younger than 65 who have certain disabilities, and people with end-stage renal disease.

Medicare is divided into four parts: Part A, Part B, Part C, and Part D:

- *Part A: Hospital Insurance:* Part A pays for most inpatient care, some inpatient skilled nursing home care, some home healthcare, and hospice care. Individuals are automatically enrolled in Part A when joining Medicare. Medicare reviews Social Security records to qualify individuals and determine the monthly premiums.

- *Part B: Medical Insurance:* Part B pays for physician services, outpatient hospital care, outpatient physical and speech therapy, some home healthcare, ambulance services, and some medical equipment and supplies. This coverage is voluntary and the monthly premium is automatically deducted from the individual's Social Security check each month.
- *Part C: Medicare Advantage Plans:* Part C governs the way Medicare benefits are provided by companies that contract with the Medicare program. Individuals who enroll in a Medicare Advantage plan generally get all of their medical services through that plan. Health maintenance organizations (HMOs) and preferred provider organizations (PPOs) that contract with Medicare will include the new (in 2006) Medicare Part D benefit. Private Fee-for-Service (PFFS) and Medical Savings Accounts (MSAs) can also contract with Medicare to provide Part A and Part B. PFFS plans have the options of including Part D; MSAs do not.
- *Part D: Medicare Prescription Drug Coverage:* Part D offers some help with prescription drugs. This coverage is voluntary and the monthly premium varies depending on the amount.

Medigap

Generally, when individuals purchase a Medigap policy, they must have Medicare Parts A and B. A Medigap policy is health insurance sold by private insurers to fill the "gaps" in Medicare.

Medicaid

Medicaid is a health program for eligible individuals and families with low incomes and resources. It is a means-tested program that is jointly funded by the states and federal government but managed by the states. This coverage was created in 1965 through Title XIX of the Social Security Act.

State Children's Health Insurance Program

The State Children's Health Insurance Program (SCHIP) was enacted by Congress in 1997 to increase health insurance coverage for low-income children.

Military and Veterans HealthCare

Military healthcare encompasses a diverse range of programs, each serving a total military population of more than 9.2 million, including active and retired personnel and their families as well as eligible veterans. TRICARE is the Department of Defense's managed care programs for beneficiaries from any of the seven services (Army, Navy, Marine Corps, Air Force, Coast Guard, Public Health Service, and National Guard).

Veterans HealthCare

The Veterans Health Administration (VHA) operates the largest integrated healthcare system and provides care to more than 5 million inpatients and outpatients. Historically, the Veterans Administration (VA) served only those with service-connected disabilities; however, the VA is now open to all veterans and has become an important safety net for many low-income veterans who would otherwise be uninsured.

Obviously, the wars the United States has been engaged in have critically affected the military system of healthcare. Although the battlefield care has made it possible for many more of our nations' heroes to survive, the physical and emotional battles are ongoing and costs for programs to help military personnel in these areas are affected.

ECONOMIC IMPACT AND GOVERNMENT RESPONSE

The government has been a payer of healthcare for the elderly and economically disadvantaged for many years, and it has been in the forefront with some initiatives to contain costs. An example of this is the early DRG reimbursement system, whereby hospitals are reimbursed based on a given diagnosis or condition and a predetermined length of stay (LOS). Although this and other cost control methods may have focused efforts on acute care hospital utilization, they did little to address the issues and problems of individuals who could benefit from case management intervention.

In its 1999 report, *To Err Is Human: Building a Safer Health System*, the Institute of Medicine (IOM) concludes that medical errors, particularly in hospital-acquired conditions, may be responsible for as many as 98,000 deaths annually, at costs of up to $29 billion. In 2007, the Leapfrog Group of more than 1,200 hospitals found that 87% did not follow recommendations to prevent many of the most common hospital-acquired conditions.[2]

The rules proposed by the Centers for Medicare and Medicaid Services (CMS, the former HCFA, or Health Care Financing Administration) expand two key initiatives that begin to link payments for healthcare services to quality of care: the Hospital-Acquired Conditions (HACs) and the Hospital Quality Measure Reporting initiatives. Medicare would no longer pay hospitals at a higher rate for the increased costs of care that resulted when a patient is harmed by one of several conditions they didn't have when first admitted, and deemed to be reasonably preventable by following generally accepted guidelines.

These include, but are not limited to decubiti, vascular catheter-associated infection, air embolism, hospital acquired injuries etc. A complete listing of the conditions and other key initiatives aimed at improving quality cost-effective care is available at the CMS Web site: www.cms.gov. CMS is proposing to expand the list of conditions which are reasonably preventable through proper care and for which Medicare will no longer pay if they are acquired during a hospital confinement. That proposed list includes, but again not limited to: surgical site infections following certain elective procedures, Legionnaire's disease, extreme blood sugar derangement, ventilator-assisted pneumonia, and other conditions also available on the CMS Web site.

CMS also noted that almost 18% of Medicare patients are readmitted to the hospital within 30 days of discharge, potentially exposing the patients and their families to additional suffering. According to the Medicare Payment Advisory Commission, readmissions cost the program $15 billion annually, with $12 billion of those costs potentially preventable.[3] In another report in 2008, data gathered from 2005 and 2006 from the National Hospital Ambulatory Medical Care Surveys (NHACS) noted that 2.3 million Emergency Department (ED) . . . 2% of all visits, were made by persons who had been hospitalized within the last 7 days.[4]

There has not, as of this writing, been a final decision on the resolution of the readmission matter, however, three potential scenarios have been proposed: adjustment in DRG payment on a performance-based methodology; direct adjustment for avoidable readmissions; public reporting of readmissions.[5]

Those case managers who are hospital-based will most assuredly be involved in these initiatives, or should, at the very least be an active member of the quality assurance committee in their facility. Examining the situations that result in these conditions or readmissions can lead to the solutions. Utilizing the core components of the case management process can be the same process employed in this problem-solving approach.

Additionally, with respect to the readmission situation, if *anything* calls attention to the need to follow patients beyond discharge, this should get folks' attention . . . it's unfortunate that it had to take a threat of non-payment to shed a spotlight on this matter.

The government contracts with various organizations to administer its health insurance programs and has been actively involved in the last several years in moving many of those participants into managed care organizations. At the federal and state levels, the government became increasingly concerned that monies to care for the growing numbers of elderly would be insufficient. These public payers also realized, as did those in the private sector, that not everyone uses the available dollars to the same degree. They recognized that several diagnostic conditions use the largest proportion of resources, which, in turn, has a direct correlation to the dollars that are expended. In an article titled "Building a Better Medicare" in *Case in Point*, the author notes that 25% of Medicare beneficiaries have the following characteristics:

- Have five or more chronic conditions
- See 14 physicians
- Fill an average of 57 prescriptions a year[6]

Those individuals who have Medicaid coverage are responsible for 18% of the total national spending on healthcare. These recipients often present with more socioenvironmental, psychosocial, and other issues than they do with medical ones, and they are frequently the patients who are the most challenging for case managers. Medicaid is "the dominant source of financing for long-term care, paying over 40% of the national bill for nursing home and long-term care . . . and is the largest source of public financing for mental health and substance abuse services."[7]

The initiatives that have been proposed by CMS, called the three Ps—prevention, prescriptions, and payments—are aimed at benefitting recipients and the entire healthcare system. Certainly, the Pay for Performance (P4P) initiative, which began in 2008, acknowledged that outcomes are improved when the physician spends more time with patients, so the E/M (Evaluation/Management) codes and their payments were revised and updated.[8]

Response to this has led to initiatives that address the most costly problems and target the population groups most likely to benefit from these efforts. To reduce costs by more effective intervention, government case management programs have typically looked at several of the following: high-risk pregnancy, high-risk newborn, sickle cell anemia, AIDS, psychiatric, cancer, and drug and alcohol patients.

In the Deficit Reduction Act of 2005, Medicaid defined and outlined the components of case management. Case management, as defined by CMS, "means services that will assist individuals eligible under the plan in gaining access to needed medical, social, educational, and other services." The components include assessment of the individual, development of a specific care plan, referral and related activities, monitoring and follow-up activities. Note that *referral* and *coordination* of the aforementioned services do not imply payment by CMS for any/all of them; additional information is available at http://www.cms.hhs.gov/MedicaidGenInfo/Downloads.[9] Case management is being incorporated into many demonstration projects and quality initiatives; this is certainly good news for case managers.

CMS is in the midst of one such initiative, a comprehensive study called the Medicare Coordinated Care Demonstration Project. As in private sector, public sector studies have shown that a relatively small number of recipients with certain chronic illnesses account for the larger portion of Medicare fee-for-service costs. The demonstration project, authorized by the Balanced Budget Act of 1997, is being conducted to determine whether private sector case management tools used by HMOs, MCOs, insurers, and providers could be applied to the fee-for-service population.

A CASE MANAGER IN THE PUBLIC SECTOR

Sherry Aliotta, RN, BSN, CCM, president and CEO of S.A. Squared, and former national president of Case Management Society of America (CMSA), who works predominantly in the public sector, finds that demand for case management is increasing notably, as it has proven to be effective in helping to secure more cost-effective care without a decline in good outcomes and the provision of services. Case management has drawn growing recognition for its success with the public sector populations, Aliotta notes. With today's tremendous financial pressures and decreasing federal and state budgetary resources, the government is turning to case management and population management to help keep Medicare and Medicaid functioning at appropriate levels.

This interest in and demand for case management has opened up new opportunities for case managers to be involved in different aspects of case management and population management, including taking their place at the table as decision makers. "Our services are perceived as value-added," comments Aliotta. "There is the clear perception that case managers have a lot to offer in terms of designing health management programs that work for these very heterogeneous and diverse populations. Medicare and Medicaid together are meant to encompass all types of people, young and old, and case managers are the key to delivering good outcomes for them."

Her mantra is, "Finding solutions that work." Aliotta has found that some strategies that are effective in the commercial environment cannot be applied to the same degree for Medicare/Medicaid populations. Her solution is to build a plan that accepts outright that persons will vary in their ability to adhere to a plan, and design accordingly, with measures to promote a quick response to events that may occur as a result of noncompliance.

This is not to infer that most of her client base is noncompliant. Rather, a majority of the people she sees are very motivated to take the best steps, to follow the suggested plan, but are challenged and sometimes thwarted by lack of access to the financial and transportation resources to achieve their goal. "If someone in my family is ill, we make the doctor's appointment, arrange for any needed testing or support equipment, pick up the medications, and address the problem," notes Aliotta. Not all of her clients can follow suit. Still, one of her public sector clients has a departmental mission statement to "Do the Right Thing": to provide for the right care at the right time in the right environment.

According to Aliotta, there is room in public sector case management to do the right things through use of alternatives to the generally accepted plan. For one client, her company designed a program that utilized a 24-hour home companion to monitor the administration of IV antibiotics and assist with tasks of daily living, rather than seeking admission to a nursing home. The option does have to be reviewed and approved, like out-of-plan solutions in the private sector, but the system is flexible enough to put such options in place.

The level of scrutiny of and accountability for case management services has increased significantly over the years. During her first review, Aliotta recalls the reviewer saying, "Case management isn't even mentioned in our survey materials," they were so far below the radar. Today, the government is looking to address regulations and standards to the practice of case management in the public sector. There is a great deal of oversight from the state and local government on any communication that goes out to the Medicare/Medicaid population, and all policies and procedures are thoroughly and stringently reviewed. The case managers work with their Compliance Departments on a daily basis to make sure they are in accordance with regulations. In her previous job, Aliotta had 2 manuals of standards; in public sector case management, there are 17 manuals.

The upside to all this is that case management has demonstrated its success with public sector clients, and now is not only requested (demanded, even), but is also one of the major players in determining and administering the healthcare programs.

CMS POPULATION GROUPS CHALLENGE MANAGED CARE INDUSTRY AND PROVIDERS

In the 1990s, increasing and somewhat aggressive marketing efforts to move older adults and economically disadvantaged individuals to managed care companies were made as the government sought to find resolution to its monetary concerns. These efforts, although initially met with resistance, became more successful, and the numbers of Medicare and Medicaid enrollees in managed care groups increased. Then, double-digit inflation in healthcare costs returned, prompting many MCOs and HMOs to move out of the Medicare/Medicaid markets.

Fortunately the market has stabilized somewhat, but because of a disproportionate share of high-cost complex patients as compared to commercial/employer groups, strategic initiatives aimed at quality and cost containment continue to be a challenge. Additionally, because of the lower reimbursement rate, many healthcare providers have discontinued providing care for the Medicaid population.

CHALLENGES FOR CASE MANAGERS

Because case management finds many of its solutions in the creative use of available benefits, such strategies are sometimes more difficult to implement in public plans. When the government is the payer, whether federal or state, approval of exceptions can be hindered due to the review process. Not being able to move cases more quickly through the system drives up costs for the government and until recently, no one in the government seemed to care.

Because Medicaid/Medicare is at risk to lose money because of unmanaged or poorly managed high-cost cases, just as private companies are, it has become a mandate for them to resolve the problems, inclusive of contract language exceptions or paying for benefits in lieu of greater exposure (costs) to the plan. In keeping with their efforts to remain profitable, today, the government actively seeks case management input in determining the management and use of public monies.

COMPLICATIONS THAT REMAIN

Although some of the cost issues are being addressed in the public sector, still others seem to be caught up in the bureaucracy and regulations that have been its historical dilemma. In our company, for instance, we are case management providers in the Medicaid model waiver program for infants and children who have complex and often life-threatening medical conditions. In addition to having medical and care need requirements, these children also must have private health insurance through a parent in order to be deemed eligible for this waiver program. Whereas most state Medicaid programs are for those in economic need, these waiver programs require that the child is denied regular Medicaid assistance, and, in fact, the family must secure this denial before being considered for the waiver program.

Each child in the program is assigned to a county-appointed case manager; the county, in turn, directs the parent to select another case manager from an approved vendor listing who will actually assume ongoing responsibility to manage the care that will be required. Our case managers face many challenges in trying to develop plans for these children. In addition to the usual activities of assessing, implementing, coordinating, evaluating, and monitoring, they need to develop detailed budgets that delineate not only each aspect of care, service, and equipment that the child will require (from MD visits, nursing care, PT, OT, and special feedings, to transportation, oxygen, and ventilators), but also enumerate just what kind of funding is expected (such as private insurance, state or county funds, or parental contribution) and the amount of dollars for each.

These care plans and the proposed budget (including the hours and dollars for the case manager's planned intervention) are then submitted for approval. The budgets are revised every three months and represent just a *portion* of the other required reports and forms. Because Medicaid reimbursement is often considerably lower than what providers can obtain from private insurance, it can be difficult to find quality providers who will accept these cases.

Although funding issues certainly complicate the management of these individuals whose benefits are derived from public funds, there are other issues that have a much greater impact on whether a case will have a successful outcome. For example, in traditional Medicare programs, the insureds are typically over the age of 65, and although there certainly are exceptions, many of them have several medical conditions. Because senior citizens are concurrently dealing with medical challenges *and* potential challenges in the healthcare system, the frustration and confusion are certainly understandable.

These frustrations, combined with other issues, place many of the elderly at significant risk for complications and poor outcomes. A good number of seniors are living alone, having lost a life partner or, perhaps, never marrying. With loss of loved ones through death or the geographic relocation of many to the warmer climates, to senior citizen communities, or to children's and friends' homes, many seniors are isolated or have little reliable, ongoing support. Homes or apartments that served them well when they were younger and stronger now present architectural barriers. Financial limitations can also be significant, with individuals making choices between food and other necessary living expenses and medical care and related expenses.

We hear of individuals who, although they have insurance through Medicare, need to pay for all of their oral prescriptions themselves (unless their plan has a drug program). Even with prescription coverage, we see growing numbers of the elderly who become so used to having to watch their dollars due to lowered incomes that they economize in this area as well. Instead of taking their medication three times a day, they reduce it to one or two times a day or take it a few times a week, thus making the drugs "last longer." Getting refills for medications is also a problem for many because of an inability to get to the pharmacy or waiting too long.

Another area of concern is one that we are seeing with growing frequency as our society ages and that is the condition of dementia and the related diagnoses of Alzheimer's and Parkinson's. Often difficult to diagnose, these disorders truly complicate the management and safety of individuals affected by them. In all but the later phases of the illness, the patient may appear and, in fact, may be physically functional. However, the individual's ability to consistently comprehend, remember, and follow medical care instructions; remember medication and dosing requirements; understand and adhere to dietary restrictions and nutrition needs; or coordinate and keep medical appointments is impaired. One can readily appreciate that the aforementioned problems would put a patient at risk, yet getting resolution is difficult because of the many restrictions, exclusions, and limitations in Medicare and Medicaid (as well as in many private insurer and payer plans). Most Alzheimer and dementia-diagnosed patients need support services rather than skilled care services, which are typically *not* covered. Yet if patients do *not* take their medications or become malnourished and dehydrated, they most assuredly will develop a medically "covered" condition.

As more seniors are moving into managed care arrangements or risk-based contracts and as it becomes financially feasible to manage the needs of individuals in the most cost-effective way and to decrease the utilization of hospital and other costly services, such problems are being addressed and resolved by case managers with improved outcomes and savings as a result. Even in situations in which the "flexing" of benefits is not possible and such support services remain uncovered, case managers are often able to serve as a broker of services by referring the frail elderly to community-based programs, such as Meals on Wheels, Alzheimer day programs, transportation, homemaker/companion assistance, and others. Such programs are often available on an "as needed" basis with payment on a sliding scale according to available funds from each citizen. More cooperation is being evidenced at the federal, state, and community levels across the country in an effort to provide care and support in the most cost-effective, least restrictive environment.

Although the elderly represent the largest group of Medicare enrollees, there are others who, because of their medical disabilities and Social Security eligibility, also qualify for medical benefits through this federal program. Because of the complexity, chronicity, and long-term needs, these individuals may also be involved in case management programs. Understandably, the issues for case managers, in addition to illness issues, will need to be addressed and resolved in this more challenging population group.

NONMEDICAL CHALLENGES INFLUENCE OUTCOMES

Perhaps the most difficult cases for case managers active in public sector programs are those we face when working with the underinsured, economically disadvantaged individuals who are in the various state-funded Medicaid programs. When children and adults have Medicaid as their insurance, they already are facing many obstacles and roadblocks in obtaining medical care. Choice of hospitals, physicians, and other providers may be limited because not all will accept Medicaid patients or because limits are placed on the number of patients to be treated for the lower reimbursement. These services are often available in clinic settings where waiting is long, care is fragmented, and follow-up is less than ideal.

Even when there is a good healthcare system in place, however, there are many other issues with Medicaid enrollees that cannot be addressed by medical care alone. Because economic need is the major criteria used for Medicaid eligibility, it seems reasonable to accept that certain other factors place many of its beneficiaries at risk. Those who are unemployed or underemployed may also have need for food, housing, clothing, and transportation. When housing is available, it is frequently substandard and unsafe due to crowding; bathroom facilities are shared by several families; there are unsanitary, often nonworking fixtures; there are no heat and limited lighting; and there is no phone service because of nonpayment. When there are also cultural differences, language barriers, and educational deficiencies, including illiteracy, one can begin to appreciate the many obstacles that would preclude a good outcome. When recipients are in rural areas, these same problems may exist but without a concentration of agencies and resources to provide the necessary assistance.

Most case managers today have some experience with these public forms of insurance and occasionally are working within several lines of insurance on the same patient. Because many people today are employed beyond the Medicare-eligible age of 65, they may be covered by their employer's health plan as their primary coverage, with Medicare as a secondary payer. A retiree over the age of 65 may have Medicare as primary coverage and the employer-sponsored plan as secondary coverage. In patients with end-stage renal disease, Medicare becomes primary 30 months following the diagnosis of this condition even if the individual is under the age of 65. Coordinating care and services for individuals with multiple lines of insurance can be confusing and frustrating, and it is extremely important to know "who's on first . . . what's on second." When the state is the payer, through Medicaid (in California, Medi-Cal), knowledge of its various regulations and requirements is also critical.

Just as in private sector case management, there is a need to identify those individuals and conditions that have potential for complex and costly problems and then develop a process of proactive intervention. Because of the conditions and factors just discussed, case managers working with these individuals will need to be especially skilled and experienced not just clinically but, equally important, in the social welfare, community resource, and financial areas. In public sector case management, there really needs to be a team approach with social workers as integral members of the team.

Perhaps the biggest challenge with the economically disadvantaged who, because of their complex medical conditions, become involved in a case management program is keeping them in the program. In conversations with case managers across the country who are struggling with this issue, "disenrollment" is becoming a major deterrent in the successful implementation of case management programs. Enrollees move from plan to plan, and many have never heard of or received case management intervention. They are often mistrustful of any efforts to "direct" or "control" them. Case management, if it is to be successful, will have to be able to meet the many challenges that these recipients present; however, the opportunities to truly make a difference with this very special population group are growing in their potential.

MILITARY CASE MANAGEMENT

Since the last edition of this book, the practice setting of case managers in the military has grown rapidly. "The conflicts in Iraq and Afghanistan have tasked the military healthcare system as never before," advises Anne M. Cobb, RNC, MSN, case management department head at the National Naval Medical Center in Washington, D.C.[10] The budgetary costs of providing disability compensation benefits and medical care to the veterans from Iraq and Afghanistan over the course of their lives is estimated to be from \$350 billion to \$700 billion.[11] Because of improvements in body armor and advances in care on the battlefield, there are, thankfully, many more survivors, but these individuals have far more severe injuries and disabilities. The military case manager has become an essential member of the multidisciplinary team that orchestrates the care and services for wounded warriors. The amputation rate for soldiers injured in these wars is 100% (!) higher than in previous wars, notes Cobb. Obviously, the decisions and care surrounding these events are stressful and emotional ones; support for the service personnel and their families is an ongoing process.

Case management in the military setting starts even before the patient arrives from the battlefield, where stabilization and urgent care are provided. The geographic location and availability of appropriate care and services often become key considerations in the development of the care plan. The soldier may be attached to a command in one state, but resides in another; family, after facing the emotionally devastating event of the injury of their loved one, want the care to be arranged close to home. The reality, however, is that the requirements of care, that is, wound care, pain management, and so forth, may be more than the family can manage. Additionally, research has shown that many combat-injury patients do better when recuperating with other military casualties. Case managers, then, provide the care coordination in distant locations, arrange temporary housing for families, coordinate spiritual and psychological counseling, and instill hope toward recovery.

During the past few years, investigations have been conducted into the care military personnel receive. There are concerns regarding the disconnects across the continuum, delays in care, poor communication, and a fragmented, convoluted system, and the role of the case manager becomes an emerging leader. Cobb concludes, "Case management is critical in easing an injured service member's recovery and post-injury rehabilitation and re-entry into civilian society, and in meeting the goal of preserving our nation's military readiness."[12]

CONCLUSION

As the public sector of healthcare continues to expand, there will be ongoing opportunities for case managers. This practice setting is one of the more demanding ones because of the bureaucratic structure of the government, the convoluted healthcare system, the financial constraints of the funding programs, and the disproportionate numbers of individuals who present with the most challenging situations and conditions. It is, however, one of the more rewarding settings because we have the unique opportunity to help those who need our assistance most. Isn't that, after all, at the heart of case management?

NOTES

1. Karen Davis and Cathy Schoen, "Testimony—Using What Works: Medicare, Medicaid, and the State Children's Health Insurance Program as a Base for Health Care Reform," September 18, 2008, http://www.commonwealthfund.org/publications/publications_show.htm?doc_id=706151 (accessed February 27, 2009).
2. Centers for Medicare and Medicaid Services, "CMS Proposes to Expand Quality Program for Hospital Inpatient Services in FY 2009" (press release), April 14, 2008, http://www.cms.hhs.gov/apps/media/press/release.asp?Counter=3041&intNumPerPage=10&checkDate=&checkKey=&srchType=1&numDays=3500&srchOpt=0&srchData=&srchOpt=0&srchData=&keywordType=All&chkNewsType=1,+2,+3,+4,+5&intPage=&showAll=&pYear=&year=&desc (accessed February 27, 2009).
3. Centers for Medicare and Medicaid Services, "CMS Proposes."
4. Burt C, McCaig L, and Smith A, "Emergency Department Visits by Persons Recently Discharged from U.S. Hospitals," *National Health Statistics Reports* no. 6 (July 24, 2008).
5. Alexander J, "CMS Issues Management Advisory Report," *Healthcare Financial Management,* May 1, 2008.
6. Mager K, "Building a Better Medicare," *Case in Point,* June/July 2007, 25–29.
7. Garrett M, "Understanding Medicaid—What Case Managers Need to Know," *Professional Case Management* 13, no. 3 (May–June 2008), 123–125.
8. Mager, "Building a Better Medicare," 25–29.
9. Garrett, "Understanding Medicaid," 123–125.
10. Cobb A, "Case Managers Care for Casualties of War," *Case in Point,* Winter 2006, 29–32.
11. Bilmes L, "Soldiers Returning from Iraq and Afghanistan: The Long-Term Costs of Providing Veterans Medical Care and Disability Benefits," KSG Faculty Research Working Paper Series (Cambridge, MA: Harvard University John F. Kennedy School of Government, January 8, 2007).
12. Bilmes, "Soldiers Returning from Iraq and Afghanistan."

Cases in Profile

HIGH-RISK PREGNANCY

Case Overview

Mrs. K, a pregnant 39-year-old, was identified for case management during her hospital admission for a cerclage for an incompetent cervix. This procedure was performed at the 17th week, when it was also discovered that the patient had developed gestational diabetes, requiring the administration of insulin twice daily. Further complicating her condition was morbid obesity, her weight was 339 pounds, and this was her ninth pregnancy. She had had five elective terminations and two spontaneous abortions. Her only child, an 18-year-old, was in college in North Carolina, and the patient lived in Brooklyn with her fiancé, also a diabetic.

Problems Identified

In addition to the aforementioned, the following problems were identified and resolved by the case manager:

1. The patient was to use a glucometer and test strips; however, the plan covered the glucometer only, with supplies to be paid for by the claimant. She was on disability with markedly decreased income and could not afford the test strips. Intervention: Case manager contacted plan administrator, obtained approval for reimbursement, following exploration of risks and potential costs without the necessary supplies.

2. Claimant was to maintain bed rest, except for bathroom privileges and visits to high-risk obstetrician every 2 weeks. Case manager learned that the claimant had walked three blocks to MD because fiancé had his driver's license suspended. Intervention: Case manager referred to social worker for funding assistance for transportation, which was obtained.

3. Claimant's blood sugars continued to be very unstable. Case manager learned claimant often skipped breakfast and then felt no need to take insulin. Also, not compliant with calls to MD three times a week to report blood sugar readings. Intervention: Case manager reinforced MD instructions, discussed risks to claimant and baby, and contacted nurse practitioner in MD office to have calls made to claimant that provided more support and closer monitoring.

4. During the sixth month, the claimant experienced cramping, diagnosed as contractions, and was not a candidate for home uterine monitoring (due to excess weight, monitor would not detect contractions). Started on Brethene with further instructions for hydration and bed rest. Case manager learned the claimant was snacking more since she was home all the time. Intervention: Case manager provided more education, and in discussion of hobbies and interests, asked if the claimant ever knitted, crocheted, etc., and learned the claimant used to "years ago." Case manager suggested resuming this hobby to keep hands and mind busy, making a baby blanket or sweater as early gift for baby (promoting commitment to unborn child).

5. Late in the sixth month, during a call to the claimant, this case manager learned she is not feeling well, had a cold several days ago, and, upon further questioning, case manager learned the claimant was having more frequent urination and some burning (did not mention during call from nurse practitioner, thought it might be from Brethene). Intervention: Case manager contacted MD's office to have claimant seen. Urinary tract infection was diagnosed; claimant was placed on antibiotics.

6. During 34th week, in weekly call to claimant, case manager learned the claimant was retaining fluid and always thirsty. To quench thirst during hot weather, she was drinking more tomato juice, adding more salt to foods, etc. Blood sugars also more unstable. Intervention: Case manager contacted MD's office and suggested nursing visits for closer monitoring of blood pressure, blood sugars, and fetal assessments; MD in agreement. Case manager arranged for services, negotiated fees, and continued to monitor claimant with calls to her, MD, and nursing agency.

Outcome

Claimant's cerclage released during 37th week and several days later delivered a healthy six-pound, two-ounce baby girl. Claimant and infant went home in 2 days (baby blanket knitted by mom finished "just in time").

Potential Charges and Savings

Without case management intervention, this patient would have had at least three hospital admissions, each one of 3 to 5 days' duration, to treat diabetic complications, urinary tract infection, premature labor episodes, or toxemia. Without our intervention, it is highly likely that a premature baby would have been born and at the very least, mother would have been hospitalized for monitoring for the last 3 to 4 weeks of her pregnancy.

  3 hospital admissions at 3 days each at $1,500/day = $13,500 for various
    complications
  3-week hospital admission at $1,500/day for monitoring = $31,500
  Total savings if premature baby was avoided = $45,000
  If premature baby had been the result, costs would be higher with a
    length of stay of 45 days in Neonatal ICU at $2,500/day = $112,500
  Total savings if preemie baby was born = $157,500

Analysis

As can be seen with this case, continuous intervention by the case manager allowed for early identification and resolution of many problems, which prevented more costly complications to the claimant and her child. The case manager was creative, persistent, and focused on the goal of a healthy baby and a safe pregnancy. This woman presented many challenges (aside from her medical problems), and the advocacy role assumed by the case manager resulted in better quality of care, excellent outcome, and demonstrated savings to the plan.

LONG-TERM CASE MANAGEMENT FOR CHRONIC DISEASE MANAGEMENT

Case Overview

An 18-year-old female was identified for case management during an admission to the hospital for seizure disorder, deliberate overdosing with Tegretol (antiseizure medication), depression, lupus, and kidney failure. Past history included cardiac surgery at age 8 and the diagnosis of lupus with progression of symptoms since age 10. This young girl's mother had died 1 year ago; her father was also hospitalized during this girl's admission for treatment of coronary disease and diabetes. He would be unable to be a care provider for his daughter, who would need home care following treatment of her serious conditions. Although this young girl had multiple problems, she was in a university children's hospital, whose healthcare team was most receptive to case management intervention.

Problems Identified

The following problems were identified and resolved by the case manager during the initial 6 months of intervention:

1. After treatment for her acute medical conditions, and before she could go home, she required inpatient treatment for her severe depression. The facility recommended was not a provider within the father's medical plan; if she were admitted here, reimbursement would be limited to 70% of the charges. The father would be unable to pay the 30% co-payment. Intervention: Case manager obtained approval from the plan administrator for reimbursement at 100% if case manager was able to negotiate a network fee. Case manager worked with CFO of facility and negotiated the approved rate.
2. After inpatient treatment of her medical and psychological conditions, it was determined that there was much anger/stress between the father and daughter, especially since the death of her mother. Counseling was recommended for both; however, the father refused to partake in sessions. There was no network provider within walking distance from the girl's home, and the father was unwilling to commit to providing the necessary transportation. Intervention: Case manager was able to locate a therapist with expertise in treating adolescents with chronic conditions, negotiated with her to accept network fee reimbursement, and negotiated with the plan to approve her in the network. In addition, the claimant was referred to a support group, located by case manager, for persons with lupus.
3. The claimant's progression of symptoms had already resulted in a kidney failure and, in an effort to reduce the severity of the progression, she would need monthly infusions of Cytoxan and weekly lab work. This girl was in her senior year of high school, had already missed much school, and further absences would jeopardize her graduation. Intervention: Case manager arranged for infusion and laboratory services after school hours and at negotiated rates.

Outcome

This girl's situation eventually stabilized and the file was closed; however, because of her prior history of noncompliance as well as low IQ, the therapist and physician were advised to contact the case manager for any further problems. Within 4 months, the claimant's symptoms had become more severe, she was having two to three seizures per day, her blood pressure had become elevated, she was showing subtherapeutic levels of medications in laboratory findings, and she was not keeping medical appointments. Both the physician and therapist contacted the case manager and the file was reopened. The case manager identified and resolved the following problems during the second phase of case management intervention, which took place over 5 months:

1. The claimant, no longer needing Cytoxan, was placed on a complex medication regimen and was being seen by a rheumatologist, neurologist, nephrologist, and psychiatrist, all of whom were changing and adjusting medications. Case manager, in reviewing medications and in conversation with MDs, patient, and her father, determined that patient once again was very depressed, overwhelmed with diet and medications, and was now dating a "nice boy" and just "wanted to be normal." Intervention: Case manager scheduled a meeting with patient, father, therapist, rheumatologist (who, at the request of case manager, agreed to act as coordinator of care with all medication changes going through him), and case manager for a Saturday morning (to accommodate patient's school requirements and father's need to not miss any more days from work with the risk of loss of medical benefits). Patient's IQ of 85 with possible neurological compromise secondary to increased seizure activity and complex medication schedule (some different doses on alternate days) were all determined to be factors contributing to noncompliance. The patient was encouraged to verbalize her concerns and desire to be "normal." She agreed to resume counseling and keep all medical appointments. Case manager worked with MD, patient, and patient's father regarding medication schedule. Dispenser/calendar system was developed and used successfully.

2. Patient's father, also experiencing medical complications, was feeling overwhelmed with care responsibilities for his daughter and had not really grieved since the death of his wife (who was closer to his daughter and was his "best friend"). Case manager learned this during calls to him and realized that he, too, needed intervention. Intervention: Case manager located a therapist near father's place of work and secured his agreement to attend "just one visit." The session was a good one and he agreed to continue. He became more compliant with his medication, diet, and visits to MD and began working in strategies to assist his daughter.

Potential Charges and Savings

For this young girl, at best several hospital admissions for seizure disorder, kidney failure, acute depression, and lupus exacerbations were avoided. Prior to our involvement, she had five hospital admissions with length of stay ranging from 7 to 19 days each. Conservative estimate of savings from her would be a minimum of $100,000. Additional savings could be realized from the minimal intervention with the father, as well.

Analysis

This case presented multiple and serious medical, psychosocial and financial issues that, without the assistance of a case manager, would have resulted in further deterioration and possible death of this young girl. Case managers should also understand from this presentation how vitally important it is to discover and address the psychosocial factors as well as family issues. Working as a member of the healthcare team, but also as a key negotiator and patient advocate, the case manager became the individual responsible for the success of this case.

PEDIATRIC ASTHMA

Case Overview

A 7-year-old boy was identified for case management when he was admitted to the hospital for the third time in 5 months for asthma, this time with an additional complication of pneumonia. This child is the oldest of three children and lives in a rural area of Mississippi with his parents. The family had just moved from Georgia, the father disabled since 1995, and the mother (the insured) employed 9 months with the current employer and provider of benefits. Prior history indicates a 5-year history of frequent asthma episodes treated in urgent care centers and emergency departments with several hospital admissions each year. The case management goal was to obtain stability of this medical condition with child and parents and to increase knowledge and compliance.

Problems Identified

During the 6 months of case management intervention, the following problems were identified and resolved by the case manager:

1. Initially, parents were very resistant to assistance from case manager. The mother, especially, was concerned that her employer

might know about all the admissions and bills, and that she might now be in danger of losing her job and medical coverage for her family. She also stated that she could not afford case management. Intervention: Case manager spent much time explaining how her son was identified for intervention, that this was part of her benefit coverage and was offered at no cost to her, and that her supervisor or managers were not involved nor would any of this be discussed with them. Finally, she provided consent, and an appointment for a visit to their home was scheduled.

2. During the home visit, the case manager noted the presence of a cat and dog as family pets, as well as carpeting in the child's room, a down comforter and pillow on his bed, and a father who smokes although he acknowledged that he was trying to stop. Intervention: Case manager discussed with parents and child that the aforementioned factors were highly probable in triggering child's asthma episodes. She recommended that nonallergic bedding be used, carpet be removed, that pets at least for the time be given to a friend, and that any smoking be done outdoors. Parents agreed and complied with requests.

3. Child had been treated by many pediatricians and family practitioners at several centers. As the case manager discussed the importance of continuity of care, the parents with much embarrassment informed her of the reason for this. Their prior insurance company required a 20% co-payment and, with the increased number of doctor visits and emergency room and hospital admissions, they were having financial problems with doctors who refused further treatment unless a payment was made at the time of their visit. Hospital emergency rooms did not require this payment, which is why the family used them more. Intervention: Case manager explained that current insurance would have a $10 co-pay for network MDs and that the case manager would intervene and arrange for assistance with the billing department. She also stressed the importance of ongoing involvement with one physician for continuity and for a better ability to evaluate and modify treatment, medications, etc.

4. The child was having clusters of episodes that the mother acknowledged she tried to treat herself with over-the-counter medications. When his temperature would start to go up, she would use the antibiotics that she "saved" from the last episode (or from another child in the family). She explained that because the antibiotics were so expensive, she tried to make them last. Intervention: Case manager explained the process of therapeutic blood levels of antibiotic steroids, bronchodilators, etc., what occurs when medications are

not taken as directed, reasons why over-the-counter preparations are contraindicated for children with asthma, etc. She also stressed that until the child's condition could be evaluated further, prompt attention by a physician needed to occur sooner rather than later. The parents related that no one had ever explained all of this to them.

5. The child had been seen by many different doctors but had never been evaluated by a pediatric pulmonologist. Because of the increasing severity of episodes, the case manager discussed this with parents and suggested that they request a referral from the present pediatrician. The parents were very reluctant to do this, because they were afraid of making the doctor angry. Intervention: Case manager, after determining parents' interest in obtaining this consult, offered to intervene on their behalf with current pediatrician. This was done and arrangements were made.

6. Following child's evaluation by a pediatric pulmonologist, it was determined that he would be a good candidate for an asthma disease management program that this group practice had available. The plan, however, had language that did not cover "educational services." Intervention: Case manager contacted plan administrator, explained child's history, financial risks to the plan (i.e., costs of continuing hospital admissions, emergency room visits, etc.), and emphasized the parents' willingness and demonstrated cooperation to date. Also advised that fees for program could be negotiated. Approval was obtained, and child and parents completed the program's initial phase of risk analysis and education and will continue to be followed indefinitely at minimal cost.

Outcome

Many escalating and potential problems were addressed during this time. Coordination among physicians, corrections of medication misuse, and asthma education all contributed to an improved and healthier lifestyle.

Potential Charges and Savings

Had case management not been involved, child had strong probability of continuing with multiple emergency department visits and several hospital admissions. Each emergency department visit was averaging $600 with 10 per year (this per mother) and 5 admissions varying in length from 5 to 10 days each. Potential charges for this child could have been between $50,000 to $60,000. For the year that included case management involvement, there were only two emergency department visits and no hospital admissions.

Analysis

With the illustration of this child's situation, case managers should be able to appreciate the value of getting "up close and personal." This was clearly a case that was being lost in the healthcare system and the financial difficulties of a family. Too often, we do not stop to uncover the reasons behind the problems and costs. As demonstrated in this case, each problem (once identified) had a relatively easy solution. Success can be attained using the sound principles of case management throughout the process. Improved outcomes, quality of care, and savings were measurable in this case, as was the parents' satisfaction as measured by a positive response to a survey sent to them.

AIDS MANAGEMENT

Case Overview

This 51-year-old male was identified for case management during his admission to the hospital for weakness of the left upper extremity and slurred speech. No definitive diagnosis was made at the time of this admission or at a subsequent admission to a different hospital 5 weeks later for the same symptomatology. His prior history was a diagnosis of HIV 10 years ago secondary to IV use of heroin. The claimant stopped the use of heroin at the time of the HIV diagnosis and up until 1 year prior to the hospital admission had received no consistent medical care. Throughout those many years, he took AZT but acknowledged that he did not take it as prescribed. There were frequent changes in physicians because of "personality clashes and other differences." Recent blood tests showed the toxoplasmosis, but CAT scans and MRIs of the brain were "inconclusive." The claimant was married. His wife was stated to be very supportive but under increasing stress because of his mood swings and angry outbursts, including threats to sign himself out of the hospital against medical advice. This man was employed as a supervisor of a trucking firm, had been working continuously (other than during these two hospital admissions), and was determined to return to work so as not to lose his benefits. Although seen by an infectious disease specialist while hospitalized, the claimant was anxious to return to his internist for ongoing care, citing that his condition was not "serious enough" to require a specialist.

Problems Identified

This case has been open for more than 1 year, and it is expected that case management intervention will be beneficial and warranted for the foreseeable future. The following illustrates just some of the problems that were identified and resolved by the case manager.

1. Claimant was being treated in local hospitals, by multiple physicians without the benefit of currently recommended drug protocol for AIDS, including protease inhibitors. Due to less-than-optimum treatment and symptoms highly probable of toxoplasmosis, his continued deterioration was likely. Claimant was extremely fearful, controlling, and in denial about his condition. He preferred to believe that he had had a mild stroke, saying, "All I need is some physical and speech therapy." Intervention: Case manager spent time establishing rapport and gaining trust of this very frightened man. She provided him with information and educational materials about the advances in the treatment of AIDS from a renowned university hospital with acknowledged expertise in this condition. She asked him to at least consider a consultation visit in order for him to be able to make an informed decision, including the option to remain with the current physician. The claimant did agree and the case manager made the arrangements and attended the appointment with him and his wife.

2. Claimant was pleased with consultation visit and treatment and attended several visits. In a follow-up call to the physician, case manager learned that he had not kept most recent appointment. Intervention: Case manager called claimant's home and was told that the trips into the city were taking too long, requiring at least a half-day from work. He was concerned that his boss was becoming less understanding and asking questions about his condition. Case manager called the physician group, explained concerns of claimant and asked for names of university-affiliated infectious disease specialists nearer to the claimant's home or place of work. Obtained names of three MDs; however, none were in the employer's plan's network. Case manager contacted plan administrator and obtained approval for physician selected by claimant.

3. Before setting an appointment with this MD, his office requested copies of hospital records (from the second most recent admissions) including MRIs, CAT scans, and laboratory tests. Claimant and his wife had difficulty in speaking to the appropriate person at each of

the hospitals, and then were told that there would be charges (payable in advance). When they called the plan's claims department to see if this would be covered, they were told "no." Intervention: Case manager contacted plan administrator, explained that not getting records would necessitate duplication of tests, further delay in treatment. Approval was obtained from the plan administrator and the hospitals agreed to submit claims for prompt payment through the case manager, who would expedite process.

4. Claimant was started on the recommended drug protocol including a protease inhibitor. His condition began to improve; however, in one of her follow-up calls to the claimant, the case manager learned that he had abruptly discontinued the protease inhibitor because of pain and left side abdominal bloating. Intervention: Remembering from her review of claimant's medical records a finding of a left adrenal tumor 1 year ago (felt to be benign but with advisory for reevaluation in order to monitor size, etc.), the case manager contacted the infectious disease specialist to discuss her concerns as well as to alert him about claimant's discontinuance of Crixovan (the protease inhibitor). Referral to an endocrinologist was made. The tumor had changed minimally but did not require surgical intervention. The claimant was placed on Viracept (another protease inhibitor, felt to have fewer side effects), which has been well-tolerated. Both MD and case manager have explained dangers involved in claimant's adjusting dosage, times, and medications without MD consultation. (The concern is that the HIV will develop immunity to these drugs, especially with the abrupt starting and stopping of the drugs.)

Outcome

Many other problems were resolved during this time. These included assisting with a return to work, referral to a support group, and ongoing advocacy for the claimant and his wife as they coped with the realities of this disease.

Potential Charges and Savings

Case management was definitely responsible for the avoidance of many charges that most certainly would have occurred. These included at least two hospital admissions (secondary to noncompliance and the resulting complications or deterioration of his condition) and duplication of testing and doctor visits as the claimant continued his pursuit of treatment from multiple physicians without appropriate expertise.

Analysis

The problems illustrated in this case are somewhat typical of those of patients dealing with life-threatening medical conditions. The desire to be in control, feelings of anxiety, and mistrust sometimes to the point of self-destruction are often seen. Patients need to be accepted where they are, and we must acknowledge their feelings while at the same time keeping them from harm's way. Continuous involvement by the case manager allowed for prompt intervention and resulted in improved, more appropriate care for this patient. Because of ongoing problems with noncompliance and real potential for further problems, this case will remain open. Activity of the case manager will be determined by the stability of the patient. Although the addition of protease inhibitors has greatly improved life expectancy for HIV patients and has changed case management, it is still more cost-effective to prevent problems than resolve them. Case management will continue to be an effective strategy in improving outcomes and demonstrating savings.

DIABETES

Case Overview

Mrs. S, a 58-year-old Caucasian female, was identified for case management during her hospital admission for a left thalamic CVA. She presented to the emergency room with complaints of numbness to the face, jaw, and right arm; dizziness; and right hemiplegia. It was noted that she had been diagnosed with type 2 diabetes 3 years prior, had not seen a physician in 1 year, and had a blood sugar on admission of 525. Mrs. S was a smoker, had a cholesterol of 221, and her triglycerides were 450. Her blood pressure in the ER was 149/99. She was not taking any medications or following any diet plan. She was divorced, and lived with her daughter, son-in-law, and grandchildren in rural Tennessee. Prior to the event, she was employed as a loader in a factory on the evening shift.

Problems Identified

The following problems were identified and resolved by the case manager:

1. Mrs. S was in need of extensive rehabilitation in order to return to her baseline functioning and return to work. Intervention: The case manager worked closely with her healthcare team and arranged for timely transition from acute care to their network participating

rehabilitation unit. When able, she was transitioned to a three times weekly outpatient program. Prior to returning to work, the case manager arranged for the occupational therapist to visit the patient's employer and evaluate her workstation and duties for safety in light of her minor residual limitations.

2. The patient had not followed a diabetic or low cholesterol meal plan in the past and did not understand the importance of it. She was started on Glucophage at the time of diagnosis, but stopped this on her own believing it to be the cause of occasional diarrhea. She was not checking her blood sugar at home. She continued to smoke and had not been educated regarding the relationship between smoking and coronary artery disease. Mrs. S was obese at 179 lbs. and a height of 5'. She had not seen a physician nor taken any medications in over 1 year. Intervention: The attending neurologist was contacted by the case manager and he agreed to consult with a network participating endocrinologist. The case manager requested the hospital's dietitian see the patient for an assessment, recommendations, and to begin teaching. The case manager obtained a prescription and letter of medical necessity for a glucometer and testing supplies, which the family picked up and brought to the rehab unit prior to discharge. This intervention allowed the claimant and her daughter to become proficient with blood sugar testing while nursing support was available. She was also instructed on drawing up and administering insulin prior to discharge. Her progress was monitored closely by communicating regularly with the dietitian and diabetes educator.

3. Mrs. S was diagnosed with coronary artery disease resulting from cardiovascular system compromise due to hyperlipidemia and hyperglycemia. A combination of high blood pressure, insulin resistance, and high levels of fats in the blood had increased her risk of heart disease and stroke significantly. If all three conditions were not brought under control, she would continue to be at high risk for future complications. The patient had never received any diabetic education, did not understand the relationship of her coronary artery disease and hypertension to diabetes, and it was felt this was the major reason for her past noncompliance. Intervention: The case manager contacted the patient at the bedside and discussed the importance of self-management education and following her physician's plan of care in order to reduce future risks. The patient verbalized understanding and a willingness to learn. The case manager, therefore, arranged for bedside education from the registered

dietitian and diabetes educator to continue on a daily basis while in the rehab unit. The patient's daughter was included in several training sessions. One follow-up skilled nursing visit was arranged by the case manager to evaluate the patient in her home environment, reinforce teaching, and answer any questions. The case manager continued to monitor the patient closely by contacting her twice weekly by phone and maintaining communication with her health-care team.

Outcome

Upon completion of her 14-day inpatient rehab stay and several-week outpatient rehab program, the patient was able to demonstrate the ability to safely perform her work duties without modification to her employer and the occupational therapist. She was allowed to return to work 4 hours per day initially and gradually transitioned to a full shift. Because she was her sole source of support, it was vital she be able to return to gainful employment.

The endocrinologist started the patient on a multidrug regimen including insulin. The physician made continuing adjustments until her blood sugars were well-controlled. After discharge, the case manager contacted the hospital's diabetes center and learned patients newly diagnosed with diabetes in their facility could attend a 2-day class free of the usual $480 fee. Orders were received and the claimant was enrolled in the class that she attended with a family member. The patient continued to see her endocrinologist every 3 months for follow-up care. She was compliant with her dietary and medication regimen, lost 14 pounds in 3 months, began a walking program, and joined a diabetes support group. The patient stopped smoking while hospitalized and remains smoke free to date. Most significantly, Mrs. S reduced her baseline HbA1c from 14.3% (goal = <7%) to 7.8% 3 months after her CVA.

Potential Charges and Savings

Without case management intervention, the claimant would have likely been discharged from rehab without having received the much needed diabetes education that was the key to her future compliance with her plan of care and avoidance of readmission to date (2 years later). It is unlikely she would have received the specialized endocrinology care, which resulted in bringing her blood sugars under control and keeping them stable, lowering her risk for repeat strokes, heart attack, and other diabetic complications. Had case management not been involved to arrange her formal diabetes class, the plan would have been billed for the class. In addition, the patient certainly would have been discharged prematurely from rehab without achieving adequate diabetes control that would have placed her at great risk for a diabetic emergency and multiple future readmissions.

Diabetes class = $480
3 hospital admissions for various complications, 5 days each at
    $1,500/day = $22,500
Associated MD fees of $100/day × 15 days = $1,500
5 emergency room visits for diabetic complications at $750/visit
    = $3,750
Total avoided charges = $28,230

Analysis

This case demonstrates the positive outcomes that can be achieved when the diabetes patient is motivated, a window of opportunity is seized, and the appropriate self-management tools are made available. Further, continuous monitoring and intervention by the case manager allowed for resolution and prevention of multiple interrelated problems that improved the patient's quality of life and reduced exposure to the plan.

ONCOLOGY MANAGEMENT

Case Overview

Mrs. H, a 58-year-old Hispanic female, was identified for case management when she was scheduled to undergo an abdominal perineal resection with creation of a permanent colostomy for adenocarcinoma of the colon. The claimant lived with her husband in Woodhaven, New York. Her husband was the insured and worked nights. She had an adult daughter living outside the home who was very supportive. The claimant was contacted and offered case management, but she declined.

Four months after her surgery, she continued to experience significant abdominal pain. She saw her surgeon for this problem and was prescribed anti-inflammatory and pain medications. He advised the claimant the pain was due to adhesions. A CAT scan was negative for tumor and did not reveal any significant pathology. The surgeon recommended she see her gynecologist for an evaluation. Meanwhile, she continued to take pain medicines. The patient saw her gynecologist 7 months after her initial surgery. She was diagnosed with a urinary tract infection and started on antibiotics. The gynecologist could find no reason for her chronic pain other than psychological issues related to the radical surgery and her husband's aversion to the colostomy. He suggested she seek counseling for this problem and started Mrs. H on antidepressants. She was scheduled for a hysteroscopy in order to visualize the uterine vault and also referred to a urologist for evaluation. The hysteroscopy with biopsies ruled out any uterine pathology.

Nine months after her initial surgery, she continued to complain of significant pain that was causing problems with her mobility. The patient began to walk with a cane. The pain was initially described as being low in the pelvis. Later, she began to complain of a burning pain in her thighs. She was referred to a neurologist who diagnosed the patient with degenerative disc disease and arthritis, which he felt was the source of her pain.

Eleven months following her initial surgery, she developed back pain in addition to the persistent burning sensations in her thighs. She was referred to a rheumatologist for evaluation. He performed an MRI, which was negative. In the interim, she was referred to an orthopedic surgeon who specialized in spinal problems. He could find no answer for the patient's chronic pain. A routine follow-up colonoscopy was performed 1 year after her surgery. The results were negative. She continued to see her urologist for worsening bladder function.

One month later, the claimant was admitted with urinary retention. She was again contacted regarding case management and this time she agreed. During this admission, a mass was identified that was compressing a ureter. Further study revealed widespread metastasis of her cancer. The case manager worked with the urologist to locate a network participating oncologist who specialized in colon cancer at a well-known metropolitan cancer center.

The case manager coordinated arrangements for a visit a few days after discharge. At that visit, participation in a clinical trial was discussed. However, after consideration, the claimant and her daughter declined. Alternatively, a plan to proceed with traditional chemotherapy was decided upon. Case management worked closely with the oncologist and his staff to arrive at a plan that allowed each chemotherapy treatment to be initiated at the cancer center and continued for 48 hours at home. The case manager made arrangements for the daughter to be trained to discontinue the infusion and perform line care. This avoided the need for an inpatient stay or skilled nursing visits. When the patient's red blood count dropped as a result of her chemotherapy, Epoetin therapy was initiated. The case manager contacted the oncologist who agreed to allow the expensive drug to be purchased through the patient's pharmacy plan and delivered to her home, as opposed to purchasing it from the cancer center at a much higher price. This intervention resulted in conservation of the patient's limited benefits and significant savings to the plan. She was started on an effective pain management regimen by the oncologist, who was familiar with her type of pain, and currently reports she is pain free. Unfortunately, the patient's prognosis is poor.

Problems Identified

The following problems were identified and resolved by the case manager:

1. Mrs. H received fragmented care for 1 year, which did not identify the source of her pain. During this time, she did not receive appropriate care for her cancer, which was spreading. In addition to pain and suffering, her benefit dollars were not used efficiently. Had the patient agreed to case management when initially offered, this unfortunate scenario might have been prevented. Intervention: After the patient agreed to case management, the admitting urologist was contacted promptly and a plan agreed upon to have the patient evaluated at a Center of Excellence by a specialist in her type of cancer.

2. The patient's chemotherapy needed to be infused over 48 hours. Intervention: To prevent an inpatient stay or skilled nursing visit, the case manager arranged for the daughter to be trained to discontinue the infusion and perform her line care.

3. The patient required expensive medication to address her low blood counts. Intervention: As an alternative to purchasing the drug at the cancer center at a price 100% above AWP, the case manager arranged to obtain the drug through a pharmaceutical house participating with the patient's pharmacy network. The drug was delivered to the patient's home, and she brought it with her to her cancer center visits for administration. This intervention resulted in significant savings to the plan and conservation of the patient's limited benefit resources.

Outcome

The patient's care became prompt, efficient, and cost-effective as a result of case management intervention. Her much needed benefit dollars were spent only for medically necessary care that was expertly coordinated through one physician and facility. Past problems with poor communication between multiple physicians were eliminated.

Potential Charges and Savings

Without case management intervention, the patient would have required, at minimum, one skilled nursing visit every 2 weeks for discontinuation of her chemotherapy infusion and line care. Over the 6-month regimen, this would amount to twelve visits. In addition, the Epoetin she received twice monthly (12 doses) would have been purchased from the cancer center at a cost 100% above AWP ($4,129.44 per dose) as opposed to 14% below AWP ($1,775.66 per dose).

Skilled nursing visits 12 avoided at $130/visit = $1,560
Drug costs avoided = $28,245.36
Total avoided charges = $29,805.36

Analysis

This case demonstrates the value of care coordinated by a case manager to avoid fragmentation, poor communication, wasted benefit dollars, and to facilitate prompt identification and intervention for health problems. Unfortunately, the patient did not have case management services for 1 year after her initial cancer surgery. If she had, it is likely the outcome would have been different and would have greatly affected her quality of life and the amount of healthcare dollars spent.

MORBID OBESITY/GASTRIC BYPASS

Case Overview

Mrs. C, a 39-year-old female, was identified for case management during precertification for a planned gastric bypass procedure. The claimant was 5'9" and weighed 370 pounds, giving her a body mass index (BMI) of 46 (a BMI of 20–25 is the ideal range for an adult, and a BMI of greater than 40 indicates a serious weight problem and carries the greatest risk for medical complications). The claimant had been overweight her entire life, and had tried numerous diets, including use of prescription weight-loss medication without demonstrable success. She had a medical comorbidity of hypertension for which she takes one prescription agent with marginal control.

She reported frequent daytime headaches and somnolence, which she attributed to poorly controlled blood pressure. The claimant also told of severe bouts of hunger during the day despite eating three full meals, often binging on high carbohydrate snacks and fast foods, and drinking approximately one liter of full calorie soda per day. Upon exertion, she experienced shortness of breath and demonstrated bilateral pitting edema to her lower extremities.

She experienced recurrent vaginal and urinary tract infections, which she suggested were caused by poor hygiene due to her large body habitus. However, she avoided medical intervention due to embarrassment about her weight and shame discussing this issue with her male primary care physician. In addition, Mrs. C stated that her physician was not supportive of her plan to undergo gastric bypass surgery, as he felt that she was a poor surgical risk and should continue conservative weight-loss measures.

Employed as a laboratory technician, she said she suffered from social anxiety for fear of ridicule and had never sought psychological counseling for treatment. She had never married and had limited social supports. The main caregiver for her elderly parents who live nearby, she lived alone in a condominium apartment.

Problems Identified

The following problems were identified and resolved by the case manager during the 12 months of intervention:

1. Of concern was the claimant's untreated social anxiety, which if not immediately addressed, would hinder her attempts at independent health management. Intervention: The case manager provided an on-site visit to the claimant's home to develop a trusting relationship with the claimant. Mrs. C voiced her frustration over many failed weight-loss attempts, and spoke of the cycle of continued weight gain and using food to self-soothe her dissatisfaction with her health and appearance. The case manager researched a psychotherapist with experience in counseling food addictions, the claimant was referred to a psychiatrist to address her anxiety disorder, and was placed on appropriate short-term medication. With ongoing telephonic support from the case manager during the initial trial of medication, the patient showed improvement in her overall mood and increased work productivity in the weeks following psychiatric intervention.

2. Referred to a bariatric surgeon by a coworker, the patient underwent an initial surgical consultation and was advised to undergo an extensive medical evaluation prior to surgical consideration. For this, she needed support and direction to locate appropriate physicians

for medical clearance. Intervention: Working collaboratively with the claimant's primary care physician, the case manager researched and recommended appropriate specialists to address the claimant's medical issues, and researched a cardiologist for the claimant. Mrs. C underwent baseline cardiac testing including a Thallium Stress Test, which did not reveal any cardiac abnormalities. She was placed on a second blood pressure medication, which effectively controlled her blood pressure.

Noting that her daytime headaches and somnolence were suggestive of sleep apnea, the case manager researched a pulmonologist for the claimant and ensured appropriate scheduling of an outpatient sleep study, which confirmed a sleep apnea diagnosis. The case manager then found a DME company that offered sleep apnea classes to assist patients with use of the equipment in a small group setting. Although initially fearful of meeting with other patients, Mrs. C received emotional backing and encouragement from the case manager to foster compliance with group attendance. She also was given appropriate training and education in appropriate CPAP use, and suitable in-home follow-up by the DME company respiratory therapist. The claimant reported compliance with use, with resultant improved sleep and decreased headaches.

3. The case manager recognized that Mrs. C's frequent vaginal and urinary tract infections countered with her increased hunger might be indicative of an underlying diagnosis of diabetes. Intervention: She collaborated with the claimant's primary care physician, who ordered a glucose tolerance test for the claimant. The test confirmed a diagnosis of type 2 diabetes mellitus, and demonstrated a Hemoglobin A1C of 8.0. The patient was referred to an endocrinologist for further intervention, placed on appropriate oral medication, and given an appropriate carbohydrate-restricted diet. The case manager started blood glucose monitoring and recommended a Nutritionist consultation to provide in-depth diabetes education. Following Nutritionist collaboration, she provided extensive dietary support to Mrs. C, recommending lifestyle modifications, including substituting diet soda and water for full-calorie soda, and reading food labels to assist with carbohydrate monitoring. She also suggested a switch to a female gynecologist, who prescribed appropriate antibiotic medication to treat the patient's urinary tract infection. The case manager also promoted good health habits by reinforcing the need for monthly breast self-examinations and an annual pap smear.

4. Excluded from consideration for the less-risky laparoscopic gastric bypass procedure due to her extremely high BMI, Mrs. C was considered for the open surgical procedure, which would have resulted in a large abdominal incision and placed her at risk for wound infection and dehiscence due to her large protuberant abdomen. As bariatric surgery has significant peri- and postoperative risks, the case manager recommended preoperative weight loss for the claimant to decrease her BMI, decrease her risk for surgical complications, and allow for consideration of a laparoscopic procedure. With improvement in the patient's social anxiety, the case manager also recommended a second try with Weight Watchers for additional support with weight loss and meal planning. At the recommendation of the case manager, Mrs. C began attending a bariatric support group to provide further information and insight regarding her planned gastric bypass surgery. Intervention: The case manager accompanied Mrs. C to her initial Weight Watchers and bariatric support group meetings, and provided ongoing encouragement to her and assistance with appropriate meal planning. The patient regularly attended both Weight Watchers and the bariatric support group meetings, and kept a written log of her meals.

    When the case manager suggested that she identify her triggers to overeating, including frustration, anger, and sadness, the patient reported that she felt overwhelmed with caring for her parents, and that her siblings were not sharing in the responsibilities. Through collaboration with the patient's treating psychotherapist, the case manager worked on solutions to empower Mrs. C to confront her siblings on parental support issues, and assisted her with developing a schedule to delegate her parents' weekly shopping excursions and medical visits equitably with her siblings.

    Following a group effort with the claimant's primary care physician and cardiologist, the case manager assisted Mrs. C in designing a realistic exercise regimen of daily walking, advising her to park her car a further distance from her office and use the stairs to her third-floor apartment instead of the elevator. Through identification of triggers to stress, a support system with weight loss, and an achievable exercise program, the patient lost 50 pounds over the course of 5 months, successfully decreasing her BMI and making possible the less risky laparoscopic surgical procedure.

5. The case remained open during the peri- and postoperative period for Mrs. C's gastric bypass procedure. Intervention: The case manager educated the claimant regarding surgical expectations and

potential postoperative complications, recommending an additional Nutritionist visit for individualized information on meal size and necessary modifications in chewing and swallowing food to prevent vomiting postoperatively. The Nutritionist's teaching was reinforced with in-depth information on the necessary protein and vitamin requirements during the initial postoperative period and beyond.

6. The patient lacked postoperative home support. Intervention: With Mrs. C's permission, the case manager contacted her sister, who offered to help her sister during her initial hospital recovery, and arranged a home care visit to instruct the patient and her sister on management of her surgical drain and surgical incision sites. Mrs. C underwent laparoscopic gastric bypass surgery as scheduled, did not experience any postoperative complications, and was able to return to full-time employment 3 weeks after her surgery.

Outcome

This case was monitored for 6 months after the successful surgery. The case manager remained in close collaboration with Mrs. C's bariatric surgeon to monitor laboratory values and identify potential hemolytic and electrolyte imbalances that might occur postoperatively and taught the patient to interpret her lab data. She was compliant with ongoing physician follow-up on a monthly basis.

The patient lost 96 pounds after her surgery, representing a total weight loss of 146 pounds since case management intervention. She no longer suffered from sleep apnea and donated her purchased CPAP machine to her local church outreach program. She continues to demonstrate an ideal Hemoglobin A1C value of 5.5 and no longer requires medication to treat diabetes. Her disease is appropriately controlled through strict carbohydrate avoidance and ongoing endocrinology management, and she has no need for blood pressure medication now. She has joined a gym, practices aerobic exercise and strength training three times per week, and anticipates reaching her target weight of 150 pounds within the next 6-to-8 months. She continues to attend Weight Watchers and a bariatric support group, and has made new friends who have shared similar experiences. On a comparably limited basis, she has stayed with psychotherapy; her antianxiety medication has been discontinued and she makes good use of her stress management system. Mrs. C has several companions with whom she often meets socially, and is building a relationship with a man. She and her siblings have placed their parents in an assisted-living facility where they enjoy socialization with senior citizens and medical monitoring.

Potential Charges and Savings

For this claimant, several hospitalizations were avoided. Prior to case management intervention, the claimant had undiagnosed sleep apnea and diabetes mellitus, and severe social anxiety that inhibited her ability to seek appropriate medical intervention. Had her medical issues not been addressed, she would have certainly experienced hospitalization due to potential problems of sleep apnea, which include cardiac arrhythmias, narcolepsy, and stroke, and her diabetes would have gone undetected for an indeterminate period of time. Conservative hospital costs would have totaled approximately $75,000. Had morbid obesity not been addressed, she would have faced increased morbidity and mortality, with lifelong costs certainly totaling at least $1 million for treatment of preventable, obesity-related complications.

In addition, had case management not been involved to provide support and direction to the claimant with regard to preoperative weight loss, the claimant likely would have undergone the more risky open surgical procedure, and been at risk for postoperative complications because of her large body habitus, and for infection due to diabetes, all while lacking social support. Case management addressed the patient's potential complications, making possible the less-invasive surgical procedure and avoiding additional hospital costs for postoperative complications of approximately $20,000.

Analysis

This case presented multiple medical and psychosocial issues that, without the assistance of a case manager, would have resulted in further deterioration and possibly death of the claimant from preventable medical issues. Instead, through development of a trusting case management relationship, the patient was able to take control of her weight and fears with resultant medical, social, and spiritual success.

PEDIATRIC: LONG-TERM FEEDING DISORDER

Case Overview

This female claimant was born at 37 weeks gestation via Cesarean section with a birth weight of 3 pounds 5 ounces and had both cardiac problems (PDA) and a diaphragmatic hernia. She remained in the NICU for nearly 3 months. Among her medical issues were having only one functioning lung, failure to thrive due to gastroesophageal reflux, and persistent retching and other feeding difficulties. She was demonstrating developmental delays.

Before entering case management, the claimant had required and undergone surgical repair of hernia, ligation of the Patent Ductus Arteriosis (PDA), Nissan Fundoplication (surgery to address chronic issues of gastric reflux) for G.I. reflux and placement of a gastrostomy button (which became her sole source for feeding and hydration). When the claimant was 20 months of age and still totally dependent on gastrostomy feedings, as well as having become completely intolerant of any food, fluid, or objects placed in her mouth (other than her pacifier), the child's parents contacted the insurer seeking approval for her inpatient admission into Columbia Presbyterian Medical Center for a high-dollar 5-day intensive behaviorally based feeding program.

The insurer wanted the program and the potential outcomes of attendance and nonattendance researched; therefore, they requested case management services. They were seeking the input of the medical case manager and the entire medical team, and recommendations provided by the case manager for approval or denial of the requested admission.

The claimant's parents had become very stressed about the child's inability to "eat normally" and were rushing in any and all directions where they believed they would find quick answers to what was potentially becoming a lifelong problem. There had been repeat hospitalizations (high dollar) related to respiratory and feeding issues. The child's parents were insistent that the insurer cover the costs of each attempt at "fixing the problems" and had threatened legal action if denial of benefits was even suggested.

The insurer was concerned that there had been duplication of services and that benefit dollars had been spent on other unsuccessful attempts to improve this child's situation. Clearly, case management was needed to oversee needs, care, and costs.

In addition, the claimant's very limited DME coverage was quickly being depleted as the physicians had put in place at home an oximeter, oxygen, and feeding pump (all non-negotiated), prior to case management being brought into the case. This needed to be addressed in retroactive negotiation to maximize the claimant's DME benefit dollars.

Problems Identified

1. The claimant's oral intolerance had become so severe that it was projected by the G.I. team that she would require gastrostomy tube feedings for an undetermined number of years and possibly into adulthood unless there were more aggressive interventions made

(beyond the Early Intervention Program services that she had already been receiving without improvement in this area).

2. Immediate research into the history of this feeding program, its clinical outcomes, and its potential for success with this claimant needed to be undertaken by the case manager so that recommendations could be made to the insurer almost immediately (as the opening in the program was made available within a short window of time and would not occur again for many months).

3. The DME providers were initially resistant to retroactive negotiations, but due to outstanding claims were eventually persuaded by the case manager to negotiate to maintain the accounts ongoing on this potentially long-term case.

4. The Columbia Presbyterian Medical Center Feeding Program was designed as an intensive "learn to eat" program with a feeding/behavioral specialist taking on the total role of teacher. The parents, although able to be present, were strictly forbidden from interfering with the process. This, like many interventions before and after this program, caused great stress for the claimant's mother as she saw this as a failure in her role as mother and caregiver to her young child.

5. The insurer requested this case manager attend a feeding session at this program for observation and recording of the quality of the intervention, etc. There was some tolerance of formula via syringe introduced into the patient's mouth, but there was also much distress on the part of the claimant and her parents. There was "some" improvement per her gastroenterologist, but the claimant was a "long way from becoming an oral eater."

6. The claimant went on to require additional interventions and other short- and long-term feeding training (all of which the insurer wanted thoroughly researched and monitored for appropriateness prior to their approval of same).

7. The claimant's slow (but generally steady) feeding and developmental progress met with some concerns by the insurer as the case continued to be high-dollar because of the costs of the DME and supplies, as well as admissions for several attempts at feeding training in various settings because the Columbia Program was no longer an appropriate site to meet her changing needs.

8. The case manager was required to monitor and process claims, research all interventions, make appropriate recommendations to the insurer, monitor height and weight via physicians, and monitor all therapies involved in the claimant's care. The case

manager was required to work closely with the family on home-based follow-up of often difficult and emotionally draining feeding sessions.

9. At one point, the mother's frustration with the time it was taking and the slowed progress in her child's accepting oral feedings caused her to overstuff her daughter's mouth with food, leading to a potential choking episode and the acute need for emergent supportive intervention with the parents. The case manager expedited a report of same to the medical team and facilitated sensitive support and teaching with the mother to avoid future episodes related to her frustration.

10. Eventually, the claimant was deemed a candidate for admission into a multiweek Intensive Feeding Program. This would train her to eat, and prepare her caregivers (both parents and extended family, as needed) to feed her, monitor her caloric intake, and break through the rigid refusal process she had developed over the years of gastrostomy feedings, still her major source of hydration and nutrition.

11. This long-term program at the Kennedy Krieger Institute was very costly and required much in the way of negotiation by the case manager to make it a program the insurer would consider. The case manager did obtain a considerable discount for the program, and the claimant was enrolled. The case manager monitored and supported the family throughout the length of the program, and for the several months of home-based follow-up required for this child's successful accomplishment of oral feeding skills.

Outcome

This child was in case management for nearly 3 years and had the benefit of the continuity of one case manager throughout that time. When the case was closed to case management, the child was attending a regular preschool with her twin brother, where she was bringing in her own choices of snack and lunch items. She remained sensitive to certain textures and taste combinations. It was believed that she would work those things out as she continued to grow, thrive, and gain weight, all by oral intake. Before closing the case, the medical team and case manager saw her through an entire winter as there was potential for complications due to respiratory problems. She did well and did not require feeding supplementation via the gastrostomy tube, and her parents had a family celebration when she "said goodbye to tubey" after all those years of dependence on it for her survival.

Potential Charges and Savings

Psychological therapy services = $14,231
Emergency room visits = $3,000
Additional hospital admissions = $26,410
Associated hospital MD charges = $7,789.75
Costs of inpatient feeding program (multiweek hospital stay) = $103,320
Feeding program physicians fees = $7,745
Total Potential Charges = $162,495.75

Note: There were likely additional charges related to family issues that resulted from this child's feeding issues, which are not documented as the family members were not the "official case management client."

Analysis

As demonstrated with this case, sometimes case management services are not only needed early in the life of a child, but also may be necessary for quite a length of time. The interventions may be necessarily continuous, the case can be closed and reopened as the child grows and the needs change, or the case may be maintained on an extended-diary basis.

The case manager was able to avoid duplication of services, entry into less than clinically successful programs and settings by this vulnerable family, repeated hospitalizations, and the potential for injury to the child due to the severity of parental frustration, which often occurs in long-term feeding disorder cases. As demonstrated, there were very high potential charges for this child, and the continued and diligent involvement of this case manager kept the family, the medical team, and the insurer all focused upon the goal of teaching this child to eat like others and to be able to gain and maintain a normal weight for her growth and development. Although the case was often challenging and frustrating because it took so long to reach the goals, the dedication of the child's family, the provision of excellent case management, and the willingness of the insurer to flex some benefits, as needed, resulted in an outstanding outcome and high-dollar savings to the insurer.

PEDIATRIC: LONG-TERM RARE RESPIRATORY DISORDER

Case Overview

This 9-month-old female infant was a direct referral for case management from a private insurer (an indemnity plan) as they sought the case manager's pediatric expertise in assessing, intervening, and monitoring the present and projected long-term needs of this young child with a rare respiratory disorder. The infant resided at home with her parents and one older sibling.

Problems Identified

1. The claimant required mechanical ventilation during any periods of sleep. Her diagnosis of Congenital Central Hypoventilation Syndrome meant that whenever she was asleep, her neurological system would "forget" to trigger spontaneous breathing. She would simply stop breathing, leaving her at risk for respiratory failure and death.
2. The claimant's father traveled the country for business much of the time and was not available as a regular care provider, further necessitating home care nursing to assist this overwhelmed mother. The case manager immediately began to form a close working relationship with the healthcare providers and the claimant's mother (primary caregiver) to gain their trust. To avoid repeated hospitalizations or a catastrophic home care event to the claimant, she began telephonic teaching to the parent regarding home care management.
3. At the time of referral for case management, the insurer had been providing home nursing care services to the young patient because physicians would not discharge her to home without home care nurses in place day and night. The claimant's insurance benefits plan did not include a home care nursing benefit but, due to the complexity of the case, the insurer provided home care nursing on a temporary basis. When the insurer attempted to decrease the number of home care nursing hours provided, the parents threatened a lawsuit. The insurer sought a medically feasible way to meet this claimant's needs while decreasing the high-dollar costs of the case.
4. To maximize the claimant's existing benefit dollars in view of the anticipated long-term nature of this medically complex case, the insurer requested that case management negotiate out-of-network charges with the only nursing agency geographically available to provide home care nursing to this child. The case manager

accomplished such negotiations, as well as retroactive negotiations of nursing care, equipment, and supply claims, and the cost of the new ventilator equipment needed to meet the needs of this growing child.

5. This case was telephonic, as the claimant and the case manager were many states apart. This case manager had to rely upon the home care nurses, physicians, and specialty caregivers, as well as the claimant's parents to accurately portray the child's medical and developmental status and needs.

6. The parents were initially distrustful of the case manager, because the insurer had brought her onto the team. Soon, they came to rely on her ability to negotiate a better quality of home care nursing while teaching them (and the extended family of caregivers) how to manage on their own for those hours being slowly weaned down by the insurer.

7. The case manager was a conduit of much important information between the parents, medical team, and insurer. Case management interventions at times took considerable hours, but resulted in better educated and less angry parents who became increasingly skilled at caring for their child at home during the nonnursing shifts. This resulted in a decrease in rehospitalizations of the child, a decrease in costs to the insurer, and freed the parents to relocate to a state where their child would be eligible for the Medicaid Model Waiver Program. During the protracted period of the parents' planned relocation, the case manager negotiated a slow tapering off of the home care nursing hours, as medically appropriate. Close support and teaching, as well as troubleshooting among all involved parties, enabled the case manager to decrease nursing care costs to the insurer without the high number of repeat hospitalizations that had been evident early in the case.

8. As the child's insurance plan did not cover air transport of the child to the new state of residency, the case manager made every attempt to secure a donated, medically safe flight for the claimant with her ventilators and all other necessary equipment. Due to legal aeronautic regulations, this was not feasible. The case manager then assisted the parents in planning medically and emotionally for the car trip, arranging for the insurer to provide rented backups to the ventilators and all the necessary precautions to expedite the claimant's safe travel across several states to her new home.

9. Home care nursing and respiratory services, provision of respiratory supplies, and all related equipment had to be put into place in the new state by the case manager in time for the family's

arrival. Close contact between the insurer and the case manager regarding the vendors involved (in-network wherever possible and negotiation of nonnetwork services, as needed) resulted in a smooth transition for this medically complex child and her family.

Outcome

Shortly after the case manager became involved in dialogue with the health-care team and the claimant's parents, there was a decrease in the rate of the child's rehospitalizations. This and the carefully managed decrease of home care nursing hours achieved considerable insurer savings. After the child was safely cared for more frequently by her parents, they became more secure in their abilities. The case manager's skill in arranging for a flexible number of home care nursing hours each week over a period of time enabled all members of the child's healthcare circle to better tolerate change and benefit limits, thus decreasing animosity while increasing compliance. By providing concrete support, education, and medically relevant relocation assistance to the parents, the case manager was able to expedite their move out of state and enroll them in the Medicaid Model Waiver Program. This resulted in a very substantial dollar savings to the insurer as the Medicaid Waiver Program then assumed the costs of all home care nursing services.

After the claimant established residency in her new state, the case manager advocated for home care nursing with the local Medicaid Waiver Program Coordinator. She secured sufficient hours to allow the parents respite and the time to care for other family members' needs, as well as those of their child with the unique respiratory issues.

After the case manager and the insurer effectively addressed home care, nursing, and supply needs, and helped establish a good relationship between the claimant and an appropriate new medical team, the client's family was able to further research the technological advances in treating their child's disorder. They have seen a medical specialist in this rare respiratory syndrome and are currently awaiting DNA assessment of the involved gene with hopes of gene manipulation to eradicate the disorder.

Potential Charges and Savings

Without case management intervention, there would likely have been a significant number of avoidable MD office visits, emergency room visits, and likely rehospitalizations. It is likely the insurer's high-dollar expenditure for 24 hour/day home care nurses would have continued, and potentially multiplied, due to the costs of a legal battle over the insurer's attempts to cut home care nursing hours had the case manager not assisted, educated, and supported the parents. Potential charges included:

Home care nursing services (avoided 8,967 hours at $38/hr) for savings = $340,764

Reduced hospital stays and/or hospital admissions avoided = $47,500

Associated MD hospital fees = $6,300

Emergency room treatments avoided = $8,550

Avoidance of unnecessary MD visits = $850

Savings on medical equipment and supplies = $22,850

Detection and elimination of erroneous billing = $2,380

Negotiation of additional out-of-network costs = $36,213

Total savings to date = $465,407

Analysis

On this case, the case manager employed many skills to manage several multifaceted problems. The family alone presented numerous challenges. To create a working foundation, the case manager needed to gain both the trust and the cooperation of the family, as well as all members of the healthcare team. She needed to keep them focused on the goal of maintaining this very fragile girl at home with her family in a medically safe, developmentally conducive, and positive environment. The case manager had to advocate for the child, parents, insurer, medical team, and home care providers, all the while keeping a close eye on the optimal care of this young child. This required great patience, skill, creativity, attention to detail, tenacity, and persuasion skills to encourage all involved to participate in what would ultimately be a win/win situation.

TRANSPLANT REJECTION OF SMALL BOWEL WITH PSYCHOLOGICAL COMPONENT

Case Overview

This 13-year-old Caucasian female was identified for on-site case management intervention during her hospital admission for transplant rejection of her small bowel with Post Transplant/Lymphoma Prolyphic Disease secondary to antirejection immunosuppression. She required Remicade IV to treat colitis. On admission to the hospital, she also presented with a urinary tract infection (UTI). Her neurogenic bladder places her at high risk for frequent UTIs. Her prior history is complex with multiple medical, financial, and socio/environmental issues identified.

At age 4, the claimant had a colon resection and ileostomy due to pseudo-obstruction of her small bowel and was evaluated for a small bowel transplant (experimental at that time but presently an approved procedure). In 1996, she subsequently developed cancerous lesions on her ribs, diagnosed as Post Transplant Lymphoma Prolyphic. In addition, she has multiple food allergies and is lactose intolerant. Our goal was to provide the child with as optimal an outcome as possible while preventing and decreasing hospital stays as they occurred.

Problems Identified

In addition to the aforementioned, the following problems were identified:

1. The claimant needed intravenous infusion of Remicade to treat her colitis; however, Remicade was not FDA-approved for her specific diagnosis. The case manager was successful in obtaining funding via the drug manufacturer for Remicade. Had case management not been involved, the claimant would have either remained hospitalized or would have been rehospitalized for colitis-related symptoms and/or continued rejection of her small bowel transplant. The medication, even though not approved for her diagnosis, was the only treatment available to place her in remission.

2. Due to the chronicity of this child's condition and other family members' medical problems, financial concerns are an ongoing issue. The claimant needed Pedialyte as an enteral supplement at night. Pedialyte was not covered by her Plan. The claimant's mother was giving it to her every other day because of financial constraints. This resulted in a hospitalization due to dehydration. Community resources were researched and funding was obtained for many of the claimant's needs (Pedialyte, diapers, food, and clothing). This resulted in decreased hospitalizations as the child was provided with adequate hydration.

3. The claimant remains at high risk for rehospitalizations because of her complex medical problems. The case manager monitored each hospital stay for medical appropriateness and provided timely implementation of services, thus decreasing length of hospital stay. The claimant required IV infusion, enteral feeding equipment, and diabetic supplies within the home setting. Home care services were implemented for both child and parental education.

4. There is a strong psychological component in this case. The claimant is depressed. Family and individual counseling is needed for all members of this family on an ongoing basis. The case manager attempted to address these issues in several ways. An extensive amount of time was spent on researching an inpatient facility that could address both the child's medical and psychological needs. The child was hospitalized and mother initially attended counseling. Unfortunately, the mother became dissatisfied with the facility and requested discharge from the facility. She eventually was noncompliant with responding to the case manager's phone calls.

Outcome

Continued case management intervention did provide early identification and timely intervention of medical problems. Hospitalizations were not only avoided, but were also decreased in length. Community resources were utilized to prevent recurrent hospitalizations for nutrition- and dehydration-related problems. Funding was obtained for Remicade. Had case management not been involved, the claimant would have been rehospitalized for colitis-related symptoms or remained hospitalized. Case management attempted to attend to the strong psychological issues but, regrettably, was not completely effective. Many of the child's problems were addressed and resolved, but without complete parental collaboration with case management, it was difficult to obtain a successful outcome for this child and, sadly, this case was closed to case management.

Potential Charges and Savings

Without case management intervention, this child would have remained hospitalized for longer lengths of stay and experienced at least one emergency room visit due to dehydration. She entered the hospital three times. CM intervention and monitoring reduced her total hospital stays by 8 days.

Decreased hospital stays by 8 days at $1,500/day = $12,000
Eliminated associated MD fees × 2 (PCP and Specialist) at $200/day × 8 days = $1,600
Avoided minimum of one ER visit = $750
Avoided rehospitalization for dehydration × 4 days = $6,000
Plus MD fees = $800

Case management monitoring of services for appropriateness, unnecessary long-term use of DME equipment (wheelchair), and associated rental fees were avoided = $850

Other savings were realized through use of in-network providers.

Total potential charges/savings = $22,000

Analysis

The problems identified in this case are typical of an individual with chronic life-threatening conditions. This child remains at high risk for complications. Both the child and family require ongoing psychological intervention and support in order to ensure a successful outcome for this child.

Unfortunately, although the psychological issues were identified and addressed, the case manager was unable to obtain a successful outcome for this child without complete parental collaboration. The child's mother refused to cooperate with the psych facility and discharged her daughter from therapy. Because of the mother's termination of contact with the case management company, the case was not open to case management, and a recommendation was made to close it. Continuous intervention by the case manager, advocating for the claimant, would have made a great difference in this outcome, and it becomes difficult and often frustrating for a case manager to let go of a case like this one.

Part VI

Continuum
Concepts

Chapter 26

Continuum of Care Initiatives

The concept of a continuum of care isn't new to case managers. We have been trying to create that since the earliest days of our practice. We recognize that the patients who become part of our caseloads oftentimes are victims of a healthcare delivery system that is too fragmented, lacking in continuity, and frequently absent of a patient-centered approach. Much of what our healthcare system offers today is wonderful and has made it possible for so many more of us to survive events and illnesses that would not have been possible a short time ago. To accomplish this, however, individuals are often seen by many different healthcare providers—no one quite knowing all of the nuances of each patient and unable because of time and other circumstances to develop trusting, caring relationships with their patients.

The incredible changes in insurance systems have also contributed to this problem. Frequently, as patients change employers, or the employer changes health plans, the physicians who were caring for patients are no longer in the "new" network, leaving patients to try to re-create years of medical history all over again with new providers who then have to start from "ground zero" to understand their new patients' complex issues. Patients going from provider to provider, hospital to hospital, or emergency rooms and walk-in medical centers for diagnostic studies and therapy encounter conflicting medical direction, multiple medications, and treatment regimens that they do not understand; these patients, for whom no one is acting as care coordinator, truly need a continuum of care. Fortunately, there's some good news on the horizon!

MEDICAL HOME MODEL

The medical home model is one of the most promising models to emerge over time. The medical home model can respond to the growing trend and demand for patient-centric, community-based care. The National

791

system needs to "redesign the manner of primary care delivery, and to re-emphasize the centrality of primary care."[1]

In February 2007, three organizations, the American Academy of Pediatrics (AAP), the American College of Physicians (ACP), and the American Academy of Family Physicians (AAFP), issued the report titled "Joint Principles of the Patient-Centered Medical Home." *Medical home* is a concept rather than a building or an office. It may be the community mental health center for those with chronic behavioral health issues, or an adult day care center for older adults, or anyplace a person may routinely access first-line care and treatment.[2]

The principles of a medical home provide for the following:

- A personal physician
- Physician-directed medical practice
- Whole-person orientation
- Care coordination
- Quality and safety
- Enhanced access
- Payment

Certainly, these principles underscore many of the core elements in case management and are also strongly aligned with advocacy and the empowerment of patients. This concept is growing in acceptance by physicians and purchasers alike, and several initiatives are in place to demonstrate its effectiveness. Because case managers are dedicated to improving outcomes while improving costs, there are opportunities for them within the medical home model. We can once again be the catalyst for change. Care coordination and case management continue to emerge in various forms; engaging the primary care physician, especially for a patient with complex conditions, has always been a challenge. Case managers can be a vital member of the medical home.

We have long recognized that episodic intervention doesn't work and that our opportunities truly to make a difference extend beyond discharge planning and need to occur in a coordinated, community-based manner. This is a callout to case managers once again to create another practice setting for themselves (see Chapter 20). The medical home model is another strategic tool that case managers can implement to address spiraling healthcare costs while broadening and expanding the range of services available to a larger population of people.

By using an integrated approach to patient care that is evidence-based and longitudinal rather than encounter- or episode-based, the medical home model responds to many of the deficiencies and disconnects in the current healthcare system. The primary physician is the essential leader of a diverse team that may include social services, behavioral health, external providers, information technology, and of course the case manager.

Eleanor Solteau, RN, BSN, CCM, in an article in *Case in Point*, notes that following Hurricane Katrina, the medical home initiative took on new meaning. In 2004, prior to Katrina a state initiative was under way for special needs children. The project was barely started, notes Solteau, when the clinic and the entire Charity Healthcare System was destroyed by the storm. Both were the primary care healthcare systems for the Medicaid population in the New Orleans area. The medical home took on new significance in reaching an already at-risk population with exponentially magnified poststorm problems and social risks. Solteau recalls, "As overwhelming as it has been to address the needs of the returning population, it would have been more so without the bare essentials of care coordination that had been laid prior to the storm."[3]

As with other emerging models, there are challenges to the implementation of this model. The following represent the biggest ones:

- *Reimbursement of care coordination activities.* Family practice/primary care practice has been in decline for many years, and a movement toward specialty practice is afoot. Between 1997 and 2005, the number of U.S. graduates entering family practice residencies declined by 50%.[4] Perhaps a reason for this move to specialties is this: "Thirty minutes spent performing a diagnostic, surgical, or imaging procedure often pays as much as a 30-minute visit with a patient with diabetes, heart failure, headache and depression. The median income of specialists in 2004 was almost twice that of primary care physicians and that gap is widening."[5]

  The Medical Home concept requires that more time is spent with patients. However, when reimbursement policies do not compensate for this time, there is little incentive for physicians to spend the time or have other professionals in their office provide this much-needed intervention. In 2008, three new codes (99441, 99442, and 99443) were added to the Current Professional Terminology (CPT) related to telephone evaluation and management services provided by a physician. Additionally, another three nonphysician codes were added for non–face-to-face telephone services. These codes represent assessment and management services to beneficiaries such as transition of care, medication reconciliation, health literacy assessment, motivational interviewing, patient education, and medical home coordination. Note that *all* of these codes were given a "Status N" rating by the Centers for Medicare and Medicaid Services (CMS), which means that they are, at present, nonreimbursable.

The Case Management Society of America (CMSA) issued a position paper during the public comment period responding and urging case managers to contact their various representatives to request funding for these codes. CMSA also prepared a template letter of support for use by members and continues to monitor this situation closely. In its public comment, CMSA notes the following: "CMSA believes that by requesting funding support for these six (6) codes, providers will be able to integrate case/care managers support of the Medical Home concept, such as the Medicare Medical Home Demonstration (MMHD), pay for performance programs, and various collaborative models of care which CMS and other regulatory agencies are discussing."

- *Information technology challenges.* Although technology is at the core of the medical home concept, many small to midsize practices have not yet invested in electronic medical records (EMR).
- *Standardization of practice.* Moving physicians away from the "I've always practiced this way" mindset into outcomes- and evidence-based practice is another element of implementation that needs to be addressed; it won't be easy!

CHRONIC CARE MODEL

Any condition that requires ongoing adjustments by the affected person and interactions with the healthcare system is termed *chronic*. Almost half of all Americans, or 133 million people, live with a chronic condition.[6] That number is projected to increase by more than 1% per year by 2030, resulting in an estimated chronically ill population of 171 million. There are acknowledged deficiencies in managing these conditions that include the following:

- Rushed practitioners not following established practice guidelines
- Lack of care coordination
- Lack of active follow-up to ensure the best outcomes
- Patients inadequately trained to manage their illnesses[7]

Once again, these issues are no surprise to case managers. There is broad recognition that to overcome these problems, which have become so much a part of our healthcare system, a transformation from a system that is essentially reactive to one that is proactive and focused on keeping patients as healthy as possible is required.[8]

More than 15 years ago, the Chronic Care Model (CCM) was developed through the efforts of Ed Wagner, MD, MPH, and colleagues at Group

Health Center for Health Studies with the support of the Robert Wood Johnson Foundation. More than 1,500 U.S. and international practices adopted the model and in "the largest roundup of evidence on how the model performs in practice confirms that it works."[9] This model differs from the commercial vendor disease management models where "high-cost" patients are encouraged to manage their own diseases better while the medical practice essentially remains the same. The CCM model recognizes that more than patients must change. It identifies the essential elements of a healthcare system that encourage high-quality chronic disease care. The elements are the community, the health system, self-management support, delivery system design, decision support, and clinical information systems. As designed, this model can be applied to a variety of chronic illnesses, healthcare settings, and target populations.

There certainly is a place for case managers in this model that "aims to transform the healthcare system from acute and chronic to proactive and planned . . . and [that is] based more on evidence about populations, less on habit."[10] We have known that the medical conditions our patients have don't just exist in one care setting, but rather extend across the continuum. Models such as the CCM respond well to this reality.

THE GUIDED CARE MODEL

The Guided Care model uses several of the successful innovations of the Chronic Care Model (CCM) and integrates them in the primary care setting. The hypothesis is that the Guided Care model of case management improves the quality of care, patients' access to care, and patients' capacity for self-care, thus resulting in improved outcomes. The Guided Care model is designed to have the following characteristics:

- Effective in practices throughout the United States
- Financially sustainable
- Attractive to physicians and nurses
- Valuable to healthcare organizations
- Popular with patients and caregivers[11]

Guided care provides case management, disease management, self-management, transitional care (the continuum concept), and caregiver support in a close partnership with the patient's primary physician.[12] As it is practiced, a Guided Care Nurse (GCN) drives the process in an office and assists three to five physicians with their patients. To be effective in this role, registered nurses can take a specially designed 3-week curriculum that teaches them the special skills they will need to practice guided care. The curriculum is designed to develop skills and confidence and includes lecture, readings, and role playing in simulated situations GCNs will likely encounter in their practice. The topics within the curriculum include using the electronic health record (EHR), health insurance, motivational interviewing, community resources, and transitional care guidelines. Qualities that make registered nurses well suited to becoming Guided Care Nurses include proficiency in communication, flexibility in complex problem solving, cultural competence, comfort with interdisciplinary care, and enthusiasm for coaching patients and families.[13]

The GCN coordinates the efforts of all of the healthcare professionals who treat guided care patients in emergency departments, hospitals, rehabilitation facilities, offices, and at home. Each patient is encouraged to contact the GCN before or during visits/admissions to emergency rooms and hospitals. The GCN then provides information to professionals about the patient, explains the GCN role, visits the patient during the hospital confinement, assists in the coordination for discharge or transfer to an alternate care setting, and remains involved through discharge and follow-up. This guided care process ensures a smooth transition between all the sites of care and among all the providers and, most important, keeps the primary physician apprised of the patient's current status.[14] One important element in this model involves the visit by the GCN on the first day the patient returns home. This insures that patients understand how to care for themselves, know how to take medications, understand what signs to watch for, and have the necessary contact information, including that of the GCN, just in case problems or questions arise.[15]

In the Guided Care model, case management is integrated with primary care. The model includes some of the previous decades' most successful innovations in managing the care of patients with multiple and chronic conditions. Comparisons will be made between guided care and traditional case management, and indeed the two approaches have some similarities. The emphasis upon transitional care and the ongoing relationship that the GCN has with primary physicians and patients render the Guided Care model a more successful and collaborative concept. Because the Guided Care model has appeal for many nurses and case managers, it is likely to attract those who might be thinking of leaving the profession as a result of the frustrations they continue to experience. Guided care may enable them to see that another path can redirect their passion and desire to really make a difference in patients' lives.

THE NATIONAL TRANSITIONS OF CARE COALITION

As patients move across the various settings in the care continuum, the opportunities for problems increase. For those individuals with multiple conditions *and* multiple providers, the situation can be extremely dangerous. Although the healthcare industry and healthcare professionals work very hard to create the best care possible, when patients transition or are transferred from one setting to another (e.g., when the patient moves from the emergency department to the ICU to an unmonitored floor) communication of important details about condition and care may be incomplete, misinterpreted, or missing. The same issues exist when patients receive care in a number of different but unrelated facilities, such as acute care hospital, rehabilitation facility, skilled nursing facility, and then possibly home care.

The complications, costs, and challenges that this issue presents to the healthcare industry are extraordinary, and the risks to patients are harm-causing incidents, poor quality of care, and unsafe conditions. In 2006, the National Transitions of Care Coalition (NTOCC), chaired and coordinated by CMSA and in partnership with Sanofi-Aventis, brought together thought leaders, professionals, patient advocates, and healthcare professionals from various settings to improve the quality of care and communication when patients are transferred from one setting or provider to another. Through their efforts, NTOCC now has 29 participating organizations and has created information and tools for consumers, professionals, policymakers, and the media. The tools facilitate communication about the essential aspects of an individual's care, are downloadable on the organization's Web site, and include the following:

- *My Medicine List:* Designed to help patients understand their medication regimens, allowing them to update it as needed and to share it with their providers as they move from setting to setting.
- *Taking Care of My Health Care:* Developed as a guide for patients and their caregivers to use as they prepare for visits to their healthcare professionals; this tool helps patients ask questions, obtain additional information, and obtain guidance on next steps.
- *Medication Reconciliation Essential Data Specifications:* This tool helps healthcare professionals collect, transmit, and receive critical medication information as patients transition across care settings.
- *Improving on Transitions of Care: How to Implement and Evaluate a Plan:* This guidebook was created as a "project in a box" to help institutions and organizations design, implement, and evaluate their own transition of care plans.[16,17]

CONCLUSION

There's a saying: "Necessity is the mother of invention." Certainly, the concepts described in this chapter are an example of that. We not only recognize that transitions of care have *not* been safe for our patients, but we accept our responsibility and have created real solutions that will make patient transitions safe, reduce unnecessary hospitalizations, and improve the quality of their care, and their lives!

NOTES

1. National Business Coalition on Health, *The Patient-Centered Medical Home: A Purchase Guide* (Washington, DC: National Business Coalition on Health, 2008).
2. Garrett M, "Understanding Medical Home—A New Opportunity for Case Managers," *Professional Case Management* 14, no. 1 (January/February 2009).
3. Solteau E, "The Patient-Centered Medical Home," *Case in Point*, June/July 2008, 30–33.
4. Bodenheimer T, "Primary Care—Will It Survive?" *New England Journal of Medicine* 358 (2008): 1064–1071.
5. Bodenheimer, "Primary Care," 1064–1071.
6. Partnership for Solutions, *Chronic Conditions: Making the Case for Ongoing Care: September 2004 Update* (Baltimore, MD: Johns Hopkins University Press for The Robert Wood Johnson Foundation, 2004).
7. Improving Chronic Illness Care, website, http://www.improvingchroniccare.org.
8. Wagner EH, Austin BT, and Von Korff A, "Improving Outcomes in Chronic Illness," *Managed Care Quarterly* 4, no. 2 (1996): 12–25.
9. Medical News Today, "Using Chronic Care Model Helps to Improve People's Health and Care," January 6, 2009, http://www.medicalnewstoday.com/articles/134538.php.
10. Medical News Today, "Using Chronic Care."
11. Boult C, Karm L, and Groves C, "Improving Chronic Care: The 'Guided Care' Model," *Permanente Journal* 12, no. 1 (Winter 2008).
12. Boyd C, Boult C, Shadmi E, et al., "Guided Care for Multi-Morbid Older Adults," *The Gerontologist* 47, no. 5 (October 2007): 697–704.
13. Aliotta S, Grieve K, Giddens J, et al., "Guided Care: A New Frontier for Adults with Chronic Conditions," *Professional Case Management* 13, no. 3 (May/June 2008).
14. Aliotta et al., "Guided Care."
15. Boult et al., "Improving Chronic Care."
16. National Transitions of Care Coalition, website, http://www.ntocc.org.
17. Powell S, "Safe Transitions Are a Team Sport," *Professional Case Management* 13, no. 5 (September/October 2008).

Additional Resources

ACADEMIC/EDUCATIONAL RESOURCES

The following offer case management certificate programs, majors, or graduate-level programs:

Adelphi University
School of Nursing
Garden City, NY 11530
(516) 877-4510
http://nursing.adelphi.edu

Baylor University
School of Nursing
3700 Worth Street
Dallas, TX 75246
(214) 820-3361
www.baylor.edu/nursing

Brigham Young University
550 SWKT, P.O. Box 25436
Provo, UT 84602-5436
www.nursing.byu.edu
(801) 422-4173

Carlow College
3333 Fifth Avenue
Pittsburgh, PA 15213
(800) 333-2275
www.carlow.edu/

Davenport University
Warren Campus
4801 Oakman Boulevard
Dearborn, MI 48126
(734) 943-2800
www.davenport.edu

George Mason University
College of Nursing & Health
  Science
4400 University Drive
Fairfax, VA 22030
(703) 993-1000
cnhs@gmu.edu

Grand Valley State University
CM Certificate Program
1 Campus Drive
Allendale, MI 49401
(616) 331-2025
www.gvsu.edu/

Greenville Technical College
Buck Mickel Center
216 S. Pleasantburg Drive
Greenville, SC 29607
Continuing Education/Health
  Sciences-Nursing
(864) 250-8800
www.gvltec.edu

**Indiana University-Purdue
  University Fort Wayne**
IPFW Continuing Education
2101 E. Coliseum Boulevard
Fort Wayne, IN 46805-1499

Continuing Studies
(260) 481-6828
www.ipfw.edu/dcs

Lewis University
One University Parkway
Romeoville, IL 60446-2200
(815) 838-0500

Michigan State University
College of Nursing
A100 Life Sciences Building
East Lansing, MI 48824-1317
(517) 432-8135
http://humanmedicine.msu.edu

Pace University
Case Management Institute
School of Nursing
961 Bedford Road, Room L17
Pleasantville, NY 10570
(914) 773-3359

Pacific Lutheran University
School of Nursing
Tacoma, WA 98447-0003
(253) 535-7324

Saint Peter's College
Department of Nursing
2641 Kennedy Blvd.
Jersey City, NJ 07306

Samuel Merritt College
College of Nursing
370 Hawthorne Avenue
Oakland, CA 94609
(510) 869-6511

San Francisco State University
School of Nursing
1600 Holloway Avenue

San Francisco, CA 94132
mahaw@sfsu.edu

Seton Hall University
S. Orange Avenue
South Orange, NJ 07079

Sonoma State University
Department of Nursing
1801 E. Cotati Avenue
Rohnert Park, CA 94928
(707) 664-2643

State University of New York-HSCB
Box 22
Brooklyn College of Nursing
450 Clarkson Avenue
Brooklyn, NY 11203-2098
Director of the Center for Nursing
  Research
(718) 270-7605

University of Alabama
Capstone College of Nursing
Box 870358
504 University Boulevard
Tuscaloosa, AL 35487-0358
http://nursing.ua.edu/

University of Arizona
College of Nursing, Building 203
1305 North Martin
P.O. Box 210203
Tucson, AZ 85721-0203
(520) 626-6154
preed@nursingarizona.edu

University of Kentucky
College of Nursing
315 College of Nursing Building
Lexington, KY 40536-0232
(859) 323-3851

**University of Maryland/
Baltimore County**
4815 Maple Grove Road
Hampstead, MD 21074

University of St. Francis
500 Wilcox Street
Joilet, IL 60435
(815) 740-3400

University of San Diego
Philip Y. Hahn School of Nursing
5998 Alaca Park
San Diego, CA 92110-9885
(619) 260-4600
www.sandiego.edu/academic/
   nursing/

University of Southern Indiana
School of Nursing and Health
   Professions
8600 University Boulevard
Evansville, IN 47712-3597
(877) 874-4584

University of Virginia
McLeod Hall
15th Street, SW
Charlottesville, VA 22903-3395
(434) 924-0211

University of Wisconsin-Madison
School of Nursing
600 Highland Avenue-K6/140
   Clinical Science Center
Madison, WI 53792-2455
(608) 263-5180

Vanderbilt University
Godchaux Hall 207
461 21st Avenue

Nashville, TN 37240
(615) 322-3800

Villanova University
College of Nursing
800 Lancaster Avenue
Villanova, PA 19085-1690
(610) 519-4900

Canada

McMaster University
1280 Main Street W
Hamilton, Ontario
Canada
L8S 4L8

University of Toronto
Department of Nursing
50 George Street
Toronto, Ontario
Canada
M5S 3H4

Australia

University of Melbourne
Level 1, 723 Swanston Street
Carlton, Victoria, 3053
Australia
011 (613) 8344-9400
www.nursing.unimelb.edu.au/
   contact

University of South Australia
GPO Box 2471
Adelaide, South Australia, 5001
Australia
011 (618) 8302-0114
CM courses offered external mode

ADDITIONAL CREDENTIALS (SEE CHAPTER 7)

American Association of Managed Care Nurses (for the CMCN credential—Certified Managed Care Nurse)
(804) 747-9698
www.aamcn.org

American Case Management Association (for the ACM—accredited case manager credential for hospital/health system case managers)
www.acma.org

Certification of Disability Management Specialists Commission (CDMS Commission for the CDMS credential)
1699 East Woodfield Road, Suite 300
Schaumburg, IL 60173
(847) 944-1335
www.cdms.org

Certified Brain Injury Specialist (CBIS)
American Academy for the Certification of Brain Injury Specialists
Brain Injury Association of America
1608 Springhill Road, Suite 110
Vienna, VA 22182
(703) 761-0750

Certified Professional Utilization Review (CPUR)
McKesson Empowering Healthcare
One Post Street
San Francisco, CA 94104
(415) 983-8300
www.mckesson.com

Commission for Case Management Certification (CCMC for the CCM credential)
National Office: 15000 Commerce Parkway, Suite C
Mount Laurel, NJ 08054
(847) 818-1967
www.ccmcertification.org

Commission on Rehabilitation Counselor Certification (CRCC) for the CRC credential
1699 E. Woodfield Road, Suite 300
Schaumburg, IL 60173
(847) 944-1325
www.crccertification.com

National Association of Certified Care Managers (for the CMC credential: Care Manager Certified) affiliated with National Association of Professional Geriatric Care Managers
3275 W Ina Road, Suite 130
Tucson, AZ 85741
(520) 881-8008
www.caremanager.org

National Board for Certification in Continuity of Care
1350 Broadway, Suite 1705
New York, NY 10018
(212) 356-0691
nbcc.net/history.htm

Rehabilitation Nursing Certification Board (for the CRRN credential)
4700 W. Lake Avenue
Glenview, IL 60025-1485
(800) 229-7530
www.rehabnurse.org

OTHER PROGRAMS

CARE2LEARN.COM
www.care2learn.com
(866) 242-8451

CMSA WebED
www.cmsa.org/Education/WebED/

Continuing Ed for Certified Health Professionals
www.aaa.ceus.com
(866) 850-5999

The Center for Case Management (CCM)
6 Pleasant Street
South Natick, MA 01760
(508) 651-2600
www.cfcm.com

Consultants in Case Management Intervention Associates (CCMI Associates)
1163 New Boston Road
Francestown, NH 03043
(603) 547-2245

Creative Health Care Management Inc.
1701 American Boulevard East, Suite 1
Minneapolis, MN 55425
(800) 728-7766
www.chcm.com

HealthCare Resource Group
12525 Lambert Road
Whittier, CA 90606
(562) 945-7224
CM certificate course

International Foundation of Employee Benefit Plans
18700 W. Bluemound Road
P.O. Box 69
Brookfield, WI 53008-0069
(414) 786-6710
Offers videotapes, audio cassettes

Professional Resources in Management Education (PRIME)
1820 SW 100 Avenue
Miramar, FL 33025
(954) 718-6055
www.primeinc.org

Registered Nurse Case Manager
www.rncasemanager.com

Social Worker Case Manager
www.swcasemanager.com

Note: Also check into educational symposia presented at regional and national conferences.

ASSOCIATIONS

AHRQ (Agency for Health Care Research and Quality)
540 Gaither Road, Suite 2000
Rockville, MD 20850
(301) 427-1364
www.ahrq.gov

The ALS Association, National Office
27001 Agoura Road, Suite 250
Calabasas Hills, CA 93101
(818) 880-9007

Alzheimer's Association
225 N. Michigan Avenue – Fl 17
Chicago, IL 60601
(800) 272-3900
www.alz.org

American Association of Occupational Health Nurses, Inc.
2920 Brandywine Road, Suite 100
Atlanta, GA 30341
(770) 455-7757
www.aaohn.org

American Association of Preferred Provider Organizations
1101 Connecticut Avenue, NW, Suite 700
Washington, DC 20036
(202) 429-5133

American Board for Occupational Health Nurses
201 East Ogden, Suite 114
Hinsdale, IL 60521
(630) 789-5799
www.abohn.org

American Board of Disability Analysts
345 24th Avenue No., Suite 200
Nashville, TN 37203
(615) 327-2984

American Burn Association
625 N. Michigan, Suite 2550
Chicago, IL 60611
(800) 548-2876

American Cancer Society
P.O. Box 29427
Atlanta, GA 30359
www.cancer.org
(800) ACS-2345

American Diabetes Association
1660 Duke Street
Alexandria, VA 22314
(703) 549-1500
(800) 232-3472
www.diabetes.org

American Heart Association
7272 Greenville Avenue
Dallas, TX 75231-4596
(800) 242-8721

American Hospice Foundation
2120 L Street, NW, Suite 200
Washington, DC 20037
(202) 223-0204

American Hospital Association
1 North Franklin
Chicago, IL 60606
Phone: (312) 422-3000
Fax: (312) 422-4796
www.aha.org

American Institute of Outcomes Care Management
1215 Lambert Road
Whittier, CA 90606
Phone: (562) 945-9990
Fax: (562) 698-2339
www.aiocm.net

American Lung Association
61 Broadway, 6th Floor
New York, NY 10006
(212) 315-8700

American Medical Association
515 North State Street
Chicago, IL 60610
(800) 621-8335 (copies)
(312) 464-4706 (information)

American Nurses Association
8515 Georgia Avenue, Suite 400
Silver Spring, MD 20910-3492
(800) 274-4ANA
www.ana.org

American Organization of Nurse Executives (AONE)
Washington, DC, Headquarters
    Liberty Place
325 Seventh Street, NW
Washington, DC 20004
Phone: (202) 626-2240
Fax: (202) 638-5499
Alternate phone: (312) 422-2800
    (Chicago office)

Association of Rehabilitation Nurses
4700 W. Lake Avenue
Glenview, IL 60025
(800) 229-7530

Blue Cross and Blue Shield Association
225 North Michigan Avenue
Chicago, IL 60601
(297) 440-6345

Case Management Society of America
6301 Ranch Drive
Little Rock, AR 72227
(501) 227-5444
www.cmsa.org

Choice in Dying
1035 30th Street, NW
Washington, DC 20007
(202) 338-9790

Disease Management Association of America
701 Pennsylvania Avenue, NW
Suite 700
Washington, DC 20004
(202) 737-5980
www.dmaa.org

Employee Benefit Research Institute
1100 13th Street, NW, Suite 878
Washington, DC 20005
www.ebri.org
(202) 659-0670

Health Insurance Association of America
601 Pennsylvania Avenue, NW
South Building, Suite 500
Washington, DC 20004-1204
Phone: (202) 778-3200
Fax: (202) 331-7487
www.hiaa.org

Health Research and Educational Trust (HRET)
1 North Franklin, 30th Floor
Chicago, IL 60606
Phone: (312) 422-2600
Fax: (312) 422-4568
www.hret.org

Joint Commission
One Renaissance Boulevard
Oakbrook Terrace, IL 60181
(630) 792-5800 for CM
    seminars/cities
www.jcaho.org

The Leapfrog Group
c/o Academy Health
1150 17th Street, NW, Suite 600
Washington, DC 20006
(202) 292-6713
www.leapfroggroup.org/

National Academy of Certified
Care Managers
P.O. Box 669
244 Upton Road
Colchester, CT 06415-0669
(800) 962-2260

National AIDS Hotline
(800) 232-4636
(800) 342-AIDS (general
information, recording)

National Association for
Healthcare Quality (NAHQ)
4700 West Lake Avenue
Glenview, IL 60025
(800) 966-9392
www.nahq.org

National Association for
Home Care
228 Seventh Street, SE
Washington, DC 20003
(202) 547-7424
www.nahc.org

National Association of People
with AIDS
8401 Colesville Road, Suite 505
Silver Springs, MD 20910
(240) 247-0880
www.napwa.org

National Association of Social
Workers
750 First Street, NE, Suite 700
Washington, DC 20002

(202) 408-8600
www.naswdc.org

National Brain Injury Foundation
www.biausa.org

National Cancer Institute
International Cancer Information
Center
Building 82, Room 123
Bethesda, MD 20892
(301) 496-2794
(800) 422-6237
www.cancer.gov

National Center for Policy
Analysis
12770 Colt Road, Suite 800
Dallas, TX 75243-1739
(972) 386-6272
www.ncpa.org

National Committee for Quality
Assurance
1100 13th St., Suite 1000
Washington, DC 20035
(202) 955-3500
www.ncqa.org

National Council State Boards for
Nursing (NCSBN)
www.ncsbn.org

National Hospice Foundation
1700 Diagonal Road, Suite 625
Alexandria, VA 22314
(703) 516-4928
www.nationalhospicefoundation.org

National Institutes of Health
9000 Rockville Pike
Bethesda, MD 20892
(301) 496-4000
www.nih.org

National Insurance Consumers
  Helpline
(800) 942-4242

National Multiple Sclerosis
  Society
www.nationalmssociety.org

National Rehabilitation
  Association
633 South Washington Street
Alexandria, VA 22314
(703) 836-0850
www.nationalrerab.org

New York Business Group
  on Health
61 Broadway, Suite 2705
New York, NY 10016-8804
(212) 252-7440
www.nybgh.org

Office of Minority Health
  Resource Center
Resource Center
P.O. Box 37337
Washington, DC 20013
(240) 453-2882
www.omhrc.gov

Susan G. Komen Breast Cancer
  Foundation
5005 LBJ Freeway, Suite 250
Dallas, TX 75244
(877) GO-KOMEN
www.komen.org

URAC (American Accreditation
  HealthCare Commissions)
1220 L Street, NW, Suite 400
Washington, DC 20005
(202) 216-9006
www.urac.org

Viatical Association of America
(407) 894-3797
www.viatical.org

Washington Business Group
  on Health
Y-Me National Breast Cancer
  Organization
50 F Street NW, Suite 600
Washington, DC 20001
(201) 628-9320
www.wbgh.org

JOURNALS AND MAGAZINES

AAOHN Journal
6900 Grove Road
Thorofare, NJ 08086-9447
(770) 455-7757
www.aaohn.org

Advance for Nurses
2900 Horizon Drive
King of Prussia, PA 19406
(800) 355-5627
www.advancefornurses.com

Alternative Healthcare Management
www.althealthcaremag.com

*Alternative Therapies in Health and
  Medicine*
www.alternative-therapies.com

Alzheimer's Care Quarterly
www.acqjournal.com

Business & Health (electronic
  version only)
www.businessandhealth.com

Business Insurance
www.businessinsurance.com

CareManagement
256 Post Road East, Suite 204
Westport, CT 06880-3617
(203) 454-1333

Caring
www.caringonline.org

Case Management Advisor
(800) 688-2421
www.ahcpub.com

Case in Point (Official Magazine of CMSA)
Dorland Health
A Coutexo Media Company
P.O. Box 25128
Salt Lake City, UT 84125
(800) 784-2332

CE-Today for Nurse Practitioners
CEU-Online, Inc.
(603) 432-7099
www.np.ce-today.com

Continuing Care
(856) 793-1557
www.ccareonline.com

Employee Benefit News
1325 G Street NW, Suite 970
Washington, DC 20005
(202) 504-1122
www.benefitnews.com

Harvard Women's Health Watch
www.health.harvard.edu

Health Monitor
www.healthmonitor.com

Home Health Care Consultant
www.mmhc.com/hhcc

Home Healthcare Nurse
www.nursingcenter.com

Home Health Care Dealer/Provider
www.hmetoday.com

HomeCare
www.homecaremag.com

Hospice
www.hospicenet.org

National Home Infusion
  Association
205 Dangerfield Road
Alexandria, VA 22314-2833
(703) 549-3740
www.nhianet.org

Journal of Case Management
(412) 787-9301

Journal of Hospice and Palliative Nursing (JHPN)
www.jhpn.com

Journal of Pain and Palliative Care Pharmacotherapy: Advances in Acute, Chronic and End of Life Symptom Control
30 S. 2000 E, Room 258
University of Utah
Salt Lake City, UT 84112-5820
alipman@pharm.utah.edu

Journal of Rehabilitation
www.nationalrehab.org

Managed Care Interface
(914) 337-7878
www.accessmylibrary.com

Managed Care Quarterly
200 Orchard Ridge Drive
Gaithersburg, MD 20878
(800) 638-8437
www.aspenpublishers.com

Medical Economics
24950 Country Club Boulevard,
   Suite 200
North Olmsted, OH 44070
(440) 243-8100
www.memag.com

Modern Healthcare
360 N. Michigan Avenue
Chicago, IL 60601
(312) 649-5350
www.modernhealthcare.com

McKnight's Long-Term Care News
(847) 784-8706
www.mcknightsonline.com

The Nations Health
800 I Street NW
Washington, DC 20001
www.apha.org/publications
(202) 777-2438

The NIH Record
9000 Rockville Pike
Bethesda, MD 20892
(301) 496-2125
http://nihrecord.od.nih.gov

Nursing Economics
East Holly Avenue
Box 56
Pitman, NJ 08071-0056
(856) 256-2300
www.ajj.com/services/pblshng/nej/

Nursing Management
1111 Bethlehem Pike
Spring House, PA 19477-1114
(215) 646-8700
www.nursingmanagement.com

Professional Case Management
Official Journal of CMSA
Lippincott Williams & Wilkins, Inc.
16522 Hunters Green Parkway
Hagerstown, MD 21740

Rehab Management
(310) 642-4400
www.rehabpub.com

Rehab & Community Care
   Management
101 Thorncliffe Park Drive
Toronto, Ontario, M4H 1M2, Canada
(416) 421-7944

Rehabilitation Nursing
4700 W. Lake Avenue
Glenview, IL 60025-1468
(800) 229-7350
www.rehabnurse.org

The Remington Report
30100 Town Center Drive, Suite 0-421
Laguna Niguel, CA 92677-2064
(800) 247-4781
www.remingtonreport.com

RNdex Information Products
Information Resources Group, Inc.
El Dorado Hills Business Park
5000 Windplay Drive, Suite 4
El Dorado, CA 95762
(800) 200-6040

Risk & Insurance Magazine
747 Dresher Road, Suite 500
Horsham, PA 19044-0980
(215) 784-0860

Risk Management Publishing
655 3rd Avenue
New York, NY 10017
(212) 286-9364

The Self-Insurer
P.O. Box 1237
Simpsonville, SC 29681
(800) 851-7789
www.siia.org

NEWSLETTERS

Case Management Advisor
P.O. Box 740059
Atlanta, GA 30301
(800) 688-2421
www.ahcmedia.com

The Case Report
CMSA
6301 Ranch Drive
Little Rock, AR 72223
(501) 225-2229
www.cmsa.org

CMSA @ At Work For You
CMSA
8201 Cantrell, Suite 230
Little Rock, AR 72227
(501) 225-2229
www.cmsa.org

Disease Management Advisor
1123 Zonolite Road, Suite 17
Atlanta, GA 30306-2016
(800) 650-6787
www.nhionline.net

Disease Management Digest
256 Post Road East, Suite 204
Westport, CT 06880-3617
(203) 454-1333

*EBRI Issue Brief and Employee
  Benefit Notes*
The Johns Hopkins University
  Press

701 West 40th Street, Suite 275
Baltimore, MD 21211
(410) 516-6964

The Elder Care Connector
www.homeinstead.com

E-News (electronic newsletter)
End of Life Physician Education
  Resource Center
Medical College of Wisconsin,
  MEB Room 3235
8701 Watertown Plank Road
Milwaukee, WI 53226
(414) 456-4353
www.eperc.mcw.edu

Home Care Case Management
3525 Piedmont Road, NE, Bldg. 6,
  Suite 400
Atlanta, GA 30305
(800) 688-2421

Inside Case Management
4343 North Clarendon, Unit 1616
Chicago, IL 60613
(773) 281-8492

Joint Commission Perspectives
1515 W. 22nd Street, Suite 1300 W.
Oakbrook, IL 60523
(877) 223-6866
www.jcrinc.com

Intramural Research Highlights
U.S. Department of Health and
  Human Services
(866) 284-4107

*Last Acts Policy Newsletter
  (e-newsletter)*
Robert Wood Johnson Foundation
P.O. Box 2316
Route 1 and College Road
East Princeton, NJ 08543

(877) 843-7953
www.lastacts.org

NAHC Report
National Association For
  Homecare
228 7th Street SE
Washington, DC 20003
www.nahc.org
(202) 547-7424

NARPPS Newsletter
313 Washington Street, Suite 302
Newton, MA 02158

Nurses' Notes (official newsletter of
  American Association of
  Managed Care Nurses)
www.aamcn.org

NRA Newsletter
633 South Washington Street
Alexandria, VA 22314
(703) 836-0850

PharmaFacts for Case Managers
256 Post Road East, Suite 204
Westport, CT 06880-3617
(203) 454-1333

Rehabilitation Review
1498 Old Fannin Road
Brandon, MS 39047
(601) 991-0030
www.rehabreview.com

Research Activities
Agency for Health Care Research
  and Quality
U.S. Department of Health and
  Human Services
540 Gaither Road, Suite 2000
Rockville, MD 20852
www.ahrq.gov
(301) 427-1364

Reference Guides

Aventis Pharmaceuticals Inc. 2003. *Managed Care Digest.* Bridgewater, NJ. (www.managedcare digest.com/HMOPPO.jsp)

Banja, J. 2004. *Medical Errors and Medical Narcissism: Bioethical Explorations* (working title). Sudbury, MA: Jones and Bartlett Publishers.

Benefits Source Book. Updated annually. (Annual guide to research data, products, and services for employee benefit management.) Marietta, GA: Employee Benefit News, Enterprise Communications.

Berkow, R., and A. Fletcher, eds. 1987. *The Merck Manual of Diagnosis and Therapy.* 15th ed. Rahway, NJ: Merck Sharp & Dohme.

Blancett, S., and Flarey, D. 1996. *Handbook of Nursing Care Management.* Gaithersburg, MD: Aspen Publishers, Inc.

Blum, L. 1993. *Free Money for Health Care: A Financial Aid Directory for Patient Care and Patient Services.* Gaithersburg, MD: Aspen Publishers.

Carpenito, L. J. 1993. *Handbook of Nursing Diagnosis.* 5th ed. Philadelphia, PA: J.B. Lippincott.

Castle Connolly Staff (Compiler) et al. 2003. *America's Top Doctors: The Best in American Medicine (America's Top Doctors,* third edition), Castle Connolly Medical, Ltd.

Castleman, M. 2000. *Blended Medicine: The Best Choices in Healing.* Emmaus, PA: Rodale Press.

Cohen, E. L., and T. Cesta. 1997. *Nursing Case Management: From Concept to Evaluation.* 2d ed. St. Louis, MO: Mosby-Year Book.

Complete Directory of People with Learning Disabilities, 1997/98. Updated annually. Lakeville, CT: Grey House Publishing.

Conner, C., ed. 1997. *Health Care Fraud and Abuse Compliance Manual.* Gaithersburg, MD: Aspen Publishers.

Cress, C. 2007. *Handbook of Geriatric Care Management.* 2d ed. Sudbury, MA: Jones and Bartlett Publishers.

Cress, C. 2009. *Care Managers: Working with the Aging Family.* Sudbury, MA: Jones and Bartlett Publishers.

Crimando, W., and T. F. Riggar, eds. 1996. *Utilizing Community Resources: An Overview of Human Services.* Boca Raton, FL: St. Lucie Press.

Curaflex Health Services. 1991. *Home Infusion Therapy Resource Guide.* Ontario, CA.

D'Avanzo, C. E., and E. M. Geissler. 2003. *Cultural Health Assessment,* third edition. St. Louis, MO: Mosby-Year Book.

Dell Orto, A. E., and P. W. Power. 1994. *Head Injury and the Family: A Life and Living Perspective.* Boca Raton, FL: St. Lucie Press.

Dietrick, H. J., and V. H. Biddle. 1990. *The Best in Medicine: Where to Find the Best Health Care Available.* New York, NY: Harmony Books.

Driving Down Health Care Costs: Strategies and Solutions 1997. Updated annually. New York, NY: Panel Publishers.

Edelstein, E., ed. 1992. *Blue Book American Druggist: Annual Directory of Pharmaceuticals.* New York, NY: Hearst Corporation.

The Editors of Prevention Magazine Health Books (Editor) et al. 1997. *New Choices in Natural Healing: Over 1,800 of the Best Self-Help Remedies from the World of Alternative Medicine.* Emmaus, PA: Rodale Press.

Field, T. F., and L. P. Norton. 1990. *ADA Resource Manual for Rehabilitation Consultants.* Athens, GA: Elliott & Fitzpatrick.

Fiesta, J. 1983. *The Law and Liability: A Guide for Nurses.* New York, NY: John Wiley & Sons.

Fincham, J. E., and A. I. Wertheimer, eds. 2000. *Pharmacy and the U.S. Health Care System,* second edition. Binghamton, NY: Haworth Press.

Garner, J. C. 1998. *Health Insurance Answer Book.* New York, NY: Panel Publishers.

Goor, R., and N. Goor. 1992. *Eater's Choice.* 3rd ed. Boston, MA: Houghton Mifflin Co.

Griffin, K. 1995. *Handbook of Subacute Health Care.* Gaithersburg, MD: Aspen Publishers, Inc.

Griffith, P. D. M. 1993. *The Managed Care Resource Manual for Obstetrics.* Marietta, GA: Healthdyne Perinatal Services.

Health and Medical Care Directory. 1988. Niagara Falls, NY: Yellow Pages of America.

Health Insurance Association of America. Updated annually. *Source Book of Health Insurance Data.* Washington, DC.

Healthcare Consultants of America. 2003. *2003 Physicians Fee and Coding Guide.* Augusta, GA.

Hilden, J. M., D. R. Tobin, and K. Lindsey. 2003. *Shelter from the Storm: Caring for a Child with a Life-Threatening Condition.* Boulder, CO: Perseus Publishing.

HMO/PPO Directory. 1995. Montvale, NJ: Medical Economics Co.

Inlander, C. B., and K. Morales. 1993. *Getting the Most for Your Medical Dollar.* New York, NY: Pantheon Books.

Isaacs, S. L., and A. C. Swartz. 1992. *Consumer's Legal Guide to Today's Health Care.* New York, NY: Houghton Mifflin.

Jenkins, M., and Henne, R., eds. 1996. *The National Directory of Managed & Integrated Care Organizations.* Wall Township, NJ: Health Resources Publishing.

Karaffa, M. C., ed. 1992. ICD-9-CM: *International Classification of Disease.* 9th rev., 4th ed. Los Angeles, CA: Practice Management Information Corporation.

Kirschner, C. G., et al. 1992. *Physicians' Current Procedural Terminology (CPT).* 4th ed. Chicago, IL: American Medical Association.

Kongstvedt, P. R. 2001. *The Managed Health Care Handbook.* 4th edition. Sudbury, MA: Jones and Bartlett Publishing, Inc.

Larson, D. E., ed. 1990. *Mayo Clinic Family Health Book.* New York, NY: William Morrow. Updated annually.

Lesko, M., et al. 1993. *What to Do When You Can't Afford Health Care.* Kensington, MD: Information USA.

MacKenzie, L., and A. Lignor, eds. 1993. *The Complete Directory for People with Learning Disabilities.* Lakeville, CT: Grey House Publishing.

The Managed Care Yearbook. 1994. Wall Township, NJ: American Business Publishing.

Medical Interface. 1993. *Executive Managed Care Directory.* Bronxville, NY: Medicom International.

Medical Society of the State of New York. 1990. *Medical Directory of New York State.* 62d ed. Lake Success, NY. (Check local library for state organizations publishing similar directories.)

Melonakos, K. 1990. *Saunders Pocket Reference for Nurses.* Philadelphia, PA: W. B. Saunders.

Mercier, L. R. 1991. *Practical Orthopedics.* 3rd ed. St. Louis, MO: Mosby-Year Book.

Meyer, D., and P. Vadasy. 1996. *Living with a Brother and Sister with Special Needs.* 2d ed. Seattle, WA: University of Washington Press.

National Association of Rehabilitation Professionals in the Private Sector. Updated annually. *National Directory of NARPPS.* Brookline, MA.

National Association of Social Workers. Updated annually. *NASW Register of Clinical Social Workers.* Washington, DC.

National Cancer Institute. 1997. Washington, DC.

Breast Cancer Screening Program Makes Good Business Sense (F370).

Establishing Workplace Breast Cancer Screening Programs: Blueprint for Action (F368).

What You Need to Know About Breast Cancer (95-1556).

Advanced Cancer: Living Each Day (93-856).

Chemotherapy and You: A Guide to Self-Help During Treatment (94-1136).

Facing Forward: A Guide for Cancer Survivors (3-2424).

The 2003–2004 National Directory of Brain Injury Rehabilitation Services. 2003. McLean, VA: Brain Injury Association.

The National Housing Directory for People with Disabilities. 1993. Lakeville, CT: Grey House Publishing.

Nicholl, L. H. 2001. *Nurses' Guide to the Internet,* 3rd edition. Philadelphia, PA: Lippincott Williams & Wilkins.

The Official ABMS Directory of Board Certified Medical Specialists 1998. 30th ed. 1998. New Providence, NJ: Reed Elsevier, Inc.

PDR: Physician's Desk Reference. Updated annually. Montvale, NJ: Medical Economics Co.

PDR Drug Interactions and Side Effects Index. Updated annually. Montvale, NJ: Medical Economics Co.

PDR for Nonprescription Drugs. Updated annually. Montvale, NJ: Medical Economics Co.

Pell, A. R. 1987. *Making the Most of Medicare: A Guide Through the Medicare Maze.* New York, NY: Prentice Hall.

Powell, S., and D. Ignavaticus. 2001. *CMSA Core Curriculum for Case Management.* Philadelphia, PA: Lippincott Williams & Wilkins.

Raymond, F. 1997. *Surviving Alzheimer's: A Guide for Families.* Forest Knolls, CA: Elder Books.

Reed, P. 1998. *The Medical Disability Advisor: Workplace Guidelines for Disability Duration.* 3d ed. Denver, CO: Reed Group, Ltd.

Robbins, D. A. 1996. *Ethical and Legal Issues in Home Health and Long-term Care.* Gaithersburg, MD: Aspen Publishing, Inc.

Roche, L. 1997. *Coping with Caring: Daily Reflections for Alzheimer's Caregivers.* Forest Knolls, CA: Elder Books.

Romano, J. 1998. *Legal Rights of the Catastrophically Ill and Injured: A Family Guide,* 2d edition. Norristown, PA: Rosenstein & Romano, P.C.

Rossi, P. 1999. *Case Management in Healthcare.* Philadelphia, PA: W. B. Saunders Company.

Rothenberg, M. A., and C. F. Chapman. 1989. *Dictionary of Medical Terms.* 2d ed. Hauppauge, NY: Barron's Educational Series.

Sapienza, J. 2002. *Urgent Whispers: Care of the Dying.* Eugene, OR: LLX Press.

St. Coeur, M., ed. 1996. *Case Management Practice Guidelines.* St. Louis, MO: Mosby-Year Book.

Schull, P., ed. 1996. *Professional Guide to Symptoms.* 2d ed. Springhouse, PA: Springhouse Publishing.

Schneider, J. S., and Lidsky, T. I. 1999. *The Doctor's Always In: A Guide to 1000+ Best Health and Medical Information Sites on the Internet.* Cherry Hill, NJ: Neuroinformatics Inc.

Schwartz, G. E., et al. 1989. *The Disability Management Sourcebook.* Washington, DC: Washington Business Group on Health and Institute for Rehabilitation and Disability Management.

Shephard, B. D., ed. 1997. *The Complete Guide to Women's Health.* 3d rev. ed. New York, NY: Plume Books.

Sherman, B. S., ed. 1988. *Directory of Residential Facilities for Emotionally Handicapped Youth.* 2d ed. Phoenix, AZ: Oryx Press.

Sherman, C. D., Jr., ed. 1990. *World Oncology Directory and Source Book.* Milan: World Directories Ltd. (Contact Charles D. Sherman, Jr., Highland Hospital, Rochester, NY 14620)

Shrey, D. E., and M. Lacerte. 1995. *Principles and Practices of Disability Management in Industry.* Boca Raton, FL: St. Lucie Press.

Spratt, J. R., Hawley, and R. Hoye, eds. 1997. *Home Health Care.* Boca Raton, FL: St. Lucie Press.

Stanhope, M., and R. N. Knollmueller. 1992. *Handbook of Community and Home Health Nursing.* St. Louis, MO: Mosby-Year Book.

Substance Abuse Residential Treatment Centers for Teens. 1990. Phoenix, AZ: Oryx Press.

Taber, C. W. 1961. *Taber's Cyclopedic Medical Dictionary.* 8th ed. New York, NY: McGraw-Hill.

Thorn, K. 1990. *Applying Medical Case Management: AIDS.* Canoga Park, CA: Thorn Publishing.

Tierney, L. M., Jr. et al., eds. 1997. *Current Medical Diagnosis and Treatment.* Updated annually. Norwalk, CT: Appleton & Lange.

Tobin, D. R. 1998. *Peaceful Dying: The Step-by-Step Guide to Preserving Your Dignity, Your Choice, and Your Inner Peace at the End of Life.* Boulder, CO: Perseus Book Group.

Wolinsky, H., and Wolinsky, J. 2001. *Healthcare Online for Dummies.* New York, NY: Hungry Minds, Inc.

U.S. Department of Health and Human Services. 1990. *AIDS and the Workplace: Resources for Workers, Managers, and Employers.* Washington, DC: U.S. Government Printing Office.

U.S. Department of Health and Human Services. Updated annually. *Guide to Health Insurance for People with Medicare.* Washington, DC: U.S. Government Printing Office.

Wasserman, D. 1996. *Physician's Fee Reference.* 13th ed. West Allis, WI: Yale.

Weiner, R. S., ed. 1997. *Pain Management.* Boca Raton, FL: St. Lucie Press and the American Academy of Pain Management.

Wong, M. M., ed. 1995. *1995 National Directory of Bereavement Support Groups and Services.* Forest Hills, NY: ADM Publishing.

Note: For ICD-9 and other code references, see Chapters 9 and 11; for ethics references, see Chapter 6; for provider references, see Chapter 2; for special camps and facilities for specific disease states, see Chapter 2; for end-of-life references, see Chapter 17.

SEMINARS/CONFERENCE SPONSORS

(Also see Other Programs section earlier in this appendix.)
Call for upcoming offerings.

Academy of Certified Case Managers
256 Post Road East
Suite 204
West Port, CT 06880
(203) 454-1333

American Association of Health Plans
601 Pennsylvania Avenue, NW
South Building, Suite 500
Washington, DC 20004
(202) 331-7487

American Association of Managed Care Nurses
4435 Waterfront Drive, Suite 101
Glen Allen, VA 23060
(804) 747-9698

American Health Consultants
P.O. Box 105109
Atlanta, GA 30353-0161
(800) 688-2421

Annual National Managed Health Care Congress
NMHCC
100 Winter Street, Suite 4000
Waltham, MA 02154
(617) 487-6700
(There are also regional managed health care conferences offered throughout the year.)

Casa Colina Centers for Rehabilitation
255 East Bonita Avenue
P.O. Box 6001
Pomona, CA 91769-6001
(909) 596-7733

Center for Bio-Medical Communication, Inc.
433 Hackensack Avenue
9th Floor
Hackensack, NJ 07601
(201) 342-5300

CMSA Annual Conference and Educational Forum
Case Management Society of America
6301 Ranch Drive
Little Rock, AR 72223
(501) 225-2229

Federal Publications, Inc.
1120 20th Street, NW
Washington, DC 20036
(800) 922-4330
(202) 337-7000

Global Business Research, Inc.
151 West 19th Street, 8th Floor
New York, NY 10011
(212) 645-4226

**Institute for International
    Research**
71 West 23rd Street, 8th Floor
New York, NY 10010
(212) 845-4400

**International Business
    Communications**
USA Conferences, Inc.
225 Turnpike Road
Southborough, MA 01772-1749
(508) 481-6400

International Business Forum
575 Broadway
Massapequa, NY 11758
(516) 765-9005

**Joint Commission on
    Accreditation of Healthcare
    Organizations**
1 Renaissance Boulevard
Oakbrook Terrace, IL 60181
(630) 792-5000

Magee Rehabilitation Hospital
1513 Race Street
Philadelphia, PA 19102
(215) 587-3000

**National Health Lawyers
    Association**
1120 Connecticut Avenue, NW,
    Suite 950
Washington, DC 20036
(202) 833-1100

**Rehabilitation Hospital of
    Colorado Springs**
325 Parkside Drive
Colorado Springs, CO 80910
(719) 630-8000

**Rehabilitation Institute
    of Chicago**
Education and Training Center
345 East Superior
Chicago, IL 60611
(312) 908-6179

Rehabilitation Management, Inc.
7144 North Harlem, Suite 241
Chicago, IL 60631
(312) 763-5600

Rehabilitation Training Institute
P.O. Box 4116
Winter Park, FL 32793-4116
(800) 431-6687

Self-Insurance Exchange, Inc.
25251 Paseo de Alicia, Suite 200
Laguna Hills, CA 92653
(714) 768-0334

**Self-Insurance Institute of
    America, Inc.**
P.O. Box 15466
Santa Ana, CA 92735
(714) 261-2553

SkillPath Seminars
6900 Squibb Road
P.O. Box 2768
Mission, KS 66201-2768
(800) 873-7545

Strategic Research Institute
500 Fifth Avenue
New York, NY 10110
(212) 302-1800
(800) 599-4950

The University of Vermont
Burlington, VT 05405
(802) 656-3131

www.uvm.edu/
Continuing Education

URAC
1220 L Street NW, Suite 400
Washington, DC 20005
(202) 216-9010
www.uraq.org

**Washington Business Group
   on Health**
777 North Capitol Street, NE,
   Suite 800
Washington, DC 20002
(202) 408-9320

Glossary

MEDICAL AND INSURANCE TERMINOLOGY

accident and health (A & H). Accident and health coverage is a feature of all group insurance except group life insurance. It is also referred to as accident and sickness, casualty, and disability coverage. The insurance industry's new general term is *health insurance.*

accident and sickness (A & S). Accident and sickness coverage, although sometimes used as synonymous with accident and health coverage, usually refers to weekly indemnity insurance (loss-of-time, short-term disability income coverage). See loss-of-time benefits.

accumulation period. The maximum length of time an individual has to incur covered expenses that satisfy a required deductible.

active life reserve. The reserve for potential disability claims on currently insured active (not disabled) lives.

actively-at-work requirement. A form of individual evidence of insurability, because the insured's health must be at least sound enough for him or her to be actively at work at his or her usual place of employment on the date the insurance takes effect. Because this definition is impractical for dependents, there is usually a provision that if a dependent is confined in a hospital on the date the insurance would otherwise become effective, the effective date of his or her insurance will be deferred until his or her release from the hospital.

activities of daily living (ADLs). Activities in the nonoccupational environment arising from daily living needs (e.g., mobility, personal hygiene, dressing, sleeping, eating, and skills required for community living).

adjustor. A person who handles claims (also referred to as a *claims service representative*).

appeal. A formal request to reconsider a determination not to certify an admission, extension of stay, or other medical service.

appeal committee. A management group not involved in initial claims decisions; it reviews denials (partial or full) when appealed by the claimant. It is an employee's right (as mandated by ERISA) to have a full and fair review of his or her case when a service is denied. The appeal committee reviews the claims file, the documentation of the denial, and the plan provision that was used to deny. It is the "court of last resort" and requires complete documentation to uphold a denial.

appropriateness of care. Care is considered appropriate if it is the right kind of care rendered in a proper setting.

assessment. The ongoing process of analyzing and integrating data obtained from the patient and family, relevant treatment providers, caregivers, and funding sources in order to identify the present plan of care, current and anticipated needs, and problems or obstacles that may be resolved through case management intervention.

assurance (insurance). The spreading of risk among many, with the likelihood that some will suffer a loss. The term *assurance* is more common in Canada and Great Britain; the term *insurance* is more common in the United States.

attending physician. The physician with primary responsibility for the care provided to a patient in a hospital or other health care facility.

authorization to pay benefits. A provision in a medical claim form by which the insured directs the insurance company to pay any benefits directly to the provider of care on whose charges the claim is based.

automatic reinsurance. A type of reinsurance in which the insurer must cede and the reinsuring company must accept all risks within certain contractually defined areas (also called *treaty reinsurance*). The reinsuring company undertakes in advance to grant reinsurance to the extent specified in the agreement in every case in which the ceding company accepts the application and retains its own limit.

benefits. The amount payable by an insurance company to the claimant, assignee, or beneficiary under a specific coverage.

bill audit. The review of hospital, physician, durable medical equipment, and health care service provider bills for inaccuracies or overbilling.

business alliances. Groups of business companies allied together to reduce health care costs by jointly purchasing medical services.

capitation. A method of payment for health services in which the health care provider is paid a fixed amount for each person over a specific amount of time regardless of the actual number or nature of services provided to each person.

caregiver. A family member, volunteer, or medical professional charged with providing care in the home setting.

carrier. The insurance company or other entity that agrees to pay the losses. A carrier may be organized as a company (stock, mutual, or reciprocal) or as an association of underwriters (e.g., Lloyds of London).

case reserve. The dollar amount stated in a claims file that represents an estimate of the amount still unpaid.

certification. A determination by a utilization review organization that an admission, extension of stay, or other medical service has been provided and qualifies as medically necessary and appropriate under the medical review requirements of the applicable health benefit plan.

claim. A request for payment of reparation for a loss covered by an insurance contract.

claimant. The person filing the claim to whom benefits are to be paid by the claims administrator.

claims administrator. Any entity that reviews and determines whether to pay claims to enrollees, physicians, or hospitals on behalf of the health benefit plan. Payment determinations are made on the basis of contract provisions, including those regarding medical necessity, and other factors. Claims administrators may be insurance companies, self-insured employers, management firms, Third Party Administrators, or other private contractors.

claims cost control. Efforts made by an insurer both inside and outside its own organization to restrain and direct claims payments so that health insurance premium dollars are used as efficiently as possible.

claims reserves. Funds reserved by an insurer to settle incurred but unpaid claims; may also include reserves for potential claims fluctuation.

claims service representative. A person who investigates losses and settles claims for an insurance carrier or the insured. *Adjustor* is a synonymous, although less preferred, term.

clinical experience. Expertise gained through professional clinical practice (e.g., any combination of direct patient care in a specialty area, home health, or general clinical area for which the applicant is licensed or certified).

coinsurance. A provision under a health insurance policy whereby the consumer assumes a percentage of the costs of covered services.

complementary and alternative medicine (CAM). The use of complementary and alternative care treatments is still considered controversial or "unorthodox" in some quarters; however, especially given the increased cultural diversity of our patient populations, they are among the most appropriate healing techniques for certain patients. Classified as mind/body/spirit treatment, holistic medicine, and Eastern medicine, these alternative approaches can refer to acupuncture, guided imagery, dietary therapy, Chinese medicine, spiritual healing, herbal remedies, homeopath, meditation, craniosacral therapy, chiropractic care, massage including Reiki, fertility treatments, paranormal healing, Tai Chi, and Yoga, among others.

comprehensive major medical insurance. A form of major medical expense insurance (written with an initial deductible) that can substitute for separate policies providing basic hospital, surgical, and medical benefits.

concurrent insurance. Insurance of a person under two or more policies providing similar or identical coverages (usually avoided in group insurance).

concurrent review. A form of utilization review that tracks the progress of a patient during treatment; conducted on-site or by telephone.

contingency reserve. A reserve established to share among all policyholders the cost to the insurer of unpredictable catastrophic losses.

coordination of benefits (COB). A method of integrating benefits payable under more than one group health insurance plan so that the insured's benefits from all sources do not exceed 100% of his or her allowable medical expenses. Another method, based on a strict benefit-by-benefit (or "carve-out") calculation, could result in zero payment by an insurer other than the one that pays benefits first.

co-payment. The portion of a claim or medical expense that a claimant must pay out of pocket.

cost-based or cost-related reimbursement. One method of payment of medical care programs by third parties, typically Blue Cross plans or government agencies, for services delivered to patients. In cost-related systems, the amount of the payment is based on the costs to the provider of delivering the service. The actual payment may be based on any one of several different formulas, such as full cost, full cost plus an additional percentage, allowable costs, or a fraction of costs. Other reimbursement schemes are based on the charges for fraction of costs, on the charges for the services delivered, or on budgeted or anticipated costs for a future time period (prospective reimbursement).

cost containment. The control of the overall cost of health care services within the health care delivery system. Costs are contained when the value of the resources committed to an activity are not considered to be excessive.

coverage. (1) The aggregate of risks insured by a contract of insurance; (2) a major classification of benefits provided by a group policy (e.g., term life, weekly indemnity, major medical); (3) the amount of insurance or benefits stated in the group policy for which an insured is eligible.

covered charges. Charges for medical care or supplies that, if incurred by an insured or other covered person, create a liability for the insurance under the terms of a group policy.

cultural and linguistic competence in health. A set of congruent behaviors, attitudes, and policies that come together in a system, agency, or among professionals that enables effective work in cross-cultural situations.

defensive medicine. The increased use of laboratory tests, hospital admissions, and extended lengths of stays in hospital by physicians for the principal purpose of forestalling the possibility of malpractice suits by patients and providing a good legal defense in the event of such lawsuits.

diagnosis-related groups (DRGs). Groupings of patients by discharge diagnosis to measure a hospital's output. These are used for analysis and monitoring of the hospital's resource utilization performance and costs.

direct contract model. A health plan that contracts directly with private practice physicians rather than through an independent practice association or medical group.

direct costs. Administration costs directly attributable to particular group cases and excluding any share of overhead expenses.

disability. A condition that makes an individual unable to earn full wages by doing the work performed when the individual was last employed.

disability benefit. A payment that arises because of total or permanent disability of an insured; a provision added to a policy that provides for a waiver of premium in case of total and permanent disability.

disability income insurance. A form of health insurance that provides periodic payments to replace income when an insured person is unable to work as a result of illness or injury.

discharge planner. The individual who assesses a patient's need for treatment after hospitalization in order to help arrange for the necessary services and resources to effect an appropriate and timely discharge.

discharge planning. The process that assesses a patient's need for treatment after hospitalization in order to help arrange for the necessary services and resources to effect an appropriate and timely discharge.

e-Health. A term that applies to the use of electronic technologies and telecommunications in the practice of clinical health care, patient and professional health-related education, public health, and health medicine. It includes the fields of telemedicine, teleHealth, medical informatics, electronic patient records, supply chain management, and biotechnologies.

enrollee. The individual who has elected to contract for or participate in a health benefit plan for him- or herself or his or her dependents.

exclusion. A specific illness or treatment that is expressly not covered by a plan or insurance contract.

exclusive provider organization (EPO). A form of PPO in which any services rendered by a nonaffiliated provider are not reimbursed, and the entire cost must be paid out of pocket by the claimant. EPO providers are usually reimbursed on a fee-for-service basis according to a negotiated discount or fee schedule.

fee-for-service. A form of reimbursement in which physicians and hospitals are paid a "reasonable or customary" fee for a unit of service; also, a system for the payment of professional services in which the practitioner is paid for the particular service rendered rather than receiving a salary for services provided during scheduled work or on-call hours.

gatekeeper. A primary care provider who authorizes all specialist referrals. Use of gatekeepers is an essential feature of HMOs.

group model HMO. An HMO that contracts with a group of physicians who are paid a set salary per patient to provide a predetermined range of services.

group practice. Three or more physicians who deliver patient care, jointly use medical equipment and personnel, and divide income by a predetermined formula.

Guided Care Model. Guided Care is a new solution to the growing challenge of caring for older adults with chronic conditions and complex health needs. A Guided Care Nurse, based in a primary care office, works with patients and their families to improve their quality of life and make more efficient use of health services. The nurse assesses patient needs, monitors conditions, educates and empowers the patient, and works with community agencies to ensure that the patient's healthcare goals are met.

health benefit plan. Any public or private organization's written plan that insures or pays for specific health or medical expenses on behalf of enrollees and/or covered persons.

Health Care Financing Administration (HCFA). An administrative body of the federal government that oversees all aspects of health financing.

health insurance. Protection that provides payment of benefits for covered sickness or injury; includes various types of insurance, such as accident protection, disability income, medical expenses, and accidental death and dismemberment coverage.

Health literacy. The ability to understand health information and to use that information to make good decisions about your health and medical care.

health maintenance organization (HMO). An organization that provides health care for a geographic area and that accepts responsibility for delivering an agreed-upon set of health maintenance and treatment services to a voluntarily enrolled group. An HMO collects a predetermined periodic payment paid in advance on behalf of each individual enrolled.

holistic medicine. A trend in medicine that emphasizes that the system must extend its focus beyond the physical aspects of disease or particular organs. It is concerned with the whole person and the interrelationships between the emotional, social, spiritual, and physical implications of disease and health.

home health care. Health care provided in the home to aged, disabled, sick, or convalescent individuals who do not need institutional care. The most common types of home care include visiting nurse services and speech, physical, occupational, and rehabilitation therapy. These services are provided by home health agencies, hospitals, or other community organizations.

home health services. Health care services provided to a patient in his or her own home by health care personnel.

hospice. A health care program whose purpose is to provide care, compassion, and support for those patients in the final stages of illness and close to death.

hospital alliances. Groups of hospitals allied together to reduce costs by sharing common services and developing group purchasing programs.

impairment. An inability or lessened ability to perform work duties because of a work-related injury or disease.

indemnity. The security against possible loss or damage; a predetermined reimbursement amount paid in the event of a covered loss.

independent medical exam (IME). A medical exam used by insurers to determine an individual's diagnosis, need for continued treatment, degree and permanency of disability, or ability to return to work.

independent practice association (IPA). An HMO that contracts with physicians who see HMO patients in their own private offices. Physicians are reimbursed on a capitated or a fee-for-service basis.

initial evaluation. The assessment conducted by a case manager following case referral. Medical, psychological, social, vocational, educational, and economic factors are explored to ascertain the best course of action for achieving rehabilitation and the feasibility of rehabilitation.

injury. Harm to a worker that requires treatment and/or compensation under workers' compensation.

inside limits. Internal control limits within the structure of overall benefits or the benefit plan; they are utilized to establish a maximum amount for a procedure, service, confinement, disability, calendar year, and so on.

job description. A detailed description of the duties, tasks, and requirements of a job, including specific physical and mental qualifications for performance. A job description is an important tool for analyzing an insured's potential to return to his or her pre-injury job and for ascertaining transferable skills.

legal reserve. The minimum reserve a company must keep to meet future claims and obligations as calculated under a state insurance code.

long-term care. The health care provided to individuals who do not require hospital care but who do need nursing, medical, and other health care services provided over time.

long-term disability income insurance. The insurance issued to a group or an individual to provide a reasonable replacement of a portion of income lost due to a serious, prolonged illness.

loss control. The efforts by insurers and insureds to prevent accidents and reduce losses through the maintenance and upgrading of health and safety procedures.

loss expenses. The part of an expense (such as legal allocation fees) paid by an insurance company directly to the plaintiff in settling a particular claim.

loss-of-time benefits. The benefits paid to help replace earned income lost through inability to work because of a disability caused by accident or illness. Weekly indemnity insurance is the type of insurance that provides such benefits.

loss ratio. The ratio of losses to premiums for a given period.

loss reserve. The dollar amount designated as the estimated cost of an accident at the time the first notice is received.

malingering. The practice of feigning illness or inability to work in order to collect insurance benefits.

malpractice. Improper care or treatment by a physician.

managed care. A system of health care delivery aimed at managing the cost and quality of access to health care. Managed care is used by

HMOs, PPOs, and managed indemnity plans to improve the delivery of services and contain costs.

maximum benefit (overall maximum benefit). The maximum amount any one individual may receive under an insurance contract.

Medicaid. The state public assistance programs open to persons of any age whose financial resources are insufficient to pay for health care. Provided under Title XIX of the Social Security Act of 1986.

Medical Home. The medical home is a concept or model of care delivery that includes an ongoing relationship between a provider and patient, around the clock access to medical consultation, respect for the patient/family's cultural and religious beliefs, and a comprehensive approach to care and coordination of care through providers and community services.

Medicare. The hospital insurance and supplementary medical insurance systems for the aged and disabled created in 1965 by amendments to the Social Security Act.

modified job. The predisability job adapted for the insured in such a manner that it can be performed within prescribed physical or mental limitations.

modified open panel plan. A service approach to the provision of group legal insurance in which any lawyer who agrees to accept a predetermined fee schedule and other procedural requirements may provide covered legal services to a member of a plan.

network model HMO. An independent practice association of group practices as opposed to solo physicians.

nondisabling injury. An injury that may require medical care but does not result in loss of working time or income.

nonduplication clause. A clause that excludes expenses incurred to the extent that an employee or dependent receives benefits under any type of policyholder-sponsored insurance plan.

nonexempt (nonexempt employees). A classification of employees designating those employees subject to overtime compensation and working time limits under the federal Labor Standards Act.

nonoccupational insurance. Insurance that does not provide benefits for an accident or sickness arising out of a person's employment.

occupancy rate. A measure of inpatient health facility use determined by dividing available bed days by patient days. It measures the average percentage of a hospital's beds occupied and may be institutionwide or limited to one department or service.

occupational therapy (OT). A program of prescribed activities that focuses on coordination and mastery and is designed to assist the insured to regain independence, particularly in activities of daily living.

orthotics. The field that specializes in using orthopedic appliances, braces, and other devices to support weight, prevent or correct deformities, or improve the function of movable parts of the body.

overinsurance. Insurance exceeding in amount the probable loss to which it applies. Overinsurance, which can be a serious problem, is controlled in group medical care coverage by the contractual use of nonduplication of benefits provisions (e.g., coordination of benefits).

partial disability. A condition resulting from an illness or injury that prevents an insured from performing one or more regular job functions.

per diem cost. Literally, cost per day. Refers, in general, to hospital or other inpatient institutional costs for a day of care. Hospitals occasionally charge for their services using a per diem rate derived by dividing total costs by the number of inpatient days of care given. Per diem costs are, therefore, averages and do not reflect the true cost for each patient. Thus, the per diem approach is said to give hospitals an incentive to prolong hospital stays.

period of disability. The period during which an employee is prevented from performing the usual duties of his or her occupation or employment or during which a dependent is prevented from performing the normal activities of a healthy person of the same age and sex. More than one cause (accident or sickness) may be present during or contribute to a single period of disability.

permanent and total disability. A disability that will presumably last for the insured's lifetime and that prevents him or her from engaging in any occupation for which he or she is reasonably fitted.

physician advisor. A physician who represents a claims administrator or utilization review organization and who provides advice on whether to certify an admission, extension of stay, or other medical service as being medically necessary and appropriate.

point-of-service (POS) plan. Evolved from the preferred provider organization concept, point-of-service plans are customized managed care plans often offered by larger companies. These plans combine employee choice and customized care with tight medical management and local utilization.

preadmission authorization (or precertification). The practice of requiring those covered by a health care plan to telephone a claims department prior to hospitalization, outpatient surgery, or other significant medical procedure. In most cases, a two-week notification period is requested, with allowances made for emergency treatment, for which a report within 48 hours of hospital admission is generally required.

preexisting condition. A physical or mental condition of an insured that manifested itself prior to the issuance of the individual policy or for which treatment was received prior to such issuance.

preferred provider organization (PPO). A system of health care delivery in which a third-party payer contracts with a group of medical care providers who furnish services at lower than usual fees in return for prompt payment and a certain volume of patients. The discounted fee structure is usually of a fee-for-service type.

preventative care. Care directed at preventing disease or its consequences (e.g., through immunization and early detection). Promotion of health through improving the environment or altering behaviors, especially through health education, has gained prominence and is an important strategy used, for example, by HMOs, primary care centers, and others.

primary care. Basic health care provided by physicians, general practitioners, internists, obstetricians, pediatricians, and midlevel practitioners that emphasizes a patient's general health needs as opposed to specialized care. Includes basic or initial diagnosis and treatment, health supervision, management of chronic conditions, and preventative health services. Appropriate referral to consultants and community resources is an important facet of primary care.

probationary period. The length of time a person must wait from the day of his or her entry into an eligible class or application for coverage to the date his or her insurance becomes effective. Also sometimes referred to as the *service period* or *waiting period.*

profile. A longitudinal or cross-sectional aggregation of medical care data. A patient profile lists all of the services provided to a particular patient during a specified period of time. Physician, hospital, or population profiles are statistical summaries of the pattern of practice of individual physicians or hospitals or the medical experience of specific populations. Diagnostic profiles, a subcategory of physician, hospital, or population profiles, focus on a specific condition or diagnosis.

proposal. A quotation submitted to a prospective group insurance policyholder by the insurance company through an agent, broker, or group representative. This quotation outlines the benefits available under the proposed plan and the costs to both employer and employee. This is an important visual sales aid.

protocols. The generally accepted procedures and methods for the delivery of medical care.

provider. A licensed health care facility, physician, or other health care professional that delivers health care services.

rate. The charge per unit of payroll used to determine workers' compensation or other insurance premiums. The rate varies according to the risk classification of the policyholder.

rating. The application of the proper classification rate and other factors that may be used to set the premium rate for a policyholder. The three principal forms are manual, experience, and retrospective rating.

reconsideration. An initial request for additional review of a utilization review organization's determination not to certify an admission, extension of stay, or other medical service. A reconsideration request is called an *expedited appeal* by some utilization review organizations.

rehabilitation. The restoration of a totally disabled person to a meaningful occupation. A provision in some long-term disability policies provides for a continuation of benefits or other financial assistance while a totally disabled insured is being retrained or attempting to resume productive employment.

reinsurance carriers. Insurers for the insurers. See stop-loss insurance.

reserve general. (1) An amount representing actual or potential liabilities that is kept by an insurer to cover debts to policyholders; (2) an amount allocated for a special purpose. Note that a reserve is usually a liability and not an extra fund. On occasion, a reserve may be an asset, such as a reserve for taxes not yet due.

retrospective review. Another form of utilization review that allows insurers and employers to maintain records of physicians' practice patterns, hospital length of stay averages, and typical treatment patterns for specific diagnoses and thereby build a database to help analyze "standard and reasonable" procedures and costs.

review criteria. The written policies, decision rules, medical protocols, or guides used by a utilization review organization to determine certification (e.g., appropriateness evaluation protocols [AEPs] and intensity of service, severity of illness, discharge and appropriateness [ISD-A] screens).

second surgical opinion (SSO). When there is a complex medical picture, when questionable treatment is under way, or when elective surgery is recommended, a second surgical opinion is often requested by the insurer, employer, or patient. Some of the elective surgeries leading to an SSO request are often unnecessary, such as the removal of adenoids, bunions, gallbladder, and tonsils or open-heart, knee, or hip surgery.

settlement options. The provisions (stated or intended) in insurance contracts that allow an insured or beneficiary to receive benefits in other than a lump sum payment.

short-term disability income insurance. The insurance that pays benefits during the time a disability exists to a covered person who remains disabled for a specified period not to exceed 2 years.

staff model HMO. An HMO that employs physicians who operate out of their own facilities or clinics but who receive a salary from the HMO.

stop-loss insurance. The insurance taken by employer groups to cover the financial responsibility of health benefit payments that exceed an established threshold. A company might have health care benefits of $1,000,000 per covered life, with a threshold set at $100,000 with a reinsurer. This means there is coverage for a patient with claims of $150,000 or $250,000, but the company only pays the first $100,000 out of its group coverage and is reimbursed dollar for dollar by the stop-loss carrier for any costs over the threshold up to $1,000,000.

subrogation. In the health insurance context, subrogation is the contractual right of the plan or carrier, where state law permits, to succeed to the rights of the covered person in relation to a claim against a third party. This means that the insured party gives up the right to sue the negligent party. This right is given to the insurance company because it has paid a claim on the insured's behalf. If the insured suffers damages over and above those covered by his or her policy, he or she can sue the third party.

targeted review. A review process that focuses on specific diagnoses, services, hospitals, or practitioners rather than on all services provided or proposed to be provided to enrollees.

third-party administration. The administration of a group insurance plan by some person or firm other than the insurer or the policyholder.

Third Party Administrator (TPA). The companies that work with insurance firms, handling all the administrative tasks involved in processing claims. Employers who have become self-insurers, taking on the responsibility of funding their own benefit plans, may use a TPA or they may oversee the payment of claims themselves, via a self-insured, self-administered plan.

third-party payment. The payment of health care by an insurance company or other organization so that the patient does not directly pay for his or her services.

transferable skills. The skills an insured has acquired through occupational or vocational endeavors that may be applied with minimal training in another occupation.

usual, customary, and reasonable (UCR). Health insurance plans often pay a physician's full charge if it does not exceed his or her usual charge, if it does not exceed the amount customarily charged for the service by other physicians in the area, or if it is otherwise reasonable.

utilization. Utilization is commonly examined in terms of patterns or rates of use of a single service or type of service (hospital care, prescription drugs, physician visits). Measurement of utilization of all medical services in combination is usually done in terms of dollar expenditures. Use is expressed in rates per unit of population at risk for a given period (e.g., number of admissions to a hospital per 1,000 persons over 65 years of age per year).

utilization review (UR). The process of reviewing medical services for necessity, appropriateness, and efficiency to ensure that a patient is not given care that exceeds medical need and, thereby, reduces the number of unnecessary or inappropriate health care services. It includes review of admissions, length of stay, discharge, and services ordered and provided and is conducted on a preadmission, concurrent, and retrospective basis.

utilization review organization. An entity that conducts utilization review and determines certification of an admission, extension of stay, or other medical service.

vocational evaluation. A professional analysis of the insured's work potential, integrating information about physical capabilities, mental aptitudes, interests, personality motivation, transferable skills, and environmental considerations.

workers' compensation. The social insurance system for industrial and work injuries regulated in certain specified occupations by the federal government.

workers' compensation law. A statute imposing liability on employers to pay benefits and furnish care to employees injured and to pay benefits to dependents of employees killed in the course of and because of their employment.

LEGAL TERMINOLOGY

agency. A relationship between two parties in which the first party authorizes the second to act as agent on behalf of the first. It usually implies a contractual arrangement between two parties managed by a third party, an agent.

agent. A party authorized to act on behalf of another and to give the other an account of such actions.

appeal. The process whereby a court of appeals reviews the record of written materials from a court proceeding to determine if errors were made that might lead to a reversal of the trial court's decision.

assumption of risk. A doctrine based on voluntary exposure to a known risk. It is distinguished from contributory negligence (which is based on carelessness) in that it involves the comprehension that a peril is to be encountered as well as the willingness to encounter it.

claimant. One who asserts a right or demand in a legal proceeding.

claims-made policy. A professional liability insurance policy that covers the holder for a period in which a claim of malpractice is made. The alleged act of malpractice may have occurred at some previous time but the policy insures the holder when the claim is made.

compensation. An act that a court orders (including money that a court or other tribunal orders to be paid) by a person whose acts or omissions have caused loss or injury in order to recompense the injured party with respect to the loss.

confidential communications. Certain classes of communications that the law will not permit to be divulged; in general, such communications pass between persons who stand in a confidential or fiduciary relationship to each other (or who, because of their relative situation, owe a special duty of secrecy and fidelity).

cross-examination. The questioning of a witness during a trial or deposition by the party opposing those who asked the person to testify.

damages. The money awarded by the court to someone who has been injured (plaintiff) that must be paid by the party responsible for the injury (defendant). Normal damages are awarded when the injury is considered to be slight. Compensatory damages are awarded to repay or compensate the injured party for the loss that was incurred. Punitive damages are awarded when the injury is found to have been committed maliciously or in wanton disregard of the plaintiff's interests.

defendant. The person against whom an action is brought because of an alleged responsibility for violating one or more of the plaintiff's legally protected interests.

deposition. A sworn pretrial testimony given by a witness in response to oral and written questions and cross-examination. The deposition is transcribed and may be used for further pretrial investigation. It may also be presented at the trial if the witness cannot be present.

disability. In a legal context, the term means incapacity for the full enjoyment of ordinary legal rights.

discovery. A pretrial procedure that allows the plaintiff's and defendant's attorneys to find out about matters relevant to the case, including information about what evidence the other side has, what witnesses will be called, and so on. Discovery devices for obtaining information include depositions and interrogatories to obtain testimony, requests for documents and other tangible evidence, and requests for physical or mental examinations.

evidence. Any species of proof or probative matter, legally presented at the trial of an issue, by the act of the parties and through the medium of witnesses, records, documents, tangible objects, and the like, for the purpose of inducing beliefs in the minds of the court or jury as to the truth of their contention.

expert witness. A person who has special knowledge of a subject about which a court requests testimony. Special knowledge may be acquired by experience, education, observation, or study but is not possessed by the average person. An expert witness gives expert testimony or expert evidence. This evidence often serves to educate the court and the jury in the subject under consideration.

fiduciary relationship. A legal relationship of confidentiality that exists whenever one person trusts or relies on another, such as a doctor–patient relationship.

fraud. A false representation of a matter of fact (whether by words or conduct, by false or misleading allegations, or by concealment of that which should be disclosed) that deceives and is intended to deceive another so that person shall act upon such representation to his or her legal injury.

guardian ad litem. A person appointed by the court to safeguard a minor's legal interest during certain kinds of litigation.

imputed negligence. Malpractice due to negligent practice of a person taught.

in loco parentis. The Latin phrase meaning "in the place of the parent." The assumption by a person or institution of the parental obligations of caring for a child without adoption.

indemnify. To secure against loss or damage; to give security for the reimbursement of a person in the event of an anticipated loss to that individual.

injury. Any wrong or damage done to another, either to the individual's person, rights, reputation, or property. Consists of damages of a permanent nature.

interrogatories. A series of written questions submitted to a witness or other person having information of interest to the court. The answers are transcribed and are sworn to under oath.

liability. The legal responsibility for failure to act, thus causing harm to another person, or for actions that fail to meet standards of care, so causing another person harm.

liaison. A nurse who acts as an agent between a patient, the hospital, and the patient's family and who speaks for the entire health care team.

litigation. A contest in a court for the purpose of enforcing a right.

malfeasance. The performance of an unlawful, wrongful act.

malpractice. A professional person's wrongful conduct, improper discharge of professional duties, or failure to meet standards of care, which results in harm to another person.

misfeasance. An improper performance of a lawful act, especially in a way that might cause damage or injury.

motion. A request to the court to take some action or a request to the opposing side to take some action relating to a case.

negligence. The failure to act as an ordinary prudent person; conduct contrary to that of a reasonable person under similar circumstances.

nonfeasance. A failure to perform a task, duty, or undertaking that one has agreed to perform or that one had a legal duty to perform.

petition. An ex parte application to a court asking for the exercise of the court's judicial powers in relation to some matter that is not the subject for a suit or action, or a request for the authority to undertake an action that requires the sanction of the court.

plaintiff. A person who brings a suit to court in the belief that one or more of that individual's rights have been violated or that a legal injury has occurred.

professional corporation (PC). A corporation formed according to the law of a particular state for the purpose of delivering a professional service.

professional liability. A legal concept describing the obligation of a professional person to pay a patient or client for damages caused by the professional's act of omission, commission, or negligence. Professional liability better describes the responsibility of all professionals to their clients than does the concept of malpractice, but the idea of professional liability is central to malpractice.

professional liability insurance. A type of liability insurance that protects professional persons against malpractice claims made against them.

release. The relinquishment of a right, claim, or privilege by a person in whom it exists or to whom it accrues, to the person against whom it might be demanded or enforced.

remedy. The means by which a right is enforced or the violation of a right is prevented, redressed, or compensated.

res ipsa loquitur. Literally, "the thing speaks for itself." A legal doctrine that applies when the defendant was solely and exclusively in control at the time the plaintiff's injury occurred, so that the injury would not have occurred if the defendant had exercised due care. When a court applies this doctrine to a case, the defendant bears the burden of proving that he was not negligent.

respondeat superior. Literally, "let the master respond." This maxim means that an employer is liable in certain cases for the consequences of the wrongful acts of its employees while the employee is acting within the scope of his or her employment.

right of conscience law. A legal equivalent to freedom of thought or of religion.

right of privacy. The right of individuals to withhold their person and property from public scrutiny, if so desired, as long as it is consistent with the law of public policy.

right to access law. A law that grants a patient the right to see his or her medical records.

right to die law. A law that upholds a patient's right to choose death by refusing extraordinary treatment when the patient has no hope of recovery. Also referred to as the *natural death law* or *living will law.*

settlement. An agreement by the parties to a transaction or controversy that resolves some or all of the issues involved in a case.

standards of care. In a malpractice lawsuit, those acts performed or omitted that an ordinary, prudent person in the defendant's position would have done or not done; a measure by which the defendant's alleged wrongful conduct is compared.

statute. The written act of a legislative body declaring, commanding, or prohibiting an action (in contrast to unwritten common law).

statute of limitations. A statute that sets forth limitations of the right of action for certain described causes (e.g., declaring that no suit can be maintained on such cases of action unless brought within a specified period of time after the right came into existence).

subpoena. A process commanding a witness to appear and give testimony in court.

tort. A private or civil wrong outside of a contractual relationship.

tort-feasor. A wrongdoer who is legally liable for the damage caused.

uniform anatomical gift act. A law of the type existing in all 50 states that allows anyone over 18 to sign a donor card willing some or all of his or her organs after death.

waiver. The intentional or voluntary relinquishment of a known right.

wrongful death statute. A statute of the type existing in all states that provides that the death of a person can give rise to a cause of legal action brought by the person's beneficiaries in a civil suit against the person whose willful or negligent acts caused the death. Prior to the existence of these statutes, a suit could be brought only if the injured person survived the injury.

wrongful life action. A civil suit usually brought against a physician or health facility on the basis of negligence that resulted in the wrongful birth or life of an infant. The parents of the unwanted child seek to obtain payment from the defendant for the medical expenses of pregnancy and delivery, for pain and suffering, and for the education and upbringing of the child. Wrongful life actions have been brought and won in several situations, including malpracticed tubal ligations, vasectomies, and abortions. Failure to diagnose pregnancy in time for abortion and incorrect medical advice leading to the birth of a defective child have also led to malpractice suits for a wrongful life.

ACRONYMS AND ABBREVIATIONS

A & H	accident and health
A & S	accident and sickness
AAOHN	American Association of Occupational Health Nurses
ABOHN	American Board for Occupational Health Nurses
A-CCC	Continuity of Care Certification, Advanced

ACCM	Academy for Certified Case Managers
ADA	Americans with Disabilities Act of 1990
ADB	accelerated death benefit
ADEA	Age Discrimination in Employment Act
ADL	activities of daily living
AEP	appropriateness evaluation protocol
AIDS	acquired immunodeficiency syndrome
AMA	American Medical Association
ANA	American Nurses Association
ANYOCC	any occupation (used in long-term disability policies)
ASO	administrative services only
CAM	complementary and alternative medicine
CARF	Commission on Accreditation of Rehabilitation Facilities
CAT	computerized axial tomography
CCM	Certified Case Manager
CCMC	Commission for Case Management
CDC	Centers for Disease Control
CDH	consumer-driven health care
CDMS	Certified Disability Management Specialist
CDMSC	Certification of Disability Management Specialists Commission
CIRS	Certified Insurance Rehabilitation Specialist
CIRSC	Certification of Insurance Rehabilitation Specialists Commission
CLAS	National Standards on Culturally and Linguistically Appropriate Service in Health Care
CM	Case Manager
CMAC	Case Management Administrator, Certified
CMC	Care Manager Certified (from NACCM)
CMC	Case Manager, Certified (from AIOCM)
CMC-A	Case Manager Associate
CMCN	Certified Managed Care Nurse
CMS	Centers for Medicare and Medicaid Services (formerly HCFA, Health Care Financing Administration)
CMSA	Case Management Society of America
COB	coordination of benefits
COBRA	Consolidated Omnibus Budget Reconciliation Act of 1986
COHN	Certified Occupational Health Nurse
COHN/CM	Certified Occupational Health Nurse/Case Manager
COHN-S	Certified Occupational Health Nurse-Specialist

COHN-S/CM	Certified Occupational Health Nurse-Specialist/Case Manager
CPHQ	Certified Professional in Health Care Quality
CPT	Current Procedural Terminology (used in code designations)
CRC	Certified Rehabilitation Counselor
CRRN	Certified Rehabilitation Registered Nurse
C-SWCM	Certified Social Worker Case Manager
DME	durable medical equipment
DRG	diagnosis-related group
EPO	exclusive provider organization
ERISA	Employee Retirement Income Security Act of 1974
FDA	Federal Drug Administration
FMLA	Family and Medical Leave Act of 1993
FRER	Foundation for Rehabilitation Certification Education & Research
HBV	Hepatitis B virus
HCFA	Health Care Financing Administration (now CMS, Centers for Medicare and Medicaid Services)
HCO	health care organization
HEDIS	Health Plan Employer Data and Information Set
HHA	home health agency
HHC	home health care
HIA	health insurance alliance
HIPAA	Health Insurance Portability and Accountability Act of 1996 (also called the Kassebaum-Kennedy Act)
HIPCs	health insurance purchasing cooperatives
HISOCC	his occupation (used in long-term disability policies)
HIV	human immunodeficiency virus
HMO	health maintenance organization
ICD-9	International Classification of Disease, 9th edition
IDFN	integrated delivery and financing network (an IDS)
IDFS	integrated delivery and financing system (an IDS)
IDN	integrated delivery network (an IDS)
IDS	integrated delivery system
IOM	Institute of Medicine
IPA	independent practice arrangement
ISD-A	intensity of service, severity of illness, discharge and appropriateness
JCAHO	Joint Commission on Accreditation of Healthcare Organizations
LPN	Licensed Practical Nurse

LTD	long-term disability
LVN	Licensed Vocational Nurse
MCO	managed care organization
MSA	Medical Savings Account
MSO	managed services organization
OMH	Office of Minority Health
OT	occupational therapist or occupational therapy
PBM	pharmacy benefits management
PCP	primary care physician
PHO	physician–hospital organization
PhRMA	Pharmaceutical Research and Manufacturers of America
PIP	personal injury protection (auto policy clause)
POS	point-of-service
PPO	preferred provider organization
PPS	prospective payment system
PRO	professional review organization
PSDA	The Patient Self-Determination Act
PSRO	professional standards review organization
PT	physical therapist or physical therapy
R & C	reasonable and customary
RN-NCM	Registered Nurse-Nurse Case Manager
SNF	skilled nursing facility
SNV	skilled nursing visit
SHMOs	social health maintenance organizations
SPD	summary plan description
STD	short-term disability
TEFRA	Tax Equity and Fiscal Responsibility Act of 1982
TPA	Third Party Administrator
TPN	total parenteral nutrition
URAC	Utilization Review Accreditation Commission, also doing business as the American Accreditation HealthCare Commission
WC	workers' compensation

The glossary includes terms adapted or reprinted from *A thru Z: Managed Care Terms*, with permission of Medicom International and Novartis, © 2001; *Managed Healthcare*, with permission of Logical Health Care Solutions Corporation, © 2000; *Managed Care: What It Is and How It Works*, second edition, by Peter R. Kongstvedt, with permission of Jones and Bartlett Publishers, Inc., © 2004; *Home Care: An Emerging Solution to the Nation's Health Care Crisis*, with permission of Olsten

Appendix C

Case Management and Health Care Web Sites

Alternative Medicine

Alternative Medicine Foundation
http://www.amfoundation.org/

Alternative Health News Online
http://www.altmedicine.com/

CAMline
http://www.camline.org/index2.htm

Complementary Medical Association
http://www.the-cma.org.uk/

Health Care Information
Resources
Alternative Medicine section
http://www-hsl.mcmaster.ca/
tomflem/altmed.html#gen

Behavioral Health

www.psychiatry24x7.com (ADHD,
Autism, Dementia, Depression, etc.
NOTE: Special login for Health
Care Professions)

Cultural Competency

AHRQ (Agency for Health Care
Research and Quality) Minority
Health Research

www.ahrq.gov/research/minorix
.htm

Cross Cultural Health Program
www.xculture.org

Diversity RX
www.diversityrx.org

Office of Minority Health
www.omhrc.gov

Transcultural Nursing Society
www.tcns.org

Death and Dying/End of Life

DignityResources.com is a new
web site that provides financial
education and related resources
for people facing serious or
life-threatening illness.
www.dignityresources.com

Dying Well
www.dyingwell.org

End of Life Education for Nurses
www.aacn.nche.edu/elnec

Growth House
www.growthhouse.org
Resources for bereavement and
grief, death and dying, death with

dignity, euthanasia, hospice, palliative care, suicide, terminal illness, AIDS, and HIV

Last Acts
http://www.lastacts.org

Partnership for Caring
www.partnershipforcaring.org

e-Health

eHealth Initiative
www.ehealthinitiative.org

eHealth International
The Journal of Applied Health Technology
www.ehealthinternational.org

eHealth Magazine
www.e-healthmag.com

HIV/AIDS

www.aidsinfonyc.org

www.AidMeds.com
For people living with HIV, to help make empowered treatment decisions; AIDS drug database

AIDS Treatment Data Network (ATDN)
www.atdn.org
1-800-734-7104

For most recent Standards of Care

www.aids-etc.org

www.aidsinfo.nih.gov

For drug interactions; treatment, testing and resources
HIV Medication Guide
www.hivmedicationguide.com

www.GayHealth.com

Hospice/Palliative Care

American Academy of Hospice and Palliative Medicine
www.aahpm.org/

The Hospice Association of America
www.hospice-america.org

Hospice Net
www.hospicenet.org

International Association for Hospice and Palliative Care
www.hospicecare.com

The National Hospice and Palliative Care Organization
www.nhpco.org/

Palliative Education Resource Center
www.eperc.mcw.edu/

The Zen Hospice Project
www.zenhospice.org

Other Sites

About.com
www.about.com

Alzheimer's Association
www.alz.org
www.alz.org/we_can_help (has listings of best of the best web sites for treatment, caregivers, statistics, stages, etc.);

Alzheimers.com
www.alzheimers.com

Best Doctors
www.bestdoctors.com

Centers for Disease Control and Prevention
www.cdc.gov

Center for Medicare & Medicaid Services
www.cms.hhs.gov

HealthAtoZ
www.healthatoz.com

Health Communities
www.healthcommunities.com

HealthFinder
www.healthfinder.gov

Intelihealth
www.intelihealth.com

Mayo Clinic Health Oasis
www.mayohealth.org

MedicineNet
www.medicinenet.com

Medline
www.medline.com

MedScape
www.medscape.com

National Family Caregivers Association (NFCA)
www.nfcacares.org

National Institutes of Health
www.nih.gov/health

National Library of Medicine
www.nlm.nih.gov

National Organization for Rare Diseases
www.rarediseases.org

Partnership for Solutions (PFS)
For people with chronic conditions
www.partnershipforsolutions.org

Strength for Caring
www.strengthforcaring.com

WebMD
www.webmd.com

Index

A

Abortion, confidentiality and, 92
Abramson, John, 645
Academy of Certified Case Managers
    (ACCM), 516
Accelerated benefits (life insurance), 77
Accidental dismemberment clauses
    (life insurance), 77
Account managers, in claims
    departments, 382
Accountability for case management
    services, 747
Accreditation Manual for Hospitals
    (JCAHO), 85, 90
Acculturation, 592–593
Acute phase, determining appropriate
    setting for, 289–290
Acutrim, 587
Adaptive Sports Center, 29
Adherence, 631–632
Adipex-P (Phentermine), 586
Administrative-services only (ASO)
    contracts, 37
"Advance Directive Information," 666
Advance directives, 663, 666–667.
    See also Do-not-resuscitate
    (DNR) orders
    checklist for, 668
Advanced Utilization Managers
    (UMC-A), 179

Advertising. *See* Business of case
    management
Advertising, direct-to-consumer. *See* DTC
    drug marketing
Advertising standards (CCMC), 159
Advisory forms, 233. *See also* Forms
    Case Management Intervention, 238
    Stop-Loss Notification, 239
Advocacy
    defined, 153–154
    professional conduct regarding, 147
African Americans, 592, 603
    end-of-life issues and, 603
    family values, 604–605
Agency for Health Care Policy and
    Research (AHCPR), 109,
    308–309, 331
Agency for Healthcare Research and
    Quality (AHRQ), 109,
    308–309, 592
Agent Orange Veterans' Disabled
    Children's Benefits Act (2003),
    113–114
Aging populations, 651–654
Aid to Families with Dependent
    Children, 67
AIDS. *See also* HIV
    Bergalis v. CIGNA Dental Health Plan
    (1991) and, 106
    case management and, 693
    case profile, 763–766

confidentiality and, 92
consent forms and, 94–95
viatical settlements and, 74
Alaska Natives, 592, 619–620
Albireo, 642
Alcohol abuse treatment, 92. *See also*
    Substance abuse
Aliotta, Sherry, 746–748
Allowances, benefit plan, 38–39
Alprazolam (Xanax), 644
Alternative care, 28–31, 429–430
Alternative Health News Online, 28
Alternative Medicine Foundation, 28
Alzheimer's disease, 651, 652
    insurance policies for, 76
AMA. *See* American Medical
    Association (AMA)
American Academy of Family Physicians
    (AAFP), 792
American Academy of Pediatrics
    (AAP), 792
American Academy of Physical Medicine
    and Rehabilitation Code of
    Conduct, 138
American Accreditation HealthCare
    Commission, 8
American Association of Occupational
    Health Nurses (AAOHN), 175
    Standards of Occupational and
    Environmental Health
    Nursing, 310
American Board for Occupational Health
    Nurses, Inc. (ABOHN), 177, 177–178
American Board of Managed Care
    Nursing, 181–182
American Cancer Society, 720
American College of Physicians (ACP), 792
American Hospital Association, 85, 308
    patient's bill of rights, 87–89, 91
American Indians. *See* Native Americans
American Institute of Outcomes Case
    Management (AIOCM), 10,
    178, 182
American Managed Care and Review
    Organization, 308
American Medical Association (AMA),
    126–128, 308, 309
    *Cultural Competence
    Compendium*, 612

on health literacy, 627
on obesity, 572
American Medical Society
    Foundation, 637
American Nurses Association
    (ANA), 180
    Code of Ethics, 310
    on obesity, impact of, 574
American Nurses Credentialing Center
    (ANCC), 175, 180, 182
American Obesity Association, 573, 583
Americans with Disabilities Act
    (ADA, 1990), 14, 110
America's Best Hospitals, 30
America's Top Doctors, 30
Amfebutamone (Bupropion), 586
Amyotrophic lateral sclerosis (ALS),
    353, 706, 723
Anxiety Disorders Association of
    America, 702
ANYOCC (any occupation), 62–63, 292
Apple-shaped bodies, 577
Approval of case management plans,
    300–308
Armenian culture, 603–604
Arthritis, 652
Arthritis case management, 353
Ask Me 3, 638
Aspen Achievement Academy, 28
Assessments. *See also* Evaluation
    defined, 154
    disability, 232
    health literacy, 628
    high-risk, 225, 229
    information gathering and, 220
    pediatric, 225
    of staff, 537, 538
    workers' compensation, 231
Assimilation, cultural, 592–593
Associations, multiple-employer benefit
    plans and trusts and, 72
Assurance. *See* Quality assurance programs
Asthma case management, 353, 760–763
AstraZeneca, 642
At risk fees, 374
Attorneys
    communications with, 210–212
    denial of case management services by,
    285–286

initial phone contact with, 281–287
types of cases involving, 281
Auto insurance, 59, 232
Autonomy of patient, definition of, 129, 154

B

Babies, premature, 713–715, 723
Back pain case management,
     318–320, 353
Bad faith actions, 102, 106
Balanced Budget Act (1997), 111
Banja, John D., 139, 142–143, 148–149, 150,
     581–582
Bariatric surgery, 587–589
Behavioral health, 697–702
     disease management programs, 701
     obesity and, 577, 585
     partnering with professionals in, 699–701
     resources on, 701–702
Behavioral/motivational activities, 315
Beneficence, definition of, 154, 171
Benefit dollars. *See also*
     Cost-containment
     case management needs assessment
          on, 229
     determining appropriate use and flow
          of, 289–290
     in workers' compensation, 292
Benefit restrictions (caps). *See* Restrictions,
     benefit plan
Benzodiazepine, 644
Benzphetamine (Didrex), 586
Bergalis, Kimberly, 106
Bergalis v. CIGNA Dental Health Plan
     (1991), 106
Best Hospitals in America, The, 30
"Best in practice" plans, 351
Bextra (valdecoxib), 643
Bill audits. *See also* Case Management
     Audit Tool
     cost containment and, 6–7
"Birthday rule," 225
Black Americans. *See* African Americans
Blanchard, Kenneth, 150
Blue Cross and Blue Shield Association, 308
Blue Cross and Blue Shield of
     Minnesota, 610

BMI (body mass index), 576
Board of Medical Specialties, 32
Body mass index (BMI), 576
Boling, Jeanne, 91, 100, 663
Bontril (etrazine tatrate), 586
bonus programs, ethics and, 137
Borden, Marian Edelman, 29
Brain injuries, long-term care for, 723
Breast Cancer Patient Protection
     Act, 112
Breast cancer screenings, 581
Breast reduction surgery, 587–588
Bupropion, 586
Bureau of Health Professions
     (BHPr), 105
Burnout, case manager, 213–215
Business & Health, 7–8
Business background, 11. *See also* Financial
     planning background
Business cards, 195
Business community, 520–524
Business of case management. *See also* Staff,
     case management
     business community and, 520–524
     competition and niches for, 514–517
     generating, 524–532
          business goals, new, 527
          marketing materials, 526–527
          reaching decision makers, 531–532
          referral sources, 525–526
          relationships with referral sources,
               530–531
     hiring additional staff, 532–539
     networking and professional community
          for, 517–520
Business of health care, case manager
     ethical responsibilities and, 136–138
Business plans
     elements in, 510–513
     pricing market for, 513–514

C

Caesarean section, inpatient coverage
     after, 111
California v. State Care Health Plan, 107
Camp Bloomfield, 29
Camp Le Mar, 29

Camp Sweeney, 29
Campinha-Bacote, Josepha, 614
Cancer
    case profile, 769–772
    health literacy and, 629
    home care and, 706
    insurance policies for, 75–76
    long-term care for, 723
    screenings, obesity and, 581
Candidate's Knowledge Assessment Tool,
        540–541
Capitation systems, 370–371,
        372–374, 427
Caps, 60
Cardiopulmonary resuscitation, 668,
        680–683
Cardiovascular disease
        management, 353
Care continuum. *See* Continuum of care
Care Continuum Alliance, DMAA, 573–574
Care Manager Certified (CMC), 10, 179
*Care Managers Working with the Aging
        Family*, 653
Care maps, 351
CareMedical Systems, 608
Caretakers, gathering information about,
        257–258
Caring Connections program, 670
Carpal tunnel case scenario, 317–318
Carr, Janet, 710–713
Carve-out services
    fee-setting and multiple, 374–375
    managed care and negotiating for, 428
Case in Point, 150
Case management. *See also* Case managers;
        Case profiles; Certified case
        managers (CCMs); Home care;
        Integrated case management;
        Long-term cases/care plans; Public
        sector case management; Staff, case
        management
    business plan for, 510–513
    case samples with and without, 334–338
    checklist for, 368–370
    checklist for legal issues in, 122–125
    claims investigations *versus*, 204–205
    communicating concept of, 333
    continuum of care, 791–798
    definitions of, 12–13, 144, 153

delivery system and report cards
        of, 40–43
    direct-to-consumer, 691–695
    establishing system for, 349, 351–353
    evaluation of, 507–508, 510
    financial analysis of, 442
    of financial issues, 416
    legal issues in, 99–107
    licensure and liability, 81–85. *See also*
            Liability issues
    managed care *versus*, 6–9
    pharmaceutical knowledge and, 644,
            646–648
    as profession, 3–4
    redefining, 505–508
    role and functions of, 13–16
    sample description of services for
            employee/patient
            populations, 340
    scenarios
        carpal tunnel scenario, 317–318
        low back pain scenario, 318–320
        not-fit-for-duty scenario, 323–324
        slip/fall incident scenario,
                320–321
        substance abuse scenario, 321–323
    scope of duties for, 4–5
    timing for, 345–347
    work format and process of, 217–324
        action plan coordination, 308–311
        approvals for, 300–308
        case finding and targeting, 233–236
        employer group information sheet,
                226–229
        evaluation, 312–313
        flowchart for, 218
        follow-up, 311–312
        independent medical and second
                opinion exams, 273–278
        information gathering and
                assessment, 220
        planning, 287–291
        referral source communication,
                221–233
        repetition of, 313–314
        reporting, 291–300
        R.I.P. interview method, 220–221
        specific activities, 314–316
        staying on point, 316

talking with other professionals,
278–287
talking with the family, 250–258
talking with the patient, 236–250
talking with the treating physician,
258–264
Case Management Administrator, Certified
(CMAC), 180
Case Management Advisor, 148, 610
ethical issues in, 150
on telephonic case management, 273
Case Management Audit Tool, 233, 240–241
Case Management Identification
Worksheet, 233, 234
Case Management Identification Worksheet
Guidelines, 233, 237
Case Management Intervention advisory
form, 238
Case Management Practice Guidelines,
148, 310
*Case Management Resource Guide,
The*, 30
Case Management Society of America.
See CMSA
Case Manager Associate (CMC-A),
10, 179, 182
Case Manager, Certified (CMC), 175,
178–179
Case Manager Practice (CMSA)
for cost-benefit analysis worksheets, 436,
437–441
for female-to-male negotiation, 420
for negotiating, 421
for provider agreement forms, 431,
433–434
service, equipment, and supplies
placement, 422–423
voluntary managed care, 308, 309–310
for writing progress reports, 309
Case Manager, The
"Consensus Paper of the 2003 Physician
and Case Management
Summit," 258
disclosure of medical error, 143
"Laws, Liabilities & Legislation"
feature, 115
obesity "Special Focus," 572, 581
Case managers. *See also* Case management;
Certified case managers (CCMs)

aging populations, working with,
652–653
attorney questions on role of, 287
burnout in, 213–215
as change agents, 692–695
in claims departments, 379–381
as consultants, 394–397
competence of, 100, 122
education, clinical preparation, and life
experience for, 16–18
funding for, 204–205
health literacy and, 634–637
important contacts for, 19–21
legal basics for, 101
long-term cases and, 734–736
medical credentials and expertise
of, 9–12
negligence and, 102
obesity intervention
opportunities, 590
as patient advocates, 287
pharmaceutical knowledge, 644, 646–648
role of, 5–6
Case profiles
AIDS, 763–766
cancer, 769–772
carpal tunnel, 317–318
diabetes, 766–769
high-risk pregnancy, 755–757
home care as appropriate solution,
713–715
home care as inappropriate solution,
710–713
integrated case management Level I,
355–356
integrated case management Level II,
357–358
integrated case management
Level III, 359–365
long-term, 736–740
long-term chronic disease, 757–760
long-term pediatric feeding disorder,
777–781
long-term pediatric respiratory disorder,
782–785
low back pain, 318–320
morbid obesity/gastric bypass, 772–777
not-fit-for-duty, 323–324
pediatric asthma, 760–763

slip/fall incident, 320–321
substance abuse, 321–323
transplant rejection of small bowel with
    psychological component, 785–788
Causally-related incidents, 60
Cavanaugh, Jane, 610
CCM Certification Guide, 173, 175
CDC. *See* Centers for Disease Control
    and Prevention
Cellulitis case management, 346
Center for Case Management, The, 180
Center for Cross-Cultural Health, 612
Center for Telemedicine Law (CTel), 82
Centers for Disease Control and Prevention
    *The State of Aging and Health in America
    2007*, 654
Centers for Disease Control and
    Prevention (CDC)
    on drug overdoses, 644
    on obesity, 573, 574, 583
    *The State of Aging and Health in America
    2007*, 652
Centers for Medicare and Medicaid
    Services (CMS)
    on case management, 746
    challenging managed care, 748
    on obesity, 574–575, 584
    payment for quality of care, 744
    "Status N" rating, 793
Centers of Excellence, case managers
    and, 19–21
Cerebral palsy, long-term care for, 723
Certification of Disability Management
    Specialists Commission
    (CDMS), 176
    Code of Professional Conduct, 310
Certification of Insurance Rehabilitation
    Specialists Commission
    (CIRSC), 173
Certified Advanced Social Work Case
    Manager (C-ASWCM), 180
Certified case managers (CCMs), 9, 173
    continuing education for, 10
    education, clinical preparation, and life
        experience for, 17
    exam for, 174–175. *See also* Case
        managers
Certified Disability Management Specialist
    (CDMS), 175–176

Certified Managed Care Nurse (CMCN),
    181–182
Certified Nursing Case Manager, 182
Certified Occupational Health Nurse
    (COHN), 175, 177
Certified Occupational Health Nurse/Case
    Manager (COHN/CM), 177–178
Certified Occupational Health
    Nurse–Specialist (COHN-S), 177
Certified Occupational Health
    Nurse–Specialist/Case
    Manager (COHN-S/CM), 177–178
Certified Professional in Health Care
    Quality (CPHQ), 180
Certified Rehabilitation Counselor (CRC),
    175, 178
Certified Rehabilitation Registered Nurse
    (CRRN), 175, 180–181
Certified Social Work Case Manager
    (CSWCM), 10, 181
Cervical cancer screenings, 581
Cervical strain. *See* Back pain case
    management
Chalmers, Linda, 47, 54, 55
Chambers of commerce, 523
Change agent, case manager as, 692–695
Charity Healthcare System, 793
Checklists. *See also* Forms; Red flags
    advance directive, 668
    case management, 368–370
    case management business plan, 510–513
    interviewing staff candidates, 537
    legal issues, 122–125
Childbirth. *See also* Pregnancy; Premature
    babies
    inpatient coverage after, 111
Children
    asthma case profile, 760–763
    case management needs assessment
        for, 225
    home care for, 706
    long-term feeding disorder case profile,
        777–781
    long-term respiratory disorder profile,
        782–785
    patient communications with oldest or
        other, 202
    transplant rejection of small bowel with
        psychological component, 785–788

Children with Special Health Needs, 67
Children's Health Insurance Program
  (SCHIP, 1997), 112
Chinese-Americans, 607, 608, 617–618
Chronic Care Model (CCM), 794–795
Chronic disease and depression, 698–699
Chronic mental illness, 699
Cialis (tadalafil), 645
Civilian Health and Medical Program of
  the Uniformed Services
  (CHAMPUS), 109
Claims adjustors, 381
Claims departments, 379–409. *See also*
  Third-Party Administrators (TPAs)
  case management, indicators for, 387–394
  case managers as consultants to, 394–397
  computerization of, 385–387
  consultant relationships with, 405–409
  issues for, 387
  structure and operations, 381–385
    paper trail in, 384–385
    personnel roles in, 381–384
  tracking claims by group, 397–402
    hospital claims register (report),
      398–399
    quarter evaluation report, 399–401
  tracking claims by individual claims
    histories, 402–405
Claims examiners, 381–382, 382–383
Claims investigations, case management
  versus, 204–205
Claims managers, 382
Claims processors, 381–382
Claims review, incentives for,
  388–389
Claims supervisors, 382
Client, definition of, 154
Clinical Chart Auditing Professionals
  (CAPC), 179
Clinical practice guidelines,
  308–309, 309
Clinical trials, 647
Clinton, Bill, 112
Cloud, John, 670
CMSA (Case Management Society of
  America), 5. *See also* Code of
  Professional Conduct for Case
  Managers (CCMC)
  on cultural diversity, 611, 612

"Dying in America" survey, 672–674
  ethics survey, 170–172
  on Nurse Licensure Compact (NLC),
    82–84
  on reimbursement of care coordination
    activities, 794
  Standards of Practice, 309–310
  Standards of Practice for Case
    Management, 16, 148, 310
    text of, 325–328
  Statement Regarding Ethical Case
    Management Practice,
    143–144, 310
  Visioneering Case Management's Future
    meeting and, 516–517
Cobb, Anne M., 753
COBRA, 61, 108
Code of Ethics. *See* Ethical
  responsibilities
Code of Professional Conduct,
  CDMS, 310
Code of Professional Conduct for Case
  Managers (CCMC), 144, 310
  excerpts from, 161–169
  guidelines for professional
    conduct, 147
  principles of, 145
  rules of conduct, 146
Coinsurance, 60, 65
Commission for Case Manager
  Certification (CCMC), 12, 16–18,
  143–144, 173. *See also* Certified case
  managers (CCMs)
  Code of Professional Conduct, 161–169
  Rules of Conduct, 152–160
Commission on Accreditation of
  Rehabilitation Facilities
  (CARF), 31
Commission on Rehabilitation Counselor
  Certification (CRCC), 178
Common sense, ethical, 148–149
Commonwealth Fund/
  Harvard/Harris Interactive
  Survey, 199
Communicable disease case study, ethical
  responsibilities in, 131–132
Communications, 187–215
  aging populations and, 652
  burnout and, 213–215

end-of-life issues, 674–675. *See also* Dying and death
  African Americans, 603
  Korean Americans, 603
  Latino culture, 603, 684–685
  Russian culture, 686–687
  Vietnamese culture, 688–689
health literacy and, 631, 634–637
for home care cases, 716–718
with legal professionals, 210–212
multicultural differences, 591, 605–606, 617–624
  American Indians and Alaska Natives, 619–620
  Chinese culture, 617–618
  Latino culture, 621–622
  Russian culture, 627–628
with patients and families, 197–206
  chain of command in, 201–202
  as collaboration, 200–201
  confidentiality and cost issues in, 204–205
  documentation of, 205–206
  group medical cases and, 199
  impact of, 197–199
  when family becomes a patient, 202–204
with payer sources, 206–210
with physicians, 187–197
  as collaboration, 191–197
  obstacles to, 187–190
  order for, 192
  practical steps for, 195–197
  timing for initial contact, 192–195
right mind-set for, 213
subtleties of, 212–213
Community-based case management, 691–695
Competence, case managers', 100–101, 122
Competitors, learning about, 514–517
Complementary care, 28–31. *See also* Alternative care
Complementary Medical Association, 28
Compliance. *See* Patient compliance
Comprehensive Long-Term Care Act (1997), 111
Computer reports

hospital claims register, 398–399
  quarter evaluation, 399–401
Computers
  case managers' claims analysis using, 394–397
  for claims departments, 385–387
  for physician working practices database, 196
Concurrent reviews, 329, 330
  case samples with and without, 334–338
  checklist for, 368–370
  communicating concept of, 332–333
  cost containment and, 6–7
  establishing system for, 349, 350–351
  process for preadmission review and, 340–345
  summary reports for preadmission review and, 347–348
Conferences
  obtaining health care pricing information at, 417
  obtaining information about competitors at, 514–515
Confidentiality
  CCMC standards for, 157–158
  communications with patients and families and, 204–205
  disclosure and, 92, 97–98
  ethical conduct, 147
  legal issues checklist for, 123–124
  patient bill of rights on, 85–87, 91–92
  sharing patient feedback questionnaire results and, 454–456
  workers' compensation and, 51–52, 55
Connolly, John J., 30
Consent authorization forms, 93–96
  example of, 93
Consent/disclosure, 93–96, 122
Consolidated Omnibus Budget Reconciliation Act (COBRA, 1986). *See* COBRA
Consultant role, 394–397, 405–409
Consumer safety, with pharmaceutical marketing, 645–646
Consumer-driven healthcare (CDH) plans, 27, 65–67
Consumer's Guide to Top Doctors, 30
Continuing education credits, 101

"The Continuing Evolution of the
Pharmaceutical Industry: Career
Challenges and Opportunities," 641
Continuity of Care Certification, Advanced
(A-CCC), 175, 178
Continuum of care, 791–798
Chronic Care Model (CCM), 794–795
Guided Care model, 795–796
medical home model, 791–794
National Transitions of Care Coalition
(NTOCC), 797
Contracts, 98–99
legal issues checklist for, 124
sample, 118–121
Coordination, defined, 154
Coordination of benefits, 78
Co-payments, 60, 65
Correspondence. *See* Letter samples
Cortes, Dharma, 626
Cost containment, 6–7, 289–290
administrative costs of reporting
and, 293
full-service managed care organizations
and, 353
specific limit reports of claims for,
396–397
Cost-benefit analysis. *See also* Case profiles
communicating success using, 456–458
elements of, 434–441
explaining difficult situations using,
443–446
sample letter for, 444–446
table supporting, 445–446
guidelines for, 436, 437–441
patient feedback on, 447–454
sharing questionnaire results from,
454–456
quality assurance programs and, 443
reports, 376
for self-funded plan, expanded summary
of, 491–503
summaries of, 441–442
expanded, 471–490
Cost-containment. *See also* Benefit dollars;
Negotiation for services
Council on Social Work Education, 181
COX-2 inhibitors, 642–643
CPT codes. *See also* Current Procedural
Terminology

individual claims histories in order of,
402–404
retrospective reviews and, 329
Credentials
Care Manager Certified, 179
Case Management Administrator,
Certified, 180
Case Manager Associate, 182
Case Manager, Certified, 178–179
case manager's expertise and, 9–12
CCM exam, 174–175
Certified Case Manager, 173
Certified Managed Care Nurse, 181–182
Certified Occupational Health Nurse, 177
Certified Occupational Health
Nurse/Case Manager, 177–178
Certified Occupational Health
Nurse–Specialist, 177
Certified Occupational Health
Nurse–Specialist/Case Manager,
177–178
Certified Professional in Health Care
Quality, 180
Certified Rehabilitation Counselor, 178
Certified Rehabilitation Registered
Nurse, 180–181
Certified Social Work Case
Manager, 181
Continuity of Care Certification,
Advanced, 178
Federal Credentialing Program, 105
other, 182–183
prior to CCM, 175–176
Registered Nurse-Nurse Case Manager
(RN-NCM), 180
Cress, Cathy Jo, 653
Crestor (rosuvastatin calcium), 645
Critical care paths, 351–352
capitated contracts and, 427
Cross Cultural Dialogues, 614–615
Cultural and social issues, 339, 352, 591–615
aging populations, 651–654
case management services and, 352
case manager roles, 610–611
demographic differences,
591–609, 634
communication differences, 605–606
data on, 591–604
family values, 604–605

health care delivery, 606–608
  resources on, 608–609
developing cultural competency, 611–615
end-of-life issues, 674–675
  African Americans, 603
  Korean Americans, 603
  Latino culture, 603, 684–685
  Russian culture, 686–687
  Vietnamese culture, 688–689
health literacy and, 629, 634. *See also*
  Health literacy
  stigma on, 630
obesity, stigma on, 579–581
Cultural Competence Compendium (AMA), 612
Cultural competency, 609–610
  developing, 611–615
  self-test, 613
  twelve steps to, 614
Culturally and Linguistically Appropriate
  Standards (CLAS), 608
Culturally Competent Nursing Modules
  (CCNMs), 609
Culture Clues, 608, 675
  American Indians and Alaska Natives,
    619–620
  Chinese culture, 617–618
  Latino culture, 621–622, 684–685
  Russian culture, 627–628, 686–687
  Vietnamese culture, 688–689
Current Procedural Terminology CPT 2003, 219
Current Professional Terminology (CPT), 793
Customer service, legal issues checklist
  for, 125
Customer service representatives, in claims
  departments, 382
Cystic fibrosis case management, 353

D

Database of physician working practices, 196
Davis, Nancy, 607
Day treatment for obesity
  treatment, 585
Death. *See* Dying and death
Deaths from pharmaceuticals, 642–645
Decision makers, case managers and,
  531–532
Decision-making, framework of, 721

Deficit Reduction Act (2005), 746
Deloitte Center for Health Solutions, 594
Dementia case management, old-age.
  See also Alzheimer's
Demographics, U.S., 591–609
  data on, 594–604
  intercultural differences
    communication differences, 605–606
    family values, 604–605
    health care delivery, 606–608
    resources on, 608–609
Demoratz, Michael J., 608
Denial of access, 106
Dental insurance, 77
Department of Education, 627
Department of Health and Human Services
  (DHHS), 608
Depression, 652
  end-of-life pain management and, 670
  obesity and, 577
Depression, chronic, 698–699
Development of pharmaceuticals, 641–642
Dexatrim, 587
DHHS. *See* Department of Health and
  Human Services (DHHS)
Diabetes, 345–346, 353
  case profile, 766–769
Diabetes Prevention Program (DPP), 586
Diabetes Treatment Centers of America,
  Tenn., 366
Diagnosis-related groups (DRGs), 108
Diagnosis-specific benefits, 67–68
Diary system, 274, 343
Diazepam (Valium), 644
DiBenedetto, Deborah, 110
Didrex (benzphetamine), 586
Diet, 585
Diethylpropion (Tenuate), 586
Direct contracting, cost containment
  and, 6
"Directive for Service," 221
Director of case management services, 533,
  556–561
*Directory of Physicians in the United States,
  The*, 32
Direct-to-consumer (DTC) marketing,
  641–642, 645–646
Direct-to-consumer case management,
  691–695

Disability. *See also* Long-term cases/care plans
  degree of, 60
  layoffs and people on, 393
Disability insurance plans, 61–64.
  See also Salary replacement plans
  case management needs assessment and, 232
  communications with legal professionals on, 210–212
  contact with employer for case under, 279–280
Disabled Veterans Adaptive Benefits Improvement Act (2003), 114
Disabled Veterans Return-to-Work Act (2003), 114
Discharge
  AMA evidence-based principles on, 126–128
  legal responsibilities in, 102–105
Discharge planning coordinators, contact with, 279
Discipline, 691–692
Disclosure. *See also* Consent/disclosure
  CCMC standards for, 157
  confidentiality and, 92, 97–98
  of medical errors, 141–143
Discover magazine, 643
Disease management, 45
  case management and, 8
  checklist for, 368–370
  communicating concept of, 332
  cost containment and, 7
  establishing system for, 349, 353–354, 366–368
  sample letter introducing program to client employee, 367
  timing for, 345–347
Disease Management Association of America (DMAA), 571–572
Disease-specific insurance policies, 75–76
Disease-specific societies, home care support by, 720
DiversityRx, 612
Documentation. *See also* Reports
  case management reports as, 293–295
  of communications with patients and families, 205–206

"Doing Well by Doing Good" (Gosfield and Reinertsen), 258
Do-not-resuscitate (DNR) orders, 663, 668–670
  guide for patients and families on, 680–683
Double "H" Hole, 29
Drawing pictures for patients, 635
Drolet V. Healthsource, 107
Drug abuse treatment, 92. *See also* Substance abuse
Drug benefits for senior citizens, 113
Drug treatments for obesity, 585–586
DTC case management, 691–695
DTC drug marketing, 641–642, 645–646
Dual relationships, 159
Dying and death. *See also* Terminally ill patients
  author's experience, 657–662, 675–678
  checklist for, 668
  CMSA survey on, 672–674
  cultural diversity, 674–675
    African Americans, 603
    Korean Americans, 603
    Latino culture, 603, 684–685
    Russian culture, 686–687
    Vietnamese culture, 688–689
  DNR orders, 668–670
  end-of-life issues, 662–663
  examining personal feelings, 663
  hospice care, 671
  pain management, 670–671
  palliative care, 671–672
  preparation for, 664–668
  sample health care proxy, 667
  sample living will, 664–666

E

Easter Seals, 67, 720
Eckerd Alternative Treatment Program, 28–29
Economic disadvantage, 751. *See also* Public sector case management
Economic impact. *See also* Cost containment; Cost-benefit analysis; Health care costs
  aging U.S. population, 653–654

direct-to-consumer drug marketing,
    645, 647
of health literacy, 626
late-stage drug development, 641–642
of obesity, 574
Education
    case manager, 10
    on red flag, 393
Effectiveness, long-term cases and, 735–736
Elderly
    aging populations, 651–654
    health literacy of, 629
    as long-term cases, 731–732
    moving to managed care companies, 748,
        750–751
E-mail, for communications with
        physicians, 196
Employee Retirement Income Security Act
        (ERISA, 1974), 36, 56, 108
Employers
    communications on risk management
        with, 206–210
    contact with, 280
    initial phone contact with, 280–281
    right to know *versus* need to know
        for, 96–97
Empowerment, ethical, 148
Encouraging questions from patients, 636
Encyclopedia of Associations, 720
Endocrine Society, 587
End-of-life (EOL) issues, 662–663, 669
Enthoven, Alain, 26
Ephedrine, 587
Esomeprazole magnesium (Nexium), 645
Ethical conduct, codes of, 143–149, 310
Ethical responsibilities, 129–150
    case study with communicable disease,
        131–132
    case study with HIV+ pregnant mother,
        133–135
    case study with substance abuse,
        132–133
    CCMC Code of Professional Conduct for
        Case Managers (excerpts), 161–169
    CCMC Rules of Conduct, 152–160
    CMSA ethics survey, 170–172
    literature on, 149–150
    obesity treatment, 581–583
    patient rights and, 130–143

medical errors, 141–143
    pharmaceutical marketing and, 647
Ethnic minorities. *See entries at* Cultural
"Ethnicity and Attitudes Toward Patient
    Autonomy" (1995), 604
Etiology of obesity, 577–578
Etrazine tatrate (Bontril), 586
Euthanasia, 662
Evaluation. *See also* Assessments
    of case management departments,
        507–508, 510
    of claims departments by quarter, 399–401
    defined, 154
    Initial Evaluation Guidelines, 250, 251–252
    Initial Evaluation Worksheet, 250, 253–256
        sample, 302–304
    script samples for initial patient,
        241–245, 252, 253–256, 257
    of staff, 562, 563
Evidence-based medicine, 31
Exclusions, 60
Exclusive provider organizations (EPOs), 23
Extracontractual services, 375

F

Facility Review for Case Managers, 463–464
Families
    communications with, 197–206
        chain of command in, 201–202
        as collaboration, 200–201
        confidentiality and cost issues in,
            204–205
        documenting, 205–206
        group medical cases and, 199
        impact of, 197–199
        when family becomes a patient,
            202–204
    implications of long-term cases for,
        732–734
    long-term care and changes in, 729
    multicultural differences, 604–605
    sharing medications, 634
    talking about case management with,
        250–258
Family and Medical Leave Act (FMLA,
    1993), 110
Fastin (Phentermine), 586

FDA (Food and Drug Administration), 586
Federal Credentialing Program (FCP), 105
Federal Employees Health Benefits
    Program (FEHBP), 109
Federal Patient Self-Determination Act
    (1990), 109–110
Fee-for-service systems, 370–371, 372–374
Feelings
    about dying in America, 663
    long-term cases and transference of, 735
Fee-setting, 224, 370–376. *See also* Payment
        arrangements
    under capitation systems, 370–371,
        372–374
    cost-benefit analysis reports for
        education in, 376
    under fee-for-service systems, 370–371,
        372–374
    marketplace volatility and, 371
    multiple carve-outs in, 375
    per-case, 375–376
    under at risk fee systems, 374
Feuer, Louis, 421
Fidelity, definition of, 129
Financial activities, case management, 315.
        See also Negotiation for services
Financial analysis, 442. *See also* Cost-benefit
        analysis
Financial funding problems, 339
    case management services and, 352
    long-term care and, 729, 734
    with public sector case management,
        748–751
Financial planning background. *See also*
        Business background
    for case managers, 64
Flaum, Margaret, 366
Flowcharts, case management work
        format, 218
Food & Friends, 720
Food and Drug Administration (FDA),
        586, 642
Forms. *See also* Checklists; Letter samples;
        Worksheets
    advisory, 233. *See also* Forms
        Case Management Intervention, 238
        Stop-Loss Notification, 239
    Candidate's Knowledge Assessment
        Tool, 540–541

Case Management Audit Tool,
        240–241
    Case Management Identification
        Worksheet, 233, 234
    Client Satisfaction Survey, 449–450
    competencies for unit-based nurse case
        managers, 564–565
    Consent Authorization, 93
    Employer Group Information Sheet,
        226–229
    Facility Review for Case Managers,
        463–464
    health care proxy, 667
    Initial Assessment Form, 594, 595–596
    Initial Evaluation Worksheet, 250,
        253–256
        sample, 302–304
    interview evaluation, 562
    living will, 664–666
    Medical Authorization Release, xpost
        Medical Authorization
        Release form
    Options Unlimited Recruitment Form,
        542
    Plan of Care Form, 597–602
    Preinvolvement of Case Management
        questionnaire, 451
    Program Questionnaire for Case
        Managers, 459–462
    provider agreement, 431, 432–433,
        433–434
    Provider Service Agreements, 465–470
    questionnaires for case management by
        treating physicians,
        264, 272
    Request for Service, 405, 406
    summary evaluation scale (for
        employment selection and
        compliance), 563
    TPA claims review sheet, 407
    Written Agreement, 118–121
Fortune magazine, 627
Fowler Healthcare Affiliates, Inc., 731
"Fractured family syndrome," 733
Fraudulent claims, computerization
        and, 387
Friedman, Emily, 140
Friends, sharing medications, 634
Furberg, Curt, 643

G

Gainer, Sandra, 30
Galanti, Geri-Ann, 605–606
GAO (U.S. Government Accountability
    Office), 645
Gastric bypass case profile, 772–777
Gatekeeper PPOs, 65
GCNs (guided care nurses), 795–796
Gender, health literacy and, 630
Genetics, in treatment of obesity, 587
Geriatric care managers, 652–653
Geriatric continuums, 731
Geriatric Interdisciplinary Team Training
    Resource Center, 611
Getting Past No (Ury), 419
Getting to Yes (Ury), 419
Gilda's Club, 29
GlaxoSmithKline, 642
Gosfield, Alice G., 99–100
    on AHCPR practice guidelines, 310
    on doctor–patient relationship, 258
    on OBRA, 108
    on *Wickline* decision, 102
    on *Wilson* decision, 104
Government Accountability Office, 645
Government response-funded insurance.
    See Public sector case
    management
Graham, Garth N., 608
Graying of U.S. population, 651–654
Gross, Cary P., 643
Gross, Jane, 607
Group medical insurance plans,
    60–61
    case management needs assessment and,
        231–232
    claims analysis for, 397
    communications with, 206–210
    marketplace volatility among, 371
    red flags for, 393
    report format for, 293
    scope of reports generated from, 292
    second-opinion exams for, 274, 276
    socioenvironmental issues and, 293
Guardians, legal, patient communications
    and, 201–202
Guided Care model, 795–796
Guided care nurses (GCNs), 795–796
Guidelines

Case Management Identification
    Worksheet, 233, 234
Case Management Practice, 310
    for case management referral, 351

H

Harvard School of Public Health, 638
HCOs (health care organizations), 23
Health benefit plans, 45
Health Care Consumer Advisory Board, 111
Health care consumer categories, 594–595
Health care costs, 413–414
    historical overview of, 414–418
    obtaining information about, 417, 418
    tracking information about, 418
Health Care Financing Administration
    (HCFA). *See also* Centers for
    Medicare and Medicaid Services
    (CMS)
Health care organizations (HCOs), 23
Health care providers, case managers
    and, 19
Health care proxies, 664, 666
    sample, 667
Health Care Quality Improvement Act
    (HCQIA, 1986), 108
Health care surrogates, 666
Health Centers Consolidation Act
    (1996), 111
Health Enhancement Research
    Organization, 702
Health Insurance Association of America
    (HIAA), 308
Health Insurance Portability and
    Accountability Act (HIPAA, 1996),
    55, 110
    confidentiality under, 92
    Patient Privacy regulations in, 112
    workers' compensation and, 51–52
Health insurance purchasing cooperatives
    (HIPCs), 26
Health literacy, 625–638
    case manager's role, 634–637
    categories and levels of, 626–628
    day-to-day considerations, 628–631
    manifestations, 631–634
    need for, 625–626
    resources on, 637–638

Health Literacy: A Prescription to End Confusion, 626, 627
Health Plan Data and Information Set (HEDIS), 31
Health Resources and Services Administration (HRSA), 105
Healthcare Integrity and Protection Data Bank (HIPDB), 105
Healthcare Quality Certification Board, 180
HealthGrades, 32
Health-maintenance organizations (HMOs)
   capitated fee systems of, 370–371
   case managers and, 5–6, 21–22
   cost containment programs of, 7
   self-insurance and, 37
Healthy People 2010, 627
Hemophilia, 353
Hewitt Associates, 343
High-cost equipment or services, 342, 416
High-risk cases, needs assessment for, 225, 229
Hip replacement, preadmission review for, 341
Hirschler, Ben, 641–642
HISOCC (his occupation), 62–63, 292
Hispanic Americans, 595–603, 604.
   See also Cultural and social issues
HIV. *See also* AIDS
   ethical responsibilities to pregnant mother with, 133–135
   health literacy and, 630
Home care, 705–721
   as appropriate solution, 713–715
   case managers as pivotal link in, 708–710
   consumer demand and ambivalence on, 707–708
   feedback and communication with, 716–718
   as inappropriate solution, 710–713
   ongoing support for, 715–716
   payment concerns with, 718–721
   policies with, 76–77
Home health care agencies, relationships with, 419
Home medical equipment, relationships with suppliers of, 419
Hoskins, Iffath Abbasi, 607
Hospice care, 671
Hospital claims register, analysis of computer-generated, 398–399

Hospital medical records, review of, 279
Hospital Quality Measure Reporting initative, 744
Hospital-acquired conditions (HAC), 575, 744
Hospitalists, case managers and, 19
Hospitals, case managers and specialized, 20
Hourly fees, 375
How to Find the Best Doctors, 30
Hughes v. Blue Cross of Northern California (1989), 104
Huntington's disease, 651
Hurricane Katrina, 793
Hyatt, Thomas K., 98, 99

I

"I Can Cope" programs, 720
ICD-9 codes, 218–219, 402–404
ICD-9-CM 2002: International Classification of Diseases, 9th Edition, Clinical Modification (Volumes 1 and 2), 219
ICD-9-CM Spiral Expert for Physicians, Volumes 1 and 2, 2002 International Classification of Diseases, 9th Revision, Clinical Modification, 219
Immigrants, 592–594
   health literacy and, 629
Implementation, defined, 154
Improving on Tranditions of Care tool (NTOCC), 797
Imus Ranch, 29
Indemnity plans, 37, 59–60
Independence, 691–692
Independent case managers, 508–510
Independent medical exams (IMEs), 7, 273–278
   sample letter to arrange for, 275–276
Independent practice arrangements (IPAs), 21, 22
Indians (American). *See* Native Americans
Industry directions. *See also* Credentials
Infections, understaffing and, 4
Information, in interviews, 220
Informed consent. *See* Consent authorization forms
Initial Assessment Form, 594, 595–596
Initial contact. *See* Case management, work format and process of

Initial Evaluation Guidelines, 250, 251–252
Initial Evaluation Report Guidelines,
    301–302
Initial Evaluation Worksheet, 250, 253–256
    sample, 302–304
Inpatient programs for obesity treatment, 585
Institute of Medicine (IOM)
    CMSA Standards of Practice *versus*,
        309–310
    on good clinical practice guidelines, 309
    on health literacy, 627
    Leapfrog Initiative and, 41
    on medical errors, 743
Insurance providers
    administrative and customized services
        of, 39–40
    auto, 59
    basic benefits administration by, 36–39
    case managers and, 5–6, 35–36
    communications with, 206–210
    consumer-driven healthcare plans, 65–67
    coordination of benefits of, 78
    diagnosis-specific benefits, 67–68
    disability plans, 61–64
    group medical plans, 60–61
    indemnity plans, 59–60
    multiple-employer benefit plans and
        trusts, 72–73
    nontraditional policies of, 75–77
    point-of-service plans, 64–65
    precertification or preadmission reviews
        by, 330
    product lines of, 45
    scope of reports generated from, 292
    self-funded plans *versus*, 68–71
    stop-loss plans, 71–72
    viatical settlements, 73–75
    workers' compensation, 46–59
Integrated case management, 329–376
    case sample with and without, 334–338
    checklist for, 368–370
    establishing effective systems for,
        349–368
        case management services, 351–353
        concurrent review services, 350–351
        disease management services,
            353–354, 366–368
        preadmission review services, 349–350
    fee structure for, 370–376

introduction to client groups and plan
    participants, 332–333
Level I example, 30-year-old African-
    American male, 355–356
Level II example, 55-year-old white
    female, 357–358
Level III example, 58-year-old white
    female, 359–365
preadmission and concurrent review
    process, 340–345
sample description for employee/patient
    populations of, 340
sample letter acknowledging
    prenotification and explanation of,
    339
sample letter introducing disease
    management program to client
    employee, 367
summary reports for, 347–348
timing for, 345–347
Integrated delivery and financing network
    (IDFNs), 23
Integrated delivery and financing system
    (IDFSs), 23
Integrated delivery network (IDNs), 23
Integrated delivery systems (IDSs), 23
Interactions with Healthcare Professionals
    (PhRMA, 2002), 130
Internal Revenue Service (IRS), 583
*International Classification of Diseases, 9th
    Edition, Clinical Modification*
    (ICD-9-CM), 218–219
International Herald Tribune, 641
Interqual, care guidelines of, 331
IRS (Internal Revenue Service), 583

J

Jamin, Denise, 603
Job descriptions. *See also* Staff, case
        management
    director of case management services,
        556–561
    medical case managers, 550–555
    nurse reviewers, 544–549
The Joint Commission, 85
    disclosure standard for medical errors,
        142–143

"Joint Principles of the Patient-Centered Medical Home" report (2007), 792
Journal of the American Medical Association, 643
Justice, definition of, 129, 154

K

Kassebaum-Kennedy Act, 110. *See also* Health Insurance Portability and Accountability Act
Katrina (hurricane), 793
Keffer, M. Jan, 140
Kid Care, 112
KidSource, 29
King, Marilou M., 104, 106
Knudson, Leslie, 646
Kohut, Heinz, 582
Korean Americans, 608
    end-of-life issues and, 603
    family values, 604–605
Krauskopf, Lewis, 641–642

L

Labor relations. *See also* Employers; Unions
    not-fit-for-duty case scenario, 323–324
Languages spoken, 591, 606–607
Laser-out agreements, 428. *See also* Carve-out services
Late-stage drug development, 641–642
Latino culture. *See also* Cultural and social issues
    communication, 621–622
    end-of-life issues and, 603, 684–685
    U.S. demographics, 592
Leapfrog Group, 743
Leapfrog Initiative, 41
Legal guardians, patient communications and, 201–202
Legal professionals. *See also* Attorneys
    communications with, 210–212
Legal responsibilities, 81–116
    adequate information and, 98
    bad faith actions and, 106
    case management and, 99–107
    consent/disclosure and consent authorization forms, 93–96, 122

contracts and letters of agreement, 98–99, 124
    day-to-day practices and, 114–115
    discharge and, 102–105, 126–128
    documentation of negotiated services and, 429
    emerging case law, 106–107
    getting legal information and, 115–116
    issues checklist, 122–125
    medical errors, 141–143
    medical records retention and, 96
    negligent referral, 105–106
    right to know *versus* need to know and, 96–97
    sample written agreement, 118–121
Legislation, 108–114
Length of stay, 342, 343
Lenzer, Jeanne, 643
Letter samples. *See also* Checklists; Forms
    acknowledging prenotification of hospital admission and case management process, 339
    to attorney who has denied services, 285–286
    claims contact, 408
    on client cost concerns with comparative analysis, 444–446
    to insured for high-risk pregnancy management, 242
    introducing disease management program to client employee, 367
    of introduction for services for insured's child, 243
    of introduction for services through Third Party Administrator, 245
    of introduction for workers' compensation case, 244
    of introduction to treating physicians, 264
        to be sent with questionnaires, 267, 268, 269–270, 271–272
        for neonatal case, 265–266
    to new client without telephone, 241
    to physician to arrange independent medical exam, 275–276
    to physician to arrange second-opinion exam, 275–276
    provider agreement, 431, 432–433
    on quality assurance when patient has passed away, 447, 452

on quality assurance with
questionnaire, 448
Letters of agreement, 98–99
for provider services, 465–470
sample, 118–121
Levitra (vardenafil), 645
Liability issues, 81–85, 288–289, 308. *See also*
Legal responsibilities
Licensure, 81–85
Life insurance, 73–75, 77
Lilly, 645
Limitations, 60
Limited provider panels, PPOs and, 22
Limiting information given to patients, 636
*Linthicum v. Nationwide Life Insurance
Company* (1986), 104
Lipase inhibitors, 586
Liposuction, 587
Literacy. *See* Health literacy
Literacy competency, 609–610
Living wills, 664–666
Llewellyn, Anne, 671, 673–674
Locke, Steven E., 698
Lonamin (Phentermine), 586
Long Island Center for Ethics, 138
Longevity, increase in U.S., 651–654
Long-term cases/care plans, 76–77, 723–740.
See also AIDS; HIV
alternative funding sources for, 730–731
changes in, 728–729
chronic disease profile, 757–760
elderly individuals as, 731–732
example of, 736–740
implications for case managers in,
734–736
implications for families in, 732–734
importance of ongoing involvement in,
726–727
informing the client about, 724–725
level of involvement in, 725–726
management of, 291
needs assessment for, 225, 229
negotiating for services, 729–730
pediatric feeding disorder profile,
777–781
Long-term disability (LTD) plans, 61–62
layoffs and people on, 393
medical expenses and, 292–293
as wage-replacement plans, 63
Low back pain case scenario, 318–320

Lowery, Sandra, 539
Low-income populations. *See*
Socioeconomic factors
Ludwig, David S., 573

M

Ma huang, 585
Malpractice, 102, 634
Mammograms, 628
Mammoplasty (reduction), 587–588
Managed care, 23–26. *See also* Health
maintenance organizations
billing for case management *versus*, 521
case management *versus*, 6–9
voluntary guidelines for coordination
of, 308
workers' compensation and, 50–51
Managed care organizations (MCOs), 7, 22
bonus programs and case manager
ethical responsibilities, 137
communications with, 206–210
health literacy and, 629
precertification or preadmission reviews
by, 330
workers' compensation and, 58–59
Managed competition, stages of, 26–28
Managing case management departments.
See also Business of case
management; Staff, case
management
evaluation of, 507–508
need for, 505–506
Marketing materials
Options Unlimited Patient Brochure,
528–529
for pharmaceuticals, 641–642, 645–646
preparation of, 526–527
Mastectomy coverage, 112
McKesson Health Solutions, Colo., 366
Meals on Wheels, 720
Meaney, Mark, 129, 139–140
Medicaid, 14, 742, 745, 751–752.
See also Public sector case
management
case management components, 746
health literacy and, 629
Medical activities, case management,
314–315

Medical associations, local and national, 32–33, 612
Medical Authorization Release form, 250, 256
Medical case managers, 533, 550–555
Medical directives, 666
Medical Directory of New York State, 32
Medical Disability Advisor, The (Reed), 392
Medical equipment, relationships with suppliers of, 419
Medical Error and Medical Narcissism (Banja), 150
Medical errors, ethics and, 141–143
Medical history, gathering information about, 248
Medical home model, 791–794
Medical Malpractice/Tort Reform, 113
Medical professionals, initial phone contact for personal consultation with, 278–280
Medical records, 96. *See also* Documentation; Reports
Medical Safety Review Boards, 646
Medical Savings Accounts (MSAs), 110
Medical societies, local and national, 32–33, 612
Medicare, 14, 647, 741–742. *See also* Public sector case management
diagnosis-specific benefits and, 67–68
health literacy and, 629
obesity treatment, 574–575, 584
readmittance of patients, 744
Title IX of Social Security Amendments (1983), 108
Medicare Catastrophic Coverage Act (MCCA, 1998), 109
Medicare Coordinated Care Demonstration Project, 111, 746
Medicare Error Response team, 142
Medicare Patient Choice and Access Act (1997), 111
Medicare+ Choice plans, 111
Medication Reconciliation Essential Data Specifications tool (NTOCC), 797
Medications. *See* Pharmaceuticals; Prescription drugs
Medigap policies, 77, 742
Medline, National Library of Medicine, 309
Medstat, 702
Meier, Diane, 670

Mental health
confidentiality of records, 92
end-of-life pain management and, 670
health literacy and, 630
obesity and, 577
Mental Health Infosource, 702
Mental Health Parity Act (1996), 113
Mercer Health & Benefits, 7
Merck & Company, 642
Merck Company Foundation, 652
Methadone, 643
Metrics for obesity, 575–577
Mexican Americans. *See* Hispanic Americans
Military healthcare, 743, 752–753
Milliman and Roberts (M&R) cataract guideline, 310
Milliman Care Guidelines, 331
Minimum premiums, 38
Minorities, ethnic. *See entries at* Cultural
Misconduct, reporting, 156
Model Hispanic Health Programs: Prevention, Treatment, Training and Research, 595–603
Models for case management, 791–796
Monitoring, defined, 154
Morbid obesity/gastric bypass case profile, 772–777
Moreo, Kathleen, 258, 607
Moshe v. Rush-Presbyterian St. Luke's Hospital (1990), 106
Mullahy, Catherine, 138, 657–662
Muller, Lynn S., 101
Multiculturalism. *See* Cultural and social issues
Multiple conditions, 339, 352, 723
Multiple sclerosis, 353, 706, 723, 733
Multiple-employer benefit plans and trusts, 72–73
My Medicine List tool (NTOCC), 797

N

Nash, David B., 258
Nassau County Medical Center patients bill of responsibilities, 89–90
National Academy of Certified Care Managers, 179
National Alliance for the Mentally Ill, 701

National Assessment of Health Literacy
(NAAL), 627
National Association for Healthcare
Quality, 180
National Association of Psychiatric Health
Systems, 701
National Association of Rehabilitation
Professionals in the Private Sector
(NARPPS), 175
National Association of Social Workers
(NASW), 10, 181
Code of Ethics, 310
National Board for Certification in
Continuity of Care, 178
National Center for Pain and Palliative
Care Research, 670
National Coalition for Patients Rights, 92
National Committee for Quality Assurance
(NCQA), 31, 331
National Council of State Boards of
Nursing (NCSBN), 82
National Culturally and Linguistically
Appropriate Standards (CLAS), 608
National Guideline Clearinghouse, 100
National Health and Nutrition Examination
Survey (NHANES), 573
National Heart, Lung, and Blood Institute,
576, 583, 643
National Hispanic Medical Association
(NHMA), 595
National Home Infusion Therapy
Association, 706
National Hospice Foundation, 662
National Hospital Ambulatory Medical
Care Surveys (NHACS), 744
National Institute for Literacy, 638
National Institute of Mental Health, 702
National Institutes of Health (NIH), 331,
574, 576, 644
dietary guidelines, 585
National Jewish Center for Immunology
and Respiratory Medicine, Colo.,
366–367
National Library of Medicine, Medline
service, 309
National Naval Medical Center, 753
National Pain Care Policy Act (2003), 670
National Practitioner Data Bank
(NPDB), 105

National Quality Measures
Clearinghouse, 331
National Transitions of Care Coalition
(NTOCC), 797
Native Americans, 592, 607, 619–620
Native Hawaiians, 592
Nazay v. Miller (1991), 106
NCLEX (National Council Licensure
Exam – RN) exam, 82
Negligence, 101–102
Negligent referral
legal responsibilities in, 105–106
liability issues in, 288–289
Negotiation for services
common female-to-male obstacles and
solutions, 420
documenting, 428–434
home care and, 720–721
legal issues checklist for, 124–125
long-term care and, 729–730
managed care and, 24, 26, 426–428
with capitated contracts, 427
carve-out services from, 428
nuances of, 424–426
skills for, 418–424
Networking, 517–520
Neuromuscular disease, case management
of chronic, 353
New England Journal of Medicine, 669
New York State, patient bill of rights of,
86–87
Newborns' and Mothers' Health Protection
Act (1999), 111
Nexium (esomeprazole
magnesium), 645
Next Generation Pharmaceutical, 646
NHANES (National Health and Nutrition
Examination
Survey), 573
"No-Brainer Test of Ethical
Behavior," 149
Nonmaleficence, defined, 154
Nonmalfeasance, definition of, 129
Nonmedical language, using, 635
Not-fit-for-duty case scenario, 323–324
Novartis Pharmaceuticals, 646
Nurse licensure, 82
Nurse Licensure Compact (NLC), 82–84
Nurse reviewers, 533, 544–549

Nurses
  corporate structure and, 506
  follow-up calls as part of concurrent
    review by, 343
  home-visit programs by, 343
  hospital staff, as information sources, 279
  shortage and responsibilities of, 4
Nursing home policies, 76–77

O

Obesity, 571–591
  etiology, 577–578
  metrics for, 575–577
  scope of, as epidemic, 572–575
  treatment, 578–590
    availability and funding of, 583–584
    ethics issues, 581–583
    intervention opportunities for case
      managers, 590
    perceptions, 578–579
    stigma of, 579–581
    strategies for, 585–590
Obesity/gastric bypass case profile, 772–777
Objectivity in ethical practices, 148–149
Oby-Cap (Phentermine), 586
Occupation-specific policies, 76
Office for the Forum on Quality and
  Effectiveness, 308
Office of Minority Health (OMH), 608–609,
  609, 638
*Official Abms Directory of Board-Certified
  Medical Specialists, The*, 32
Off-label pharmaceutical use, 647–648
Older adults
  aging populations, 651–654
  health literacy of, 629
Omnibus Budget Reconciliation Act
  (OBRA), 108, 109
Open-access HMOs, 65
Options Unlimited Patient Brochure, 528–529
Oraflex, 645
Organ donation, 666
Osteoporosis, 652
OTC weight loss treatments, 586–587
Out of contract services, 375, 719
Outpatient programs for obesity
  treatment, 585

Overdosed America, 645
Over-the-counter weight loss treatments,
  586–587
Overweight. *See* Obesity
Oxycontin (oxycodone), 643, 644

P

Pacific Islanders, 592
Pain, end-of-life management of, 670–671
Palliative care, 671–672
Panniculectomy, 587
Paper trail, in claims departments, 384–385
Parkinson's disease, 652
Part A, Medicare, 741–742
Part B, Medicare, 742
Part C, Medicare, 742
Part D, Medicare, 742
Patient advocates, 287
Patient bill of responsibilities, 89–90
Patient bill of rights, 85–92. *See also* Patient
  bill of responsibilities
  of American Hospital Association, 87–89
  from New York state, 86–87
Patient compliance
  communication with physicians
    on, 196
  telephonic *versus* in-person case
    management and, 266
Patient Protection Act (1997), 111
Patient Right to Know Act, 92, 112
Patient rights, ethics involving, 130–143
  medical errors, 141–143
Patient Self-Determination Act (PSDA,
  1990), 663
Patients
  aging populations, 651–654
  communications with, 197–206
    chain of command in, 201–202
    as collaboration, 200–201
    confidentiality and cost issues in,
      204–205
    documenting, 205–206
    group medical cases and, 199
    impact of, 197–199
    methods to improve, 635–637
    when family becomes a patient,
      202–204

feedback on cost-benefit analysis from, 447–454
health literacy, 625–638
  case manager's role, 634–637
  categories and levels of, 626–628
  day-to-day considerations, 628–631
  manifestations, 631–634
  need for, 625–626
  resources on, 637–638
sharing questionnaire results from, 454–456
surveys of, 447
talking about case management with, 244–246, 251–252, 253–256
Patients bill of responsibilities. *See also* Patient bill of rights
"Patterns of Abuse Among Unintentional Pharmaceutical Overdose Fatalities," 643
Pay for Performance (P4P) initative, 745
Payment arrangements, 430, 718–721. *See also* Fee-setting
Peale, Norman Vincent, 150
Pear-shaped bodies, 577
Per-case fees, 375–376
Pew Research Center, 592
Pfizer Clear Health Communication Initiative, 638
Pfizer Inc., 642
Pharmaceutical Research and Manufacturers of America (PhRMA), 130
Pharmaceuticals, 113, 638
  adherence to prescriptions, 631–632
  deaths from, 642–645
  gathering information about, 248
  maintaining current knowledge on, 646–648
  marketing direct to consumers, 641–642, 645–646
  sharing prescriptions, 634
  treatment of obesity, 585–586
Pharmacy benefits, 354
Pharmacy Benefits Management (PBM), 7
Phentermine (Lonamin, Oby-Cap, Fastin, and Adipex-P), 586
Physician and Case Management Summit, 258
Physician-assisted suicide, 663, 670

Physician-hospital organizations (PHOs), 22
Physicians. *See also* Independent medical exams (IMEs); Letter samples; Second-opinion exams
  communications with, 187–197
    as collaboration, 191–197
    obstacles to, 187–190
    order for, 192
    practical steps for, 195–197
    timing for initial contact, 192–195
  hospitalists, case managers and, 19
  on obesity treatment, 579
  talking about case management with, 258–264
    initial phone contact for personal consultation, 259–260
    initial phone contact for telephone consultation, 260, 260–262
    questionnaires for, 264, 272
    sample script for personal consultation, 261–262
Physicians Practice Digest, 196
Pictures, drawing for patients, 635
Plain language, using, 635
Plan, case management, 220, 287–291
Plan administrators, in claims departments, 382
Plan of Care Form, 597–602
Planning, defined, 154
Plateaus, in long-term cases, 728
Point-of-service plans (POSs), 6, 7, 37, 64–65
Postacute healthcare facilities, 20
Power of attorney, 202
Power of Ethical Management (Blanchard and Peale), 150
The Practical Guide: Identification, Evaluation, and Treatment of Overweight and Obese Adults, 585
Preadmission review
  case samples with and without, 334–338
  checklist for, 368–370
  communicating concept of, 332
  cost containment and authorization for, 7
  establishing system for, 349–350
  industry norms for fees, 371
  process for concurrent review and, 340–345
  summary reports for concurrent review and, 347–348

PreCert, case management and, 8
Precertification, 330
Preexisting conditions, 60
Preferred provider organizations (PPOs), 6,
    7, 21–22, 25, 37
Pregnancy
  ethical responsibilities with HIV and,
    133–135
  high-risk, 443–446
    claims department red flags and, 388
    as disease management candidate, 353
    profile case, 755–757
    sample letter to insured for
      management of, 242
    preadmission review for, 341–342
Premature babies, 713–715, 723
Prescription drugs, 113. *See also*
    Medications; Pharmaceuticals
  abuse of, 644
  adherence, 631–632
  direct-to-consumer (DTC) marketing,
    641–642, 645–646
  Medicare coverage, 742
  sharing, 634
Presenteeism, 574, 698
Privacy practices
  CCMC standards for, 157–158
  ethical conduct, 147
Proactive behavior, 691–692
Professional associations, 517–520, 612
Professional Case Management, 150
Professional relationships, ethical, 147
Professional responsibility, ethical, 147
Professional review organizations
    (PROs), 108
Program Questionnaire for Case Managers,
    459–462
Progress report, sample, 306–307
Prospective reviews, 329, 330
ProStrakan Group, 642
Provider agreement forms, 431, 433–434
Provider-sponsored organizations
    (PSOs), 111
Psychiatric disorders, 652. *See also*
    Behavioral health
Psychosocial factors, gathering information
    about, 249
Public sector case management, 741–754.
    See also Medicaid; *under* Medicare

case managers and, 746–748
  challenges for, 748
  complications remaining in, 748–751
  economic impact and government
    response, 743–746
  funding sources, 741–743
  military case management, 752–753
  nonmedical challenges, 751–752

Q

Quality assurance programs, 443.
    See also National Committee for
    Quality Assurance
  letter sample when patient has passed
    away, 447, 452
  letter sample with questionnaire, 448
Quality of care, managed care and, 24
Quarter evaluation, 399–401
Questionnaires. *See* Forms; Surveys
Questions, encouraging from patients, 636

R

R&D, pharmaceutical, 641–642
Rapport, in interviews, 220–221
Reading lists, for families with
    long-term cases, 733–734
Recordkeeping, CCMC standards for,
    157–158
Recruiting staff, 539–543
  Options Unlimited Recruitment Form
    for, 542
Red flags
  case management services and, 351
  development of, 387, 405
  for different insurance lines, 389–391, 392
    AccuClaim, 390–391
    CareSolutions, 389–390
  for long-term care, 723–724
  teaching aids for recognizing, 394
Red Flags List, Case Management, 233,
    235–236
Reduction mammoplasty, 587–588
Reed, Presley, 392
Referral sources
  attorney requests for reports for, 287

case managers and, 39, 217
for cases, 219–220
legal issues checklist for, 122–123
needs determination process with, 221–233
for new business, 525–526
report frequency and length for, 292
as resource for physicians, 196
Regent Atlantic Capital, LLC, 641
Registered Nurse, Certified, 182
Registered Nurse-Nurse Case Manager (RN-NCM), 180
Registered nurses, 9. *See also* Nurse reviewers; Nurses
Rehabilitation counselors, 9
Rehabilitation Nursing Certification Board, 175, 180
Rehabilitation phase, 289–290, 425–426
Reimbursement of care coordination activities, 794
Reinersten, James L., 258
Reinsurance, 38
Relationships, ethical, 147
Repeating information to patients, 636
Report cards, 40–41
Reports, 291–300. *See also* Communications; Documentation
attachments to, 295–296
attorney requests for, 287
CCMC standards for, 158
as communication tool, 291–293
format for, 296
frequency of, 293–294
guidelines for writing, 305–306
presentation of alternatives in, 297
as professional documentation, 294–295
sample of, 306–307
scope for, 294
timeliness of, 296–297
Request for Service form, 405, 406
Research, CCMC standards on, 160
Research, pharmaceutical, 641–642
Research conduct, ethical, 147
Reserving the dollars, in workers' compensation, 292
Restrictions, benefit plan, 38, 229
Resuscitation, 668, 680–683. *See also* Do-not-resuscitate (DNR) orders
Retrospective reviews, 7, 329, 330

Review services, 329–330
R.I.P. interview method, 220–221
Risk management, 125, 368, 386–387
Rofecoxib (Vioxx), 643
Rogers v. Cigna HealthCare (2001), 107
rosuvastatin calcium (Crestor), 645
Rules of Conduct, CCMC, 152–160
Russian culture
communication, 627–628
end-of-life issues and, 686–687

S

Safety issues, with pharmaceutical marketing, 645–646
Safety Management Teams, 646
Salary replacement plans, 230
Sanofi-Aventis SA, 642
Schantz, Stephen J., 106
Scheutzow, Susan, 91, 97
Scope of practice, case managers, 152–153
SCORE, 524
Script samples. *See also* Telephonic case management
for initial contact with an employer, 280
initial evaluation or assessment, 246–250, 253–256
for initial phone contact with an attorney, 281–282
with medical professionals to set up personal consultation, 278
for obtaining approval, 300, 307
personal visit with doctors, 259–262
talking with doctor's receptionist, 259–260
talking with family, 250–258
talking with referral source, 222–223, 225, 229, 231–232
telephone call for initial patient visit, 251–252
telephone call for physician consultation, 260
Second surgical opinions (SSOs), 7
Second-opinion exams, 273–278
Self-assessment as case manager, 691–692
Self-insurance, 37
Self-realization, 691–692
Seniors

aging populations, 651–654
health literacy of, 629
Sensitivity, cultural. *See* Cultural
competency
Sex, health literacy and, 630
Sexually transmitted diseases, 92
Shame-free environment for patients,
636–637
Sharing medications, 634
Short-term disability (STD) plans, 61–62,
62, 393
Shriners, diagnosis-specific benefits of, 67
Side-effects from approved
pharmaceuticals, 642, 644–645
Significant others, patient communications
and, 202
Sills, Judith, 646
Slip/fall incident scenario, 320–321
Slowing down communications, 635
Social issues. *See* Cultural and social issues
Social Security Amendments (1983), Title IX
on Medicare, 108
Social welfare caseworkers, 9–10
Social workers, medical, 9–10, 279, 700
Socioeconomic factors
gathering information about, 249–250
health literacy and, 629
Software
case management screening, 219
claims department, 385–387
Solicitation, CCMC standards on, 160
Solteau, Eleanor, 793
Specialized care providers, 19–21
Specific limit reports, 395
Spinal injuries, long-term care for, 723
Spouses, patient communications and,
201–202
Staff, case management, 532–539
case situation assessment—asthma, 538
case situation assessment—
pregnancy, 538
competencies for, 564–565
educational background for, 535
interview evaluation form, 562
life experience for, 535–536
Options Unlimited Recruitment Form, 542
position descriptions
director of case management services,
556–561

medical case managers, 550–555
nurse reviewers, 544–549
professional background for, 534–535
scenarios for assessing potential, 537
search for, 539–543
summary evaluation scale, 563
Staff-model health maintenance
organizations, 21
Standards of care, 31–33, 100–101, 122
Standards of Occupational and
Environmental Health Nursing
(AAOHN), 310
Standards of practice
CMSA, 16, 309–310, 325–328
IOM on guidelines for, 309
URAC, 16
Standards of Practice for Case
Management, 16, 148, 310
text of, 325–328
State Children's Health Insurance Program
(SCHIP, 1997), 111, 742
*The State of Aging and Health in America
2007*, 652, 654
"Status N" rating, 793
Stereotypes, in communication, 190–191
Stigma
health literacy, 630
obesity, 579–581
Stop-loss coverage, 38, 71–72
Stop-Loss Notification, 239
Storti, Craig, 614–615
Stress, health literacy and, 629–630
Strickland, Tom, 46, 49, 52
Study to Understand Prognosis and
Preferences for Outcomes and Risks
of Treatment (SUPPORT, 1995), 669
Subacute healthcare facilities, 20–21
Substance abuse, 132–133, 321–323, 354
Summer Fun (Borden), 29
Surgical treatments for obesity, 587–589
*Survey of Health Care Consumers
(2008)*, 594
Surveys
Client Satisfaction, 449–450
"Dying in America," 672–674
on ethics by CMSA, 170–172
on patient-physician
communications, 199
Sympathomimetic drugs, 586

T

tadalafil (Cialis), 645
Taft-Hartley Act, 72–73
Taking Care of My Health Care tool
(NTOCC), 797
Tax Equity and Fiscal Responsibility Act
(TEFRA, 1982), 108, 111
Teach-back technique, 636
Technology, home care and, 706
Tegaserod maleate (Zelnorm), 645
Telephonic case management, 14,
264–273
Initial Evaluation Report Guidelines,
301–302
for initial visit with patient, 253–256
Tenuate (diethylpropion), 586
Terminally ill patients. *See also* Dying
and death
advance directives for, 663, 666–667.
See also Do-not-resuscitate
(DNR) orders
checklist for, 668
viatical settlements and, 73–75
Third-Party Administrators (TPAs), 37.
See also Claims departments
case managers and, 5–6, 405–409, 521
precertification or preadmission reviews
by, 330
sample letter of introduction for services
through, 245
traditional insurance *versus*, 70–71
Thompson, Tommy, 584
Time availability, health literacy
and, 630
Time limits, needs assessment and, 223
To Err Is Human, 743
Touch, 606
Towers Perrin 2002 Health Care Cost Survey
Report of Key Findings, 7
tPA, 642
Training in cultural sensitivity, 611–615
Transcultural C.A.R.E. Associates, 614
Transference of feelings, long-term cases
and, 735
Transplant rejection of small bowel with
psychological component,
785–788
Travel time, 223, 246

TRICARE, 743
Trust, health literacy and, 631
12-step program for cultural
competency, 614
*2003 ICD-9-CM: International Classification of
Diseases, 9th Edition, Clinical
Modification*, 219
*2008 Survey of Health Care
Consumers*, 594

U

UCare Minnesota's Senior Health
Options, 610
Underinsured individuals, 751
Unions, 72, 323–324. *See also* Workers'
compensation
United Way, 720
University of Chicago, 644
University of Washington Medical Center,
608, 674
Unprofessional behavior, 159
UnumProvident Corporation, 574
URAC (Utilization Review Accreditation
Commission), 8, 16–17, 55, 354
Case Management Standards, 609
Urinary incontinence, 652
Ury, William, 419
U.S. Census Bureau, 591–592, 651
U.S. Department of Education, 627
U.S. Department of Health and Human
Services (DHHS), 608
U.S. Government Accountability
Office, 645
U.S. Preventive Services Task Force, 583
Utilization review, 39–40, 45
ability of physicians to render care
and, 106
case management and, 8
cost containment and, 7
as element in health care package, 331
introduction to client groups and plan
participants of, 332–333
legal responsibilities in discharge and,
103–104
types of, 329
without preadmission review,
341–342

V

Vacation Camp for the Blind, 29
Valdecoxib (Bextra), 643
Valium (diazepam), 644
Value Health Sciences, Santa Monica, Calif., 331
Vardenafil (Levitra), 645
Vehicle insurance. *See* Auto insurance
Veracity, definition of, 129, 154
Veritas Health Solutions, 698
Veterans, insurance for, 113–114, 743
Veterans Health Administration (VHA), 743
Viatical settlements, 73–75
Vicodin (hydrocodone bitartrate and acetaminophen), 643, 644
Vietnamese and Armenia Health Attitudes Survey, 603
Vietnamese culture, 603–604
  end-of-life issues and, 688–689
Vioxx (rofecoxib), 643
Visioneering Case Management's Future meeting, 516–517
Vocational activities, 316
Voluntary Health Organizations: A Guide to Patient Services, 30

W

Waist circumference, 576
Waist-to-hip ratio (WHR), 577
Warne v. Lincoln National Administrative Services Corp., 106
Weight loss. *See* Obesity
Welch, George, 47
Wellbutrin (Bupropion), 586
Western Journal of Medicine, 577
Western Pennsylvania Hospital's Summer Camp for Burned Children, 29
Wheelchairs, loaner, 720
WHR (waist-to-hip ratio), 577
Wickline v. State of California (1986, 1987), 102–103, 308
Wilson v. Blue Cross of Southern California and Blue Cross Blue Shield of Alabama and Western Medical Review (1990), 103–104
"Wonder Drugs That Can Kill," 643

Wood, Christopher, 48
Woods Ranch, 29
Workers' compensation
  case management needs assessment on injury cause and, 231
  claims analysis for, 396
  communications with legal professionals on, 210–212
  communications with providers of, 206–210
  contact with employer for case under, 279–280
  discussion of trends in, 46–49
  HIPAA, confidentiality and, 51–52
  improvements for case managers in, 58
  managed care and, 50–51
  red flags for, 392–393
  replacement salaries and, 57
  report format for, 293
  sample letter of introduction for case under, 244
  scope of reports generated from, 292
  state regulations on, 54–55, 56
  union status or job type and, 230
  work settings and, 50
Workers' Compensation Commissions, state, 55
Worksheets
  Case Management Identification, 233, 234
  cost-benefit analysis, 436, 437, 437–441
  Initial Evaluation, 250, 253–256
    sample, 302–304
World Education, Literacy and Health Initiative, 638
World Health Organization (WHO), 702
  BMI classifications, 576
World's Greatest Camp, 29

X

Xanax (alprazolam), 644
Xenical, 586

Z

Zelnorm (tegaserod maleate), 645
Zonisamide, 586
Zyban (Bupropion), 586